AF836290

Challenging Cases and Complication Management in Pain Medicine

Magdalena Anitescu
Honorio T. Benzon • Mark S. Wallace
Editors

Challenging Cases and Complication Management in Pain Medicine

Springer

Editors
Magdalena Anitescu
Department of Anesthesia and Critical Care
University of Chicago Medicine
Chicago, IL
USA

Honorio T. Benzon
Department of Anesthesiology
Northwestern University
Feinberg School of Medicine
Chicago, IL
USA

Mark S. Wallace
Division of Pain Medicine
Department of Anesthesiology
University of California San Diego School of Medicine
La Jolla, CL
USA

ISBN 978-3-319-60070-3 ISBN 978-3-319-60072-7 (eBook)
https://doi.org/10.1007/978-3-319-60072-7

Library of Congress Control Number: 2017960332

Printed on acid-free paper

This Springer imprint is published by Springer Nature
The registered company is Springer International Publishing AG
The registered company address is: Gewerbestrasse 11, 6330 Cham, Switzerland

Preface

Pain is unpleasant. Pain is serious. Pain leads to suffering. Pain needs to be treated. These facts motivate our mission as pain physicians.

As physicians, we learn early in medical school what disease means for our patients. We know that, left untreated, pain can really progress to that continuous suffering that is the disease state of chronic pain. With a sense of urgency, we treat our patients in pain, we try to heal them, and we try to comfort them, but how do we achieve the confidence that we are truly helping them?

A millennia-old symptom, pain is one of the most common complaints we hear in any doctor's office or in the hospital setting. Despite aggressive treatments, some patients develop long-lasting, refractory pain. As our therapeutic methods evolved from the old poppy seed juice to sophisticated, technologically advanced tools, so did our understanding of chronic pain.

In some instances, however, despite true progress on medical knowledge, clear understanding of pathophysiology, and application of modern interventions to tackle pain, some patients' pain sets on an unusual course.

Whether side effects of a medication, complications from interventional procedures, or unusual anatomical variations, we learn very quickly after starting our medical practice that our patients are unique. The variety of situations we do encounter in a lifetime of practicing medicine is therefore significant. And that is when clinical experience is important and in some sense becomes invaluable.

That is why, many times in the hallways of local, regional, national, and international meetings, you will find pain physicians discussing difficult cases with peers. That is why many meetings have special sessions of "Ask the Experts."

Sharing expertise, together with formal learning, ensures a true, deep, and profound progress on understanding of a topic from the incidence/prevalence to complex pathophysiology, differential diagnosis, and elaborate treatments.

That is the rationale of this current book *Challenging Cases and Complications in Pain Medicine*. In many ways, it is an extension of the discussion all of us have had during the years with our peers. Stemming from the American Society of Regional Anesthesia and Pain Medicine Fall Annual Meeting sessions of "Ask the Experts," this book is meant to be a review of problems, common and uncommon, that may arise in clinical pain practice. Most importantly, it is meant to contribute to the understanding of unanticipated clinical situations. It aims also to enhance readers' medical knowledge through the scholarly contribution to the "discussion" section of each chapter.

In this book, to access the pain physician community's collective knowledge and experience, the chapters were assigned to practitioners from both academic and private practices. Each chapter starts with a description of a clinical scenario. In order to avoid patient source identification, each of these scenarios represents a combination of at least two clinical cases. All those clinical situations, however, are based on real-life cases as described by the physicians contributing to the chapter. Thus the entire book represents the collective clinical experience of the authors.

Following the case descriptions, the discussion section of each chapter offers a comprehensive review of the topic brought up by the case description. The reviews are written based on the most current evidence-based literature and give the reader an updated reference on the subject described.

This book does not aim to discuss all topics of pain management; however, employing scholarly expertise from known academicians in the country as well as established practitioners, we hope this collection will be an accessible and broad reference for common and uncommon problems that starting practitioners as well as experienced ones may come across in their day-to-day pain practice.

Finally, we would like to emphasize the importance of continuing learning; as we complete our training, our professional journey is really just at the beginning of the road. While during residency and fellowship we do learn the basis of our profession, it is during our formative initial years of independent practice as physicians that we actually begin to grow and to use decision-making skills learned during our training.

As the mother of one of the editors, an accomplished Romanian ophthalmologist, once told her, you can teach your trainees a clinical manual skill relatively easy. It is the identifying and optimal treating of complications related to that task that takes a lifetime of learning. In some ways, we may say that true learning of how to really treat our complex pain patients only starts with ending our formal fellowship training.

We hope that our readers will enjoy this review book and find relevant information useful both in clinical practice and for advancing and acquiring medical knowledge. We also hope that, with this book, clinicians will be better equipped in identifying and treating possible complications related to pain medicine interventions.

As pain is unpleasant and may lead to suffering, with this book and what it contains, we aim to help our colleagues in finding the best pain regimen and cure for their patients, as well as help patients to ease their pain and suffering and achieve a better quality of life through treatments that could possibly minimize complications.

Chicago, IL, USA — Magdalena Anitescu, M.D., Ph.D.
La Jolla, CA, USA — Mark S. Wallace, M.D.
Chicago, IL, USA — Honorio T. Benzon, M.D.

Contents

Contributors

Magdalena Anitescu, M.D., Ph.D. Department of Anesthesia and Critical Care, University of Chicago Medical Center, Chicago, IL, USA

Benjamin R. Beal, M.D. Department of Pain Medicine, UCSD Medical Center, San Diego, CA, USA

Rena Beckerly, M.D. University of Illinois, Chicago, IL, USA

Honorio T. Benzon, M.D. Department of Anesthesiology, Northwestern University Feinberg School of Medicine, Chicago, IL, USA

Mark J. Burish, M.D., Ph.D. Department of Neurosurgery, University of Texas Health Science Center, Houston, TX, USA

Jeffrey Chen, M.D., M.H.S. Center for Pain Medicine, University of California San Diego, San Francisco, CA, USA

Qian CeCe Chen, M.D. NYU School of Medicine, Dept. of Anesthesiology, Perioperative Care and Pain Medicine, New York, NY, USA

Sheetal Kerkar DeCaria, M.D. Department of Anesthesia, University of Chicago, Chicago, IL, USA

David M. Dickerson, M.D. Department of Anesthesia and Critical Care, University of Chicago, Chicago, IL, USA

Dalia Elmofty, M.D. Department of Anesthesia and Critical Care, University of Chicago, Chicago, IL, USA

Timothy Furnish, M.D. Department of Anesthesiology, University of California, La Jolla, San Diego, CA, USA

David Gordon, M.D. Section of pain management, Department of Anesthesia, University of California at San Francisco, Chicago, SF, USA

Johal Gurbir Prestige Pain Centers, Carteret, New Jersey, USA

Jeffrey Hopcian, M.D. University Suburban Health Center, Cleveland, OH, USA

Kenneth Ike, M.D. Department of Anesthesiology, Stanford University School of Medicine, Stanford, CA, USA

R.C.W. Jones III, M.D., Ph.D. Department of Anesthesiology, Center for Pain Medicine, University of California San Diego, San Diego, CA, USA

John Kenny, M.D. Department of Anesthesia, University of Chicago, Chicago, IL, USA

Irina Khrenova, M.D. Department of Anesthesiology and Perioperative Care, University of California San Francisco—UCSF, UCSF Pain Management Center, San Francisco, CA, USA

Randall W. Knoebel, Pharm.D., B.C.O.P. Department of Pharmacy, University of Chicago Medicine, Chicago, IL, USA

Katherine Kozarek, M.D. Department of Anesthesia and Critical Care, University of Chicago, Chicago, IL, USA

Alina Lazar Department of Anesthesia and Critical Care, University of Chicago Medical Cente, Chicago, IL, USA

Gemayel Lee, M.D. Center for Pain Medicine, University of California San Diego, La Jolla, CA, USA

Imanuel Lerman, M.D. Department of Anesthesiology, Center for Pain Medicine, University of California San Diego, San Diego, CA, USA

Daniel Levin, M.D. Department of Anesthesia and Critical Care, University of Chicago Medical Center, Chicago, IL, USA

Neil Malhotra, M.D. Expert Pain Physicians, Pain and Wellness Center, Orland Park, IL, USA

Nitin Malhotra, M.D. Expert Pain Physicians, Pain and Wellness Center, Orland Park, IL, USA

Khalid M. Malik, M.D. Department of Anesthesiology, University of Illinois, Chicago, IL, USA

Tariq Malik, M.D. University of Chicago Hospitals, Chicago, IL, USA

Ryan Mattie, M.D. Division of Pain Medicine, PGY-5, Department of Anesthesia and Perioperative Care, University of California at San Francisco, San Francisco, CA, USA

Christina C. Moore, M.D. Department of Anesthesia, Medical College of Wisconsin, Milwaukee, WI, USA

Mikiko Murakami, D.O. Department of Anesthesiology, Center for Pain Medicine, University of California San Diego, San Diego, CA, USA

Geeta Nagpal, M.D. Department of Anesthesiology, Northwestern University, Feinberg School of Medicine, Chicago, IL, USA

Ramana K. Naidu, M.D. Pain Physician and Anesthesiologist Mt Tam Orthopedics, Medical Director of Pain Management for Marin General Hospital Novato, CA, USA

Kenneth Justin Naylor, M.D. Mercy Pain Management, Mercy Hospital, Washington, MO, USA

Ariana Nelson, M.D. Department of Anesthesiology and Perioperative Care, UC Irvine School of Medicine, Irvine, CA, USA

Kristen Noon, M.D. Department of Anesthesiology, Center for Pain Medicine, University of California San Diego, San Diego, CA, USA

Alexander Papp, M.D. Department of Psychiatry, University of California San Diego, San Diego, CA, USA

Vijal Patel Department of Anesthesia, University of Chicago, Chicago, IL, USA

Mario De Pinto, M.D. Department of Anesthesiology and Perioperative Care, University of California San Francisco—UCSF, UCSF Pain Management Center, San Francisco, CA, USA

Gregory Polston, M.D. UC San Diego Health—Perlman Medical Offices, La Jolla, CA, USA

Lawrence R. Poree, M.D., M.P.H., Ph.D. Department of Anesthesia and Perioperative Care, Division of Pain Medicine, University of California San Francisco, San Francisco, CA, USA

Omar R. Qureshi, M.D. Advanced Pain Management, Stoneham, Bedford, MA, USA

Joseph Rabi, M.D. Pain Treatment Centers of Illinois, Orland Park, IL, USA

Maunuk V. Rana, M.D. Associate Professor, Department of Anesthesiology and Critical Care, The University of Chicago Medical Center, Burr Ridge, Chicago, IL, USA

Meghan E. Rodes, M.D. Northwestern University Feinberg School of Medicine, Chicago, IL, USA

Matthew V. Satterly, M.D. Western Anesthesia Associates, St Louis, MO, USA

Paul M. Scholten, M.D. Pain Management Center, Shirley Ryan AbilityLab, Chicago, IL, USA

Andrea Shashoua University of Chicago Medical Center, Chicago, IL, USA

Bradley Silva, M.D. Department of Anesthesia and Critical Care, University of Chicago, Chicago, IL, USA

Shaan Sudhakaran, M.D. Department of Anesthesia and Critical Care, University of Chicago Medical Center, Chicago, IL, USA

Lucia Daiana Voiculescu, M.D. NYU School of Medicine, Dept. of Anesthesiology, Perioperative Care and Pain Medicine, New York, NY, USA

R. Lee Wagner, M.D. Scripps Green Hospital, La Jolla, CA, USA

David R. Walega, M.D. Feinberg School of Medicine Northwestern University, Chicago, IL, USA

Mark S. Wallace, M.D. Division of Pain Medicine, Department of Anesthesiology, University of California San Diego, San Diego, CA, USA

Ajay Wasan, M.D., M.Sc. Department of Anesthesiology, University of Pittsburgh School of Medicine, Pittsburgh, PA, USA

Simon Willis, M.D. Department of Physical Medicine and Rehabilitation, Medstar Georgetown University Hospital/National Rehabilitation Hospital, Washington, DC, USA

Brad Wisler, M.D. Active Duty Air Force anesthesiologist and pain physician, Wright Patterson AFB, Dayton, OH, USA

Sophy Zheng, M.D. Department of Anesthesia and Critical Care, Northwestern University, Feinberg School of Medicine, Chicago, IL, USA

Part I

Non-interventional Pain Therapy

1 Opioid Overdose

Gregory Polston

1.1 Case Description

A 54-year-old male is brought to an emergency room via ambulance. He is obtunded and is breathing shallowly. He responds minimally to stimulation. His wife states that "he was sleepy today but had more pain than usual." She calls for the ambulance when he stopped breathing. His past medical history is significant for multiple back surgeries, which have left him with chronic pain. His wife says his pain has gotten worse over the past few months. She also reports that he takes multiple medications for his pain, including opioids, but she does not know which specific names or doses. He has a longstanding relationship with his current pain physician, and his wife believes that he may have recently had his opioid medication increased, although she is not certain.

His blood pressure is 90/72, heart rate is 105, and respiratory rate is 6. Oxygen saturation is 92%, and oral temperature is 38 °C. The patient is not able to answer questions or follow commands, although he is arousable with sternal stimulation. Physical exam shows normal pupils that are round, equal in size, and reactive to light. A full body exam shows no signs of trauma or needle marks. No topical patches are found on his body. Breath sounds are shallow but clear. The abdomen is soft, and bowel sounds are absent.

Emergency staff begin delivering oxygen. IV access is obtained, and blood is drawn and sent to the lab. Because an opioid overdose is suspected, the patient is given 0.4 mg of naloxone intravenously. His respiratory rate increases, and his oxygen saturation improves, but he is still confused and not fully able to follow commands.

A review of the state online prescription monitoring system shows monthly opioid prescriptions from one provider. His last opioid prescription was 4 days ago and shows that oxycodone CR was increased from 20 mg p.o. b.i.d. to oxycodone CR 40 mg p.o. b.i.d. Oxycodone/acetaminophen 10/325 p.o. q.i.d. was also dispensed on the same date and at the same dose as the previous month. This document also shows a prescription for alprazolam 0.5 mg #30 2 months ago.

His wife states that the patient is compliant regarding his medication and is careful to not take them in a way other than prescribed. He has seen a psychiatrist in the past for depression, but his wife does not believe that he has been overly depressed or anxious recently. He has no prior histories of overdoses or suicide attempts.

Fifteen minutes after being given the naloxone dose, the patient becomes groggier, and his saturation levels start to decrease. A repeat dose of 0.4 mg of naloxone is given. Again, oxygen saturation quickly improves, and he becomes more awake.

A finger stick blood sugar test is 90, and a urine immunoassay is positive for oxycodone and negative for benzodiazepines and illicit drugs.

Over the next 4 h, he slowly becomes more awake. He receives three more doses of naloxone. The patient improves and is able to maintain his oxygen saturation on 2 L via a nasal cannula. It is determined that he does not need an IV infusion of naloxone, but he is admitted for overnight observation.

The patient later admits that he took two extra doses of oxycodone CR, along with one alprazolam on the morning before his emergency admission because his pain was really bad. He was discharged the next morning and sent home with two doses of naloxone with a nasal spray adaptor for rescue. Both he and his wife were given instructions on how to recognize the signs of an overdose and how to use this medication. He was instructed to follow up with his pain physician as soon as possible.

1.2 Case Discussion

The United States is currently experiencing an epidemic of opioid dependence, abuse, and overdose involving prescription opioids and illicit use of heroin. It has become increasingly clear that this epidemic is the result of increased availability of

G. Polston, M.D.
UC San Diego Health—Perlman Medical Offices,
9350 Campus Point Drive, La Jolla, CA 92037, USA
e-mail: gpolston@ucsd.edu

M. Anitescu et al. (eds.), *Challenging Cases and Complication Management in Pain Medicine*,
https://doi.org/10.1007/978-3-319-60072-7_1

prescription opioids. The incidence of opioid overdoses has more than quadrupled in the United States since 1999 [1]. In fact, the prevalence of opioid-related overdoses is so great that it is now the leading cause of unintentional deaths. Currently, nearly half of all drug overdoses involved prescription opioids. Additionally, many speculate that the current heroin epidemic is the result of increased prescribing of opioids for pain because an overwhelming number of new heroin users report that, before abusing heroin, they first abused prescription opioids.

1.3 Clinical Findings (Table 1.1)

The possibility of drug overdose should be considered in any person with altered mental status, especially in patients prescribed or suspected to have access to opioids. Patients can present with symptoms ranging from coma, somnolence, confusion, and lethargy to euphoria, agitation, and unusual behavior [2].

Respiratory depression, with rates less than eight per minute, and decreased tidal volume are always present and should be a primary finding with this diagnosis. A respiratory rate of less than 12 in a patient who is not asleep strongly suggests acute intoxication. Decreased bowel sounds are also common due to the paralysis of smooth muscles. Miosis, which is a common side effect of opioids, is believed to occur via the Edinger-Westphal nucleus but is not always seen during an overdose. This inconsistency occurs because not all opioids cause constriction of the pupil (e.g., meperidine), and the use of other medications such as sympathomimetics or anticholinergics may make pupils appear normal or even dilated [3].

Other signs and symptoms include hypothermia and hypoglycemia due to exposure and delayed presentation to health-care providers. If the victim has taken opioids that can prolong QTc (most frequently methadone), dysrhythmias are possible. Seizures can occur with tramadol and tapentadol through serotonergic effects. In the fall of 2015, the FDA issued a warning about a large increase in the number of fentanyl-related seizures and fatalities. It was thought that this increase was due to illicit use of non-pharmaceutical fentanyl containing high doses of fentanyl which was also mixed with heroin and or cocaine [1].

Table 1.1 Clinical findings in opioid overdose

Respiratory depression (RR < 8 breaths/min)
Alerted sensorium (sedation)
Absent bowel sounds
Constricted pupils (inconsistent finding)
Compartment syndrome
Rhabdomyolysis
Hypothermia (if exposure occurs)
Signs of aspiration
Dysrhythmias (QTc prolongation)
Seizures (tramadol/tapenadol/meperidine/non-pharmaceutical fentanyl)
Signs of other non-opioid drug use/overdose (most overdoses have multiple classes)
Signs of illicit drug use (needle tracks, endocarditis)
Pulseless/pulmonary edema (end stages)

If hypoxia continues after intubation and mechanical ventilation, pulmonary edema needs to be ruled out. The primary reason why pulmonary edema develops is because of reduced intrathoracic pressure secondary to inspiration against a closed glottis. It has also been hypothesized that rapid naloxone administration precipitates pulmonary edema by causing a significant increase in afterload secondary to a surge in catecholamines. The reasoning is that this increase in pressure could then lead to interstitial edema and alveolar filling. This theory, however, is questioned by some. They argue that pulmonary edema develops after circulation is restored in the lungs that are damaged due to the arrest [4, 5].

Another common reason for difficulties with respiration is aspiration. It is important to remember that aspiration can also occur with any poisoning, especially when multiple drugs are involved.

After stabilization of respiration and circulation, the physical examination should also include palpation of all muscle groups to rule out compartment syndromes. In addition, if there is concern that a patient, out of fear of criminal arrest, may have hidden opioids on his person, a rectal or vaginal exam should be considered. The body should be examined for medication patches. They should be removed immediately, and the skin should be washed with soap and cool water. Abdominal x-rays can be considered if the patient is suspected of smuggling swallowed drug packets.

1.4 Laboratory Findings

Serum glucose is a required initial test since hypoglycemia can mimic an overdose and is quickly correctable. Electrolytes, serum creatine phosphokinase, and creatine kinase can be tested when there is concern about rhabdomyolysis and myoglobinuria. One should also consider obtaining an acetaminophen level if there is any concern of potential use. Salicylate testing is not necessary without clinical suspicion or an unexplained anion gap [4].

Urine drug screens have little clinical value in the initial resuscitation and should not delay the delivery of naloxone. A positive result from a urine test only detects what medications have been taken over a period of time. Therefore, positive results in a urine screen may not be a causal factor. In addition, treatment is based on opioids as a class and not as an individual drug.

1.5 Treatment of Opioid Overdose

Restoration of ventilation and oxygenation is the priority. Basic life support and trauma resuscitation protocols should take precedence before an antidote is considered. If an overdose is suspected, attempts should be made to determine what drug was ingested. If one can ascertain when the drug was taken, the manner in which the drug was taken, as well as the amount of drug taken, this information will play a role in tailoring the resuscitation. By way of example, serum half-lives of opioids can vary significantly from a few hours to nearly 60 h for methadone. There are wide ranges in individuals, due to genetic differences and the patient's chronicity of exposure to opioids. For suspected prescription overdoses, reviewing the patient's medical records and accessing state prescription monitoring programs can provide valuable and detailed information. Treatment of illicit drug overdoses can be an unpredictable task due to the uncertainty of potency in the drug taken as well as the potential presence of other adulterating drugs [6].

Naloxone is a synthetic derivative of oxymorphone. It can be given via parenteral or intranasal methods or through an endotracheal tube. It is a competitive antagonist with affinity at the μ, δ, and κ receptors and has no risk of respiratory depression or abuse. Dosing of naloxone is empiric. Its onset of action, when given intravenously, is 1–2 min. It peaks by 10 min and has a half-life of 30–80 min.

The most often recommended initial dose is 0.04 mg intravenously, and based on the individual response, it is increased every 2–5 min. If given nasally, volumes should not exceed 1 mL per nostril because higher volumes will not be absorbed. It is important to note that dosing decisions should be based on return of respiration and not on reversal of sedation. This is because complete reversal runs the risk of precipitating a violent opioid withdrawal and destabilizing the patient. Further, if the patient is taking prescription opioids for pain, complete reversal through naloxone will lead to the return of symptoms being treated. Carbon dioxide monitoring may be a more accurate monitor of the level of respiration and make the titration of naloxone easier.

Another formulation to prevent the opioid overdose has been rapidly gaining acceptance in clinical practice. Evzio is a product that contains two single-use auto-injectors, each containing 0.4 mg naloxone that is usually prescribed together with a white and black trainer (Fig. 1.1).

Naloxone causes the release of catecholamines, which can precipitate acute withdrawal leading to tachycardia, hypertension, abdominal cramping, vomiting, diarrhea, and agitation. These symptoms can be especially dangerous in patients with cardiovascular disease and in neonates born to opioid-dependent mothers. Naloxone must be used with caution in patients with seizures, and its use must be avoided in treatment of suspected meperidine-induced seizures.

Fifteen milligrams of naloxone is considered the upper limit, but no maximum dose has been established. An apneic patient without a pulse may receive higher initial doses. Patients who are opioid dependent may also require higher

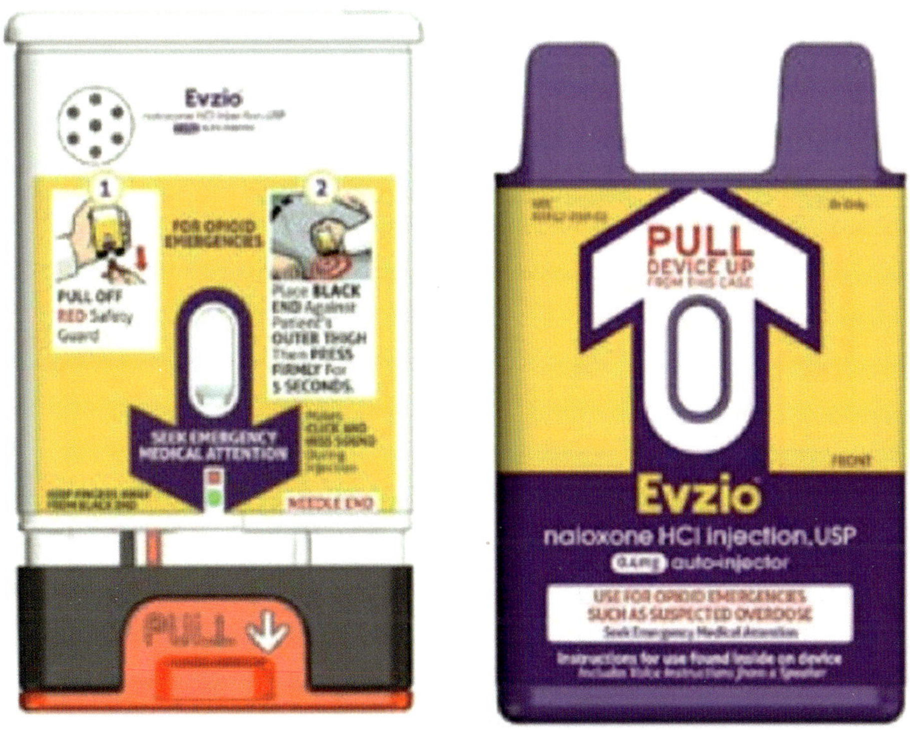

Fig. 1.1 Evzio is a product that is supplied with two auto-injectors, each containing 0.4 mg naloxone and a black and white trainer. It is increasingly prescribed for patients on long term and high doses of opioid medication to likely prevent overdose

doses. Initial improvements in respiration, especially in patients who are not opioid naïve, are frequently transient, making the need for readministration of naloxone necessary. Naloxone infusions should be considered if multiple doses are required and the patient continues to relapse. The concentration and rate of the naloxone infusion are again based on the patient's respiration. But as a general guide, begin by giving two-thirds of the initial naloxone dose every hour and then titrate down as respiration is restored.

Naloxone's only adverse effect is inducing withdrawal in an opioid-dependent patient. If the dose given during the resuscitation "overshoots" the reversal and signs of opioid withdrawal develop, do not attempt to counteract this error by giving the patient more opioids. This is because the half-life of naloxone is usually much shorter, and giving more opioids will only compound the problems of respiratory depression later. In addition to the previously stated danger, complete reversal can also cause the patient to become very agitated and combative. This in itself can be an emergency due to safety concerns for the patient as well as health-care providers. There are also case reports of patients who have left the hospital against medical advice despite having a great risk of relapsing. Slower and more controlled emergence is always safer. This is in part why lower initial doses of naloxone are recommended [4].

If naloxone fails to change or improve symptoms, other conditions or causes should be considered. Similar presentations to an opioid overdose include head trauma, cerebrovascular accidents, electrolyte abnormalities, and sepsis.

Suction of gastric contents can be considered, but clinically it has limited effects, and activated charcoal is not beneficial if ingestion occurred more than an hour before admission. In rare refractory cases, cerebrospinal fluid lavage can be considered. This is most common in a patient who has overdosed from an intrathecal opioid pump. In patients with elevated temperatures, aspiration or endocarditis from intravenous drug use should be considered. Sending a patient for dialysis is not recommended due to opioid's large volume of distribution (1–10 L/kg). Seizures are associated with tramadol, tapentadol, propoxyphene, and meperidine. Partial opioid agonists and mixed opioid agonists/antagonists such as buprenorphine may require high doses and longer infusions of naloxone.

In the case of opioid overdose, pulmonary edema is not due to fluid overload. Therefore, the use of diuretics should not be given and can in fact worsen associated renal failure. Rhabdomyolysis, myoglobin-induced renal failure, and compartment syndromes secondary to prolonged immobility in a comatose patient complicate resuscitation and need individualized treatment. Before the dose of acetaminophen in opioid combination products was reduced by FDA mandate, liver failure was frequently found in prescription opioid-related overdoses. Today the incidence is less likely. Nevertheless, this should be ruled out if there is any question about ingestion of acetaminophen. It is also important to remember that acetaminophen toxicity may not become clinically apparent until after the initial resuscitation is completed [7].

When heroin is the only drug involved in an overdose, single doses of naloxone have been shown to be the only intervention needed, due to similar half-lives of these two drugs. But with methadone or other sustained release opioids, prolonged infusions of naloxone may be needed.

Remember too that naloxone will not block the respiratory effects of other non-opioid sedatives. For example, the respiratory depression caused by benzodiazepines or alcohol will not be changed with delivery of naloxone. But empiric use of flumazenil for suspected combined opioid and benzodiazepine overdose is not recommended. There is the possibility of a withdrawal seizure or loss of the protective effect of benzodiazepines in a patient who has also ingested a pro-convulsant drug. Opioids are clinically much stronger respiratory depressants then GABA agonists. Therefore, the need to reverse benzodiazepines may not be necessary for successful resuscitations [8]. Also not recommended in the treatment of drug overdoses is the use of stimulants, ice baths, or "smelling salts" to reverse or "wake up" an obtunded patient.

1.6 Risk Factors for Overdose (Table 1.2)

Groups with increased risk for opioid overdose include non-Hispanic whites, those with a history of chronic pulmonary disease, substance abuse, mental health issues, and low socioeconomic status. A history of a prior overdose and frequent emergency room visits are also independent risk factors [9, 10]. Children and elderly patients are more vulnerable to overdose and more likely to experience a poor outcome. Overdoses in children are more problematic due to their smaller body weight and differences in their immature metabolisms. The elderly differ in that they are more likely

Table 1.2 Risk factors for opioid overdose

White non-Hispanic
Age < 35 years (more likely heroin)
Age > 65 years (more likely prescription opioids)
Liver disease
Kidney disease
Pulmonary disease
Cardiac disease
Sleep apnea
Psychiatric history
Substance abuse
Prior overdose
Recent increase in prescription opioid dose
Total daily dose >50 MME[a]
Concurrent use of sedatives and/or stimulants
Recent release from incarnation

[a]Morphine milligram equivalents per day

to have renal insufficiency, chronic obstructive disease, altered liver function, or sleep apnea [10, 11].

Men, despite their much higher rates of abuse and dependence, are only slightly more likely than women to die from an overdose. In both sexes, the highest rates of death secondary to both heroin and prescription opioids occur between the ages of 19 and 35 years. After the age of 35, overdose is more likely due to prescription opioids.

Total opioid dose per day is an independent risk factor that has been seen in multiple studies. The use of extended release/long-acting prescription opioids (ER/LA) can increase the risk of overdose due to higher total doses and prolonged effects. Concurrent use of benzodiazepines or other sedatives with prescription opioids increases the risk of both nonfatal and fatal overdoses. It is also worth noting that recently released prisoners are at high risk for overdoses due to loss of tolerance during incarceration.

1.7 Unique Aspects of Opioid Metabolism

Tolerance to respiratory depression is slower to develop than other opioid side effects [12]. Tolerance is also not complete and can vary with time. This means that patients who are prescribed opioids over longer periods of time, even while taking the same dose, are still at risk for overdose. Further, when total daily opioid dose increases to counteract tolerance to analgesic effects, tolerance to respiratory depression may not have changed to the same degree. This may explain why overdoses are frequently seen shortly after even small dose increases. This same concern is present in individuals who abuse opioids because the tolerance to euphoric effects also develops more quickly than tolerance to respiratory depression.

Tolerance to opioids is not completely mediated by μ receptors, and conditioning and learning also plays a part in tolerance. Taking opioids in new environments has shown to lower tolerance and increase the risk of overdose [3]. In one study, a disproportional number of heroin overdoses occurred in locations where the addict had not used this drug before [13]. Whether this applies to prescription opioid overdoses is not known, but this type of conditioning and learning plays a role in pain behavior.

The pharmacokinetics of opioids can be greatly altered during an overdose. Therefore, relying on normally expected clearance times and half-lives can be very dangerous. Ingestion of a large number of pills can lead to altered absorption as well as delayed gastric emptying. Further, if enzymatic elimination is overwhelmed, small amounts of opioid absorption can lead to large increases in plasma concentrations. Elimination will also switch from a percentage decrease in drug levels to a constant fixed amount. These factors can increase the severity and length of respiratory depression.

Because individual opioids metabolize differently, the risk of overdose also varies with the individual drug [14]. For example, heroin, a prodrug, is first metabolized to 6-monacetylmorphine (6 MAM) and then to morphine. Morphine is slow to cross the blood-brain barrier, but 6 MAM quickly penetrates it. Thus, heroin, by crossing the blood-brain barrier as 6 MAM, is metabolized to morphine within the central nervous system. This means that morphine, a long-acting respiratory depressant, has greater penetration of respiratory centers via heroin than when it is taken on its own. This leads to a greater risk of respiratory depression with heroin. Another example of how metabolism can alter risk can be seen in examining the clearance of methadone. The primary step in eliminating methadone from the body is *N*-demethylation via cytochrome P450 3A4. Inhibition of this enzyme by other medications or individual variation will significantly delay the removal of this drug and increase the potential for oversedation.

References

1. CDC Health Alert Network October 26, 2015, 0815 EDT (08:15 AM EDT) CDCHAN-00384. http:// http://emergency.cdc.gov/han/han00384.asp. Accessed 10 July 2016.
2. Dunn KM, Saunders KW, Rutter CM, et al. Opioid prescriptions for chronic pain and overdose: a cohort study. Ann Intern Med. 2010;152(2):85–92.
3. Paulozzi LJ, Kilbourne EM, Shah NG, et al. A history of being prescribed controlled substances and risk of drug overdose death. Pain Med. 2012;13(1):87–95.
4. Boyer EW. Management of opioid analgesic overdose. N Engl J Med. 2012;367(2):146–55.
5. Gomes T, Mamdani MM, Dhalla IA, Paterson JM, Juurlink DN. Opioid dose and drug-related mortality in patients with nonmalignant pain. Arch Intern Med. 2011;171(7):686–91.
6. Bohnert AS, Valenstein M, Bair MJ, et al. Association between opioid prescribing patterns and opioid overdose-related deaths. JAMA. 2011;305(13):1315–21.
7. Dasgupta N, Funk MJ, Proescholdbell S, Hirsch A, Ribisl KM, Marshall S. Cohort study of the impact of high-dose opioid analgesics on overdose mortality [published online September 1, 2015]. Pain Med. doi:10.1111/pme.12907.
8. Sivilotti ML. Flumazenil, naloxone and the 'coma cocktail'. Br J Clin Pharmacol. 2016;81(3):428–36. Epub 21 Sept 2015.
9. Gwira Baumblatt JA, Wiedeman C, Dunn JR, Schaffner W, Paulozzi LJ, Jones TF. High-risk use by patients prescribed opioids for pain and its role in overdose deaths. JAMA Intern Med. 2014;174(5):796–801.
10. Liang Y, Turner BJ. Assessing risk for drug overdose in a national cohort: role for both daily and total opioid dose? J Pain. 2015;16(4):318–25.
11. Zedler B, Xie L, Wang L, et al. Risk factors for serious prescription opioid-related toxicity or overdose among Veterans Health Administration patients. Pain Med. 2014;15(11):1911–29.
12. White JM, Irvine RJ. Mechanisms of fatal opioid overdose. Addiction. 1999;94(7):961–72.
13. Siegel S. Pavlovian conditioning and heroin overdose: reports by overdose victims. Bull Psychon Soc. 1984;22(5):428–30.
14. Bohnert AS, Logan JE, Ganoczy D, Dowell D. A detailed exploration into the association of prescribed opioid dosage and overdose deaths among patients with chronic pain [published online January 22, 2016]. Med Care. doi:10.1097/MLR.0000000000000505.

2 Polypharmacy and Drug-Drug Interactions: Methadone

Randall W. Knoebel and David M. Dickerson

2.1 Case Presentation

A 69-year-old male presents to the pain clinic with a history of seronegative rheumatoid arthritis, multiple lumbar spine surgeries for radiculopathy, chronic myalgias, cervicalgia, and recently diagnosed antecedent acute myelogenous leukemia (AML). He suffers from severe neck and low back pain that at one time responded to oxycodone and fentanyl patch and triggers point injections with steroid, local anesthetic, and botulinum toxin, and physical therapy. Unfortunately, his symptoms have progressively worsened, deteriorating his ability to function. He was referred to the pain clinic after an emergency department visit for refractory pain symptoms. He had tried, without relief, NSAIDS, acetaminophen, gabapentin, amitriptyline, tizanidine, cyclobenzaprine, baclofen, and hydrocodone. Pain not only impaired his function significantly but also was affecting his sleep, relationships, and mood. His range of motion was unremarkable, but he was diffusely tender across his upper back and upper pelvis. Numbness and weakness were absent.

The patient was prescribed oral methadone 5 mg every 8 h with immediate-release hydromorphone for breakthrough pain. Oxycodone was discontinued; baclofen and a short course of diclofenac were initiated. His pain and function improved in the following days and weeks. Methadone was gradually titrated to 7.5 mg orally every 8 h and denied side effects from the therapy. During this time, he was enrolled on a clinical trial for the treatment of his AML using a combination of azacitidine, high-dose cytarabine, and mitoxantrone. His therapy was complicated by persistent neutropenic fevers and radiographic evidence identifying a probable invasive fungal pneumonia, at which time voriconazole therapy was initiated. The oncology clinic decreased the tamsulosin dose while the patient was taking voriconazole. The potential for an interaction with methadone was not noted or discussed with the patient or prescribing pain physician. During the following 2 weeks, the patient's control of pain continued to improve, but he and his wife reported increased and progressive sedation, fatigue, and cognitive dysfunction. The decision was made to halve the methadone dose during voriconazole treatment. Within a week the patient experienced a resolution of the aforementioned side effects. His pain remained well controlled, and AML remission permitted a 2-month vacation to Florida. Unfortunately, the patient's AML relapsed 3 months later and shortly thereafter succumbed to an episode of severe sepsis.

2.2 Discussion

Methadone is a synthetic opioid discovered in Germany in 1937 and approved by the US Food and Drug Administration (FDA) in 1947 for a number of pain-related syndromes. It is available as a racemic mixture of the L-stereoisomer, levomethadone, responsible for the mu, kappa, and delta opioid binding and a D-stereoisomer, dextromethadone, responsible for blocking the NMDA receptor [1]. This unique pharmacology partially explains methadone's apparent increased potency when administered to patient's already taking another opioid. Furthermore, methadone seems to offer a broader coverage of multidimensional pain syndromes—including ones only partially responding to opioids. In recent year, methadone has garnered interest based on its unique pharmacology, potential efficacy in difficult to treat pain syndromes, and low cost. Yet unique challenges are posed by dosing a medication with an uncertain potency, a long and variable half-life, and numerous pharmacokinetic and pharmacodynamic drug-drug interactions.

R.W. Knoebel, Pharm.D., B.C.O.P.
Department of Pharmacy, University of Chicago Medicine, Chicago, IL, USA
e-mail: Randall.Knoebel@uchospitals.edu

D.M. Dickerson, M.D. (✉)
Department of Anesthesia and Critical Care, University of Chicago, Chicago, IL, USA
e-mail: DDickerson@dacc.uchicago.edu

M. Anitescu et al. (eds.), *Challenging Cases and Complication Management in Pain Medicine*,
https://doi.org/10.1007/978-3-319-60072-7_2

Methadone is readily absorbed after oral administration with approximately 85% of the dose reaching the bloodstream, three times that of morphine [2]. Unlike other opioids, methadone has a rapid and extensive drug elimination phase (α-elimination) from the bloodstream into the adipose tissue (analgesic period) followed by a slow and variable elimination phase (β-elimination) that does not contribute to additional analgesia but attenuates withdrawal [3]. Delayed β-elimination may result in drug accumulation and toxicity [4]. Methadone is highly bound to α-1 acid glycoprotein (AAG), a plasma protein and acute phase reactant. As a result nonprotein bound (active) drug fluctuates during times of stress, opioid dependence, malignancy, and coadministration of other highly protein-bound medications [5, 6]. Methadone's metabolism is highly reliant on the hepatic cytochrome enzyme system primarily CYP3A4 and, to a lesser extent, CYP2B6, CYP2D6, and CYP1A2, resulting in two biologically inactive metabolites via *N*-demethylation [7]. High reliance upon the CYP system, particularly CYP3A4, predisposes methadone to a myriad of drug-drug interactions.

The World Health Organization reports that drug interactions are a leading cause of morbidity and mortality [8]. Although methadone represents less than 5% of all opioid prescriptions dispensed in the United States each year, it is identified in more than a third of opioid-related deaths with drug interactions frequently being implicated [9, 10]. A drug-drug interaction is the pharmacologic or clinical response to the coadministration of two or more drugs or substances beyond that expected from the known effects of the drugs given individually resulting in a synergistic, antagonistic, or idiosyncratic outcome [11]. Drug interactions are pharmacokinetic, if a drug alters the absorption, distribution, or elimination of a second drug, or pharmacodynamic, if multiple drugs act on the same receptor, site of action, or physiologic system [11].

Pharmacokinetic interactions are influenced by the degree to which a drug reduces (inhibits) or increases (induces) the activity of the target enzyme. CYP3A4 inhibitors are classified as either strong, moderate, or weak, based on the increase in exposure they cause in sensitive CYP3A4 substrates (Table 2.1). In our patient, methadone, a CYP3A4 substrate, was coadministered with voriconazole, a strong CYP3A4 inhibitor. Systemic exposure of methadone increased when metabolism of methadone was impaired, resulting in the increased and progressive sedation, fatigue, and cognitive dysfunction. Pharmacodynamic interactions such as the potential to cause QTc prolongation and additive respiratory depression or sedation should be considered when initiating or maintaining a patient on methadone.

Table 2.1 Classification of CYP3A4 inhibitors

Strong CYP3A4 inhibitors (cause ≥ fivefold increase in AUC of sensitive CYP3A4 substrate)	*Moderate CYP3A4 inhibitors* (cause ≥ 2 but < fivefold increase in AUC of sensitive CYP3A4 substrate)	*Weak CYP3A4 inhibitors* (cause >1.25 but <fold increase in AUC of sensitive CYP3A4 substrate)

Prolonged QTc interval and ECG abnormalities have been reported in methadone-treated patients leading to the development of torsades de pointes and sudden death [12]. Torsades de pointes (TdP) is often caused by drugs that block potassium current channels in cardiac myocytes or in patients with a prolonged QT interval (>500 ms elevates risk). Methadone blocks the cardiac human ether-a-go-go related gene (HERG) potassium channel producing negative chronotropic properties [13]. Many factors contribute to QT interval prolongation and subsequent progression to TdP, such as age, female gender, hypokalemia, severe hypomagnesemia, bradycardia, recent conversion from atrial fibrillation, congestive heart failure, subclinical long QT syndrome, baseline QT interval prolongation, ion-channel polymorphisms, and concomitant medications [14]. The relative impact of each of these risk factors is unknown, but all must be considered before methadone or another therapy is started that increases the risk for QT prolongation. The effect on the QT interval is dose related and robust in patients taking greater than 100 mg orally everyday or with lower doses in cocaine users [15]. Preexisting QT prolongation appears to be a serious risk factor for drug-induced arrhythmia and remains the most consistent predictor in the development of TdP [16]. The international regulatory guidance for drug development suggests a gender-independent categorical threshold for QT prolongation of 450 ms [14]. In patients with long QT syndrome, a QTc interval >500 ms was associated with an odds ratio for syncope or sudden death of 4.2 [17]. Therefore, methadone should not be prescribed for patients with a QTc of >500 ms at any time. Alternative opioids should be considered in patients with a baseline QTc >450 ms, assuming all modifiable risk factors have been corrected.

When considering a patient's candidacy for methadone treatment, initial assessment must include concomitant medications, the use of illicit substances, personal and family history of structural heart disease, and personal history of arrhythmia. Additionally, a review of a recent ECG evaluating the QTc interval is recommended for patients with baseline risk factors for prolongation of the QTc interval prior to initiating methadone therapy. Obtaining an ECG for such evaluation may be necessary. Figure 2.1 provides a stepwise approach for safely initiating methadone therapy. Concomitant medications should be evaluated for their ability to influence methadone's metabolism through CYP3A4 as well as potential to cause overlapping toxicity (i.e., somnolence or respiratory depression) or QTc prolongation. If a drug-drug interaction is identified, consider discontinuation or reduction of the dose of the offending medication. Once methadone is initiated, close

Fig. 2.1 Methadone initiation and monitoring algorithm

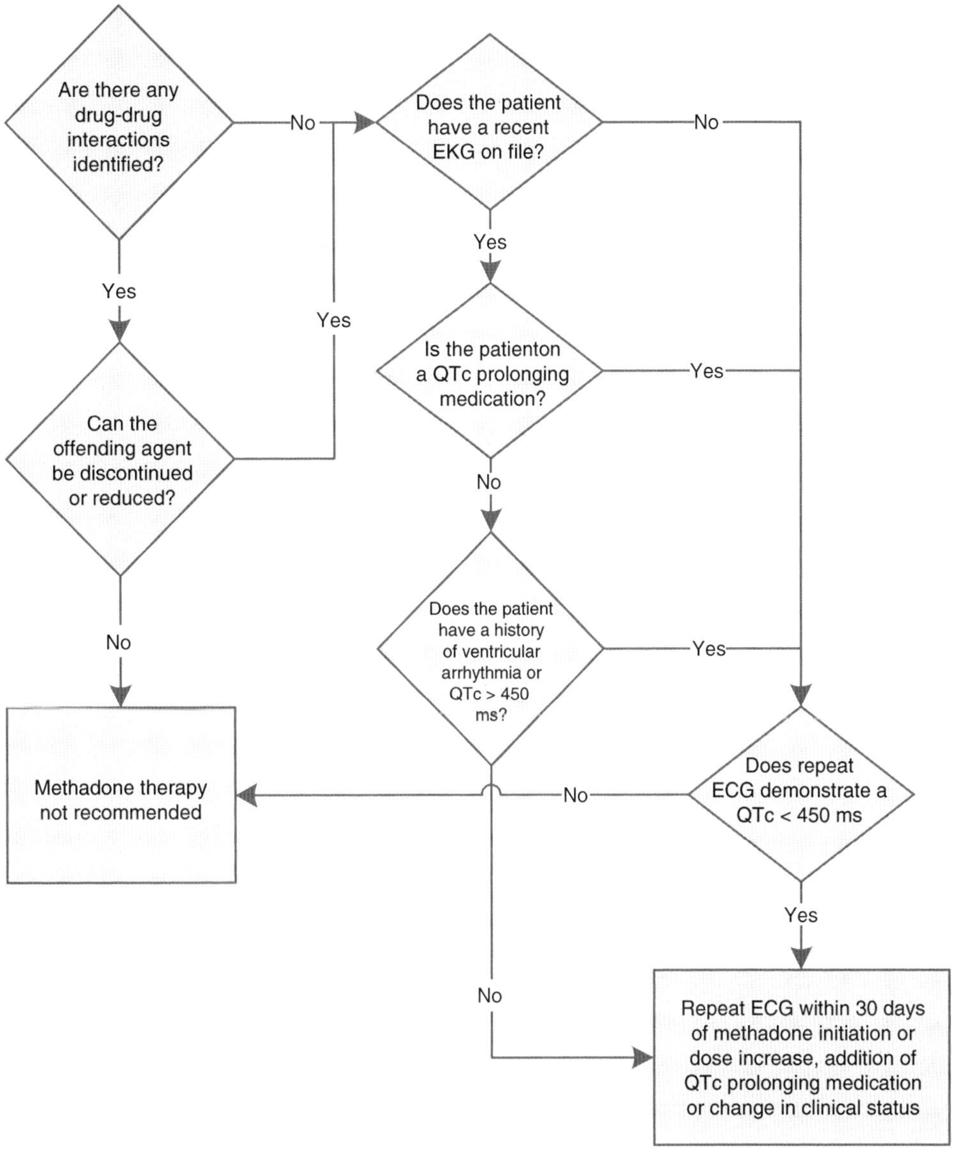

monitoring is necessary. Overdose symptoms are typically not observed after a single dose but tend to accumulate over several days' dosing [18]. After monitoring for potential interactions, the methadone dose may be adjusted. When CYP inducers or inhibitors are coadministered, heightened monitoring is required [17]. Table 2.2 lists the medications with known interactions with methadone. Because novel therapeutics are continually emerging (44 drugs were granted FDA approval in 2014), the potential for drug-drug interactions increases necessitating vigilance and consultation with a medication expert. Additionally, the vast majority of patients receiving methadone are also on other drugs for associated comorbidities or pain. Thus polypharmacy should be considered the rule rather than the exception. A number of approaches to mitigate the risks for drug-drug interactions have been suggested [19]: (1) At each visit, review with the patient each medication being taken and document the medication and dose. (2) Advise the patient to contact you if any physician has made any additions or changes to their medication regimen. (3) Educate the patient about potential side effects and potentially lethal side effects. (4) Educate the patient that street drugs, over-the-counter medications, and herbal supplements can accentuate drug-drug interactions and increase the risk of side effects. (5) Initiate the susceptible drug at a low dose and increase the dose gradually after assessing response. (6) Keep the dose of the inhibitor low or increase slowly. (7) Consider utilizing drugs that are metabolized by multiple P-450 enzymes rather than one CYP system. (8) Be aware of which drugs are strong inhibitors of the CYP system. (9) Therapeutic drug monitoring is indicated if relationship exists between drug-level and toxicity. (10) Utilize a computer software program to identify drug-drug interactions or consult with a pharmacist or medication expert. And perhaps, most importantly, patients should be educated to fill all medications at the same pharmacy, so that the pharmacist can identify potential drug interactions.

Table 2.2 Clinically significant methadone drug-drug interactions

Drug	Effects on methadone levels	Effects on QTc interval	Sedative or respiratory depressant effects
Antibiotics			
Ciprofloxacin	Increased		
Clarithromycin	Increased	Increased	
Erythromycin	Increased	Increased	
Itraconazole	Increased		
Ketoconazole	Increased		
Fluconazole	Increased		
Voriconazole	Increased		
Posaconazole	Increased		
Rifampin	Decreased		
Anticonvulsants			
Carbamazepine	Decreased		
Phenytoin	Decreased		
Antihistamines			
Diphenhydramine			Increased
Promethazine			Increased
Antipsychotics			
Quetiapine	Increased	Increased	
Barbiturates			
Phenobarbital	Decreased		Increased
Benzodiazepines			
Alprazolam			Increased
Clorazepate			Increased
Diazepam			Increased
Estazolam			Increased
Flurazepam			Increased
Lorazepam			Increased
Midazolam			Increased
Triazolam			Increased
Zopiclone			Increased
Zolpidem			Increased
HIV medications			
Abacavir	Decreased		
Nevirapine	Decreased		
Delavirdine	Increased		
Efavirenz	Decreased		
Ritonavir-lopinavir	Decreased		
Nelfinavir	Decreased		
Amprenavir	Decreased		
Atazanavir	Decreased		
Selective serotonin reuptake inhibitors			
Fluvoxamine	Increased		
Nefazodone	Increased		
Paroxetine	Increased		
Tricyclic antidepressants			
Amitriptyline		Increased	
Desipramine		Increased	
Imipramine		Increased	
Nortriptyline		Increased	
Protriptyline		Increased	
Urinary alkalinizers			
Bicitra	Increased		
Polycitra	Increased		
Verapamil	Increased		
Other			
Aprepitant	Increased		
Cimetidine	Increased		
Cocaine	Decreased	Increased	
Disulfiram	Increased		
Ethanol	Decreased		Increased
Grapefruit juice or whole fruit	Increased		
Omeprazole	Increased		
St. John's wort	Decreased		

Key Points

- Methadone while highly effective poses unique challenges due to a long and variable half-life and numerous drug-drug interactions.
- Close patient monitoring is imperative particularly in the days following methadone initiation, dose increase, or initiation of concomitant medications known to influence methadone's metabolism.
- Evaluation of the QTc interval is recommended for all patients prior to starting methadone therapy and within 30 days of methadone initiation or dose increase.

References

1. Gaertner J, Voltz R, Ostgathe C. Methadone: a closer look at the controversy. J Pain Symptom Manag. 2008;36(2):e4–6.
2. Gourlay GK, Cherry DA, Cousins MJ. A comparative study of the efficacy and pharmacokinetics of oral methadone and morphine in the treatment of severe pain in patients with cancer. Pain. 1986;25:297–312.
3. Bruera E, Sweeney C. Methadone use in cancer patients: a review. J Palliat Med. 2002;5(1):127–38.
4. Ettinger DS, Vitale PJ, Trump DL. Important clinical pharmacologic considerations in the use of methadone in cancer patients. Cancer Treat Rep. 1979;63:457–9.
5. Garrido MJ, Aguirre C, Troconiz IF, et al. Alpha 1-acid glycoprotein (AAG) and serum protein binding of methadone in heroin addicts with abstinence syndrome. Int J Clin Pharmacol Ther. 2000;38(1):35–40.

6. Baumann P, Tinguely D, Schopf J. Increase of alpha 1-acid glycoprotein after treatment with amitriptyline. Br J Clin Pharmacol. 1982;14:102–3.
7. Sullivan HR, Smits SE, Due SL, et al. Metabolism of d-methadone: isolation and identification of analgesically active metabolites. Life Sci. 1972;11:1093–104.
8. Lepakhin VK. World Health Organization Web site. Safety of medicines: a guide to detecting and reporting adverse drug reactions. 2002. http://whqlibdoc.who.int/hq/2002/WHO_EDM_QSM_2002.2.pdf. Accessed 14 Nov 2015.
9. Shields LB, Hunsaker JC III, Corey TS, Ward MK, Stewart D. Methadone toxicity fatalities: a review of medical examiner cases in a large metropolitan area. J Forensic Sci. 2007;52:1389–95.
10. Webster LR, Cochella S, Dasgupta N, et al. An analysis of root causes for opioid-related overdose deaths in the United States. Pain Med. 2011;12:S26–35.
11. Crowther NR, Holbrook AM, Kenwright R, Kenwright M. Drug interactions among commonly used medications. Can Fam Physician. 1997;43:1972–81.
12. Stimmel B, Lipski J, Swartz M, Donoso E. Electrocardiographic changes in heroin, methadone and multiple drug abuse: a postulated mechanism of sudden death in narcotic addicts. Proc Natl Conf Methadone Treat. 1973;1:706–10.
13. Krantz MJ, Lewkowiez L, et al. Torsades de Pointes with very-high-dose methadone. Ann Intern Med. 2002;137(6):501–4.
14. Roden DM. Drug-induced prolongation of the QT interval. NEJM. 2004;350:1013–22.
15. Kornick CA, Kilborn MJ, Santiago-Palma J, et al. QTc interval prolongation associated with intravenous methadone. Pain. 2003;105:499–506.
16. Soyka LF, Wirtz C, Spangenberg RB. Clinical safety profile of sotalol in patients with arrhythmias. Am J Cardiol. 1990;65(2):74A–81A.
17. Chou R, Weimer MB, Dana T. Methadone overdose and cardiac arrhythmia potential: findings from a review of the evidence for an American Pain Society and College on Problems of Drug Dependence clinical practice guideline. J Pain. 2014;15(4):338–65.
18. Baxter LE Sr, Campbell A, DeShields M, et al. Safe methadone induction and stabilization. J Addict Med. 2013;7:377–86.
19. Perkins NA, Murphy JE, Malone DC, Armstrong EP. Performance of drug-drug interaction software for personal digital assistants. Ann Pharmacother. 2006;40(5):850–5.

Opioid Withdrawal

3

Mark S. Wallace and Alexander Papp

3.1 Case Description

A 63-year-old male presents to the pain clinic for a new patient evaluation. At age 40, he was in a motorcycle accident and sustained a left brachial plexus avulsion injury. He reports constant burning and shooting pains into his left upper extremity. Current pain level is 8/10 with a range of 6–10/10. He reports that the left arm feels cooler than the right with color changes and some involuntary muscle movements. He denies allodynia or hyperalgesia. He has tried multiple medications including anticonvulsants, antidepressants, benzodiazepines, and various opioids. He is currently taking sustained release oxycodone 30 mg four times per day with oxycodone 30 mg six to eight times per day. On review of records from his primary care physician who is prescribing the opioids, there are multiple entries of the patient running out early, noncompliance, and excessive demands for higher doses. The patient admits that the opioids are not really effective in treating his pain and would like to get off but every time he tries to reduce the dose, he experiences severe withdrawal syndrome. He has never tried to slowly taper them. He expresses a desire to get off of them stating that he feels like they are an "albatross" around his neck.

Review of systems is positive for a sleep disturbance, fatigue, anxiety, and depression.

Physical exam reveals significant weakness in the entire left upper extremity. Temperature is about 3 °C cooler than the right. Skin color is slightly pale. There is no allodynia or hyperalgesia. Neck shows pain with extension and rotation with some paraspinous muscle tenderness.

Problem list and diagnosis include:

1. Neuropathic pain secondary to brachial plexus avulsion
2. Opioid dependence
3. Depression
4. Anxiety

Cervical spine MRI shows severe multilevel disk degeneration with multilevel spinal stenosis, left > right.

Treatment plan is discussed with the patient and consists of the following steps:

1. Initiate an opioid taper.
2. Refer to psychology.
3. Refer to addiction psychiatrist for a Suboxone detoxification if indicated.
4. Start bedtime dose of gabapentin with titration increase.

The patient was given an opioid taper schedule with a return visit in 1 week. He calls the clinic after 4 days stating he is out of his opioid and was self-medicating due to pain increase.

3.2 Case Discussion

3.2.1 Biology of Opioid Tolerance, Dependence, and Withdrawal

Opioid tolerance, dependence, withdrawal, and addiction are the result of changes in the brain resulting from chronic opioid exposure. Most pain patients taking opioids chronically will develop tolerance and dependence resulting in withdrawal syndrome with abrupt cessation. This is in contrast to addiction which involves intense drug craving and compulsive use. Opioid withdrawal is one of the most

M.S. Wallace, M.D. (✉)
Division of Pain Medicine, Department of Anesthesiology, University of California San Diego, San Diego, CA, USA
e-mail: mswallace@ucsd.edu

A. Papp, M.D.
Department of Psychiatry, University of California San Diego, San Diego, CA, USA

M. Anitescu et al. (eds.), *Challenging Cases and Complication Management in Pain Medicine*,
https://doi.org/10.1007/978-3-319-60072-7_3

powerful factors driving opioid dependence and addiction. There is no fine line between opioid dependence and addiction as many patients on chronic opioids exhibit behaviors suggesting addiction. Are the patients addicted, or are they trying to avoid the withdrawal syndrome? This creates a complexity that causes great challenges in using this class of drug to treat chronic pain.

Opioid withdrawal is the result of adaptations on multiple areas of the brain including the mesolimbic (midbrain) reward system, ventral tegmental system (VTA), nucleus accumbens (NAc), locus ceruleus, and periaqueductal gray. Activation of the mesolimbic system by the opioids generates signals in the VTA resulting in the release of dopamine (DA) from the NAc resulting in feelings of pleasure. Neurons in the LC produce noradrenaline (NA) which upon release will stimulate wakefulness, breathing, blood pressure, and general alertness. Opioids suppress NA release resulting in drowsiness, respiratory depression, and low blood pressure. The PAG is rich in opioid receptors and endogenous opioid peptides and mediates many physiological functions. This suggests that the PAG plays a key role in dependence and withdrawal syndrome [1, 2].

Opioid withdrawal only results in patients who consume opioids over a long period and who have developed tolerance. Tolerance refers to the decrease in effectiveness of the opioid with continuous use. Different organ systems show differential levels and rates of tolerance. Pupillary miosis shows little or no tolerance; constipation, nausea, analgesia, respiratory depression, low blood pressure, and sedation show moderate tolerance, and euphoria shows rapid tolerance. Over time, tolerance can develop to the pleasure, and opioid abusers continue to consume the opioids not for the pleasure but to avoid the withdrawal syndrome. Interestingly, this feeling of pleasure is blunted in the presence of pain thus chronic pain patients consuming opioids do not necessarily experience the pleasure; however, tolerance to the analgesic effects results in the need for higher doses, dependence, and severe withdrawal with abrupt cessation. It is unclear why there is this differential tolerance between systems, but it is thought to result from differences in functional receptor reserve. In other words, miosis requires a lower receptor activation than analgesia. Opioid tolerance involves multiple levels of the nervous system including mu-receptors, intracellular signaling mechanisms, and supraspinal sites. The effects of chronic opioid exposure on receptors is controversial. Mechanisms proposed include receptor internalization and dephosphorylation, but there is no firm consensus [3, 4]. Intracellularly, chronic opioid exposure initiates adaptive counter regulatory changes resulting in return of neurotransmitter release to more normal levels. Thus higher doses are required to achieve more neurotransmitter release [5]. This adaptation will occur in the areas of the brain described above resulting in tolerance.

In the presence of the tolerance to the opioids described above, the LC neurons will adjust by increasing their level of activity and offset the suppressive effects of the opioids resulting in the patients feeling normal. However, with abrupt cessation, there is a dramatic increase in NA release resulting in the withdrawal syndrome [5].

3.2.2 Opioid Withdrawal Syndrome

Abrupt cessation of an opioid or administration of an opioid antagonist in patient receiving chronic opioids will result in signs and symptoms of withdrawal including abdominal cramping, diarrhea, rhinorrhea, sweating, elevated heart rate, increased blood pressure, irritability, dysphoria, hyperalgesia, and insomnia. These symptoms are the result of a norepinephrine surge in the brain [5]. The onset and duration of the withdrawal will vary depending on the pharmacokinetics of the opioid. Abrupt cessation of morphine will result in withdrawal syndrome within 24 h and lasting 7–10 days. Methadone, which has a much longer half-life, will have more of a slower and sometimes less intense withdrawal syndrome. Sustained or controlled release opioids will have a delayed onset after full release of the opioid. Patients who experience a withdrawal syndrome are often misled into assuming they need the opioids forever. Administration of an antagonist will result in immediate withdrawal syndrome. Although opioid withdrawal is usually not life threatening, acute withdrawal after antagonist administration has been reported to result in neurogenic pulmonary edema, acute respiratory distress syndrome, respiratory failure, and death [6]. If administering an antagonist to reverse sedation and respiratory depression, it is recommended that dosing be given incrementally. However, in the case of respiratory arrest and unconsciousness, a full dose should be administered.

Opioid withdrawal usually goes through three phases. Phase 1 (acute withdrawal) begins about 12 h after the last dose of opioid (up to 30 h for methadone), peaks around 3 days, and lasts for about 5 days. Symptoms include depression, insomnia, nausea, vomiting, diarrhea, and abdominal cramps. Phase 2 lasts about 2 weeks as the body is adjusting the imbalance in brain neurotransmitters caused by the chronic opioids. Symptoms include chills, dilated pupils, and leg cramps. Phase 3 is the least severe and lasts anywhere from 1 week to 2 months. Symptoms include anxiety, restlessness, and insomnia (http://balboahorizons.com/wp-content/uploads/2013/06/Opiate-Withdrawal-Timeline-Infographic.png).

3.2.3 Assessment of Opioid Withdrawal

The DSM-5 criteria for opioid withdrawal are as follows:

1. Either of the following:
   (a) Cessation of (or reduction in) opioid use that has been heavy and prolonged (several weeks or longer)
   (b) Administration of an opioid antagonist after a period of opioid use
2. Three (or more) of the following, developing within minutes to several days after criterion A:
   (a) Dysphoric mood
   (b) Nausea or vomiting
   (c) Muscle aches
   (d) Lacrimation or rhinorrhea
   (e) Pupillary dilation, piloerection, or sweating
   (f) Diarrhea
   (g) Yawning
   (h) Fever
   (i) Insomnia
3. The symptoms in criterion B cause clinically significant distress or impairment in social, occupational, or other important areas of functioning.
4. The signs or symptoms are not due to another medical condition and are not better accounted for by another mental disorder, including intoxication or withdrawal from another substance [7].

There are several validated scales used to assess opioid withdrawal severity. The most commonly used tool is the clinical opioid withdrawal scale (COWS) which is an 11-item scale administered by a clinician. The total score is the sum of all 11 items (5–12 = mild, 13–24 = moderate, 25–36 = moderately sever, more than 36 = severe withdrawal) [8]. The objective opioid withdrawal scale (OOWS) contains 13 physically observable signs, rated present or absent, based on a timed period of observation of the patient by a rater (maximum score is 14). The subjective opioid withdrawal scale (SOWS) contains 16 symptoms whose intensity of the patient rates on a scale of 0 (not at all) to 4 (extremely) (1–10 = mild, 11–20 = moderate, 21–30 = severe withdrawal). The main differences between these scales are that the COWS combines both clinician observation of signs and patient report of symptoms, the OOWS relies only on signs, and the SOWS relies only on symptoms [9].

3.2.4 Whom Should Be Withdrawn from Opioids?

Due to high dependence, the opioids are one of the few classes of drugs that require a commitment once started. Stopping the therapy can be extremely challenging, labor intensive, and time-consuming. As a general rule, opioids should not be abruptly discontinued; however, in the noncompliance patient, abuser, or diverter, abrupt cessation is acceptable. Unlike alcohol or benzodiazepines, acute opioid withdrawal is not life threatening.

It is assumed that all patient receiving adequate pain control and are compliant should continue to receive the opioid indefinitely. However, this is being challenged due to the negative effects of opioids on other organ systems and health. Therefore, even in these patients, recurring consideration for tapering should be introduced to the patient. Many patients who think they need the opioids for life discover that once off, their pain is not that severe and they feel better. Holidays from the opioids provide a period to observe quality of life on and off the drug. There is no clear consensus on this approach, and it should be considered on a case-by-case basis.

However, for patients that are clearly not benefiting from the opioid therapy, reporting high levels of pain, noncompliant, exhibiting drug seeking behaviors, and experiencing unacceptable side effects, a strict plan for tapering the opioid should be initiated.

3.2.5 Approaches to Opioid Tapering

Once the decision is made to stop the chronic opioid use, the patient must be counseled and educated on the reasons behind the decision. It must be made clear to the patient that the therapy is being abandoned, not the patient. Discuss alternatives to treating their pain with non-opioids, integrative therapies, injections, exercise, and psychosocial support. If you present a picture that you are still there for them, they are more likely to cooperate and succeed. However, at the same time, you must remain firm on the decision to taper, and that noncompliance with the taper will not be tolerated. Do not be held hostage for patients that are not compliant, especially when tapering due to noncompliance or abuse issues. Outline a step-by-step plan for the patient which could be a one step of uneventful taper off, a second step of treating severe withdrawal symptoms with adjuvants, a third step of stopping the taper and referring for buprenorphine therapy, a fourth step of referral to an inpatient detoxification center if available, and a fifth step of abrupt cessation if noncompliant.

Most opioids can be reduced by 10–20% per week. For patients taking long-acting opioids, a portion of the long-acting opioid can be converted to short acting with a taper of the short acting until complete. This process can be repeated

Table 3.1 Opioid taper example

Week	Morphine ER dose	Morphine IR dose
1	100 mg TID	30 mg TID
2	100 mg TID	15 mg QID
3	100 mg TID	15 mg BID
4	100 mg BID	30 mg TID
5	100 mg BID	15 mg QID
6	100 mg BID	15 mg BID
7	30 mg TID	30 mg TID
8	30 mg TID	15 mg QID
9	30 mg TID	15 mg BID
10	15 mg TID	15 mg TID
11	15 mg TID	7.5 mg QID
12	15 mg TID	7.5 mg BID
13	Stop	15 mg TID
14		7.5 mg QID
15		7.5 mg BID
16		Stop

Patient on 100 mg sustained release morphine TID with 30 mg morphine immediate release 4 times/day

Table 3.2 Medications used for treating opioid withdrawal symptoms

Withdrawal Symptoms	Medication
Nausea and vomiting	• Metoclopramide 10 mg QID prn
	• Prochlorperazine 5 mg QID prn
	• Ondansetron 4–8 mg BID prn
Diarrhea	• Atropine and diphenoxylate (Lomotil®) 1–2 tablets TID prn
	• Loperamide (Imodium®) 1–2 tablets BID prn
Skeletal muscle cramps	Quinine 300–600 mg at nighttime prn
Muscle and joint aches	• Nonsteroidal anti-inflammatory agents
	• Acetaminophen
Anxiety*	• Clonidine 0.1 mg BID, titrate up to 0.3 mg TID as needed and tolerated
Insomnia	• Gabapentin 300–900 mg at bedtime
	• Pregabalin 75–300 mg at bedtime

*For the anxiety symptoms during opioid withdrawal, benzodiazepines can be useful during the taper but should be used cautiously; upon completion of the opiod taper, benzodiazepines should be also strictly tapered off.

until off the opioid. Depending on the compliance of the patient, weekly or monthly visits and refills are acceptable (Table 3.1).

3.2.6 Management of Opioid Withdrawal Symptoms

If given a slow taper (about 10% per week), most patients will only experience mild withdrawal symptoms. However, some patient will experience severe withdrawal symptoms requiring adjuvants and possible referral for outpatient or inpatient detoxification with buprenorphine. The use of buprenorphine in the treatment of opioid withdrawal generally limits the need for symptomatic medications. However, given the current status of buprenorphine regulation, many practices do not have access and will require attempts at symptomatic treatment of withdrawal symptoms. There are a range of symptomatic medications appropriate for use in opioid withdrawal (Table 3.2). Clonidine is the most commonly used medication for opioid withdrawal as it counteracts the norepinephrine surge that results from opioid cessation. As clonidine is an antihypertensive, it should be used cautiously in patients with low blood pressure and/or heart rate. It is usually administered in conjunction with other agents used to treat symptoms such as nausea, diarrhea, abdominal and muscle cramping, and insomnia. Patients with poor oral intake or vomiting should be monitored for dehydration.

3.2.7 Buprenorphine Detoxification

For patients who cannot tolerate the withdrawal symptoms of the opioid taper, buprenorphine induction and detoxification may be indicated. Buprenorphine is partial μ-receptor agonist and a kappa-receptor antagonist. This results in less analgesia, sedation, euphoria, and respiratory depression than with the full agonists. As a partial agonist, buprenorphine has a "ceiling effect" of the agonist effects at higher dose thus improving safety. It has a high affinity for the opioid receptor and will displace full agonist opioids with less affinity from the receptor. Because buprenorphine does not stimulate the receptors as much as the full agonist, this displacement can result in opioid withdrawal symptoms. Therefore, buprenorphine is initiated when the patient is experiencing opioid withdrawal symptoms (e.g., at least 4 h after the use of a short-acting opioid or 24 h after use of a long-acting opioid such as methadone). In this so-called induction phase, the patient is observed in office for a few hours, and buprenorphine is given in every 30–60 min until the withdrawal symptoms are gone.

Buprenorphine has a poor oral bioavailability necessitating transmucosal or transdermal delivery. A transdermal 7-day patch is FDA approved to treat pain. An oral transmucosal preparation combined with naloxone (Suboxone®) is available. Since Suboxone is approved to treat office-based opioid addiction, the naloxone has been added to discourage intravenous use of the drug. To initiate and stop opioid withdrawal symptoms, 2 mg is typically used and then titrated up to 8–24 mg/day. Because of the ceiling effect, doses above 32 mg are unlikely to provide any further benefit. The effect peaks in 1–4 h after the initial dose with a very long half-life of 24–60 h. Thus it can be administered as a single daily dose although some prefer twice a day dosing and some patients can extend dosing to every other day. Once stable, the dose can be reduced by 2 mg every 1–3 days in inpatients or 2 mg every week in outpatients. Once a patient is free of withdrawal symptoms after induction on certain dose of buprenorphine, they usually go through a stabilization period (called the "maintenance phase") before they are tapered off buprenorphine. Although opioid withdrawal symptoms tend to be less with a buprenorphine taper, if they occur, the medications summarized in Table 3.2 can be used [10].

3.2.8 Buprenorphine Regulations

Prior to the Drug Addiction Treatment Act of 2000 (DATA 2000), medication-assisted treatment of opioid addiction was authorized only in specialized outpatient treatment programs, (OTPs, colloquially known as "methadone clinics"). The activities of such clinics are regulated by the Controlled Substances Act of the United States Code which restricts the MAT of opioid addiction to those types of facilities. It stipulates strict rules for the administration of methadone or levo-alpha-acetylmethadol (LAAM), both schedule II drugs. DATA 2000 enabled qualified physicians to obtain a "waiver" from those requirements and provide MAT in general office settings, including the dispensation or prescription of specifically approved schedule III, IV, and V medications.

The waiver can be obtained from the Substance Abuse and Mental Health Services Administration (SAMHSA). Only DEA-registered physicians can obtain such waivers, not other prescribers, such as nurse practitioners. Any of the following will qualify a physician:

- Being board certified in the subspecialty of addiction psychiatry
- Holding an addiction certification from the American Society of Addiction Medicine [11]
- Having completed a minimum of 8 h training for the treatment and management of opioid use disorders, provided by qualified organizations

There are also a few more, infrequent, qualifying criteria detailed in the DATA 200 document.

The following buprenorphine-containing products are FDA approved for the MAT of opioid addiction:

- Buprenorphine only sublingual tablet (Subutex® and its generic equivalents)
- Buprenorphine + naloxone sublingual film (Suboxone® and its generic equivalents)
- Buprenorphine + naloxone transmucosal patch (Bunavail® and Zubsolv®, no generic equivalents exist)

There are other buprenorphine-containing products (namely, injectable or transdermal formulations) that are approved only for the treatment of pain.

Buprenorphine-containing products are schedule III drugs, and prescriptions for them can be refilled up to five times, as per DEA guidelines. If state rules happen to be stricter, the stricter rules apply.

Qualified physicians are assigned a special DEA number which must be used on every prescription written for a buprenorphine-containing product if it is given for the treatment of opioid dependence: (If it is given for an off-label use, such as pain, this special DEA number does not have to be used).

As there are potential serious risks associated with the use of buprenorphine, the FDA requires that physicians holding a DATA 200 waiver adhere to a Risk Evaluation and Mitigation Strategy (REMS) during the course of office-based treatment of opioid dependence.

During the induction phase, the REMS requires that prescribers:

- Verify that patients meet diagnostic criteria for opioid dependence.
- Discuss the risks and benefits of the treatment with patient.
- Explain the correct ways of storing and disposing of buprenorphine-containing products.
- Prescribe only a limited amount of buprenorphine-containing products after the first visit and schedule frequent follow-ups until stabilization and maintenance.

The managing and monitoring of the treatment is often aided by "treatment contracts" patients sign at the inception of the treatment. It is a recommended but not required aspect of the REMS.

During the maintenance phase, the REMS requires that prescribers:

- Order regular drug screens including for buprenorphine metabolites (this latter to monitor for diversion). Toxicology tests for relevant illicit drugs should be administered at least monthly.
- Check on participation in professional counseling and support services by the patient.
- Schedule visits with frequencies commensurate with the stability and progress of the patient. Once a stable buprenorphine dose is reached and urine toxicology shows no signs of illicit substance use, biweekly or monthly visits can be scheduled.

Pharmacotherapy alone is typically insufficient for the treatment of opiate addiction. Studies repeatedly showed a positive correlation between the intensity of psychosocial services received and the success in the maintenance of abstinence. Therefore the REMS requires the physician either to be able provide such services or to have the capacity of referring patients to such services. Either drug abuse counseling by licensed providers or participation in self-help programs (Alcoholics Anonymous, Narcotics Anonymous, Smart Recovery) are considered sufficient, the best results for patients are provided by participating in both.

The DEA requires that physicians who conduct office-based buprenorphine treatment of opioid addiction should adhere to specific recordkeeping requirements. On random occasions the DEA visits the office of the physician and audits the charts of patients for whom buprenorphine is prescribed, for adherence to the requirements of the REMS. Keeping buprenorphine records separate is advised, but it is not required by the DEA.

Physicians who have waivers to prescribe buprenorphine for the treatment of opioid dependency can request to be listed on SAMHSA's Buprenorphine Treatment Physician Locator [12].

3.2.9 Opioid Management in the Pregnant Patient

It is generally not advised to do an aggressive taper off opioids in the pregnant women as the opioid withdrawal syndrome can have adverse effects on the fetus. However, there are many women on chronic opioids who wish to discontinue the opioids from fears of opioid dependence that the newborn will experience. Therefore, it is reasonable to attempt to gently wean the opioids. Whereas, nonpregnant patients can be weaned 10–25% per week, pregnant patients may need as low as <5% per week. Close assessment of opioid withdrawal symptoms is required. If they are mild and tolerable, the wean can be continued. Otherwise, the wean should be slowed down or stopped. In general, adding other drugs to treat the withdrawal symptoms is discouraged due to risks to the fetus. Ondansetron is a category 2 antiemetic which can be safely used. But consultation with the patient's obstetrician should be made for clearance of any drug used to treat symptoms. Currently, buprenorphine is not FDA approved to treat opioid withdrawal in the pregnant patient. If opioid withdrawal is not successful, the patient should remain on the opioids until delivery, and a neonatologist consultation should be completed before delivery to plan for treatment of the newborn's opioid withdrawal [13].

Key Points

- The chronic use of opioids results in physiological changes in the central nervous system leading to dependence, withdrawal, and possibly addiction.
- The opioid withdrawal syndrome is not life threatening but, can lead to strong resistance to opioid discontinuation in order to avoid the withdrawal symptoms.
- There is not a fine line between treating pain and addiction with chronic opioids. Although many patients may benefit from chronic use to treat pain, these patients should be carefully selected, and in some patients, the opioids will need to be aggressively removed in a controlled fashion. The patients should be aware that the therapy, not the patient, is being abandoned.
- Buprenorphine detoxification is a useful method to discontinue opioids; however, certain regulations must be followed.

References

1. Kosten TR, George TP. The neurobiology of opioid dependence: implications for treatment. Sci Pract Perspect. 2002;1(1):13–20.
2. Ouyang H, Liu S, Zeng W, Levitt RC, Candiotti KA, Hao S. An emerging new paradigm in opioid withdrawal: a critical role for glia-neuron signaling in the periaqueductal gray. ScientificWorldJournal. 2012;2012:940613.
3. Pasternak GW. Molecular biology of opioid analgesia. J Pain Symptom Manag. 2005;29(5 Suppl):S2–9.
4. Yaksh TL, Wallace MS. Opioids, analgesia and pain management. In: Brunton L, Chabner B, Knollman B, editors. Goodman and Gilman's the pharmacological basis of therapeutics, vol. 12. New York: McGraw-Hill; 2011. p. 481–525.
5. Koob GF, Le Moal M. Drug addiction, dysregulation of reward, and allostasis. Neuropsychopharmacology. 2001;24(2):97–129.
6. Hamilton RJ, Olmedo RE, Shah S, et al. Complications of ultrarapid opioid detoxification with subcutaneous naltrexone pellets. Acad Emerg Med. 2002;9(1):63–8.
7. American Psychiatric Association. Diagnostic and statistical manual of mental disorders (DSM-5®). American Psychiatric Pub; 2013.
8. Wesson DR, Ling W. The clinical opiate withdrawal scale (COWS). J Psychoactive Drugs. 2003;35(2):253–9.
9. Handelsman L, Cochrane KJ, Aronson MJ, Ness R, Rubinstein KJ, Kanof PD. Two new rating scales for opiate withdrawal. Am J Drug Alcohol Abuse. 1987;13(3):293–308.
10. Srivastava A, Kahan M. Buprenorphine: a potential new treatment option for opioid dependence. CMAJ. 2006;174(13):1835.
11. Molassiotis A, Uyterlinde W, Hollen PJ, Sarna L, Palmer P, Krishnasamy M. Supportive care in lung cancer: milestones over the past 40 years. J Thorac Oncol. 2015;10(1):10–8.
12. Center for Substance Abuse Treatment. Clinical guidelines for the use of buprenorphine in the treatment of opioid addiction. DHHS Publication No. (SMA) 04-3939 ed. Rockville: Substance Abuse and Mental Health Services Administration; 2004.
13. Patwardhan AG, Rathmell J, Viscomi CM, Bernstein IM. Managing pain during pregnancy and lactation. In: Staats P, Wallace MS, editors. Pain medicine and management: just the facts, vol. 2. New York: McGraw-Hill; 2015. p. 316–24.

Relationship of Chronic Pain and Suicide

4

Sheetal Kerkar DeCaria and Vijal Patel

4.1 Case Study

A 62-year-old female presents to pain clinic a s a new referral from her neurologist. Her chief complaint is leg pain. She has a history of bilateral lower extremity peripheral neuropathy secondary to poorly controlled diabetes. The patient describes the pain starting 10 years prior in her toes. It is now in both lower extremities extending to her mid-thigh. She describes numbness, burning, cramping, and throbbing pain. She also describes occasional debilitating migraine headaches. She is tearful and says she wants to travel to another state to kill herself. She reports reading on the Internet that euthanasia (physician-assisted suicide) was offered in California. She statea 1 day she would travel there to be "put to sleep." She reported having these thoughts for roughly 2 years now. She reports decreased energy, appetite, and activity level, as well as an inability to sleep due to pain.

She sees her psychiatrist regularly for her diagnosis of major depression; he recently increased her dose of sertraline. Between attempts to treat her chronic pain and concurrent depression, she was previously trialed on gabapentin, duloxetine, nortriptyline, amitriptyline, venlafaxine, topiramate, and cyclobenzaprine. All these medications per patient were tolerated but provided no analgesic benefit. Her neurologist recently started her on 5/325 oxycodone/acetaminophen every 4 h. She reports it improves her pain by 20%.

She smokes one pack of cigarettes per day and denies history of illicit drug or alcohol use. She has no family in the United States, was never married, and has no children. She reports having no close friends in the area and living alone. She obtained a high school degree and is currently unemployed.

Review of her lumbar MRI was unremarkable. Lower extremity EMG showed sensory axonal polyneuropathy. Her appearance is disheveled, her clothes mismatched, and her eyes are bloodshot. She is tearful throughout the exam. She fidgets in her seat and appears restless. She makes poor eye contact, and her clothes bear a strong smell of cigarette smoke. Vital signs are stable. Physical exam of lower extremities is notable for 1+ edema. Lower extremity bulk and tone are normal, strength 5/5 throughout, and she displays no fasciculations. Sensory exam of lower extremities shows diminished pinprick up to the knees; position sense and vibratory sensation are within normal limits.

Following exam, we further discussed her intentions to commit suicide. The patient stated that the pain is so bad she is "thinking of killing herself." She said "I don't think I have the guts to kill myself, but you have to help me with this pain." Her psychiatrist was contacted immediately, who reported he feels comfortable sending her home if she verbalized that she has no plan and no intent to harm herself. He would see her in clinic the following week. I asked her if she had purchased a plane ticket, and she said no she had never been on a plane and did not have money for a ticket. Patient stated she had no plan, no means, and no intent to kill herself. We reviewed the risk of overdose of her narcotics. We also started pregabalin to help with her neuropathic pain. I inquired about a prior history of suicide attempts, which she denied. We also discussed scheduling her for a sympathetic block in the next week; she stated that we had "given her so much hope."

4.2 Case Discussion

Chronic pain conditions are associated with an increased risk of suicide. Numerous studies have noted this association, with suicidal ideation approximately three times more likely in chronic pain sufferers and suicide attempt approximately two times more likely compared to those without chronic

S.K. DeCaria, M.D. • V. Patel (✉)
Department of Anesthesia, University of Chicago, Chicago, IL, USA
e-mail: sdecaria@dacc.uchicago.edu; SPatil@dacc.uchicago.edu

M. Anitescu et al. (eds.), *Challenging Cases and Complication Management in Pain Medicine*,
https://doi.org/10.1007/978-3-319-60072-7_4

pain [1–7]. In fact, a 2015 review of chronic pain and suicidality (suicidal thoughts, plans, and attempts) within Australia found that 65% of people who attempted suicide had a history of chronic pain, and after controlling for demographic, mental health, and substance use disorders, chronic pain was independently associated with higher rates of suicidality [6].

In recent years, a number of publications have attempted to study the link between chronic pain and suicide. Overall, multiple psychological processes simultaneously increase pain patients' suicide risk, including depression, pain-related helplessness, desire for escape, erosion of fear of dying, and catastrophizing [1, 2]. Pain-related catastrophizing is described as an exaggerated, negative focus on pain that is linked to feelings of helplessness and hopelessness. Their focus on pain becomes centric to all other ongoing processes, leading to feelings of being unable to escape and continuously in pain [8]. This creates a cycle to worsen depression, pain intensity, and pain-related disability [1, 8]. This also plays a role in engendering a sense of mental defeat, in which the chronic pain patient's identity has suffered a severe blow due to a loss of autonomy and human integrity due to living with chronic pain [9, 10]. This loss and suffering, i.e., mental defeat, helps drive a desire to escape from chronic pain, which could manifest as suicidality [10]. Mental defeat can be considered a larger encompassing term that reflects the deep impact that chronic pain imparts on the patient's sense of self that is not explained wholly by depression alone [10].

4.2.1 Risk Factors

When examining suicide in the chronic pain population, a number of risk factors have been identified. In reviewing publications from 1966 to 2004, Tang et al. were able to pinpoint the most common risk factors (1, Table 4.1). Family history of suicide increases this risk, with suicidal ideation being up to eight times as prevalent in chronic pain patients with a family history of suicide compared to those without such a history [11]. This correlates with general suicide risk literature, with family history being a significant risk factor for suicide ideation and attempt [12, 13]. Similarly, previous suicide attempt and the presence of comorbid depression were found to have an increased risk of suicidality in chronic pain patients (as well as in the general population) [2, 6, 9, 12–16]. Gender, however, was not in line with general population studies that show men are more likely to complete a suicide attempt. In chronic pain patients, female sufferers were more likely to engage in suicidal behaviors [6, 16]. However, this association may be due to the increased prevalence of female chronic pain patients [1, 17]. There is also a fair amount of evidence noting specific pain conditions with increased suicidality: back pain, neck pain, abdominal pain, and migraine [1, 6, 18–20]. Additionally, the longer the duration of pain, the greater the likelihood of suicidal ideation [4, 15]. While pain severity seems logical as a risk factor for suicidality, the data is thus far conflicting and as such it cannot be considered a definitive risk factor [1, 4, 18]. Finally, comorbid insomnia was found to be a significant risk factor for suicidal ideation in chronic pain patients, with greater sleep disturbance noted in suicidal individuals versus nonsuicidal [1, 11, 18]. It should be noted, however, that not *all* depressed chronic pain patients are suicidal [11, 14].

Table 4.1 Risk factors for suicide in chronic pain patients [1, 2]

1.	Family history of suicide
2.	Previous suicide attempt
3.	Comorbid depression
4.	Female gender
5.	Location of pain (back, neck, abdominal, migraine)
6.	Pain duration
7.	Comorbid insomnia

4.2.2 Do Certain Pain Medications Increase Suicide Risk?

When considering pharmacologic therapy in chronic pain patients, a number of agents are currently employed, including a variety of neuropathies (antiepileptics and antidepressants) and opioids.

Antiepileptic drugs (AEDs) frequently prescribed in the chronic pain setting include gabapentin, pregabalin, and carbamazepine. In 2008, the FDA completed a statistical analysis that resulted in a federal mandate requiring all AEDs to have labeling noting a warning of increased risk of suicide [21]. However, since then, numerous publications have refuted this broad generalization. In regard to the FDA data analysis itself, statistical significance for increased risk of suicide was noted only with topiramate and lamotrigine [21, 22]. Since then, a number of studies have been published showing AEDs commonly prescribed in the chronic pain setting are both efficacious and pose no increased risk of suicidality, with some data possibly conferring a protecting effect (by helping to control the chronic pain) [22, 23]. Rissanen et al. found no increased risk of suicidal ideation with AED users and nonusers (although this was a retrospective analysis on patients with epilepsy, not in chronic pain patients) [24]. Gibbons et al. conducted a pharmacoepidemiological study regarding gabapentin within a medical claims database in chronic pain patients and found no statistically significant increased risk of suicide attempts [25]. This data matched the FDA data analysis. While it is worthwhile to note there are studies citing increased risk of suicidality with gabapentin, specifically that by Patorno et al., this may be due to confounding factors since it is an outlier from other analyses (when reviewing the aggregate FDA analysis tables) [25, 26]. Like gabapentin, overall, pregabalin is considered low risk of suicidality. While there are three case reports of suicidal ideation and attempt after pregabalin therapy initiation, the larger data set in the FDA data analysis shows no statistically significant increase in suicidality with pregabalin, with large confidence intervals crossing 1 [21, 26–28]. However, the risk of suicidality should not be discounted entirely with AEDs. While the trend may not be statistically significant and may be at best an association, chronic pain patients have a number of risk factors for increased risk of suicidality; thus, initiation of an AED may be an appropriate time to consider screening a patient for suicidal ideation.

Selective serotonin reuptake inhibitors (SSRI's), as a class, were initially thought to increase suicidality. In recent years, clarification of this suicide risk has been made with multiple studies. In adults, there is either no difference or possibly a decreased risk of suicide risk between SSRI users and nonusers in depressed populations [29, 30]. However, in adolescents, SSRIs may increase risk of suicidality [30–32]. When examining time course, the highest risk of suicidality in both adults and adolescents occurred within the first 28 days of initiating medication or when discontinuing therapy [32]. Within the SSRI class, there were no differences noted in suicide risk [32]. When compared to tricyclic antidepressants (TCAs), such as amitriptyline, Coupland et al. noted similar rates of suicidality and self-harm in a primary care cohort of depressed patients treated with either SSRIs or TCAs [32, 33].

Opioid therapy for chronic pain has specific factors that are associated with suicidality. In fact, Fischer et al. showed that there was an increase in opioid-related mortality, as opioid prescribing increased, when examining opioid prescriptions and related mortality in Ontario over 6 years [34]. It was also noted that patients receiving higher opioid doses were at increased risk of opioid overdose, both intentionally and unintentionally [35, 36].

To limit the risk of suicide attempt while prescribing opioids, a number of recommendations have come to light. In particular, frequent drug screens are associated with decreased risk of suicide attempt, as well as follow-up within 4 weeks after beginning new opioid prescriptions [20]. Finally, avoiding (if not limiting) prescribing additional sedatives can increase the risk of adverse side effects, particularly if an overdose is taken [20, 36].

4.2.3 Need for Risk Assessments

While not every chronic pain patient is suicidal, clinicians need to be able to recognize particular risk factors that elevate the risk of suicidality as well as develop a plan to manage that risk [37].

Drug overdose is the most common method of suicide in chronic pain patients, with approximately 75% of those studied by Smith et al. to have attempted overdose on prescribed analgesics and tricyclic antidepressants [11]. Furthermore, it was noted by Tang et al. that the majority of chronic pain patients who ended their lives visited their physician within the month prior to their suicide [1]. This timeline emphasizes the importance of prevention, intervention, and risk management by the physician.

There is currently no gold standard to formally assess suicidality within chronic pain patients. Risk assessment should focus on key points of evaluating fearlessness, depression, hopelessness, mental defeat, catastrophizing, coping skills, and support system. There are multiple different assessments that have been validated on various specific risk factors. The Beck Depression Inventory and Profile of Mood States are two screening tools recommended by the Initiative on Methods, Measurements, and Pain Assessment in Clinical Trials (IMMPACT) consensus group regarding measuring emotional functioning in chronic pain trials [8]. The Beck Depression Inventory Fast Screen (BDI-FS) is another tool that has been validated in assessing depression within pain patients and was specifically designed to eliminate false positives associated with the original Beck Depression Inventory [38]. The BDI-FS)may be extremely useful in busy practices since it is a short, seven-question screen; however, it is copyrighted and thus not freely available.

Risk assessment should extend beyond depression and include key points of evaluating fearlessness, hopelessness, mental defeat, catastrophizing, coping skills, and support system. While a simple discussion with the patient may help elucidate many of these factors, specific screening measures are available. The Hospital Anxiety and Depression Scale, Beck Hopelessness Scale, Pain Self-Efficacy Questionnaire, Catastrophizing in Pain Scale, and Pain Self-Perception Scale have all been utilized to this end in academic practices [2, 9].

A strong indicator of suicide risk is that of mental defeat. Tang et al. found that mental defeat was the strongest predictor of pain interference, depression, and psychosocial disability and a key indicator of heightened suicide risk within chronic pain patients [10, 39]. To assess mental defeat, one can employ the Pain Self-Perception Scale (PSPS) (Fig. 4.1), a 24-item questionnaire used to assess mental defeat in chronic pain patients that has been validated both in English and Spanish [10, 39, 40]. The PSPS is a combination of select questions adapted from both PTSD mental defeat scale and depression defeat scale, in which patients rate a recent pain episode on a five-point scale (0 = "Not at all/Never," 1 = "Very little," 2 = "Moderately," 3 = "Strongly," 4 = "Very strongly"), to generate a total score from 0 to 96 [40]. A limitation is that no specific score cutoff has been clearly implicated as indicating a statistically significant increased suicide

Pain Self-Perception Scale

1. I feel defeated by life
2. I felt that I had lost my standing in the world
3. I felt that life had treated me like a punchbag
4. I felt powerless
5. I felt that my confidence had been knocked out of me
6. I didn't feel able to deal with things that life threw at me
7. I feel that I had sunk to the bottom of the ladder
8. I felt completely knocked out of action
9. I felt that I was one of life's losers
10. I felt that I had given up
11. I felt down and out
12. I felt I had lost important battles in life
13. I felt that there was no fight left in me
14. I felt I was losing my will power
15. I didn't care what happened to me anymore
16. I felt defeated
17. I felt less like a human being
18. In my mind, I gave up
19. I felt destroyed as a person
20. I felt like I wanted to die
21. I felt like I was losing my inner resistance
22. I felt like an object
23. I felt completely at the mercy of what was happening to me
24. I felt humiliated and that I was losing my sense of inner dignity

Fig. 4.1 Pain Self-Perception Scale. Score is based recent pain episode, evaluated on a five-point scale (0 = "not at all/never," 1 = "very little," 2 = "moderately," 3 = "strongly," 4 = "very strongly"), with chronic pain patients generally scoring greater than 30 [40]

risk. However, in the original exploration of the PSPS and in its Spanish translation validation, chronic pain patients were seen to have mean scores >30, and their scores tended to be higher than those of acute pain patients [10, 40]. This scale can also be utilized to trend a patient's psychological health over time with treatment and evaluate the need for increased suicidality risk management if their score increased.

If you are concerned about suicide risk in a patient, be forward and address it directly with the patient. Asking about a patient's potential suicidal intent does not increase risk of suicide; Dazzi et al. found that such questions may actually reduce suicidal ideation and lead to improvements in mental health [41]. The following are suggested questions you may ask to gauge your decision making (referral, hospitalization, etc.), adapted from the full Columbia-Suicide Severity Rating Scale [42, 43]:

- Have you actually had thoughts about killing yourself?
- Have you been thinking about how you might do this?
- Have you had these thoughts and had some intention of acting on them?
- Have you started to work out or worked out the details of how to kill yourself? Do you intend to carry out this plan?
- Have you done anything, started to do anything, or prepared to do anything to end your life?

Regardless of method employed, risk assessments should be performed at initial visits and periodically with follow-up visits. If a patient displays risk factors of suicide, it is important to ask them if they have active thoughts of suicide, and if so, whether they have a plan. If their answers are yes, it is prudent to involve psychiatry, and if a suicide plan has been made, one must admit the patient to a hospital.

Furthermore, key actions to consider in high-risk patients are listed in Table 4.2. The physician should provide the high-risk chronic pain patient key phone numbers and contact information in case of emergency, including 911 and National Suicide Prevention Lifeline (1-800-273-8255), which is available in English and Spanish, as well as online at www.suicidepreventionlifeline.org [7, 19]. Discuss with the patient their support network (including family, friends, and support groups), and help them formulate a plan to address access to means of suicide, such as prescription medications and firearms. Emphasize the need for behavioral health and psychiatric co-treatment for a multidisciplinary approach to managing their chronic pain. This can help in the management of comorbid depression as well as provide psychotherapeutic interventions such as coping skills to minimize catastrophizing, relaxation therapy, cognitive behavior treatment (CBT), and acceptance and commitment therapy (ACT) [37]. Irrespective of the particular psychiatric therapy approach, there should also be clear validation of the patient's

Table 4.2 Interventions to consider in high-risk of suicidality patients

–	Key emergency contacts
	National Suicide Prevention Lifeline
	1 (800) 273-8255, www.suicidepreventionlifeline.org
–	Emphasize support network (family, friends, clergy, support groups, etc.)
–	Create plan to address availability to means, including prescription medications, weapons, etc.
–	Behavioral health/psychiatric care for co-treatment (for assistance in managing depression, as well as psychotherapy)
–	Early follow-up (within 4 weeks) after initiating new prescriptions (opioids, neuropathies, antidepressants)
–	Immediate inpatient hospitalization for high suicide risk requiring intervention

pain problem by all involved in the patient's care, emphasizing it to be a genuine and difficult chronic health condition. One should also foster and nurture the patient's reasons for living [37]. Finally, continually assess the need for prompt inpatient hospitalization if deemed high suicide risk necessitating immediate intervention [7, 19].

In regard to opioids, in patients screened to be at increased risk of suicide, opioids should be avoided if possible. If required, possible prescribing strategies include dispensing small amounts of opioids at the lowest possible dose to effectively manage pain and limiting concomitant central nervous system depressants, such as benzodiazepines [20, 35, 36]. Furthermore, conduct early follow-up (3–4 weeks) after initiating new prescriptions and dose changes (opioids, neuropathies, and antidepressants), as this was shown to significantly decrease risk of suicide attempt [20, 32, 34]. Finally, as with all chronic pain patients, target potential mediators of suicide risk (insomnia, pain coping skills, etc.) and incorporate psychotherapy and psychiatric care as part of multimodal pain management therapy.

Key Point Section

- Chronic pain is independently associated with increased risk of suicidality.
- Suicidal ideation and attempt is two to three times more likely in chronic pain suffers (versus those without chronic pain).
- Multiple underlying psychological processes drive increased suicide risk, including depression, pain-related helplessness, and mental defeat.
- Risk factors for suicidality in chronic pain: family history of suicide, comorbid depression, previous suicide attempt, female gender, pain location (back, neck, abdomen, and migraine), prolonged pain duration, comorbid insomnia, and opioid prescriptions.
- Opioids are the only commonly used chronic pain medication linked to increase suicide risk.
- Regular screening and risk assessments: Beck Depression Inventory (and Beck Depression Inventory Fast Screen), Profile of Mood States, Pain Self-Perception Scales.
- Early integration of multispecialty chronic pain management, including behavior and psychiatric therapy.
- Early follow-up (within 4 weeks) after initiating new prescriptions (opioids, neuropathies, antidepressants) decrease suicide in high-risk patients.

References

1. Tang NKY, Crane C. Suicidality in chronic pain: a review of the prevalence, risk factors and psychological links. Psychol Med. 2006;36(5):575–86.
2. Hooley JM, Franklin JC, Nock MK. Chronic pain and suicide: understanding the association. Curr Pain Headache Rep [Internet]. 2014;18(8):435. http://link.springer.com/10.1007/s11916-014-0435-2. [Cited 29 Aug 2015].
3. Breslau N. Migraine, suicidal ideation, and suicide attempts. Neurology. 1992;42(2):392–5.
4. Hinkley BS, Jaremko ME. Effects of pain duration on psychosocial adjustment in orthopedic patients: the importance of early diagnosis and treatment of pain. J Pain Symptom Manag. 1994;9(3):175–85.
5. Magni G, Rigatti-Luchini S, Fracca F, Merskey H. Suicidality in chronic abdominal pain: an analysis of the Hispanic Health and Nutrition Examination Survey (HHANES). Pain. 1998;76(1–2):137–44.
6. Campbell G, Darke S, Bruno R, Degenhardt L. The prevalence and correlates of chronic pain and suicidality in a nationally representative sample. Aust N Z J Psychiatry. 2015;49(9):803–11.
7. Wang H, Ahrens C, Rief W, Schiltenwolf M. Influence of comorbidity with depression on interdisciplinary therapy: outcomes in patients with chronic low back pain. Arthritis Res Ther. 2010;12(5):R185.
8. Cheatle MD. Depression, chronic pain, and suicide by overdose: on the edge. Pain Med. 2011;12(Suppl 2):S43–8.
9. Tang NKY, Beckwith P, Ashworth P. Mental defeat is associated with suicide intent in patients with chronic pain. Clin J Pain. 2016;32(5):411–9.
10. Tang NKY, Salkovskis PM, Hanna M. Mental defeat in chronic pain: initial exploration of the concept. Clin J Pain. 2007;23(3):222–32.
11. Smith MT, Edwards RR, Robinson RC, Dworkin RH. Suicidal ideation, plans, and attempts in chronic pain patients: factors associated with increased risk. Pain. 2004;111(1–2):201–8.
12. Hawton K, Casañas i Comabella C, Haw C, Saunders K. Risk factors for suicide in individuals with depression: a systematic review. J Affect Disord. 2013;147(1–3):17–28.
13. Hawton K, van Heeringen K. Suicide. Lancet. 2009;373(9672):1372–81.
14. Fisher BJ, Haythornthwaite JA, Heinberg LJ, Clark M, Reed J. Suicidal intent in patients with chronic pain. Pain. 2001;89(2–3):199–206.
15. Treharne GJ, Lyons AC, Kitas GD. Suicidal ideation in patients with rheumatoid arthritis. Research may help identify patients at high risk. BMJ. 2000;321(7271):1290.
16. Timonen M, Viilo K, Hakko H, Särkioja T, Ylikulju M, Meyer-Rochow VB, et al. Suicides in persons suffering from rheumatoid arthritis. Rheumatology (Oxford). 2003;42(2):287–91.
17. Jackson T, Thomas S, Stabile V, Han X, Shotwell M, McQueen K. Prevalence of chronic pain in low-income and middle-income countries: a systematic review and meta-analysis. Lancet. 2015;385(Suppl 2):S10.
18. Smith MT, Perlis ML, Haythornthwaite JA. Suicidal ideation in outpatients with chronic musculoskeletal pain: an exploratory study of the role of sleep onset insomnia and pain intensity. Clin J Pain. 2004;20(2):111–8.
19. Hassett AL, Aquino JK, Ilgen MA. The risk of suicide mortality in chronic pain patients. Curr Pain Headache Rep. 2014;18(8):436.
20. Im JJ, Shachter RD, Oliva EM, Henderson PT, Paik MC, Trafton JA. Association of Care Practices with suicide attempts in US veterans prescribed opioid medications for chronic pain management. J Gen Intern Med. 2015;30(7):979–91.
21. U.S. Department of Health and Human Services, Food and Drug Administration, Center for Drug Evaluation and Research, Office of Translational Sciences, Office of Biostatistics. Statistical review and evaluation: antiepileptic drugs and suicidality. 23 May 2008.
22. Kanner AM. Are antiepileptic drugs used in the treatment of migraine associated with an increased risk of suicidality? Curr Pain Headache Rep. 2011;15(3):164–9.
23. Hesdorffer DC, Berg AT, Kanner AM. An update on antiepileptic drugs and suicide: are there definitive answers yet? Epilepsy Curr. 2010;10(6):137–45.
24. Rissanen I, Jääskeläinen E, Isohanni M, Koponen H, Ansakorpi H, Miettunen J. Use of antiepileptic or benzodiazepine medication and suicidal ideation—the Northern Finland Birth Cohort 1966. Epilepsy Behav. 2015;46:198–204.

25. Gibbons RD, Hur K, Brown CH, Mann JJ. Gabapentin and suicide attempts. Pharmacoepidemiol Drug Saf. 2010;19(12):1241–7.
26. Mutschler J, Grosshans M, Herwig U, Heekeren K, Kawohl W, Brühl A. Pregabalin-induced suicidal ideations. Pharmacopsychiatry. 2011;44(3):119.
27. Kustermann A, Möbius C, Oberstein T, Müller HH, Kornhuber J. Depression and attempted suicide under pregabalin therapy. Ann Gen Psychiatry. 2014;13(1):37.
28. Tandon V, Mahajan V, Gillani Z, Mahajan A. Pregabalin-induced self-harm behavior. Indian J Pharmacol. 2013;45(6):638.
29. Khan A, Khan S, Kolts R, Brown WA. Suicide rates in clinical trials of SSRIs, other antidepressants, and placebo: analysis of FDA reports. Am J Psychiatry. 2003;160(4):790–2.
30. Barbui C, Esposito E, Cipriani A. Selective serotonin reuptake inhibitors and risk of suicide: a systematic review of observational studies. CMAJ. 2009;180(3):291–7.
31. Gordon M, Melvin G. Selective serotonin re-uptake inhibitors—a review of the side effects in adolescents. Aust Fam Physician. 2013;42(9):620–3.
32. Coupland C, Hill T, Morriss R, Arthur A, Moore M, Hippisley-Cox J. Antidepressant use and risk of suicide and attempted suicide or self harm in people aged 20 to 64: cohort study using a primary care database. BMJ. 2015;350:h517.
33. Atkinson SD, Prakash A, Zhang Q, Pangallo BA, Bangs ME, Emslie GJ, et al. A double-blind efficacy and safety study of duloxetine flexible dosing in children and adolescents with major depressive disorder. J Child Adolesc Psychopharmacol. 2014;24(4):180–9.
34. Fischer B, Jones W, Urbanoski K, Skinner R, Rehm J. Correlations between prescription opioid analgesic dispensing levels and related mortality and morbidity in Ontario, Canada, 2005-2011. Drug Alcohol Rev. 2014;33(1):19–26.
35. Dunn KM, Saunders KW, Rutter CM, Banta-Green CJ, Merrill JO, Sullivan MD, et al. Opioid prescriptions for chronic pain and overdose: a cohort study. Ann Intern Med. 2010;152(2):85–92.
36. Madadi P, Persaud N. Suicide by means of opioid overdose in patients with chronic pain. Curr Pain Headache Rep [Internet]. 2014;18(11):460. http://link.springer.com/10.1007/s11916-014-0460-1. [Cited 29 Aug 2015].
37. Newton-John TR. Negotiating the maze: risk factors for suicidal behavior in chronic pain patients. Curr Pain Headache Rep. 2014;18(9):447.
38. Poole H, Bramwell R, Murphy P. The utility of the Beck Depression Inventory Fast Screen (BDI-FS) in a pain clinic population. Eur J Pain. 2009;13(8):865–9.
39. Tang NKY, Goodchild CE, Hester J, Salkovskis PM. Mental defeat is linked to interference, distress and disability in chronic pain. Pain. 2010;149(3):547–54.
40. García-Campayo J, Rodero B, del Hoyo YL, Luciano JV, Alda M, Gili M. Validation of a Spanish language version of the pain self-perception scale in patients with fibromyalgia. BMC Musculoskelet Disord. 2010;11:255.
41. Dazzi T, Gribble R, Wessely S, Fear NT. Does asking about suicide and related behaviours induce suicidal ideation? What is the evidence? Psychol Med. 2014;44(16):3361–3.
42. Posner K, Brown GK, Stanley B, Brent DA, Yershova KV, Oquendo MA, et al. The Columbia–suicide severity rating scale: initial validity and internal consistency findings from three multisite studies with adolescents and adults. Am J Psychiatr. 2011;168(12):1266–77.
43. Posner K, Brown GK, Stanley B, Brent DA, Yershova KV, Oquendo MA, et al. Columbia-suicide severity rating scale, Daily/Shift Screen [Internet]. 2008. http://www.cssrs.columbia.edu/documents/C-SSRSFrequentScreener.docx. [Cited 17 Sept 2015].

Torsades de Pointes After Methadone Treatment

5

Andrea Shashoua

5.1 Case Description

A 62-year-old man with alcoholic cirrhosis and hepatitis C complicated by hepatocellular carcinoma is admitted to the hospital for non-operative treatment of his cancer. The patient is brought to interventional radiology for planned chemoembolization and radiofrequency tumor ablation. His current medications include amiloride, fluoxetine, furosemide, lactulose, methadone, rifaximin, Peri-Colace, and zinc sulfate. He has no known drug allergies. He smokes every day and has a 45 pack-year history. He abstained from alcohol 3 years ago and intravenous (IV) drug abuse 25 years ago.

Before the procedure, his temperature is 95.5 °F, heart rate 79 bpm, respiratory rate 20, blood pressure 126/58 mmHg, and SpO_2 97% on room air.

An IV is started by the nurse, and the following monitors are placed: ECG, noninvasive blood pressure, and pulse oximetry. A nasal cannula is applied and conscious sedation begins with fentanyl and midazolam. The patient is anxious at the start of the procedure.

Approximately 25 min later, the nurse monitoring the patient notes frequent episodes of bigeminy on the ECG. Vital signs are stable. The interventional radiologist is made aware, and the procedure continues. Ten minutes later, the patient displays frequent short runs of what appears to be ventricular tachycardia. Vital signs remain relatively unchanged. The patient is drowsy but easily awakened. The rapid response team is called to assess the patient in the procedure room. A decision is made to proceed based on stable hemodynamics and patient disposition. Blood is drawn for basic chemistries and cardiac enzymes. A 12-lead ECG in the recovery room is planned for immediate use after the procedure.

The procedure is successfully completed 45 min later. Vital signs remained unchanged throughout, despite continued frequent bursts of ventricular tachycardia alternating with a baseline bigeminy pattern. In the post-procedure area, the patient appears comfortable and denies cardiopulmonary symptoms. Intervals of ventricular tachycardia are now longer and more frequent. ECG reveals sinus rhythm with premature ventricular contractions in a bigeminy pattern. There is a non-specific ST abnormality and a long QT interval with a corrected QT (QTc) of 596 ms. The patient is brought on a gurney to the emergency department.

An ECG reveals ventricular tachycardia, T wave abnormality with possible inferolateral ischemia, and prolonged QT interval. Heart rate is now 150–170 bpm. Blood pressure is stable. Almost immediately after administration of an IV bolus of amiodarone, normal sinus rhythm is maintained with heart rate in the 70s. Thirty minutes later, the monitor reveals frequent episodes of what appears to be a wide complex ventricular tachycardia. The cardiology service is called for evaluation and management.

Laboratory test results are as follows: potassium 3.1 mEq/L, calcium 7.7 mg/dL, magnesium 1.0 mg/dL, albumin 2.4 g/dL, total bilirubin 2.5 mg/dL, alkaline phosphatase 170 IU/L, AST 110, and ALT 56. Cardiac enzymes and troponins are negative. The cardiologist interprets the ECG as torsades de pointes with a heart rate of 180–200 bpm. An IV bolus of amiodarone and magnesium is given, followed by an infusion of both.

The patient's heart soon converts back to sinus rhythm. He is transferred to the telemetry floor where bedside two-dimensional echocardiography is performed. The echocardiogram shows no significant structural abnormalities. The patient remained asymptomatic throughout all the events described and wanted to know why he had to stay and be monitored.

Upon more detailed questioning, the cardiology service learns from the patient that he has been taking methadone every day for the last 30 years for maintenance therapy. He

A. Shashoua
University of Chicago Medical Center, Chicago, IL, USA
e-mail: ashashoua@yahoo.com

M. Anitescu et al. (eds.), *Challenging Cases and Complication Management in Pain Medicine*,
https://doi.org/10.1007/978-3-319-60072-7_5

admitted to a history of IV drug abuse and said that the only reason he hasn't relapsed is because of daily methadone. He receives methadone from an outpatient detoxification clinic and has been on the same dose for many years. He reports being told that he "hypermetabolizes" methadone and therefore needs a high dose. He was never warned of the side effects associated with his dose of methadone.

The hospital care team elects to discontinue the patient's daily medications, which are known to alter methadone's metabolism. At this point, sinus rhythm had been maintained for several consecutive hours. Since his liver function is already compromised, the team decides to stop the amiodarone infusion. Methadone is discontinued that day and the next. Morphine 2 mg IV every 2 h as needed and Ativan 1 mg IV every 4 h as needed are ordered. After 48 h without methadone, the patient becomes anxious and reports having diarrhea. He tells the physicians that he is leaving to get methadone because he doesn't want to go into withdrawal. The physicians explain about the black box warning on methadone: high doses pose cardiac risks. The process of weaning is explained, but the patient refuses to consider it. He prefers a fatal arrhythmia to relapse or withdrawal.

The hospital physician contacts the patient's methadone clinic to verify the dosage, discuss the events that occurred, and propose that the patient's methadone dose be weaned to decrease his cardiac risk. The clinic physician refuses to discuss specifics regarding the patient but says that the clinic has protocols in place to treat QT prolongation. He asks to be notified of any dosage changes that are made when the patient is discharged from the hospital.

After a long discussion with the patient about adjuncts that can be prescribed to alleviate withdrawal symptoms, he finally agrees to a slow wean from methadone. The patient is discharged home on a clonidine patch, loperamide when needed, and methadone 145 mg daily. A wearable defibrillator is given to the patient to use until the risk of recurrent arrhythmia is reduced. An appointment for follow-up with a cardiologist is scheduled for the next week.

5.2 Case Discussion

5.2.1 Methadone Uses

Methadone, legalized in the United States in 1947, is listed as a schedule II substance under the Controlled Substances Act [1]. It is available as a tablet, oral solution, and injectable liquid.

Methadone maintenance therapy is strictly regulated by the federal government, and programs must be certified by the Federal Substance Abuse and Mental Health Services Administration. Prescribers must be specifically licensed by the DEA. Methadone maintenance is associated with a decreased risk of illicit opioid use and its related complications [1–3]. Data suggest that the benefits from decreased illicit drug use outweigh the harm [4]. Less evidence exists for the benefit or harm of methadone for pain management [4]. The use of methadone for pain management increased in the early 2000s. It was an excellent alternative to other opioids because of low cost, long-acting pharmacokinetics, and favorable tolerability. Within the last decade, more attention has been given to methadone because of data indicating large increases in the number of associated deaths [5]. There are many challenges in interpreting the statistics regarding methadone-associated mortality.

5.2.2 Pharmacokinetics

Methadone is an NMDA receptor antagonist. It is at this receptor that methadone is thought to decrease tolerance and craving for opioids and combat neuropathic pain. As a mu agonist, it acts at the same receptor site as morphine and heroin. The release of clinically important neurotransmitters such as glutamate, acetylcholine, norepinephrine, and dopamine is another proposed benefit of the drug.

Because methadone is metabolized slowly and is highly fat soluble, elimination half-life can range anywhere from 15 to 60 h, longer than its duration of analgesic action [6].

Full analgesic effect is usually not reached until 3–5 days of dosing; therefore, titration and dose adjustments should be made slowly. The metabolism of methadone by individuals is highly variable because of multiple enzymatic interactions with cytochrome p450. The most important isozymes involved are CYP3A4, CYP2B6, and CYP2D6 [7]. A large variety of drugs and certain foods can induce or inhibit these enzymes, thus affecting methadone's half-life. See Table 5.1. Increases or decreases in methadone's metabolism have implications on dosing frequency, side effects, and overall drug profile. Incomplete cross-tolerance and methadone's effect on tolerance complicate conversion to alternative opioids [8].

Table 5.1 Cytochrome P-450 drug interactions

Inhibitors	Inducers
Quinidine	Phenobarbital
Cimetidine	St. John's wort
Ketoconazole	Phenytoin
Fluconazole	Carbamazepine
Metronidazole	Rifampin
Grapefruit juice	Cigarette smoking
Erythromycin	Pioglitazone
Paroxetine	Oxcarbazepine
Fluoxetine	
Amiodarone	
Simvastatin	

5.2.3 Safety Warnings

In 2006, the FDA released a public safety advisory after a trend of methadone-related deaths in patients treated for non-malignant pain [9]. A black box warning from the manufacturer was then issued. This warning identifies severe respiratory depression as the most problematic side effect of methadone. The warning also exposes the risk of fatal arrhythmia (torsades de pointes) and QT prolongation with methadone treatment. These events were reported in patients treated for pain with large, daily doses of methadone. But patients taking conventional doses for opioid detoxification and maintenance were not excluded from these risks [9, 10] (Table 5.2).

5.2.4 Cardiac Manifestations

Methadone can cause serious cardiac conduction effects, including QT interval prolongation and torsades de pointes [11]. A host of common cardiac and non-cardiac medications as well as electrolyte disturbances can prolong the QT interval. QT prolongation can be inherited as well as acquired. All forms cause abnormal repolarization leading to altered refractory periods in the heart. Patients with prolonged QT interval are especially prone to syncope or even sudden death during periods of stress or sympathetic stimulation because of deranged repolarization [12].

Table 5.2 Risk factors for QTc prolongation and torsades de pointes

QTc prolongation	Torsades de pointes
Genetic disposition	Concurrent use of one or more QT interval prolonging drugs
Electrolyte abnormalities	Congenital prolonged QT
Liver disease	QTc interval greater than 500 ms
Thyroid disease	Electrolyte abnormalities
Advanced age	History of torsades de pointes
Female gender	A-V node dysfunction and bradyarrhythmias
Structural heart disease	Ischemic heart disease and congestive heart failure
Medication induced	Advanced age
Illicit drug use	Recent conversion from atrial fibrillation

Rate-corrected QT (QTc) greater than 450 ms is considered prolonged, and >500 ms is associated with an increased risk for sudden death [13]. Generally, the QTc is slightly longer in women [14].

In a review of patients on methadone therapy, the prevalence of QTc interval prolongation ranged from 0.5 to 31% based on a threshold of >430 to 450 ms in men and >460 to 470 ms in women [10, 12, 15–18]. The proportion of patients who exceeded a QTc >500 ms ranged from 0 to 6% in six studies [10, 13, 16, 19–21]. Higher methadone doses were associated with greater prolongation of QTc interval after controlling for other confounding factors [10, 12, 18, 19, 22, 23]. Patients who took high daily doses had torsades de pointes [22, 24].

5.2.5 Torsades de Pointes

Torsade de pointes is a polymorphic ventricular tachycardia that can lead to sudden death. It is characterized by a gradual change in the amplitude and twisting of the QRS around the isoelectric line. What differentiates it from generic ventricular tachycardia is the prolonged QT interval. Quite often, the arrhythmia terminates spontaneously and comes in bursts. Because the rhythm is not usually sustained, the patient's baseline QT prolongation may be seen on the rhythm strip. In certain cases, prolongation may evolve into ventricular fibrillation. Ventricular rates can vary from 150 to 250 bpm, and patients may be completely asymptomatic (Fig. 5.1).

5.2.6 Treatment

Recognizing torsade de pointes and differentiating it from generic ventricular tachycardia is important. Certain conventional antiarrhythmic agents will be ineffective and can even exacerbate the arrhythmia. For example, group IA antiarrhythmic drugs will prolong the QT interval and thus worsen the torsades [25]. Goals of treatment are aimed at shortening the QT interval. Modalities of therapy include cardiac pacing, intravenous atropine, and isoproterenol infusion. The treatment that has gained in popularity and has proven to be extremely efficacious is intravenous magnesium sulfate. Synchronized cardioversion may be ineffective because the

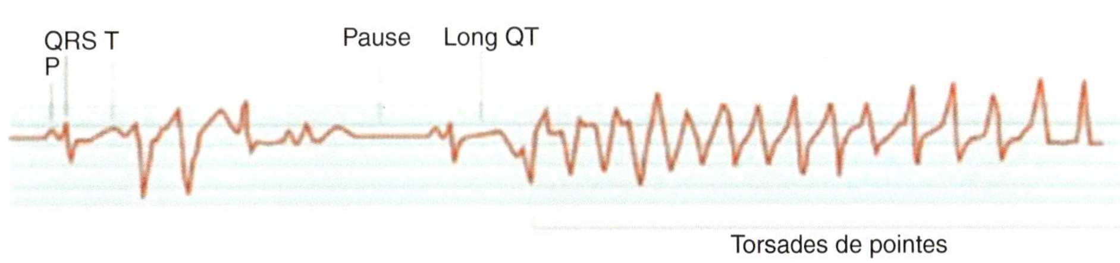

Fig. 5.1 Electrocardiogram of torsades de pointes

abnormal rhythm is polymorphic. Unsynchronized shock or defibrillation may be necessary.

5.2.7 Risk Mitigation Strategies

In 2009, to decrease the risk of cardiotoxicity with methadone treatment, the FDA published monitoring guidelines. An expert advisory panel formulated a list of six recommendations: informed consent, history, baseline ECG, QT prolongation risk assessment, drug interactions, and no doses at or greater than 120 mg/day [9].

Key Concepts

- With the increased use of methadone in pain management, the number of associated deaths has increased.
- QT interval prolongation associated with methadone use predisposes patients to cardiac arrhythmias.
- Torsades de pointes is a potentially fatal type of ventricular arrhythmia that requires precise recognition to properly treat and not exacerbate its effects.
- Understanding the unique pharmacodynamics of methadone is crucial. Its potential for interaction with multiple drugs can decrease effect or promote toxicity.
- The literature is limited to a small number of studies and case reports on the cardiac risks associated with methadone use.
- More research is needed to determine guidelines for diagnostic screening and surveillance testing (i.e., electrocardiogram), optimal dosing parameters, and risk-modifying tactics.

References

1. Caplehorn JR, Dalton MS, Haldar F, Petrenas AM, Nisbet JG. Methadone maintenance and addicts' risk of fatal heroin overdose. Subst Use Misuse. 1996;31:177–96.
2. Gronbladh L, Ohlund LS, Gunne LM. Mortality in heroin addiction: impact of methadone treatment. Acta Psychiatr Scand. 1990;82:223–7.
3. National Institutes of Health: NIH consensus panel recommends expanding access to and improving methadone treatment programs for heroin addiction. Eur Addict Res. 1999;5:50–1.
4. Chou R, Weimer MB, Dana T. Methadone overdose and cardiac arrhythmia potential: findings from a review of the evidence for an American Pain Society and College on Problems of Drug Dependence clinical practice guideline. J Pain. 2014;15:338–65.
5. Chou R. Comparative efficacy and safety of long-acting oral opioids for chronic non-cancer pain: a systematic review. J Pain Symptom Manag. 2004;26:1026.
6. General Accountability Office: Methadone-associated overdose deaths: factors contributing to increased deaths and efforts to prevent them. http://www.gao.gov/products/GAO-09-341. Accessed 16 Nov 2015.
7. Lynch ME. A review of the use of methadone for the treatment of chronic noncancer pain. Pain Res Manag. 2005;10:133–44.
8. Inturrisi CE. Clinical pharmacology of opioids for pain. Clin J Pain. 2002;18:S3–S13.
9. Anderson R, Saiers JH, Abram S, Schlicht C. Accuracy in equianalgesic dosing: conversion dilemmas. J Pain Symptom Manag. 2001;21:397–406.
10. Christie JM. Opioid prescribing: methadone risk mitigation. Anesthesia Patient Safety Foundation Newsletter. 2011;26:1–15.
11. Krantz MJ, Lewkowiez L, Hays H, Woodroffe MA, Robertson AD, Mehler PS. Torsades de pointes associated with very-high-dose methadone. Ann Intern Med. 2002;137:501–4.
12. Fanoe S, Hvidt C, Ege P, Jensen GB. Syncope and QT prolongation among patients treated with methadone for heroin dependence in the city of Copenhagen. Heart. 2007;93:1051–5.
13. Cruciani RA, Sekine R, Homel P, et al. Measurement of QTc in patients receiving chronic methadone therapy. J Pain Symptom Manag. 2005;29:385–91.
14. Chang KC, Huang CL, Liang HY, et al. Gender-specific differences in susceptibility to low dose methadone-associated QTc prolongation in patients with heroin dependence. J Cardiovasc Electrophysiol. 2012;23:527–33.
15. Athanasos P, Farquharson AL, Compton P, Psaltis P, Hay J. Electrocardiogram characteristics of methadone and buprenorphine maintained subjects. J Addict Dis. 2008;27:31–5.
16. Fareed A, Vayalapalli S, Byrd-Sellers J, et al. Onsite QTc interval screening for patients in methadone maintenance treatment. J Addict Dis. 2010;29:15–22.
17. Maremmani I, Pacini M, Cesaroni C, Lovrecic M, Perugi G, Tagliamonte A. QTc interval prolongation in patients on long-term methadone maintenance therapy. Eur Addict Res. 2005;11:44–9.
18. Mayet S, Gossop M, Lintzeris N, Markides V, Strang J. Methadone maintenance, QTc and torsades de pointes: who needs an electrocardiogram and what is the prevalence of QTc prolongation? Drug Alcohol Rev. 2011;30:388–96.
19. Katz DF, Sun J, Khatri V, et al. QTc interval screening in an opioid treatment program. Am J Cardiol. 2013;112:1013–8.
20. Peles E, Bodner G, Kreek MJ, Rados V, Adelson M. Corrected-QT intervals as related to methadone dose and serum level in methadone maintenance treatment (MMT) patients: a cross-sectional study. Addiction. 2007;102:289–300.
21. Roy AK, McCarthy C, Kiernan G, et al. Increased incidence of QT interval prolongation in a population receiving lower doses of methadone maintenance therapy. Addiction. 2012;107:1132–9.
22. Krantz MJ, Lewkowiez L, Hays H, Woodroffe MA, Robertson AD, Mehler PS. Dose-related effects of methadone on QT prolongation in a series of patients with torsades de pointes. Pharmacotherapy. 2003;23:802–5.
23. Martell BA, Arnsten JH, Krantz MJ, Gourevitch MN. Impact of methadone treatment on cardiac repolarization and conduction in opioid users. Am J Cardiol. 2005;95:915–8.
24. Justo D, Gal-Oz A, Paran Y, Goldin Y, Zeltser D. Methadone-associated torsades de pointes (polymorphic ventricular tachycardia) in opioid-dependent patients. Addiction. 2006;101:1333–8.
25. Anchersen K, Clausen T, Gossop M, Hansteen V, Waal H. Prevalence and clinical relevance of corrected QT interval prolongation during methadone and buprenorphine treatment: a mortality assessment study. Addiction. 2009;104:993–9.

Acute Delirium After Ketamine Infusion for Chronic Pain

6

Tariq Malik

6.1 Case Description

A 52-year-old male, with a history of right arm and right-sided body pain, came to the pain clinic for evaluation and management. He suffered right arm pain after a fall which broke his wrist. His fractured wrist was treated surgically, but later the pain that resulted suggested complex regional pain. He was treated with series of stellate ganglion blocks before a thoracic epidural injection. The injection was stopped because of paresthesia, but he developed right-sided pain after that. Various membrane-stabilizing drugs failed to relieve his pain. A trial of spinal cord stimulation therapy also failed. Intravenous lidocaine improved his pain but only for the duration of the infusion. After a discussion of the adverse effects and benefits of a ketamine infusion, patient agreed to this treatment. The plan was to administer 0.5 mg/kg ketamine over 30 min. In the monitoring area, a pulse oximeter, electrocardiogram, and blood pressure were applied. He was premedicated with midazolam 2 mg and ondansetron 4 mg. Approximately 10 min into the infusion, he became agitated and aggressive. His blood pressure and heart rate went up dramatically. Infusion was stopped. He remained restless and seemed completely disoriented. He developed visual hallucinations: he thought he was in a space, and the resident physician administering the infusion was an alien trying to abduct him. Attempts to calm the patient down by verbally engaging him confused him more. The patient was given an additional 2 mg midazolam. To minimize visual stimulation, lights were dimmed in the room, and a calm and quiet environment was created. During this time, he did not require physical restraints. He calmed down somewhat but remained agitated for another 10 min before getting calm down and relaxed. His mentation recovered back to baseline about 2 h after receiving ketamine and midazolam. He was discharged home when he had completely recovered from the effects of ketamine and midazolam.

T. Malik, M.D.
University of Chicago Hospitals,
5841 S. Maryland Avenue, Chicago, IL 60637, USA
e-mail: tmalik@dacc.uchicago.edu

6.2 Discussion

Chronic pain, increasing in prevalence [1], is often poorly managed. Treatment for chronic pain is based on a trial and error method with a variety of antiepileptics, antidepressants, or membrane-stabilizing drugs. Overall response to pain management with such interventions is around 30–40% [2, 3]. Chronic pain involves a number of mechanisms like phosphorylation and upregulation of the *N*-methyl-D-aspartate (NMDA) receptor, loss of descending inhibition, plastic changes in the spinal cord, and activation of immune cells in the spinal cord with the release of pro-inflammatory cytokines [4, 5].

Ketamine is a phenylpiperidine, structurally similar to phencyclidine (PCP). It crosses the blood-brain barrier rapidly and reaches equilibrium in a few minutes. Its analgesic effect far exceeds its pharmacokinetic half-life. In one study, it was estimated that the analgesic effect lasted 11 days in patients with complex regional pain syndrome who were treated for 100 h with 20–30 mg/h of *S*-ketamine [6]. Ketamine is a cytochrome P450-dependent drug, metabolized in the liver by CYP3A4, CYP2B6, and CYP2C9 to norketamine, which then is metabolized to 4-, 5-, and 6-hydroxynorketamine by CYP2A6 and CYP2B6. Norketamine is produced within minutes of intravenous administration of ketamine and may exceed the ketamine concentration particularly after long-term infusion [7]. Norketamine and various hydroxyl-norketamines are eliminated, after glucuronidation in the liver, through the kidney and bile [8]. Inhibitors of the CYP enzymes that metabolize ketamine increase ketamine plasma concentrations; however, induction of the CYP system has a limited effect

M. Anitescu et al. (eds.), *Challenging Cases and Complication Management in Pain Medicine*,
https://doi.org/10.1007/978-3-319-60072-7_6

because hepatic clearance of ketamine is high at baseline. Ketamine concentrations decline rapidly once the infusion is terminated. Norketamine concentrations tend to exceed the ketamine concentration once the infusion is terminated. The role of these various ketamine metabolites in affecting chronic pain is unknown. A human study on the effect of variations in norketamine concentration on acute ketamine analgesia revealed no or even a negative effect on acute pain relief, an issue that becomes important when ketamine is infused for a long time [9].

Currently there is no consensus on the use of ketamine in treating various chronic pain conditions. More than 30 randomized clinical trials have evaluated ketamine for the treatment of various chronic pain conditions in the last 10 years (Table 6.1). While ketamine has proved effective in complex regional pain syndrome (CRPS), other conditions such as chronic refractory headache and unrelenting chronic low back may benefit from this treatment with sustained pain relief of up to 3 weeks (Fig. 6.1) [10]. The effectiveness of ketamine seems to be duration dependent, but evidence is limited. Generally, doses used for CRPS are 20–30 mg/h for 100 h or for 4 h daily for 10 days, giving 6 weeks to 3 months of pain relief. Despite improvement in pain relief, functionality is not improved. Adverse effects in the cardiovascular or central nervous system (CNS) accompany ketamine infusion.

The most important CNS effects are psychotropic. Psychedelic effects are dose dependent but are not uncommon even at the low doses used in the treatment of chronic pain (20–30 mg/h). In a study in healthy volunteers, ketamine caused distortion of reality, auditory hallucinations, paranoid ideas, anxious feelings (panic attacks) an inability to control thoughts, derealization in time and space, visual hallucinations, and increased awareness of sound and color. An intense feeling of a high was felt, which some described

Table 6.1 Conditions where ketamine infusions were reported as effective in the last 10 years as described in the literature

Migraine
Cancer pain
Neuropathic pain
Chemo-induced neuropathic pain
Chronic neuropathic pain
Fibromyalgia
CRPS
Ischemic limb pain
Traumatic nerve injury pain
Phantom limb pain
Postherpetic neuralgia
Spinal cord injury pain
TMJ pain
Trigeminal neuralgia
Whiplash injury pain

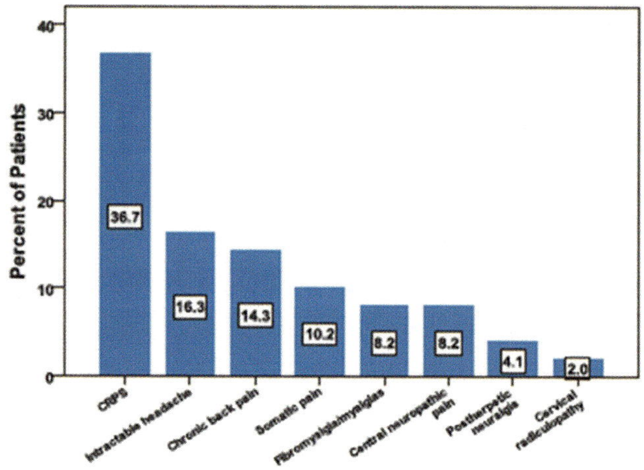

Fig. 6.1 Patients suffering from a variety of chronic refractory conditions reported effective pain relief in a retrospective cohort followed retrospectively for 5 years. The graph below shows percentage of patients suffering from those conditions in this series of 49 individuals [10]

as extremely unpleasant; others expressed an intense feeling of euphoria. Other CNS adverse effects are dizziness, blurred vision, vertigo, nausea/vomiting, dysphasia, nystagmus, nightmares or vivid dreams, impaired motor function, and memory deficits [11, 12]. These effects decrease rapidly after termination of ketamine administration, although unpleasant dreams may persist up to three nights afterward. In clinical studies the incidence of psychological or psychedelic effects, although common, is still low. Sedation is most common during the infusion; the incidence of other effects is approximately less than 5% [10, 13].

Adverse effects were overall considered mild by patients in a retrospective study where subanesthetic doses of ketamine was administered over 30–60 min (Table 6.2) [10].

Prevention of psychedelic effects may not be possible, but the effects may be attenuated with coadministration of benzodiazepines or an alpha 2-adrenergic receptor agonists (e.g., clonidine) [14]. Clonidine may have the added benefit of counteracting the cardiovascular stimulatory effects of ketamine. The effects on memory are short term. To diminish the possibility of overt CNS-related adverse effects, all patients should have a psychiatric evaluation before ketamine treatment to rule out schizophrenia (and related disorders) or bipolar and post-traumatic stress disorder. Ketamine is now being evaluated for the treatment of PTSD and depression. Patients in a manic phase or with poorly managed PTSD are not a good candidate for ketamine treatment as they are at higher risk to suffer from the adverse effects. Patients with a history of drug abuse should be excluded from ketamine treatment because ketamine is itself highly addictive.

Ketamine has a direct negative inotropic effect and an indirect stimulatory effect on the cardiovascular system [15]. The sympathetic system is activated from the systemic

Table 6.2 Common side effects reported by patients undergoing ketamine infusions for refractory chronic pain states

	Patient group: *N* (%) of patients		
	CRPS (*N* = 18)	Non-CRPS (*N* = 31)	Total (*N* = 49)
Any event	9 (50.0%)	14 (45.2%)	23 (46.9)
Agitation	1 (5.7%)	1 (3.2%)	2 (4.1%)
Confused state	1 (5.7%)	2 (6.5%)	3 (6.1%)
Disorientation	0 (0.0%)	1 (3.2%)	1 (2.0%)
Dissociation	0 (0.0%)	1 (3.2%)	1 (2.0%)
Feeling cold	0 (0.0%)	1 (3.2%)	1 (2.0%)
Hallucination	1 (5.7%)	4 (13.2%)	5 (10.2%)
Hypertension	4 (22.2%)	2 (6.5%)	6 (12.2%)
Nausea	1 (5.7%)	1 (3.2%)	2 (4.1%)
Nystagmus	0 (0.0%)	1 (3.2%)	1 (2.0%)
Paresthesia	0 (0.0%)	1 (3.2%)	1 (2.0%)
Pharyngolaryngeal pain	0 (0.0%)	1 (3.2%)	1 (2.0%)
Restlessness	1 (5.7%)	0 (0.0%)	1 (2.0%)
Sedation	2 (11.1%)	2 (6.5%)	4 (8.0%)
Somnolence	0 (0.0%)	1 (3.2%)	1 (2.0%)
Tachycardia	1 (5.7%)	0 (0.0%)	1 (2.0%)
Vertigo	0 (0.0%)	1 (3.2%)	1 (2.0%)
Vomiting	2 (11.1)%	1 (3.2%)	3 (6.1%)

Overall hallucinations and hypertension seemed to be reported more often by the patients [10]
One patient may have experienced more than one adverse event
CRPS complex regional pain syndrome

release of catecholamines, inhibition of the vagal nerve, inhibition of norepinephrine uptake at peripheral nerves and nonneuronal tissues (such as the myocardium), and norepinephrine release from sympathetic ganglia. Myocardial depression happens at a high-dose ketamine infusion or during repeated infusions. Cardiovascular stimulation occurs at a low-dose ketamine infusion and is characterized by tachycardia and systemic and pulmonary hypertension and increases in cardiac output and myocardial oxygen consumption. Monitoring is required when treating chronic pain patients with cardiovascular disease with a low-dose ketamine. The use of clonidine or beta-blockers to improve hemodynamics after ketamine treatment has not been studied.

Drug-drug interactions can never be discounted. There is a long list of drugs that inhibit CYP-450 enzymes and can increase the level of ketamine in the blood. CYP3A4, more important than the others, is the target of most inhibitors. A review of a patient's medication list will help prevent an unexpected high level of ketamine in blood and weight if weight is used to calculate the dose for administration.

Ketamine-induced psychological excitement is best managed with benzodiazepines, administered before the start of infusion. If adverse effects appear moderate in intensity, they can be managed conservatively by minimizing visual or auditory stimulation. If a patient interacts verbally despite hallucinating and is not completely disoriented, frightened, or experiencing a panic attack, a conservative approach will succeed. Violence or aggression is always a potential and psychotropic side adverse effect that should be promptly treated with extra doses of benzodiazepines. Quite often the nature of the hallucination and the reaction of patient to it will indicate whether the situation will become violent. In such cases, the ketamine infusion is stopped promptly. Vital signs should be monitored. Heart rate and blood pressure return to baseline as psychotropic effects wane. Both rarely require intervention, and if they do, they are treated with intermittent doses of a short-acting beta-blocker. Heart rate and blood pressure are used to determine the amount of the dose and frequency of administration.

After any such episode, the history of a patient should be reviewed, especially focusing on psychological history (schizophrenia, bipolar, PTSD) and medication history (for CYP450 inhibitors). To prevent an overdose of ketamine, the original drug vial and infusion bag should be analyzed, especially if the patient had an uneventful previous ketamine infusion.

Managing acute delirium
1. Stop the infusion
2. Minimize stimulation
3. Talk to patient if oriented in place and person
4. Treat hypertension and heart rate if patient has cardiac disease
5. Use short-acting benzodiazepine (midazolam) to sedate the patient
6. Rule out dose or drug error
7. Rule out any drug-drug interactions by reviewing medication history
8. Refer for psychiatric evaluation if not already done to rule out any still undiagnosed problem
9. Adjust the ketamine dose downward for future infusion
10. Discontinue ketamine treatment if treatable reason can be found for acute delirium

Conclusion

Ketamine is safe drug when used in low, clinically recommended doses to manage chronic pain. It can cause CNS depression or excitation depending upon the medications a patient intakes and preexisting psychological states. A patient with significant psychological issues should have a psychiatric evaluation before a ketamine infusion. Ketamine dose should be carefully calculated to avoid dose error. To prevent drug-drug interactions that may cause an unexpected high level of ketamine in the blood, a patient's medication history should be avoided by carefully reviewed. Adverse reactions are treated promptly. Some patients are not suited for this therapy; for others dose must be adjusted downward.

References

1. Nahin RL. Estimates of pain prevalence and severity in adults: United States, 2012. J Pain. 2015;16(8):769–80.
2. Dworkin RH, O'Connor AB, Audette J, et al. Recommendations for the pharmacological management of neuropathic pain: an overview and literature update. Mayo Clin Proc. 2010;85:S3–14.
3. Finnerup NB, Otto M, McQuay HJ, Jensen TS, Sindrup SH. Algorithm for neuropathic pain treatment: an evidence based proposal. Pain. 2005;118:289–305.
4. Petrenko AB, Yamakura T, Baba H, Shimoji K. The role of N-methyl-D-aspartate (NMDA) receptors in pain: a review. Anesth Analg. 2003;97:1108–16.
5. Marchand F, Perretti M, McMahon SB. Role of immune system in chronic pain. Nat Rev Neurosci. 2005;6:521–32.
6. Dahan A, Olofsen E, Sigtermans M, et al. Population pharmacokinetic-pharmacodynamic modeling of ketamine-induced pain relief of chronic pain. Eur J Pain. 2011;15:258–6.
7. Domino EF. Taming the ketamine tiger. Anesthesiology. 2010;113:876–86.
8. Hijazi Y, Boulieu R. Contribution of CYP3A4, CYP2B6, and CYP2C9 isoforms to N-demethylation of ketamine in human liver microsomes. Drug Metab Dispos. 2002;30:853–8.
9. Olofsen E, Noppers I, Niesters M, Kharasch E, Aarts L, Sarton E. Estimation of the contribution of norketamine to ketamine-induced acute pain relief and neurocognitive impairment in healthy volunteers. Anesthesiology. 2012;117:353–64.
10. Patil S, Anitescu M. Efficacy of outpatient ketamine infusion in refractory chronic pain syndromes: a 5 year retrospective analysis. Pain Med. 2012;13(2):263–9.
11. Bowdle AT, Radant AD, Cowley DS, Kharash ED, Strassman RJ, Ray-Byrne PP. Psychedelic effects of ketamine in healthy volunteers. Anesthesiology. 1998;88:82–8.
12. Pomarol-Clotet E, Honey GD, Murray GK, et al. Psychological effects of ketamine in healthy volunteers. Phenomenological study. Br J Psychiatry. 2006;189:173–9.
13. Cverck P. Side effect of ketamine in the long-term treatment of neuropathic pain. Pain Med. 2008;9:253–7.
14. Bergman SA. Ketamine: review of its pharmacology and its use in pediatric anesthesia. Anesth Prog. 1999;46:10–20.
15. Sigtermans M, Dahan A, Mooren R, et al. S(+)-ketamine effect on experimental pain and cardiac output: a population pharmacokinetic-pharmacodynamic modeling study in healthy volunteers. Anesthesiology. 2009;111:892–903.

Cardiac Dysrhythmia After Lidocaine Infusion

7

Andrea Shashoua

7.1 Case Description

A 75-year-old woman had pain and tingling on the right side of her face for 2 days before an eruption of a painful rash. Her primary care physician diagnosed herpes zoster infection. The antiviral medication valacyclovir was prescribed for a week. Acetaminophen and nonsteroidal anti-inflammatory drugs were suggested for her pain. A few days later, the patient reported more intense pain from the rash and inquired about alternative pain medications. Tramadol 50 mg every 8 h as needed was prescribed.

At a 1-month follow-up, the zoster vesicles were crusted and drying, and the erythema and inflammation were almost gone. The woman stated that tramadol did not relieve her pain, which was burning and tingling on her face and scalp. Even a light touch from her hand or the wind seemed to cause excruciating pain. The physician prescribed gabapentin and oxycodone as needed for pain.

Three months later, the patient returned visibly distressed. She had discontinued the medications because they made her feel sedated and ill. The area of pain had increased in size, intensity, and chronicity. During the visit, she cried and said that she could no longer put on makeup or socialize with friends. She reported weight loss and difficulty performing daily activities. At this point, the patient is referred to an outpatient pain clinic at a large academic hospital.

The patient's medical history includes coronary artery disease, right bundle branch block (RBBB), atrial fibrillation, congestive heart failure, nonalcoholic steatohepatitis, remote history of seizure, controlled hypertension, and gastroesophageal reflux disease.

Her medications include aspirin, amiodarone, atorvastatin, lisinopril, Dilantin, fluvoxamine, and cimetidine. She has no known drug allergies. Her height is 5′3″ and her weight is 43 kg. Vital signs are as follows: blood pressure 108/72 mmHg, heart rate 64 bpm, respiratory rate 18, and SpO_2 96% on room air.

The patient, who is accompanied by her daughter, appears to have a flat affect. Her responses to questions are appropriate, but answers are limited to just a few words. Her daughter asks the pain physician if there is anything that can be done immediately to help ease the mother's pain. The family is concerned about the mother's deteriorating mood, for which she is taking an antidepressant.

The pain physician suggests a trial of intravenous (IV) lidocaine infusion. After consent is obtained, an IV line is placed, and the patient is connected to monitors: a 3-lead electrocardiogram, pulse oximeter, and noninvasive blood pressure cuff. The dose is calculated based on ideal body weight. A lidocaine bolus of 1.5 mg/kg is administered over 5 min. The clinic does not have infusion pumps, so the drip rate is calculated to infuse 3 mg/kg over 30 min. During the infusion, the patient reports feeling tired but remains alert. At the end of the treatment, she becomes dysarthric, and her mental status changes abruptly. After a few minutes, she is nonverbal and unresponsive to commands or painful stimuli. Her eyes remain open with a fixed gaze. Vital signs remain stable and relatively unchanged.

Given these acute changes, a cerebrovascular accident is suspected. The hospital stroke team is notified, and the patient is brought to radiology for computed tomography of the head. Afterward she is brought to the emergency department (ED). Upon arrival to the ED, the patient is hooked up to monitors and a 12-lead electrocardiogram (ECG). The ECG shows regular wide complex bradycardia at a rate of 37 bpm. A RBBB and left anterior fascicular block are present. Atropine is administered, and her heart rate increases to 64 bpm. Blood work is drawn for cardiac enzymes, a basic metabolic panel, complete blood count, and lidocaine level. Within 20 min of arriving to the ED, the patient's mental status begins to normalize. Cardiac enzymes and chemistry test results are normal, but serum lidocaine level is 7.0 μg/mL (normal values 1.5–5.0 μg/mL). A bolus of Intralipid (20%

A. Shashoua
University of Chicago Medical Center, Chicago, IL, USA
e-mail: ashashoua@yahoo.com

M. Anitescu et al. (eds.), *Challenging Cases and Complication Management in Pain Medicine*,
https://doi.org/10.1007/978-3-319-60072-7_7

fat emulsion) of 1.5 mL/kg is given IV. Repeat ECG performed 30 min later shows normalizing QRS morphology and resolution of bradycardia. The patient is admitted to telemetry for observation, and cardiology is consulted. She is discharged within 48 h with no other acute events.

Three weeks later, she reports significant improvement in her pain and asks if the infusion can be repeated. After consultation with the cardiologist, the patient is admitted to telemetry for IV lidocaine infusion. The bolus and infusion doses are decreased to 1 mg/kg and 2 mg/kg, respectively, over 60 min. She tolerates the treatment well without complications.

Table 7.1 Cytochrome P450 drug interactions

Inhibitors	Inducers
Quinidine	Phenobarbital
Cimetidine	St. John's wort
Ketoconazole	Phenytoin
Fluconazole	Carbamazepine
Metronidazole	Rifampin
Grapefruit juice	Cigarette smoking
Erythromycin	Pioglitazone
Paroxetine	Oxcarbazepine
Fluoxetine	
Amiodarone	
Simvastatin	

7.2 Case Discussion

7.2.1 Clinical Usage of Intravenous Lidocaine

The analgesic effect of systemic lidocaine for postoperative pain was first reported in 1961 [1]. In the 1980s, systemic lidocaine treatment attenuated central pain, which had been recalcitrant to most traditional medications [2]. Non-opiate intravenous infusions have been used to alleviate pain from chronic conditions such as fibromyalgia, phantom limb pain, neuropathic pain, complex regional pain syndrome, diabetic neuropathy, postherpetic neuralgia, and central pain conditions associated with spinal cord injury or stroke [3, 4].

Clinical and experimental data have shown that changes in expression of voltage-gated sodium channels affect the pathogenesis and duration of neuropathic pain [5]. Activation of sodium channels after nerve injury leads to ectopic, maladaptive neuronal discharges. Drugs that block sodium channels, such as lidocaine, can be therapeutic in doses lower than doses that impair nerve impulse propagation. Controlled clinical studies have demonstrated efficacy for intravenous lidocaine for neuropathic and acute nociceptive pain [6]. Infusions are typically delivered over the course of 30–60 min. Recommended monitors are ECG, noninvasive blood pressure, and pulse oximeter. The plasma concentration necessary to relieve pain is much less than that needed to overcome nerve conduction [5]. As with most therapies for pain, dose requirements, response, and side effects vary among individual patients.

7.2.2 Pharmacokinetics

Lidocaine has a biphasic elimination profile. The initial half-life can be up to 30 min because of protein binding and redistribution. In general, terminal half-life can be up to 2 h, as with continuous IV infusions. Half-life is prolonged in patients with liver dysfunction. Dosing must be modified in patients who have medical conditions that alter the liver's ability to clear lidocaine or change its volume of distribution. The parent compound is broken down rapidly into active metabolites, which are more toxic than the parent and have a half-life of 2–10 h [7, 8], prolonging symptoms. Lidocaine doses and infusion rates also should be reduced in patients with congestive heart failure because of lower volume of distribution and hepatic blood flow [9].

Lidocaine is rapidly eliminated by the liver. The rate of metabolism depends on rate of blood flow to the liver. The cytochrome P450 family of enzymes is essential for lidocaine metabolism. The isoenzymes that are important are 3A4, 1A2, 2C19, and 2D6. Lidocaine clearance can be reduced or increased by drugs that inhibit or induce CYP3A4 activity, respectively. Toxic levels of lidocaine may result when given concurrently with a variety of medications [10, 11] (Table 7.1).

7.2.3 Factors Increasing Lidocaine Toxicity

- Older age
- Decreased body weight
- Acute myocardial infarction
- Congestive heart failure
- Impaired hepatic function
- Concomitant use of P450-inhibiting drugs
- Pulmonary disease
- Preexisting A-V node dysfunction or sick sinus syndrome
- Hypercarbia or acidosis

7.2.4 Cardiovascular Effects

Local anesthetics decrease blood pressure and heart rate through alterations in electrical excitability of the heart, dilation of blood vessels, and inhibition of sinoatrial node firing. All local anesthetics have the potential to induce cardiac dysrhythmias. The negative inotropic action of local anesthetics is dose dependent, depresses myocardial contractility, and decreases cardiac output. Typical effects include widening of the QRS complex and lengthening of the PR interval [12].

The earliest signs of systemic toxicity are usually caused by blockade of inhibitory central nervous system pathways for unopposed excitatory nerve activity. Subjective symptoms include dizziness, confusion, tinnitus, difficulty focusing, shivering, tremors, and possible seizures. Symptoms of central nervous system depression, such as sedation, lack of responsiveness, and potential respiratory depression, follow soon after. These signs are rapidly reversed with discontinuation of the drug. Tissues with the highest aerobic demand and least tolerance for hypoxia, such as the heart, the lungs, and the central nervous system, are most vulnerable to the toxic effects of local anesthetics [5–7].

Initially, low serum levels of local anesthetic slightly increase cardiac output, blood pressure, and heart rate from increased sympathetic activity and vasoconstriction. As the blood levels rise, peripheral vasodilation of vascular smooth muscle and lower peripheral vascular resistance leads to hypotension and lower cardiac output [13]. Local anesthetic-induced arrhythmias can manifest as conduction delays, from prolonged PR interval to complete heart block, sinus arrest, and asystole. Conduction defects with IV lidocaine infusions are more prone to occur with preexisting bundle branch blocks [14, 15] (Table 7.2).

Lidocaine has little effect on normal sinoatrial (SA) node activity but can cause severe bradycardia in patients with SA node dysfunction (i.e., sick sinus syndrome). This effect can be intensified by medications such as digitalis, phenytoin, or amiodarone (Fig. 7.1).

In patients with ischemic heart disease, the atrioventricular node can similarly be affected by lidocaine. Ventricular dysrhythmias, such as simple ectopy, torsades de pointes, and fibrillation, may result.

Combined or alone, these conditions can lead to cardiac arrest [16, 17].

Table 7.2 Published randomized, placebo-controlled, or comparative trials for intravenous lidocaine infusions

Condition	Author	IV lidocaine infusion	Results
Central pain	Attal et al.	5 mg/kg, 30 min	Lidocaine > placebo
	Finnerup et al.	5 mg/kg, 30 min	Lidocaine > placebo
	Kvarnstrom et al.	2.5 mg/kg, 40 min	Lidocaine = placebo
Peripheral neuropathic pain	Viola et al.	5 and 7.5 mg/kg, 4 h	Lidocaine > placebo
	Kastrup et al.	5 mg/kg, 30 min	Lidocaine > placebo
	Backonja et al.	1, 3, and 5 mg/kg/h, 6 h	Lidocaine > placebo
Postherpetic neuralgia	Rowbotham	5 mg/kg, 60 min	Lidocaine > placebo
	Baranowski et al.	1 and 5 mg/kg, 2 h	Lidocaine = placebo
CRPS	Wallace et al.	Targeted plasma concentrations 1, 2, and 3 μg/mL, 20 min	Lidocaine = placebo
	Tremont-Lukats et al.	1, 3, and 5 mg/kg, 6 h	Lidocaine > placebo at 5 mg/kg dose
Fibromyalgia	Sorenson et al.	5 mg/kg, 30 min	Lidocaine = placebo

Reproduced and modified with permission from the American Society of Interventional Pain Physicians [3]

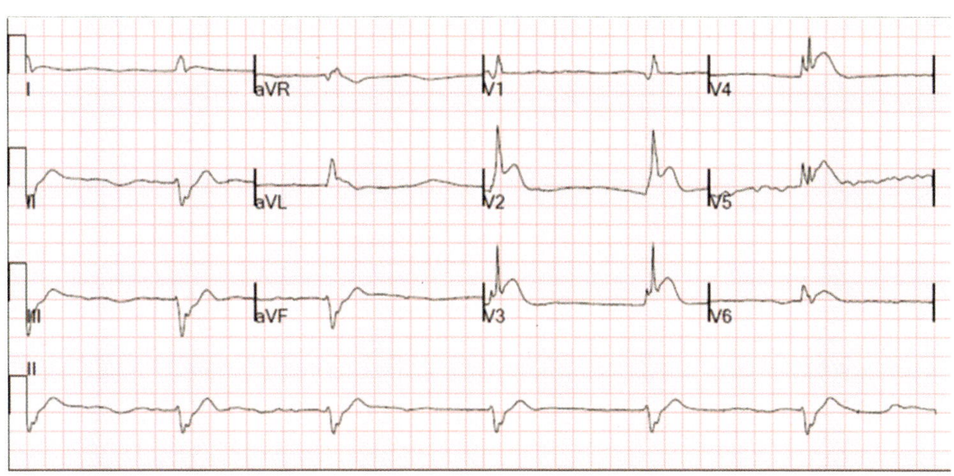

Fig. 7.1 Wide complex bradycardia

7.2.5 Differential Diagnosis

- Cerebrovascular accident
- Myocardial infarction
- Anaphylaxis

7.2.6 Treatment

- Early recognition.
- Discontinuation of infusion.
- ABCs (airway, breathing, circulation) and hyperventilation.
- Advanced cardiac life support.
- Discontinue calcium channel blockers and beta-blockers.
- Vasopressin not recommended.
- Epinephrine can induce or exacerbate dysrhythmia.
- Lipid emulsion bolus of 1.5 mL/kg followed by an infusion of 0.25 mL/kg/min for at least 10 min. Consider rebolusing and increasing infusion if circulatory stability is not established (propofol is *not* an adequate alternative).
- Cardiopulmonary bypass if the patient is unresponsive to lipid emulsion [18, 19].

Key Concepts

- Intravenous lidocaine is used to treat certain acute and chronic pain conditions.
- A patient's comorbidities and medications affect lidocaine metabolism.
- Monitor blood pressure, heart rate, rhythm, and oxygen saturation throughout infusion.
- Infusion pumps are recommended for standardization and to decrease error.
- Early recognition of signs of toxicity should prompt decrease in or discontinuation of infusion.
- Toxic responses may be difficult to identify in patients with multiple complicated medical problems.
- Resuscitative equipment and medications should be readily available.

References

1. Bartlett EE, Hutaserani Q. Lidocaine (xylocaine) for the relief of postoperative pain. J Am Med Womens Assoc. 1962;17:809–15.
2. Boas RA, Covino BG, Shahnarian A. Analgesic responses to i.v. lignocaine. Br J Anaesth. 1982;54:501–5.
3. Kosharskyy B, Almonte W, Shaparin N, Pappagallo M, Smith H. Intravenous infusion in chronic pain management. Pain Physician. 2013;16:231–49.
4. Challapalli V, Tremont Lukats IW, McNicol ED, Lau J, Carr DB. Systemic administration of local anesthetic agents to relieve neuropathic pain. Cochrane Database Syst Rev. 2005;CD003345.
5. Bryant CA, Hoffman JR, Nichter LS. Pitfall and perils of intravenous lidocaine. West J Med. 1983;139:528–30.
6. Pfeifer HJ, Greenblatt DJ, Koch-Weser J. Clinical use and toxicity of intravenous lidocaine. A report from the Boston Collaborative Drug Surveillance Program. Am Heart J. 1976;92:168–73.
7. Jonville AP, Barbier P, Blond MH, et al. Accidental lidocaine overdosage in an infant. J Toxicol Clin Toxicol. 1990;28:101–6.
8. Bursell B, Ratzan RM, Smally AJ. Lidocaine misinterpreted as a stroke. West J Emerg Med. 2009;4:292–4.
9. Thompson PO, Melmon KL, Richardson JA, et al. Lidocaine pharmacokinetics in advanced heart failure, liver disease, and renal failure in humans. Ann Intern Med. 1973;78:499–508.
10. Ha HR, Candinas R, Stieger B, et al. Interaction between amiodarone and lidocaine. J Cardiovasc Pharmacol. 1996;28:533–9.
11. Hogan Q. Local anesthetic toxicity: an update. Reg Anesth. 1996;21(6S):43–50.
12. Block A, Covino B. Effect of local anesthetic agents on cardiac conduction and contractility. Reg Anesth. 1982;6:55–61.
13. Marriott JL, Phillips K. Profound hypotension and bradycardia after a single bolus of lidocaine. J Electrocardiol. 1974;7:79–82.
14. Kunkel F, Rowland M, Scheinman M. The electrophysiologic effects of lidocaine in patients with intraventricular conduction defects. Circulation. 1974;49:894–9.
15. Gupta P, Lichstein E, Chadde K. Lidocaine-induced heart block in patients with bundle branch block. Am J Cardiol. 1974;33:487–92.
16. Cheng T, Wadhwa K. Sinus standstill following intravenous lidocaine administration. JAMA. 1973;223:790–2.
17. Lichstein E, Chadda K, Gupta P. Atrioventricular block with lidocaine therapy. Am J Cardiol. 1973;31:277–81.
18. Weinberg G. Current concepts in resuscitation of patients with local anesthetic cardiac toxicity. Reg Anesth Pain Med. 2002;27(6):568–75.
19. Weinberg GL. Lipid infusion therapy: translation to clinical practice. Anesth Analg. 2008;106(5):1340–2.

Alternative Treatments for Local Anesthetic Systemic Toxicity: Therapeutic Hypothermia After Bupivacaine-Induced Cardiac Arrest

8

Shaan Sudhakaran and Magdalena Anitescu

8.1 Case Description

A 39-year-old female (50 kg, American Society of Anesthesiologists physical status 3) was admitted to the ambulatory surgery center for a left total wrist arthroplasty. Her medical history was significant for congestive heart failure (LVEF of 23%) from nonischemic cardiomyopathy, mixed connective tissue disease, and renal failure. Surgical history included multiple upper extremity surgeries (for connective tissue disease) under regional anesthesia without complications (Table 8.1).

The patient agreed to a brachial plexus block via an axillary approach after a detailed discussion of the risks, benefits, and alternatives of regional anesthesia.

After standard American Society of Anesthesiologists-recommended monitors were applied, intravenous midazolam (1 mg) and fentanyl (50 mcg) were administered. The left axilla was identified, and the area around the axillary artery was prepped and draped for the procedure.

After application of an electric nerve stimulator, a 22-gauge, 2-inch B-bevel echogenic needle was inserted superior to the palpated axillary artery. When median nerve activity was identified by wrist flexion at 0.32 mA, 20 mL of 0.5% bupivacaine with 1:200,000 epinephrine was injected with negative aspiration every 5 mL over a period of 90 s. No adverse cardiovascular effects (increase in heart rate by more than 20%) were observed during the injection. At the conclusion of the block, the patient became nonresponsive. Initial small fluttering of her eyelids progressed in 30 s to a generalized tonic-clonic seizure.

Resuscitation measures were initiated with 100% oxygen by bag mask ventilation. Additional intravenous midazolam (2 mg) did not stop the seizure activity, and the patient continued tonic-clonic movements for another 2 min when 50 mg propofol abruptly interrupted the event. The patient was nonresponsive but hemodynamically stable with baseline blood pressure, heart rate, and rhythm for approximately 5 min. At that point, ventricular tachycardia progressed to ventricular fibrillation.

The possible differential diagnoses considered were acute cardiac ischemia, local anesthetic allergic reaction, and local anesthetic systemic toxicity (LAST). Neither acute ischemia nor allergic reaction was seriously considered given the timeline of the event.

Table 8.1 Pertinent medical history and preoperative evaluation

Medical history	*Preoperative assessment*
CHF	*EKG*—sinus rhythm with occasional premature ventricular complexes
Mixed connective tissue disease	*Echocardiogram*—severe decrease in LV function (LVEF 21%); severely dilated left ventricle, left atrium (no thrombus), right atrium; mild mitral regurgitation; mild decrease RV function
History of pericardial effusion	
Hodgkin's lymphoma—age 16	
Polyseptic arthritis—Methicilline resistant Staphyloccocus Aureus	
Chronic renal insufficiency/anemia	
Medications	***Airway assessment***
Omeprazole	Mallampati class I
CellCept	Otherwise unremarkable
Plaquenil	
Diovan	
Coreg	
Lipitor	
Calcium/vitamin D	
Epogen	
Restoril	
Prednisone	
KCl	

S. Sudhakaran, M.D. • M. Anitescu, M.D., Ph.D. (✉)
Department of Anesthesia and Critical Care, University of Chicago Medical Center, Chicago, IL, USA
e-mail: ssudhakaran@dacc.uchicago.edu; MAnitescu@dacc.uchicago.edu

M. Anitescu et al. (eds.), *Challenging Cases and Complication Management in Pain Medicine*,
https://doi.org/10.1007/978-3-319-60072-7_8

Suspicion of LAST led to quick action with immediate attention to airway, breathing, and circulation. In the absence of lipid emulsion, an advanced cardiac life support was initiated.

The patient's trachea was intubated with a 7.0 endotracheal tube (grade I view), and chest compressions were started. The patient received a total of 3 mg epinephrine, 40 units vasopressin, and 3 rounds of defibrillation. Quality chest compressions were maintained continuously for 10 min. Spontaneous circulation and sinus rhythm returned with intermittent premature ventricular complexes. The patient was hemodynamically stable yet remained unconscious.

In attempts to preserve her neurological function, therapeutic hypothermia was initiated by placing ice bags in the axilla, groin, and neck. Cool fluid was administered through the right internal jugular triple-lumen catheter. These measures quickly achieved core body temperature values of 34.0 °C measured upon arrival to cardiac intensive care unit, 15 min later. The patient remained unconscious without a shivering response. No sedation or neuromuscular blocking agents were given. Four hours after arrest, the patient began to move her extremities and was able to follow commands. The therapeutic hypothermia protocol was discontinued. The patient's trachea was extubated the next morning on 2 L nasal cannula with oxygen saturation of 99%. The patient was discharged home with full neurologic recovery 4 days after the event with no sequelae. She returned 3 weeks later for wrist surgery under general anesthesia without complications (Fig. 8.1).

8.2 Case Discussion

Regional anesthesia is an effective and important tool for various surgical procedures. Devastating cardiovascular and neurologic complications result if concentrated local anesthetic is not injected correctly. Intravascular injection of local anesthetics during a peripheral nerve block is associated with LAST that progresses to seizures and cardiovascular collapse.

Treatment with intravenous lipid resuscitation (bolus and infusion) after local anesthetic-induced cardiac collapse that is refractory to protocols for advanced cardiac life support has been well described [1, 2]. Before it was introduced into clinical practice, lipid emulsion therapy in animal models seemed to decrease mortality [3] and improve myocardial function [4].

There is minimal evidence for preservation of neurological function and cardiac function after LAST. In the absence of readily available intravenous lipid emulsion, LAST can be fatal. Hypothermia decreases morbidity after return of spontaneous circulation in patients with cardiac arrest [5], making this therapy attractive for prevention of neurologic dysfunction in witnessed cardiac collapse.

8.2.1 Therapeutic Hypothermia: Historical Facts

In 1803, Russian surgeons covered patients in snow to induce hypothermia as a resuscitative method. In 1812, Napoleon's physicians used hypothermia to preserve injured limbs and

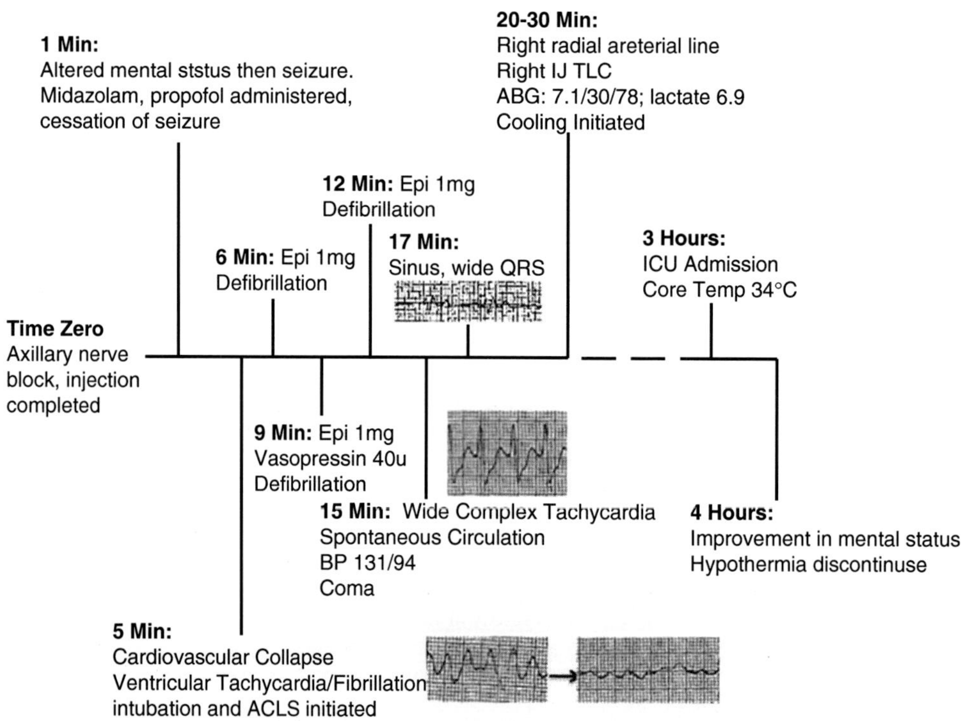

Fig. 8.1 Timeline of events with cardiac rhythm strips, from personal library

as an anesthetic adjuvant during amputations. In 1937, neurosurgeon Temple Fay cooled his patients to 32 °C to prevent tumor cells from multiplying [6]. He called this technique "general refrigeration" and proved that malignant cells are actually more susceptible to cold than normal ones, opening the door for this technique in cancer palliation.

Therapeutic hypothermia improved perioperative outcomes during cardiac and neurological surgery over the next 20 years. Between 1960 and 1990, the technique was partially abandoned because of arrhythmogenicity and less clearance of staphylococcal bacteria.

Therapeutic hypothermia reduces oxygen requirements and thus preserves cardiac and neurological function. In the 2000s, the American Heart Association and European Resuscitation Council recommended therapeutic hypothermia as a treatment for out-of-hospital cardiac arrest.

8.2.2 Accidental Intravascular Injection of Local Anesthetics

Accidental intravascular injection of local anesthetic during regional anesthesia techniques and its consequence, LAST, have been amply described. There are many methods to minimize the risks. Frequent negative aspirations during local anesthetic injection, dose restrictions, and epinephrine additives in local anesthetics have limited the risk of vascular uptake. In the early 1980s, stimulator needles assisted in detecting proximity to targeted nerves. Ultrasound-guided blocks have become ubiquitous in regional anesthetics for visualizing anatomy and local anesthetic spread in real time. In our patient with weakened connective tissue from long-term use of glucocorticoids and with documented underlying mixed connective tissue disease, intravascular uptake was possible even with the use of ultrasound imaging.

Early signs and symptoms of LAST, caused primarily by blockade of inhibitory pathways in the cerebral cortex, include agitation, lightheadedness, slurred speech, altered mental status, visual changes, hypertension, and tachycardia. These symptoms are the results of unopposed excitatory nerve activity. Moderate toxicity, manifesting by central nervous system excitation, cardiac arrhythmias, contractile depression, and conduction blockade progress to hypotension, bradycardia, ventricular arrhythmias, and complete cardiovascular collapse. Bupivacaine is the most cardiotoxic local anesthetic because of its strong attraction to myocardial sodium channels and delayed dissociation with lipophilic properties. In our patient, the severity of the cardiovascular collapse may have been exacerbated by the underlying cardiomyopathy. Our patient showed signs of vascular uptake and LAST despite serial negative aspirations and an epinephrine additive to bupivacaine to detect vascular uptake.

Initially, intravascular injection of local anesthetic minimally increases systemic vascular resistance and cardiac output. As local anesthetic builds up, smooth muscle relaxation produces vasodilation, and cardiac output decreases when local anesthetic binds to myocytes. The witnessed cardiac arrest in our patient may have been fatal had all of the 20 mL of bupivacaine been placed into the axillary artery. The brachial plexus block was performed with the assistance of a stimulator needle but without ultrasound guidance or readily available lipid emulsion.

8.2.3 Lipid Emulsion Rescue Medication for LAST

The current use of lipid emulsion (Intralipid 20%, Fresenius Kabi, Hamburg, Germany) for LAST came from an unexpected finding in the 1990s. Noting the cardiotoxic effects of bupivacaine in patients with carnitine deficiency, Weinberg et al. showed the protective effects of lipid infusions in rats and dogs with bupivacaine-induced arrhythmias [3, 7]. Lipids act as a "sink" for local anesthetic. In the early 2000s, lipid therapy emerged to target patients for overdose of lipophilic local anesthetic drugs. The currently used lipid emulsion formulation contains 20% soybean oil, 1.2% egg yolk phospholipids, 2.25% glycerin, and water. It has an osmolarity of 350 mOsm/kg water and 260 mOsm/kg lipid emulsion.

When LAST is suspected, a 1.5 mL/kg bolus is administered over 1 min (about 100 mL for a 70 kg patient). Then an infusion of 0.25 mL/kg/min for approximately 500 mL over 30 min is given [8]. The infusion is continued for at least 10 min after hemodynamic stability is attained. All dosing weights are based on lean body mass. A repeat bolus every 5 min may be given 1–2 times for persistent asystole. If hypotension persists, infusion rate can be increased to 0.5 mL/min and continued for at least 30 min. The maximum recommended total dose over the first 10 min is 10 mL/kg. Treatment begins at the first signs of neurologic or cardiac toxicity.

8.2.4 Therapeutic Hypothermia: Pathogenesis and Protective Effects

Although not studied to treat LAST, hypothermia has been used extensively in unconscious patients after cardiac arrest to preserve neurological function. Since the first description of therapeutic hypothermia over 200 years ago, more efficient and controlled cooling protocols have reduced complication rates.

Decreasing body temperature to 32–34 °C has a protective effect on the cerebral function by decreasing the cerebral metabolic rate. Cooling leads to cerebral vasoconstriction and lower intracranial pressure to lessen the risk of seizures. The effects of neuroprotection are best in ischemic neuronal injuries after cardiovascular collapse.

Myocardial protection is an additional effect of therapeutic hypothermia. Mild decreases in the core body temperature are associated with a lower heart rate and greater systemic vascular resistance to increase coronary perfusion during chest compressions. Reducing body temperature reduces the defibrillation threshold to terminate ventricular fibrillation [9]. Therapeutic hypothermia proves beneficial not only for reliable neuroprotection but also for cardiac protection against ischemic-reperfusion injury responsible for most "post-resuscitation" myocardial failure and ischemic brain damage.

Therapeutic hypothermia has been shown to be advantageous for neurologic recovery [10] and survival benefits [11] after witnessed out-of-hospital cardiac arrest from ventricular fibrillation. In one case, therapeutic hypothermia was used for a 28-year-old patient who was arrested from a cocaine overdose. Cardiotoxicity from the cocaine was related to its sodium channel antagonism. The patient had complete neurologic recovery despite profound lactic acidosis [12].

There remain many challenges for the use of therapeutic hypothermia as a treatment for LAST. There are no standardized protocols for this technique [13]. Debate centers on the best induction of cooling [14]. The most basic tools (cooling blankets, ice packs) are cost-effective [15]; however, the cost can be overwhelming for more advanced cooling technologies.

Cooling temperature may be revised from previous extremes. In a recent multinational, multicenter study, benefits of cooling patients to 36 °C versus 33 °C were compared in patients after cardiac arrest. The investigators found that in unconscious survivors of out-of-hospital cardiac arrest of presumed cardiac causes, hypothermia at a target temperature of 33 °C did not confer additional neuroprotective benefit as compared with targeted temperature of 36 °C [16].

Cardiopulmonary bypass must be considered when LAST is resistant to standard protocols. This treatment requires preparation and reliance on a specialized team.

Conclusions

Although not routinely used in the resuscitation protocol in cardiac arrest for local anesthetic systemic toxicity, therapeutic hypothermia offers a unique advantage in isolated cases where cardiac comorbidities predispose patients to fatal events. Possible use of hypothermia may be beneficial in remote locations with limited supplies and resources such as in frontline combat hospitals. With new guidelines that target hypothermia to 36 °C, the technique is even easier to achieve.

Timely institution of surface (ice packs), invasive (cold intravenous fluids) cooling methods and aggressive resuscitation measures ensured complete neurologic and cardiac recovery for our patient. An otherwise fatal outcome from complex comorbidities in the absence of pharmacological antidote was prevented.

Key Points

- Intravenous lipid rescue is the standard of care for local anesthetic systemic toxicity and should be readily available during all regional anesthetics.
- Bupivacaine is the most cardiotoxic local anesthetic given its strong affinity for myocardial sodium channels.
- Post-cardiac arrest hypothermia to 32–34 °C improves cardiac and neurologic recovery in witnessed out-of-the hospital cardiac arrest.
- Therapeutic hypothermia to milder values of 36 °C may preserve neurological function during local anesthetic systemic toxicity when lipid emulsion is not readily available.

References

1. Litz RJ, Roessel T, Heller AR, Stehr SN. Reversal of CNS and cardiac toxicity after local anesthetic intoxication by lipid emulsion injection. Anesth Analg. 2008;106:1575–7.
2. Warren JA, Thoma RB, Georgescu A, Shah SJ. IV lipid infusion in the successful resuscitation of local anesthetic induced cardiovascular collapse after supraclavicular brachial plexus block. Anesth Analg. 2008;106:1578–80.
3. Weinberg G, Ripper R, Feinstein D, Hoffman W. Lipid emulsion infusion rescues dogs from bupivacaine induced cardiac toxicity. Reg Anesth Pain Med. 2003;28(3):198–202.
4. Stehr SN, Ziegeler JC, Pexa A, et al. The effect of lipid infusion on myocardial function and bioenergetics in L-bupivacaine toxicity in the isolated rat heart. Anesth Analg. 2007;104:186–92.
5. Benson DW, Williams GR Jr, Spencer FC, Yates AJ. The use of hypothermia after cardiac arrest. Anesth Analg. 1959;38:423–8.
6. Varon J, Acosta P. Therapeutic hypothermia: past, present, and future. Chest J. 2008;133(5):1267–74.
7. Weinberg GL, VadeBoncouer T, Ramaraju GA, Garcia-Amaro MF, Cwik MJ. Pretreatment or resuscitation with a lipid infusion shifts the dose-response to bupivacaine-induced asystole in rats. Anesthesiology. 1998;88(4):1071–5. [PubMed].
8. Neal JM, Bernards CM, Butterworth JF, et al. ASRA practice advisory on local anesthetic systemic toxicity. Reg Anesth Pain Med. 2010;35(2):152–61.
9. Boddicker KA, Zhang Y, Zimmerman MB, Davies LR, Kerber RE. Hypothermia improves defibrillation success and resuscitation outcomes from ventricular fibrillation. Circulation. 2005;111(24):3195–201.
10. Bernard SA, Gray TW, Buist MD, et al. Treatment of comatose survivors of out of hospital cardiac arrest with induced hypothermia. N Engl J Med. 2002;346:557–63.
11. Hypothermia After Cardiac Arrest Study Group. Mild therapeutic hypothermia to improve neurologic outcome after cardiac arrest. N Engl J Med. 2002;346:549–56.

12. Fuller ET, Milling TJ Jr, Price B, Spangle K. Therapeutic hypothermia in cocaine-induced cardiac arrest. Ann Emerg Med. 2008;51:135–7.
13. Chamorro C, Borrallo JM, Romera MA, Silva J, Balandin B. Anesthesia and analgesia protocol during therapeutic hypothermia after cardiac arrest: a systematic review. Anesth Analg. 2010;110:1328–35.
14. Sessler DI. Defeating normal thermoregulatory defenses: induction of therapeutic hypothermia. Stroke. 2009;40:e614–21.
15. Merchant RM, Becker LB, Abella BS, Asch DA, Groeneveld PW. Cost-effectiveness of therapeutic hypothermia after cardiac arrest. Circ Cardiovasc Qual Outcomes. 2009;2:4521–428.
16. Nielsen N, Wetterslev J, Cronberg T, et al. Targeted temperature management at 33°C versus 36°C after cardiac arrest. N Engl J Med. 2013;369(23):2197–206.

A Case of Serotonin Syndrome in a Patient Receiving Epidural Steroid Injection for Chronic Low Back Pain

9

Brad Wisler and Honorio T. Benzon

9.1 Introduction

Patients presenting to the pain clinic are frequently on complex analgesic regimens. Multidimensional therapies are governed by the particular pain syndrome as well as associated comorbidities including depression. While polypharmacy may assist in management of the chronic pain patient, the approach generates increased potential for harm. We present a case of a patient who developed serotonin syndrome shortly after receiving epidural steroid injection for low back pain.

9.2 Case Presentation

A 54-year-old man with chronic low back pain presented for repeat lumbar epidural steroid injection. His medical history was significant for hypertension, hyperlipidemia, morbid obesity, type II diabetes mellitus, gastroparesis, chronic sinusitis, osteoarthritis, depression, and lumbar spinal stenosis at the L3–L4 level with chronic right-sided radiculopathy. He has a surgical history of bilateral knee replacements. He smoke four to five cigarettes daily and consumes roughly 10 ounces of alcohol each week. He denies use of illicit drugs. His medications included hydrochlorothiazide, amlodipine, atorvastatin, metformin, metoclopramide, naproxen, acetaminophen, and sertraline. He frequently takes dextromethorphan for his chronic sinus infections. He was seen initially in the pain clinic 2 months prior to this visit where he received an interlaminar epidural steroid injection with good immediate response. His pain had slowly returned over a 1-month span, exacerbated by doing yard work 1 week prior to his follow-up appointment. He presented to his primary care physician who prescribed tramadol and a fentanyl patch for short-term relief until he could return to pain clinic. Upon presentation to pain clinic, a repeat interlaminar epidural steroid and local anesthetic injection at the same level, the patient received almost immediate 100% relief of his pain. While in the recovery suite, the patient began complaining of anxiety, restlessness, sweating, and tremor. Physical examination at that time showed tachycardia, hypertension, low-grade fever, clonus, and hyperreflexia. A review of medications with the patient revealed the use of tramadol and a fentanyl patch along with his chronic daily use of sertraline and metoclopramide and periodic use of dextromethorphan. Serotonin syndrome was presumed as the likely cause of his symptoms, and the patient was transferred immediately to the emergency department for confirmatory diagnosis and care, where he was admitted to the intensive care unit overnight. The patient developed progressive worsening of his shivering and muscular rigidity and developed a high-grade fever. In addition to supportive therapy, pharmacologic management including benzodiazepine and the 5-HT2A antagonist, cyproheptadine, was administered. The patient was given an initial 12 mg dose of cyproheptadine, followed by several doses of 2 mg at a time guided by symptoms. The patient improved over the next 24 h. After a thorough review of his medications, he was counseled on the risks of combining multiple serotonergic agents, and these medications were either discontinued or changed. He was discharged home the following day. His primary care physician was informed of the patient's episode.

9.3 Discussion

Serotonin syndrome is a potentially life-threatening adverse drug reaction that is a consequence of excess serotonergic activation of the central nervous system due to either medication use, drug interactions, or intentional overdose [1]. The clinical triad of mental status changes, autonomic hyperactivity, and

B. Wisler, M.D.
Active Duty Air Force anesthesiologist and pain physician, Wright Patterson AFB, Dayton, OH, USA

H.T. Benzon, M.D. (✉)
Department of Anesthesiology, Northwestern University Feinberg School of Medicine, Chicago, IL, USA
e-mail: Honorio.Benzon@nm.org

M. Anitescu et al. (eds.), *Challenging Cases and Complication Management in Pain Medicine*,
https://doi.org/10.1007/978-3-319-60072-7_9

neuromuscular abnormalities is typically seen in the condition [2, 3]. The association of neurological effects and serotonergic agents was initially described in 1960, when Oates and Sjoerdsma described ethanol-like intoxication, drowsiness, hyperreflexia, and clonus in patients given L-tryptophan during therapy with a monoamine oxidase inhibitor [4]. However, it wasn't until 1984 with the infamous Libby Zion case that the syndrome was widely recognized [5].

The incidence of serotonin syndrome is difficult to ascertain, largely because of the variable and nonspecific nature of its presentation. One can look at the Annual Report of the American Association of Poison Control Centers' National Poison Data System for insight. In the 2014 report, there were 1105 fatalities attributed to a pharmaceutical agent, where antidepressants accounted for 98 cases (9%) and ranked fifth overall, and of these 98 cases, a pro-serotonergic agent was involved in 74 (76%) [6]. It has been reported that the syndrome occurs in approximately 14–16% of people who overdose on SSRIs [7]. With the widespread use of antidepressants and the ever-growing popularity of other pro-serotonergic agents, serotonergic syndrome must remain in the differential diagnosis of the patient presenting with complex neurocognitive signs and symptoms.

The pathophysiology of the serotonin syndrome is not completely understood. Serotonin, or 5-hydroxytryptamine (5-HT), is produced from L-tryptophan in presynaptic neurons, in which it remains within vesicles until released into the synaptic cleft following axonal stimulation [8]. Reuptake mechanisms, degradation by monoamine oxidase, and feedback loops exist to keep its effect under tight control. There are a number of different serotonin receptors, including 5-HT1 to 5-HT7 [9], that which serotonin will bind. Historically, serotonin syndrome has been believed to be caused by excess stimulation of the serotonin 5-HT1A receptor [10]; however, a majority of the life-threatening effects (hyperthermia, severe hypertonicity) appear to be primarily mediated by 5-HT2A receptors. In general, three important mechanisms in relation to severe serotonin syndrome exist: inhibition of reuptake, enhanced presynaptic release, and MAO inhibition [11].

A wide variety of drugs have been associated with the serotonin syndrome. Medications that affect any of the steps in serotonin metabolism or regulation can provoke toxicity. These include monoamine oxidase inhibitors (MAOIs), antidepressants, SSRIs, opiate analgesics, over-the-counter cough medicines, antibiotics, weight-reduction agents, antiemetics, antimigraine agents, drugs of abuse, and herbal products [1]. The syndrome is classically associated with the simultaneous administration of two serotonergic agents, but it can occur after initiation of a single drug or increasing the dose of a drug in individuals who are sensitive to serotonin. SSRIs are the most common. Severe cases appear to be more likely after drug interactions, particularly MAOIs and SSRIs [12] (Table 9.1).

Table 9.1 Drugs with serotonergic activity that may contribute to serotonin syndrome

Mechanism of action	Drug category	Drug
Reuptake inhibition	Antidepressant	
	• SSRI	Fluoxetine, paroxetine, sertraline, citalopram, escitalopram
	• SNRI	Venlafaxine, desvenlafaxine, duloxetine
	• DNRI	Bupropion
	• TCA	Amitriptyline, nortriptyline, clomipramine, desipramine, doxepin
	• Serotonin modulator	Trazodone
	Others	1. Antiepileptic—valproate, carbamazepine 2. Antiemetic—ondansetron, metoclopramide 3. Bariatric—sibutramine 4. Muscle relaxant—cyclobenzaprine 5. Amphetamine —dextromethorphan 6. Analgesic—meperidine, tramadol 7. Supplement—St. John's wort, ginseng 8. Illicit—cocaine, MDMA
Serotonin metabolism inhibition	MAOI	
	• Antidepressants	Phenelzine, selegiline, isocarboxazid
	• Antimicrobials	Linezolid
	• Others	Methylene blue
Increases serotonin release	Amphetamine	Dextromethorphan, methamphetamine
	Parkinsonian	Levodopa, carbidopa-levodopa
	Illicit	Cocaine, MDMA
Increases serotonin formation	Amino acid	Tryptophan
Direct serotonin agonist	Antimigraine	1. Triptans—sumatriptan, rizatriptan 2. Ergots—ergotamine, methylergonovine
	Analgesic	Fentanyl
	Illicit	LSD
Increases sensitivity at postsynaptic receptor	Antipsychotic	Lithium

The clinical presentation is classically described as a triad of cognitive/behavioral changes (confusion, agitation, lethargy, coma), autonomic instability (hyperthermia, tachycardia, diaphoresis, nausea, vomiting, diarrhea, dilated pupils), and neuromuscular changes (myoclonus, hyperreflexia, rigidity, trismus) [13]. It is known to vary on a spectrum ranging from mild to moderate to severe including death [2]. Several sets of diagnostic criteria have been developed to define serotonin syndrome, including the Sternbach criteria [2] and the Hunter Criteria [14] (Box 9.1). In a study of the Hunter Criteria, the clinical findings that have been shown to have a statistically significant association were clonus (inducible, ocular, spontaneous), myoclonus, hyperreflexia, peripheral hypertonicity, and shivering [14]. The onset of symptoms is typically rapid; approximately 75% of patients with serotonin syndrome present within 24 h after initial use of medication, an overdose, or a change in dosing [13]. However, administration of a serotonergic agent within 5 weeks after the discontinuation of fluoxetine has been shown to initiate serotonin syndrome [15]. It does not resolve spontaneously unless the causative agents are discontinued.

Box 9.1 Comparison of Serotonin Syndrome Diagnostic Criteria

Sternbach criteria—1991	Hunter serotonin toxicity criteria—2003
Recent addition or increase in dosage of a known serotonergic agent	*In the presence of a serotonergic agent*
Absence of other possible etiologies (e.g., infection, metabolic disorder, endocrine disorder, substance abuse, withdrawal, etc.)	• If spontaneous clonus, then SS
No recent addition or increase in the dose of a neuroleptic drug	• If inducible clonus PLUS agitation or diaphoresis, then SS
The presence of ≥3 of the following clinical signs or symptoms 1. Agitation 2. Altered mental status (confusion, hypomania) 3. Ataxia/incoordination 4. Diaphoresis 5. Diarrhea 6. Fever 7. Hyperreflexia 8. Myoclonus 9. Shivering 10. Tremor	• If ocular clonus plus agitation or diaphoresis, then SS
	• If tremor plus hyperreflexia, then SS
	• If hypertonia plus temperature above 38 °C plus ocular clonus or inducible clonus, then SS

Early recognition is paramount in the management of serotonin syndrome as many cases have been shown to resolve within 24 h of initiation of therapy. First-line treatment includes prompt withdrawal of the offending agents and supportive care. Benzodiazepines are often used for agitation in mild, moderate, and severe cases. In severe cases with cardiac and respiratory system disturbances, administration of 5-HT2A antagonists, commonly cyproheptadine, may be beneficial [1]. Severe cases with hyperthermia may require endotracheal intubation, neuromuscular paralysis, and sedative agents [16].

As is illustrated in our case, a chronic pain patient presenting to the clinic may be on a multitude of agents for various conditions including pain and depression. Often these medications are prescribed from more than one physician, and the patient may not be as forthcoming with the use of every single one of his drugs. The patient is just in the pain clinic to get his injection. The pain physician must take into account the patient as a whole and use every encounter to review the associated comorbidities and treatment regimens. The patient we described was taking multiple serotonergic agents at baseline (metoclopramide and sertraline), in addition to the CYP2D6 inhibitor dextromethorphan. The possibility of a serotonin syndrome should probably have been suspected on the initial encounter. The addition of tramadol and fentanyl likely facilitated the emergence of the syndrome. Prompt recognition of the signs and symptoms and early treatment are crucial to the successful treatment of the disorder. Polypharmacy and the chronic pain patient frequently go hand and hand, and therefore, the pain physician must keep this disorder in mind in the overall management and care of these patients.

References

1. Boyer EW, Shannon M. The serotonin syndrome. N Engl J Med. 2005;352:1112–20.
2. Sternbach H. The serotonin syndrome. Am J Psychiatry. 1991;148:705–13.
3. Nierenberg DW, Semprebon M. The central nervous system serotonin syndrome. Clin Pharmacol Ther. 1993;53:84–8.
4. Oates JA, Sjoerdsma A. Neurologic effects of tryptophan in patients receiving a monoamine oxidase inhibitor. Neurology. 1960;10:1076–8.
5. Asch DA, Parker RM. The Libby Zion case: one step forward or two steps backward? N Engl J Med. 1988;318:771–5.
6. Mowry JB, Spyker DA, Brooks DE, Mcmillan N, Schauben JL. 2014 Annual report of the American Association of Poison Control Centers' National Poison Data System (NPDS): 32nd annual report. Clin Toxicol. 2015;53:962–1147.
7. Isbister GK, Bower SJ, Dawson A, Whyte IM. Relative toxicity of selective serotonin reuptake inhibitors (SSRIs) in overdose. J Toxicol Clin Toxicol. 2004;42:277–85.
8. Thanacoody R. Serotonin syndrome. Medicine. 2007;35(10):556–7.
9. Nichols DE, Nichols CD. Serotonin receptors. Chem Rev. 2008;108:1614–41.
10. Goodwin GM, De Souza RJ, Green AR, Heal DJ. The pharmacology of the behavioural and hypothermic responses of rats to 8-hydroxy-2-(di-n-propylamino)tetralin (8-OH-DPAT). Psychopharmacology. 1987;91:506–11.

11. Isbister GK, Buckley NA. The pathophysiology of serotonin toxicity in animals and humans—implications for diagnosis and treatment. Clin Neuropharmacol. 2005;28:205–14.
12. Gillman PK. A review of serotonin toxicity data: implications for the mechanisms of antidepressant drug action. Biol Psychiatry. 2006;59:1046–51.
13. Mason PJ, Morris VA, Balcezak TJ. Serotonin syndrome: presentation of 2 cases and review of the literature. Medicine (Baltimore). 2000;79:201–9.
14. Dunkley EJ, Isbister GK, Sibbritt D, Dawson AH, Whyte IM. The Hunter serotonin toxicity criteria: a simple and accurate diagnostic section rules for serotonin toxicity. QJM. 2003;96:635–42.
15. Isbister GK, Dawson A, Whyte IM, Prior FH, Clancy C, Smith AJ. Neonatal paroxetine withdrawal syndrome or actually serotonin syndrome? Arch Dis Child Fetal Neonatal Ed. 2001;85:F147–8.
16. Cooper BE, Sejnjowski CA. Serotonin syndrome: recognition and treatment. AACN Adv Crit Care. 2013;24:15–20.

The Difficult Pain Patient

10

Mark S. Wallace and Ajay Wasan

10.1 Case Description

A 55-year-old 300-pound white male presents to the pain clinic with a 20-year history of low back pain. He transferred into the health system after he switched his insurance. He is taking 300 mg/day of morphine, 40 mg/day of valium, 3 SOMA/day, and zolpidem 10 mg at bedtime. The primary care urgently referred him to the pain clinic for an evaluation. The resident physician in training sees the patient first. During the interview, the patient repeatedly tells the resident that she is wasting his time with the questions and that she should just review his medical records. He states that he is only present to receive refills for his medications and he will be on his way. The resident continues to make attempts to obtain a detailed history, and the patient responds that she is wasting his time and that he did not come to the clinic to be evaluated by the physician in training. The resident notifies the attending who meets with the patient. The attending explains the importance of a comprehensive evaluation and that in order for the clinic to help the patient, he must cooperate in the history and physical process. The patient becomes angry and starts yelling foul language and states that if he cannot get his medication, why is he here? The attending tells the patient that he is going to leave the room to review his records and will return in a moment, in hopes that this will give the patient some time to calm down. He returns and tries to resume the interview, but the patient again becomes verbally abusive and demanding that his medications be refilled and he will be on his way. He stands and approaches the attending. The attending asks him to remain seated and tells him he will contact the primary care physician and see what can be done. The attending leaves the room and asks for security to come to the clinic. Security arrives and the situation is explained to them. They are requested to remain outside the room, and the attending is going to make one more attempt to calm the patient. He returns to the room and makes another attempt to calm the patient and encourage cooperation; however, the patient continues to become more agitated and abusive.

10.2 Case Discussion

10.2.1 Introduction

Among medical specialties in the United States, pain medicine has the lowest patient satisfaction scores, as measured by Press Ganey surveys, which are widely collected in outpatient and inpatient settings. Press Ganey surveys from 4,274,639 patients from 17,685 sites nationwide between January 1, 2012, and January 31, 2012, showed average scores to be the lowest for pain management among 50 different specialties. There are many reasons why pain patient satisfaction is low including frustration among patients due to lack of effective therapies, inadequate training in pain management, expectations for pain improvement, and coexisting psychosocial abnormalities. This low degree of satisfaction is indicative of the challenges inherent in treating chronic pain and in managing patients with a chronic painful illness. A subset of these patients are particularly challenging to treat because of their pain-related behaviors which diminish the success of many treatments for chronic pain, and as providers know, this subgroup is often quite dissatisfied with their pain care. These patients are often thought of as "difficult," but the difficulty is more in understanding the most appropriate treatment approaches to this subgroup at risk for poor pain treatment outcomes. This chapter will discuss the concept of the "difficult patient" as a lens through which to better understand how to identify and manage successfully this patient subgroup.

M.S. Wallace, M.D. (✉)
Division of Pain Medicine, Department of Anesthesiology, University of California San Diego, San Diego, CA, USA
e-mail: mswallace@ucsd.edu

A. Wasan, M.D., M.Sc.
Department of Anesthesiology, University of Pittsburgh School of Medicine, Pittsburgh, PA, USA

M. Anitescu et al. (eds.), *Challenging Cases and Complication Management in Pain Medicine*,
https://doi.org/10.1007/978-3-319-60072-7_10

Up to 60% of patients treated in allopathic healthcare systems exhibit "difficult behaviors" [1]. The incidence of difficult patients is higher in pain management than other specialties leading to many healthcare providers wanting to avoid this population. Psychiatric comorbidity (including substance use disorders), self-destructive pain behaviors (such as treatment nonadherence), difficulties forming a therapeutic doctor-patient relationship, and unrealistic expectations characterize patients labeled "difficult" in pain treatment settings. For instance, depression and anxiety disorders are 2–3 times more prevalent in patients with chronic pain presenting to pain medicine specialists than in the general population, and there is a high incidence of an array of comorbid emotional disturbances, such as abnormal personality characteristics [2]. Hallmark features of many of these disorders include anger, irritability, concrete and inflexible thinking, and problems getting along with others. Each of these makes it difficult for the provider to treat the painful condition and have a treatment alliance with patient, based on trust, caring, and mutual understanding. In addition, pain patients are more likely to report idiosyncratic increases in pain with interventional therapies. Of patients that are perceived as "difficult," the majority meets DSM criteria for psychiatric disorders, such as major depression, generalized anxiety disorder, dysthymia, substance use disorder, or somatoform illness disorders (in descending order) [3]. Hence, the feeling of the provider that a patient is difficult most often reflects the presence of an underlying untreated or poorly treated psychiatric disorder.

However, even in the presence of psychiatric comorbidity, most patients with chronic pain do have an underlying physical basis for their pain, which may be amplified by overlying psychiatric conditions. The processing of pain in the brain and the consequent perception of pain are influenced by a number of factors including depression/anxiety, genetics, environmental stressors, cultural background, social/functional disability, and cognitive dysfunction. Depending on the circumstances in the individual, each of these factors can act as "amplifiers" of pain perception. A cornerstone of the psychological approaches to pain is generation of patient insight regarding these issues so that patients can diminish the negative impacts of psychosocial stressors on their painful condition. As an aside, when discussing these issues with patients, they will often say, "so you're telling me that the pain is all in my head?" A reasonable reply is, "No, I am saying that there is pain coming from your brain too." This approach couches the issue of the psychiatric components of pain into more concrete terms that a patient may relate to and diminishes the potential negative stigma and self-blame associated with patients hearing that they have a psychological problem.

The wide array of psychosocial factors have wide variations in presentation among patients, and the imbalance of these factors can turn a patient who otherwise would be reasonable to extremely difficult to manage [4]. This high individual variability makes it very challenging to provide a "one-size-fits-all" treatment plan, and thus. comprehensive, multidisciplinary assessment and individualized, multimodal care are the essence of high-quality pain treatment. It is exceedingly hard for any physician to provide this level of care for every patient they see, which also contributes to pain medicine specialists perceiving many of their patients to be difficult.

Historically, "difficult patients" have been classified as falling into one of four groups: dependent clingers, entitled demanders, manipulative help-rejecters, and self-destructive deniers. Table 10.1 summarizes these categories with suggested treatment strategies [5]. This approach has never been validated, but it is a useful starting point to begin to think about how to conceptualize what patients thought of as difficult. The approach of Groves and colleagues ties clinical scenarios to different styles of clinical interactions which may be more therapeutic. This approach does not delve into the deeper issues of why a patient may be presenting as "difficult."

As noted, there are many potential causes for patients seeming to be difficult, including the challenge of hard-to-treat pain syndromes (such as complex regional pain syndrome), leading the patient down a path of multiple treatment failures and frustration. In addition, many patients have ongoing psychosocial stressors, and others may have unrealistic expectations. However, it is not often the patient's fault as there are some physician characteristics and healthcare system-related issues that can lead to a difficult pain patient. For instance, in a physician's zeal to offer hope and optimism, they may convey to a patient that they will be 75% or

Table 10.1 Summary of Grove's difficult patient groups

Type	Identifying features	Treatment strategies
Dependent clinger	Escalating need for reassurance and over time becomes more helpless	Set limits with realistic expectations
Entitled demanders	Initially present as needy but soon exhibit aggressive and intimidating behavior	Do not react to their anger, but instead acknowledge the situation and discuss realistic expectations
Manipulative help-rejecters	Generally ungrateful for any help and are often pessimistic about treatment outcome	Paradoxically advocate adopting skeptical attitude toward treatment and schedule regular appointments
Self-destructive deniers	Tend to engage in behaviors that thwart attempts to improve their condition	Avoid vengeful feelings and punishment; instead focus on and treat underlying depression

even 100% better from the prescribed treatment (such as an epidural steroid injection). For a chronic painful condition, this approach leads inevitably to disappointment and frustration in the patient as they are the ones left dealing with the aftermath of unfilled promises from the provider. It is more appropriate to have a discussion at the initial evaluation regarding realistic expectations for treatment success, such as a 30 or 50% improvement in their condition over the next 3–6 months. Similarly, pain specialists commonly face the patient expectation that we will prescribe opioids, and often the referring physician has given the patient this message, creating unrealistic expectations. In addition, higher insurance co-pays and deductibles and restricted access to specialty care also contribute to increased patient frustration, anger, and pain, which the patient carries in with them to the initial consultation.

10.2.2 Borderline Personality Disorder

Borderline personality disorder (BPD) can be one of the most challenging patient experiences for healthcare providers. They are often difficult to diagnose and will catch the healthcare provider by surprise. They exhibit pervasive patterns of instability of interpersonal relationships, self-image, and affect with marked impulsivity. BPD patients see things as "black and white" and easily go from different extremes of emotions. BPD may amplify the pain or be the sole cause. The symptoms of BPD can occur in a variety of combinations, and individuals with the disorder have many, if not all, of the following traits: fears of abandonment, extreme mood swings, difficulty in relationships, unstable self-image, difficulty managing emotions, impulsive behavior, self-injuring acts, suicidal ideation, and transient psychotic episodes. It is important to understand that BPD patients are quite impaired and often have very little insight into their limitations. These patients often have a history of significant physical or sexual abuse as a child, predisposing them to develop BPD as a maladaptive coping mechanism to deal psychologically with the trauma. Thus, while these patients often create angry feelings within the provider, it is crucial to remember that BPD patients suffer profound mental anguish and to have empathy for their plight.

Dealing with the BPD patient can be challenging, and early recognition is important to prevent the path of costly invasive procedures that are likely to fail. The pain should be managed conservatively as response to treatment can be difficult to assess. Try to be understanding of emotional extremes, and do not react negatively, despite the anger you may be feeling. The BPD pain patient should be co-managed with a psychiatrist or psychologist. Randomized controlled trials have shown that dialectical behavioral therapy is effective in teaching BPD patients to control and not react to their emotions.

10.2.3 Affective Disorder

Affective disorder is highly prevalent among pain patients with 30–50% of pain clinic patients having an untreated major depression or anxiety disorder [2]. Affective disorder (AD) may emerge in the course of treatment, especially if the patient is not responding. AD results in poor coping and poor motivation, and the patient tends to blame the physician for lack of response to therapy. If not recognized and treated, response to pain treatment is very poor. For instance, it has been shown that high levels of depression or anxiety symptoms predict poor analgesic responses to epidurals, facet blocks, and opioids [6–8]. Preexisting psychosocial disturbances will have significant effects on the chronic pain patient's prognosis and stress the importance of exploring the psychosocial history of the patient prior to developing the pain problem.

A combination of psychotropic medications and psychotherapy is the most effective treatment. However, it is often challenging to get the patient to buy into mental healthcare as they feel the provider does not believe they have a physical problem. Try to educate the patient on the importance of embracing a biopsychosocial approach to their problem. Use language they understand, and educate on all aspects of the pain experience including physical, emotional, and social. Addressing these aspects as one is more likely to gain the patient's trust rather than addressing them in isolation.

10.2.4 Somatization

Somatization (SZ) is best thought of as a process of amplification. It is characterized by self-perpetuating somatic symptoms in the absence of organic pathology. They present with a multitude of unexplained symptoms in the presence of normal results from physical examination and diagnostic tests [9]. However, this should not be confused with the chronic pain patient who will often present with pain as their only symptom with normal laboratories and radiological studies. SZ patients tend to catastrophize, embrace the "sick role," and present with many difficult-to-diagnose symptoms. They have high disability and healthcare utilization. However, be careful in labeling patients as SZ before making reasonable attempts to make the diagnosis of their symptoms. For example, fibromyalgia (now referred to as widespread pain) may present as SZ. However, it is a recognized condition with a biological basis.

In dealing with the SZ, the time will come to have an honest discussion with the patient. Point out that you believe that the patient is experiencing the symptoms but they are not life-threatening and do not require treatment. Discussing amplification processes within the brain is helpful as well. Psychiatric consultation is important but puts the consultation in the context of a biopsychosocial approach to the patient's problem. Cognitive behavioral therapy and antidepressant medications may help. It is important to keep treatment conservative as these patients enjoy the sick role and are likely to experience idiosyncratic reactions to treatment and invasive therapies.

10.2.5 Hostile Patient

Hostile patients are common in pain clinic settings and can present a very stressful situation for staff members. These patients can become verbally and may be physically abusive. All pain clinic staff should be educated on how to deal with these patients so as not to escalate a stressful situation into an out-of-control situation. Data suggest that pain medicine physicians are at a greater risk of violence from patients than other medical specialists [10, 11].

A risk management article published by Princeton Insurance (www.riskreviewonline.com, 2002) outlines six steps for dealing with angry patients: (1) remain calm and collected, (2) handle the problem in private, (3) listen to the patient's complaints uninterrupted, (4) convey kindness and reassurance, (5) try and reach a solution, and (6) document the encounter. Wasan et al. recommend five "As" for dealing with the hostile patient: (1) acknowledge the problem, (2) allow the patient to vent uninterrupted in a private place, (3) agree on what the problem is, (4) affirm what can be done, and (5) assure follow-through [3].

However, there are times when a resolution is not possible, and extremes will be required for the safety of the staff and the patient. All clinics should have policy and procedures for summoning the police or security.

10.2.6 The Suicidal Patient

Suicidal ideation and attempts are common among chronic pain patients [2]. Many pain patients exhibit passive death wishes in which they wish they were dead but do not actively want to end their life or have a plan. Patients with suicidal intent (actively want to end their life) should be taken seriously. For those with a plan to end their life should be transferred to the emergency room for an evaluation. In these cases, it may require sending a police officer to the patient's home if suicidal intent with plan is expressed over the phone. Assessment and treatment of suicidal patients are summarized in Table 10.2 [3].

Table 10.2 Suicide assessment and treatment

• Evaluate intent and lethality
• Evaluate existence and feasibility of plan
• Identify evidence of self-destructive behavior and past attempts
• Attempt to establish an alliance with the patient
• Consider a safety contract
• Refer to mental health specialist
• If suicide intent with plan is present, escort to the emergency room
• Document communication with the patient and treatment strategies

Modified from www.rmf.harvard.edu/reference/guidelines/suicideprev/

10.2.7 Substance Abuse Disorder

A prior history of substance abuse disorder requires careful assessment and monitoring if using drugs of abuse to treat pain. First, a careful medical and psychosocial history can identify things associated with substance abuse disorder [12] (Table 10.3). Screening tools such as the Drug Abuse Screening Test (DAST), Opioid Risk Tool (ORT), and Screener and Opioid Assessment for Patients with Pain (SOAPP) are useful in assessing risk level for use of opioids. In assessing aberrant drug-taking behaviors, certain behaviors are probably more predictive of risk for true drug addiction or diversion than others. Some of the more predictive behaviors, many of them illegal, include selling prescription drugs, forging prescriptions, stealing or borrowing another patient's drugs, injecting an oral formulation, obtaining prescription drugs from nonmedical sources, concurrent abuse of related illicit drugs, multiple unsanctioned dose escalations, or recurrent prescription losses [13, 14]. There should be zero tolerance for these behaviors, and once identified, the use of drugs of abuse should be stopped. It should be explained to the patient that the therapy is being abandoned, not the patient. On the other hand, aberrant behaviors, such as aggressive complaining about needing higher doses, drug hoarding, requesting specific drugs, acquisition of similar drugs from other medical sources, unsanctioned dose escalation on one or two occasions, unapproved use of the drug to treat another symptom, or reporting unintended psychic effects, may not be as predictive for drug abuse but, rather, misuse of prescription opioids. Because some degree of aberrant behavior is common among pain patients, it is important to consider not only the type of behavior but also the frequency or number of occurrences in an individual patient when assessing a potentially problematic situation.

Regardless if the patient has a past history of drug abuse or not, always plan an exit strategy prior to starting opioids to treat chronic pain. This should include criteria for tapering (lack of pain reduction, lack of functional improvement, misuse, abuse, positive urine screen for illegal substances, noncompliance). Distinguish between abandoning the opioid

Table 10.3 Medical history findings associated with substance abuse disorders

• *Medical history*: hepatitis C, HIV, TB, cellulitis, sexually transmitted disease, elevated liver function tests
• *Social history:* motor vehicle or fire-related accidents, DUIs, domestic violence, criminal history
• *Psychiatric history:* personal history of psychiatric diagnosis, outpatient and/or inpatient treatment, current psychiatric medications, past history of substance abuse

therapy, abandoning pain management, and abandoning the patient. Clear treatment goals should be agreed upon between provider and patient prior to open prescribing (such as a 30% improvement in pain and function). Prior to prescribing, it should be made clear that opioids do not work for every painful condition or in every patient and that prescribing of opioids is considered a trial, which will be stopped if agreed-upon benchmarks are not reached. Document methods of tapering the opioid, with or without specialty assistance. It is best to put the exit strategy in writing and ask the patient to sign acknowledging understanding. If the time comes, the written document can be provided to the patient. This is a common feature of opioid treatment agreements.

10.2.8 Noncompliance

Noncompliance or nonadherence can occur with medications, rehabilitation, psychological referral, or lifestyle changes. Causes include nonacceptance of the treatment plan, unrealistic expectations, social issues (financial, time, work, transportation, etc.), or addiction. Management of nonadherence can be challenging but should be approached methodically. Realize that at some level, the patient has made a choice not to follow the provider's instructions and there may be a good reason. First, consider modifying the treatment plan which may coax the patient into accepting a slower transition into the original plan. Educate the patient on the importance of compliance with the treatment plan to a successful outcome. If the patient is unwilling to comply, it may be necessary to inform them that no further appointments will be made unless they are ready to accept the treatment plan. As a consultant, when the patient does not accept your plan, the referring physician should also need to be notified of the situation; the plan of treatment whould be described to the primary medical provider and mesures should be taken to tranfer patient care back to his/her referring MD.

Poor lifestyles are also a common cause of increase pain. Pain is more common in obese patients as well as in those who do not regularly exercise, eat appropriately, and get enough sleep. Therefore, lifestyle changes should be a part of every pain treatment plan, and compliance with these changes is just as important as compliance with medical therapies.

Noncompliance with drugs of dependency should be managed very carefully. There should be a low tolerance for noncompliance with drugs of dependency as they carry significant risks to the patient as well as to the provider's license. As discussed under the substance abuser above, a concise exit plan prior to starting the therapy makes it easier to stop the therapy. Persistent noncompliance should result in drug tapering which can be achieved with a well-defined tapering schedule to avoid withdrawal. However, patients who cannot comply with a taper should be warned that no further refills will be provided and given locations of detoxification programs. Carefully document the care in the medical records. Do not be held hostage to therapy just to avoid withdrawal.

10.2.9 Pain Patients with Secondary Gain

There are many causes of secondary gain including litigation, social turmoil, or work dissatisfaction. These patients are at a high risk of using pain medications (especially opioids and benzodiazepines) to treat emotional disturbances. Most secondary gain issues are associated with stress and anxiety, and once lifted, pain is likely to be reduced. When dealing with patients that have secondary gain issues, it must be stressed to the patient that you believe that they have pain; do not suggest that they are malingering and "milking" the issue. However, the effect of the stress and anxiety associated with the secondary gain is beyond their control. Once the stressor is removed from their life, the pain is likely to be reduced. It is advisable to avoid aggressive invasive therapies in pain patients with secondary gain. Explain to the patient that it is in their best interest to treat their pain conservatively until stressors are removed from their life after which they will be reassessed to determine a treatment plan.

Some pain patients are focused on getting disability approved which is a significant secondary gain. It is controversial whether pain in and of itself is a reason to go onto disability. In general, disability is probably counterproductive to pain treatment, and declaring disability is probably better left to specialists that can assess the need for disability in the context of functional abilities rather than pain. However, it may be reasonable to provide work restrictions and accommodations as it relates to the pain.

10.2.10 The Patient Who Wants to Be Fixed

These patients usually have unrealistic expectations and do not understand the limitations of modern medicine. They will go from provider to provider in desperate searches for a cure and often become angry when a cause and cure is not reached. Attempt an honest discussion with the patient and try to adjust expectations. Be empathetic and acknowledge their frustration. Point out that there are inadequacies in the healthcare system and medical science beyond our control.

For instance, we still cannot cure the common cold, but we can put a man on the moon. Failure to adjust expectations can lead the patient down a path of excessive treatment and failure. Try and get them to focus on what can be done, rather than what cannot be done.

10.2.11 Healthcare Provider and System Factors

Difficult pain patients are not always the fault of the patient. Healthcare providers have many different personalities, competencies, and skills that may affect patient behavior. Physicians who are less empathetic are more likely to perceive patients as difficult. Likewise, patients who perceive providers as less empathetic may react negatively and come across as difficult [15]. A study in 2001 showed that older, more experienced doctors reported fewer difficult patients and coped better with a wide variety of patients [16]. Healthcare providers should not take patient negative behavior personally and recognize that patients will react differently to the same situation. Providers should not let patient behavior drive poor decisions and should maintain a level head. Jamison recommends that there should be five components to every patient encounter so as to improve the interaction: engage, empathize, educate, enlist, and end. This is a challenge in today's healthcare market where the provider's face-to-face time with the patient is being overtaken with non-face-to-face time requirements.

In addition to provider factors, there are increasing healthcare system factors damaging the clinician-patient relationship with perceptions that both sides are being difficult. These include poor access, delays in treatment due authorization delays and denials, increasing co-pays, and overburdened clinic phone systems.

10.2.12 The Difficult Patient with Implantable Therapies

Patients with implantable therapies are less likely to become difficult as they undergo more psychological screening and treatment before deciding to implant and tend to have more of an established strong physician-patient relationship. If noncompliance or unacceptable behaviors arise, implantable therapies can still be discontinued. This is easier done with stimulation as there are no drug withdrawal issues to deal with. Discontinuing intrathecal therapy can be more challenging due to the high dependency and life-threatening withdrawal from some of the drugs used (baclofen and clonidine). If the need arises to discontinue intrathecal therapy due to behavioral issues, weekly visits should be scheduled with titration down until pump can be turned off. Explain to the patient that if they are not compliant with the visits, they will go into withdrawal. If the patient is noncompliant, at the next pump refill, turn off the pump and provide oral medications to cover drugs of dependence with a weaning schedule and a list of local detoxification programs to report to if they are noncompliant with the taper. If the patient shows up in the emergency room, explain the situation to the physician and recommend transfer to an inpatient detoxification unit. Once weaned from the intrathecal therapy, explant of the system has to have the consent of the patient. Leaving the system implanted will not harm the patient.

10.2.13 Interventional Therapies That Go Wrong

It is not uncommon for patients to report increased pain after interventional procedures. In the absence of "red flags," reassurance is the best remedy along with a short course of analgesics if necessary. In the case of serious injury, remain levelheaded and approach the case as you would any patient and do not get defensive. Do not let threats of litigation intimidate you. Remain calm and manage the patient's problem as indicated. Risk management should be notified. Carefully document the facts as it pertains to the care, but avoid long narratives and do not point fingers.

10.2.14 Dismissing the Difficult Patient

Fortunately, it is a rare occurrence to require patient dismissal. Dismissing a patient should not be taken lightly, and every practice should have a policy and procedure. First, inform the patient both face to face and in writing why they are being dismissed. If the patient is noncompliant with the treatment plan, that usually is *not* a reason to dismiss a patient. Instead, it is more appropriate to tell the patient that they are welcome to return for further assessment and treatment if they decide that they want to follow the treatment plan. Even in cases of using illegal drugs while prescribed opioids, taking the patient off of the opioids and prescribing non-opioid medications is preferred rather than dismissal from the practice. A similar analogy is in the treatment of HIV. If the patient cannot comply with a "triple cocktail," they are taken off of these medications and continue to see the provider. A clear-cut example of the need to dismiss a patient is if the patient is diverting the medications you are prescribing. If there is concern over hostility and staff safety, only a letter is needed. A 30-day notice is adequate with a referral to the local medical society for a list of other practitioners they can choose from. If the patient is receiving drugs of dependency, give them a taper schedule with a list of local detoxification programs to choose from if they are not compliant with the taper. If the patient is a part of a contracted health plan with your group, the group medical director will need to be notified and approve of the termination [3].

References

1. Hahn SR, Kroenke K, Spitzer RL, et al. The difficult patient: prevalence, psychopathology, and functional impairment. J Gen Intern Med. 1996;11(1):1–8.
2. Fishbain DA. Approaches to treatment decisions for psychiatric comorbidity in the management of the chronic pain patient. Med Clin North Am. 1999;83(3):737–60, vii.
3. Wasan AD, Wootton J, Jamison RN. Dealing with difficult patients in your pain practice. Reg Anesth Pain Med. 2005;30(2):184–92.
4. Gatchel RJ. Comorbidity of chronic pain and mental health disorders: the biopsychosocial perspective. Am Psychol. 2004;59(8):795–805.
5. Groves JE. Taking care of the hateful patient. N Engl J Med. 1978;298(16):883–7.
6. Karp JF, Yu L, Friedly J, Amtmann D, Pilkonis PA. Negative affect and sleep disturbance may be associated with response to epidural steroid injections for spine-related pain. Arch Phys Med Rehabil. 2014;95(2):309–15.
7. Wasan AD, Jamison RN, Pham L, Tipirneni N, Nedeljkovic SS, Katz JN. Psychopathology predicts the outcome of medial branch blocks with corticosteroid for chronic axial low back or cervical pain: a prospective cohort study. BMC Musculoskelet Disord. 2009;10:22.
8. Wasan AD, Michna E, Edwards RR, et al. Psychiatric comorbidity is associated prospectively with diminished opioid analgesia and increased opioid misuse in patients with chronic low back pain. Anesthesiology. 2015;123(4):861–72.
9. Barsky AJ, Borus JF. Functional somatic syndromes. Ann Intern Med. 1999;130(11):910–21.
10. Bruns D, Fishbain DA, Disorbio JM, Lewis JE. What variables are associated with an expressed wish to kill a doctor in community and injured patient samples? J Clin Psychol Med Settings. 2010;17(2):87–97.
11. Fishbain DA, Bruns D, Lewis JE, Disorbio JM, Gao J, Meyer LJ. Predictors of homicide-suicide affirmation in acute and chronic pain patients. Pain Med. 2011;12(1):127–37.
12. Mirin SM. Practice guidelines for the treatment of patients with substance use disorders: alcohol, cocaine, opioids. In: McIntyre JS, editor. American Psychiatric Association practice guidelines for the treatment of psychiatric disorders. Washington, DC: American Psychiatric Association; 2000. p. 151–9.
13. Passik SD, Portenoy RK, Ricketts PL. Substance abuse issues in cancer patients. Part 1: prevalence and diagnosis. Oncology. 1998;12(4):517–21, 524.
14. Passik SD, Portenoy RK, Ricketts PL. Substance abuse issues in cancer patients. Part 2: evaluation and treatment. Oncology. 1998;12(5):729–34; discussion 736, 741–22.
15. Ranjan P, Kumari A, Chakrawarty A. How can doctors improve their communication skills? J Clin Diagn Res. 2015;9(3):JE01–4.
16. Steinmetz D, Tabenkin H. The 'difficult patient' as perceived by family physicians. Fam Pract. 2001;18(5):495–500.

Part II

Interventional Pain Procedures: Neuraxial Procedures

Traumatic Spinal Cord Injury After Cervical Interlaminar Epidural Steroid Injections

11

Bradley Silva and Dalia Elmofty

11.1 Case Description

A 39-year-old female with a history of systemic lupus erythematosus and rheumatoid arthritis who was taking Plaquenil complained of neck pain that radiates to the left upper extremity. The pain is associated with occasional numbness and tingling. She denies any extremity weakness. The patient underwent a 6-week course of physical therapy along with a trial of gabapentin 300 mg PO TID with minimal relief. Magnetic resonance imaging of the cervical spine revealed a C6–C7 diffuse disc bulge without spinal stenosis. After progressively worsening symptoms, the patient underwent a cervical epidural steroid injection. Upon awakening from the procedure, she felt her numbness worsen and developed mild weakness in her left upper extremity. No further imaging was performed at that time. Over the ensuing months, the patient suffered from severe burning pain. She was unable to tolerate heat, cold, or air blowing on her arm. The pain was accompanied by left upper extremity weakness, swelling, atrophy, discoloration, and temperature change, along with severe fatigue. Physical examination was notable for left hypothenar muscle atrophy. Pain limits her left grip, and she has 3/5 strength of her left abductor pollicis brevis, interossei, and finger extensor muscles. Otherwise strength is 5/5 throughout. Sensation to pinprick is decreased in the left upper extremity in all dermatomes, and reflexes are reduced. The right upper extremity has 2+ deep tendon reflexes and normal sensation. A repeat magnetic resonance imaging of the cervical spine showed two small foci of increased T2 signal measuring 4–5 mm within the left dorsal aspect of the spinal cord at the level of the C6 and C7 vertebral body level. The differential diagnosis based on the history, physical examination, and diagnostic testing included the following: (1) complex regional pain syndrome from iatrogenic injury after the cervical epidural steroid injection, (2) central nervous system infection in the setting of chronic immunosuppression, or (3) progression of the underlying autoimmune condition. Infectious workup revealed cerebrospinal fluid positive for John Cunningham virus (JCV, a type of human polyomavirus) but negative for Lyme disease, West Nile, and oligoclonal bands. The patient was referred to a tertiary health-care system, for initial evaluation by a neurologist and then referral to the pain clinic. Repeat lumbar puncture was negative for JC virus or any other abnormality. An electromyogram and test of nerve conduction velocity revealed a left C8 radiculopathy but no definitive evidence for left upper extremity neuropathy or brachial plexopathy. The diagnosis was complex regional pain syndrome, likely from iatrogenic injury from the cervical epidural steroid injection.

11.2 Case Discussion

Chronic pain is a common and medically challenging condition. According to the Institute of Medicine Report from the Committee on Advancing Pain Research, 100 million Americans suffer from chronic pain, resulting in health-care costs ranging from $560 to 635 billion in 2010, which include medical and economic costs from disability and lost wages [1]. In the subspecialty of pain management, although chronic pain is multifactorial, the utilization of interventional techniques has increased dramatically over the last two decades [2]. An analysis of Medicare beneficiaries from 2000 to 2011 found that interventional techniques increased by 228% [3]. Yet there is a paucity of literature on the incidence of complications associated with these techniques.

Cervical epidural steroid injections are commonly used to treat a variety of chronic conditions, including cervical radicular pain, neck pain, spinal stenosis, degenerative disc disease, and spondylolisthesis. The most widely used routes

B. Silva, M.D. • D. Elmofty, M.D. (✉)
Department of Anesthesia and Critical Care, University of Chicago, 5841 S. Maryland Ave., M.C. 4028, Chicago, IL 60637, USA
e-mail: DElmofty@dacc.uchicago.edu

M. Anitescu et al. (eds.), *Challenging Cases and Complication Management in Pain Medicine*,
https://doi.org/10.1007/978-3-319-60072-7_11

for cervical epidural steroid injection (CESI) are interlaminar and transforaminal. In the interlaminar route, the needle is advanced through a midline or a paramedian approach, traversing the ligamentum flavum to enter the posterior epidural space. In the transforaminal route, the needle is advanced along the axis of the intervertebral foramen.

11.3 Epidemiology

Although neurologic injury from CESI is undoubtedly rare, the actual incidence in the United States is difficult to ascertain. The majority of cases are identified through the American Society of Anesthesiologists (ASA) Closed Claims database. Events, however, may be under-reported and biased as to the degree of severity because a plaintiff's attorneys often will not pursue cases in which the estimated financial recovery for damages is less than $50,000 [4]. Another problem is that the Closed Claims database does not provide the total number of CESI procedures in the United States; therefore, there is no denominator from which to derive incidence. A Swedish study sought to determine the incidence of neurologic complications after neuraxial blockades from 1990 to 1999 using a postal survey to all departments of anesthesia in Sweden [5]. The incidence of complications was 1:25,000 in obstetric epidural blockade and 1:3600 in non-obstetric epidural blockade [5]. An important caveat to these results, however, is that the complications specified were epidural abscess, meningitis, spinal hematoma, and cauda equina syndrome, including many cases in which the neurologic symptoms were either temporary or absent. A French study, in which inclusion criteria were limited to neurologic complications lasting for at least 3 months and impairment in daily living, found an incidence of 1:116,639 in obstetric epidurals and 1:65,464 in non-obstetric epidurals for the year 2000 [6].

Despite the limitations, the Closed Claims database provides overall trends in chronic pain management claims and details of the cause of injury from interventional procedures. Coinciding with the increase in interventional procedures, the percentage of chronic pain claims has increased from <5% in the 1980s, to 11% in the 1990s, to 18% of all claims from 2000 to 2007 [7]. A review of the ASA's Closed Claims database between 2005 and 2008 revealed that 22% (64/294) of chronic pain claims were associated with cervical interventional procedures [8]. Of those 64 claims, the most common event was direct needle trauma to a nerve or the spinal cord (31%, 20/64), followed by cord infarction or stroke after intra-arterial injection (14%, 9/64), dural puncture (6%, 4/64), compressive hematoma (5%, 3/64), infection or abscess (5%), high block or total spinal (5%), unintentional intravascular injection of local anesthetic (3%, 2/64), and pneumothorax (3%) [8].

11.4 Anatomy

The cervical neuraxial anatomy is predisposed to catastrophic neurologic injury. The margin for error during needle advancement diminishes away from the lumbar epidural space. The posterior epidural space ranges from 5 to 13 mm in the dorsal-to-ventral dimension, 2 to 4 mm in the thoracic posterior epidural space, and to an average 0.4 mm in the cervical posterior epidural space [9]. The loss of resistance, expected during epidural needle placement, may not occur in patients whose ligamentum flavum has not fused at the midline, a condition that is more prevalent in the upper thoracic (4–21% midline gaps at T3–T4 and above) and cervical regions (51–74% midline gaps) [10].

The spinal cord is supplied with blood via three arteries within the subarachnoid space: the single anterior spinal artery which perfuses the anterolateral two-thirds of the cord and two posterior spinal arteries which perfuse the posterior one-third of the cord. More pertinent to interventional neurologic injuries, however, are branching arteries that arise outside the meningeal layers, course into the intervertebral foramen, penetrate the dura, and reinforce the anterior and posterior spinal arteries (referred to as "spinal segmental" or "spinal medullary" arteries). These arteries are derived from the deep and ascending cervical and radicular arteries which themselves come from the vertebral artery.

11.5 Pathophysiology

Both the interlaminar and transforaminal routes can result in direct needle trauma, even though the site of injury may differ (Table 11.1). The limited width of the epidural space in the interlaminar route and the possibility of a midline gap in the ligamentum flavum make direct needle trauma to the cord possible. Unintentional lateral deviation of the needle, however, also may cause contact with the spinal nerve or the anterior or posterior ramus at the intervertebral foramen [9]. Direct contact with the spinal nerve or one of the rami in the

Table 11.1 Associated injuries from direct needle trauma during cervical epidural steroid injections

Route of needle entry	Site of injury
Interlaminar approach	1. Injury to the spinal cord
	2. Injury of spinal nerve, ventral or dorsal ramus with lateral deviation of the needle
Transforaminal approach	1. Injury to spinal nerve
	2. Injury to ventral or dorsal ramus
	3. Injury to spinal cord
	4. Injury to vertebral, ascending or deep cervical arteries

transforaminal route seems anatomically more likely (Fig. 11.1). There has been at least one case report of direct needle trauma to the spinal cord during transforaminal CESI [11]. There is also the significant risk of needle contact with an artery. Studies have shown that the vertebral artery and the ascending and deep cervical arteries lie in close proximity to needles inserted into the cervical intervertebral foramen [12]. There are case reports of vertebral artery perforation as well as traumatic aneurysm [13, 14]. Theoretically, needle contact could also cause vessel irritation leading to vasospasm and cord ischemia from reduced blood flow [9, 15].

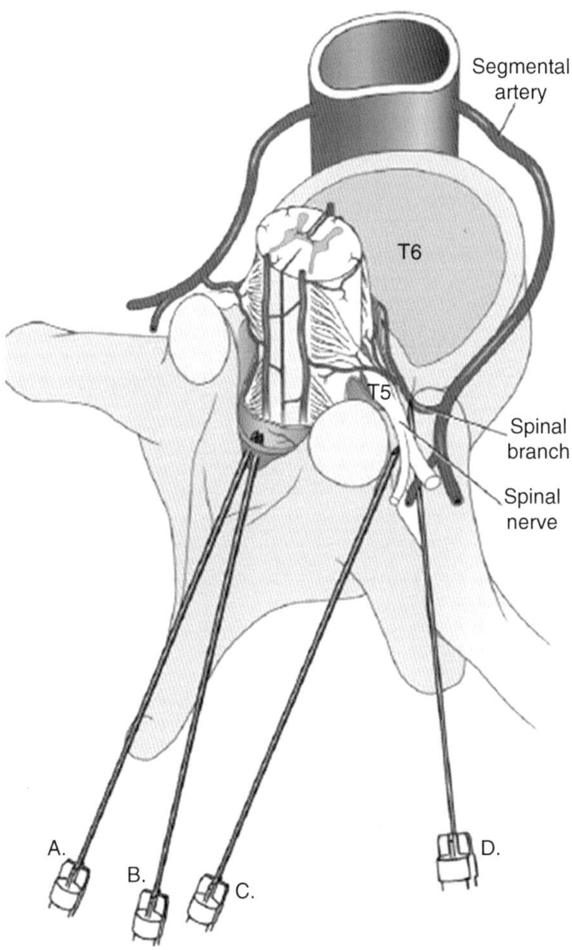

Fig. 11.1 Direct needle trauma from interlaminar and transforaminal approach. Needle A and B demonstrate a midline interlaminar approach which can directly traumatize the spinal cord. Needle C represents lateral deviation of the needle resulting in trauma to the spinal nerve, ventral or dorsal ramus. Needle D illustrates a transforaminal approach resulting in trauma to the spinal nerve, ventral or dorsal ramus, and spinal artery. Reprinted from Complications in Regional Anesthesia and Pain Medicine, Joseph M Neal, James P Rathmell, 2007, with permission Saunders/Elsevier

11.6 Clinical Presentation

Case reports illustrate the variability in the symptoms of direct needle trauma. Classic signs are severe pain, often correlating with the dermatomal pattern of the nerve contacted by the needle and radiating to one or more extremities, along with extremity paresthesia and weakness. Often, the symptoms manifest immediately upon needle penetration. There have been documented cases of fully awake patients, however, who sustained neuraxial injury but experienced no symptoms at the time of needle placement [16, 17]. Several factors influence clinical symptoms: cervical level, structure intruded (i.e., spinal cord or spinal nerve), and volume and type of injectate [18]. A higher cervical entry point may involve cranial nerves. One case report documented facial numbness after a C5–C6 interlaminar injection that was believed to be caused by direct damage to the spinal nucleus of the trigeminal nerve (which extends from the medulla to C3 or below C3) and by cephalad movement of intramedullary injectate [18].

The onset and quality of symptoms are also likely influenced by the structure that has sustained injury. Pain is more likely when extra-axial trauma affects the nerve roots or blood vessels, which are innervated by sensory neurons mediating pain [16]. On the other hand, there are no pain receptors within the spinal cord, which may render intra-axial lesions painless [16]. Pain is rarely reported with dural puncture, and symptoms may appear only after injection or from the sequelae of the needle trauma such as edema or hematoma [16].

11.7 Risk Factors

Risk factors for direct needle trauma are conditions that reduce or obscure the epidural space. Osteoporotic and degenerative processes of the spine, which become more common with advancing age, reduce the epidural space and close the intervertebral foramen [5]. Other pathologies that can compete with spinal cord and nerve roots for space are spinal stenosis, ligamentum flavum hypertrophy, and vertebral disc bulges [9, 18].

11.8 Preventative Measures

Numerous recommendations have been set forth to reduce the risk of direct needle trauma. Pre-procedural MRI or CT imaging is performed to verify adequate epidural space for needle placement at the target site [15]. Axial or sagittal cuts are measured to approximate dermal-to-epidural distance of the target interlaminar injection level, which can then be used to determine needle depth during the procedure [18]. Interlaminar CESI is performed at C7–T1 and preferably not higher than C6–C7 [15]. The cervical epidural space becomes narrower at higher cervical levels, increasing the likelihood of penetration of the dural sac and spinal cord [15]. At the C7–T1 level, medication can reach as high as the C4–C5 epidural space [18]. Low cervical targets reduce the risk of medication reaching the respiratory centers and cranial nerve nuclei in the medulla and upper cervical levels [18].

Radiographic guidance and the use of a test dose of contrast medium are essential for all CESI procedures. Interlaminar CESI should be performed under fluoroscopic guidance with anteroposterior, lateral, or contralateral oblique views to gauge the depth of needle insertion. Transforaminal CESI should be performed under fluoroscopy or digital subtraction angiography to decrease the risk of both direct needle trauma and intravascular injection [15]. The procedure should be stopped if a contrast test dose reveals a myelographic or arterial pattern [18]. A contrast pattern of a central canal stripe without flow to the lateral foramen may indicate cord injection [18].

Finally, the use of sedation during CESI continues to be debated. Those in favor of sedation point to case reports of needle trauma caused by sudden head movement, which would likely be prevented under sedation [19]. Those opposed to sedation argue that sedation could render a patient unable to report any pain or paresthesia caused by spinal cord or nerve trauma [19]. This position, however, is somewhat undermined by case reports, as described earlier, of fully awake patients reporting no unusual symptoms at the moment of traumatic needle penetration. The current consensus is to refrain from moderate-to-heavy sedation, and if light sedation is used, the patient should remain able to communicate pain or other adverse sensations or events [15].

11.9 Treatment

According to the literature, many of the factors that contribute to neuraxial injuries are unavoidable. If there are signs of injury, the procedure should be aborted, and the patient's condition should be reevaluated. Diagnostic testing should be initiated. For ischemic injuries, a magnetic resonance imaging scan is preferable over computerized tomography imaging. Magnetic resonance images may appear normal after an initial insult. After a few days, changes in the form of hyperintensities on T2-weighted images or focal cord swelling appear (Fig. 11.2). There are limited data regarding the use of corticosteroids after iatrogenic-induced direct spinal cord trauma from CESI, but corticosteroids have been shown to improve outcomes after acute traumatic spinal cord injury [20]. Methylprednisolone sodium succinate has been administered as an initial bolus of 30 mg/kg followed by an infusion of 5.4 mg/kg per hour infused for 23 h [20]. Corticosteroids are not recommended for ischemic-induced injuries of the spinal cord [9].

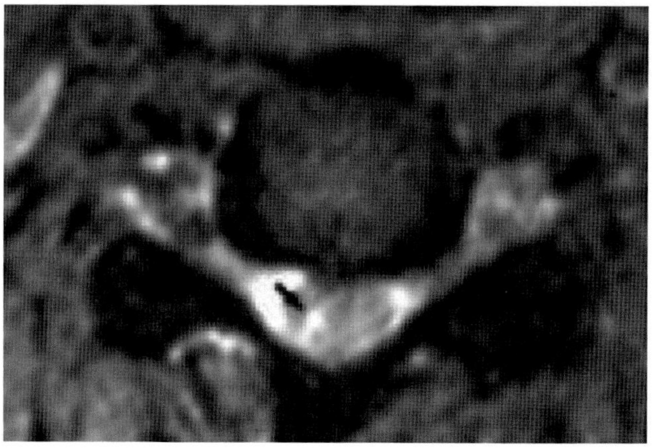

Fig. 11.2 Magnetic resonance imaging revealing a T2-weighted hyperintensity within the cord at C6 (*black arrow*). Reprinted from Journal of Neurology, Neurosurgery & Psychiatry, Volume 72, Issue 4, PA Wilkinson, A Valentine, J M Gibbs, Intrinsic spinal cord lesions complicating epidural anaesthesia and analgesia: report of three cases, 537–539, 2002, with permission from BMJ Publishing Group Ltd

Key Concepts

- Cervical interlaminar and transforaminal epidural steroid injections are performed for the interventional treatment of pain, yet there is a paucity of literature on the associated complications of the procedure.
- Awareness of potential complications associated with cervical intralaminar and transforaminal epidural steroid injections may enhance patient safety.
- The anatomic characteristics of the cervical neuraxial space predispose or contribute to its potential for sustaining needle injury.
- Refrain from deep sedation for neuraxial procedures because detecting paresthesia by the patient or the pain practitioner is diminished.
- If unanticipated sensory or motor deficits persist after an interventional procedure, imaging may be indicated. Magnetic resonance imaging is preferable to computerized tomography imaging for ischemic injuries.
- Corticosteroids may be beneficial for direct spinal cord trauma, but not for ischemic injuries of the cord.

References

1. Institute of Medicine Report. Relieving pain in America: a blueprint for transforming care, prevention, education, and research. Washington, DC: The National Academic Press; 2011.
2. Rowbotham DJ. Advances in pain. Br J Anaesth. 2001;87:1–2.
3. Manchikanti L, Falco FJ, Singh V, et al. Utilization of interventional techniques in managing chronic pain in a Medicare population: analysis of growth pattern from 2000 to 2011. Pain Physician. 2012;15(6):E969–82.
4. Gallagher RM. Chronic pain: a public health problem? Clin J Pain. 1998;14:277–9.

5. Moen V, Dahlgren N, Irestedt L. Severe neurological complications after central neuraxial blockades in Sweden 1990-1999. Anesthesiology. 2004;101:950–9.
6. de Sèze MP, Sztark F, Janvier G, Joseph PA. Severe and long-lasting complications of the nerve root and spinal cord after central neuraxial blockade. Anesth Analg. 2007;104:975–9.
7. Metzner J, Posner KL, Lam MS, Domino KB. Closed claims' analysis. Best Pract Res Clin Anaesthesiol. 2011;25:263–76.
8. Rathmell JP, Michna E, Fitzgibbon DR, Stephens LS, Posner KL, Domino KB. Injury and liability associated with cervical procedures for chronic pain. Anesthesiology. 2011;114:918–26.
9. Neal JM, Kopp SL, Pasternak JJ, Lanier ML, Rathmell JP. Anatomy and pathophysiology of spinal cord injury associated with regional anesthesia and pain medicine. Reg Anesth Pain Med. 2015;40:506–25.
10. Lirk P, Kolbitsch C, Putz G, et al. Cervical and high thoracic ligamentum flavum frequently fails to fuse in the midline. Anesthesiology. 2003;99:1387–90.
11. Lee JH, Lee JK, Seo BR, Moon SJ, Kim JH, Kim SH. Spinal cord injury produced by direct damage during cervical transforaminal epidural injection. Reg Anesth Pain Med. 2008;33(4):377–9.
12. Huntoon M. Anatomy of the cervical intervertebral foramina: vulnerable arteries and ischemic injuries after transforaminal epidural injections. Pain. 2005;117:104–11.
13. Rozin L, Rozin R, Koehler SA, et al. Death during transforaminal epidural steroid nerve root block (C7) due to perforation of the left vertebral artery. Am J Forensic Med Pathol. 2003;24:351–5.
14. Wallace MA, Fukui MB, Williams RI, Ku A, Baghai P. Complications of cervical selective nerve root blocks performed with fluoroscopic guidance. Am J Roentgenol. 2007;188:1218–21.
15. Rathmell JP, Benzon HT, Dreyfuss P, et al. Safeguards to prevent neurologic complications after epidural steroid injections: consensus opinions from a multidisciplinary working group and national organizations. Anesthesiology. 2015;122:974–84.
16. Tsui BC, Armstrong K. Can direct spinal cord injury occur without paresthesia? A report of delayed spinal cord injury after epidural placement in an awake patient. Anesth Analg. 2005;101(4):1212–4.
17. Bernards CM, Hadzic A, Suresh S, Neal JM. Regional anesthesia in anesthetized or heavily sedated patients. Reg Anesth Pain Med. 2008;33:449–60.
18. Maddela R, Wahezi SE, Sparr S, Brook A. Hemiparesis and facial sensory loss following cervical epidural steroid injection. Pain Physician. 2014;17:E761–7.
19. Abbasi A, Malhotra G, Malanga G, Elovic EP, Kahn S. Complications of interlaminar cervical epidural steroid injections: a review of the literature. Spine. 2007;32(19):2144–51.
20. Bracken MB. Steroids for acute spinal cord injury. Cochrane Database Syst Rev. 2012;10:CD001046.

Total Spinal After Cervical Epidural Steroid Injection

12

Meghan E. Rodes

12.1 Case Description

A 48-year-old male presents to the pain clinic for evaluation of neck pain and left arm pain of 2 months' duration. The pain began after lifting and disposing of some heavy garbage bags. He reports pain in his left neck, radiating into his left shoulder, front of his chest, in the back of his upper arm and forearm. He notes associated numbness and tingling in his left hand, worst in the middle digit, and reports that he has dropped items on occasion due to weakness of his grip. Thus far he has initiated a physical therapy program and has tried nonsteroidal anti-inflammatory drugs (NSAIDs) without much relief of his pain. Physical examination is significant for diminished (4/5) strength in his left triceps and flexor carpi radialis and diminished sensation to light touch in the middle of his left hand and left triceps reflex 1+. He underwent magnetic resonance imaging (MRI) of the cervical spine, which was notable for a shallow broad-based posterior disk bulge with a superimposed left foraminal disk protrusion, resulting in mild spinal canal stenosis and moderate left neural foraminal stenosis at C6–C7 (see Figs. 12.1, 12.2, and 12.3). He also underwent electromyography (EMG), which revealed increased insertional activity, fibrillation potentials and positive sharp waves, moderately increased motor unit action potential duration, and moderately reduced motor unit action potential recruitment in the left triceps and left flexor carpi radialis muscles, consistent with an acute on chronic left C7 radiculopathy. The patient was referred to the pain clinic by a neurosurgeon for CESI for the diagnosis of cervical radiculopathy. This procedure was discussed with the patient as a pain management strategy, and he was counseled on the risks of the procedure including bleeding, infection, nerve injury including permanent paralysis, death, headache, worsening of pain, adverse effects of medication, and allergic reaction to medication. The patient fully understood the potential adverse effects and risks of the procedure and to proceed to the emergency department immediately if any serious reactions or symptoms should occur. He consented for CESI. The patient was brought into the fluoroscopy suite and positioned prone on the examination table, with his arms at his side. Continuous pulse oximetry and noninvasive blood pressure (NIBP) monitors were applied. A time-out was performed, confirming this patient was having CESI and that he was not allergic to latex, local anesthetic, steroids, or contrast media. The site was prepped with chlorhexidine gluconate and a sterile drape applied. The cervical spine was imaged under fluoroscopy in an anterior-posterior (AP) view, with the C7–T1 interspace identified. Local infiltration with lidocaine 1% 3 mL was performed. A 20-gauge Tuohy needle was then inserted through the local anesthetic wheal and advanced under AP view toward the C7–T1 interspace using a loss of resistance (LOR) to saline technique. Loss

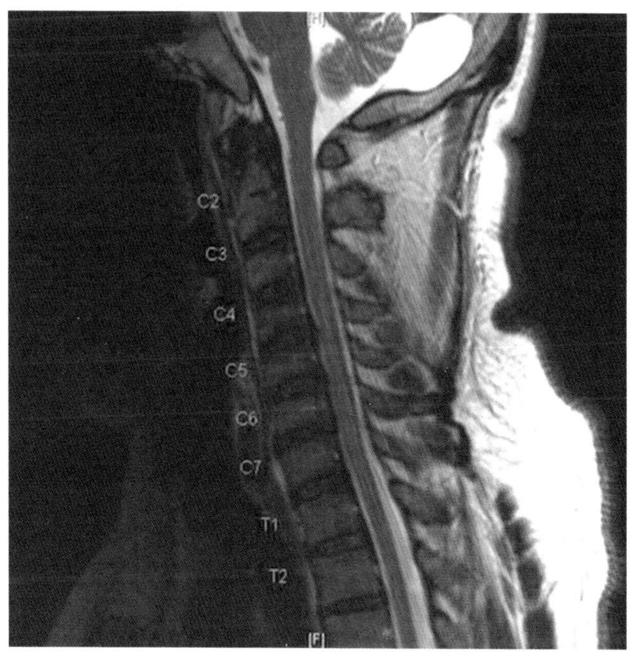

Fig. 12.1 Sagittal T2 MRI with cervical spinal levels identified; note the limited CSF signal (bright white on T2) in the cervical spine as compared with the thoracic spine

M.E. Rodes, M.D.
Northwestern University Feinberg School of Medicine
251 E. Huron St. F5-704, Chicago, IL 60611, USA
e-mail: meghan.rodes@northwestern.edu

M. Anitescu et al. (eds.), *Challenging Cases and Complication Management in Pain Medicine*,
https://doi.org/10.1007/978-3-319-60072-7_12

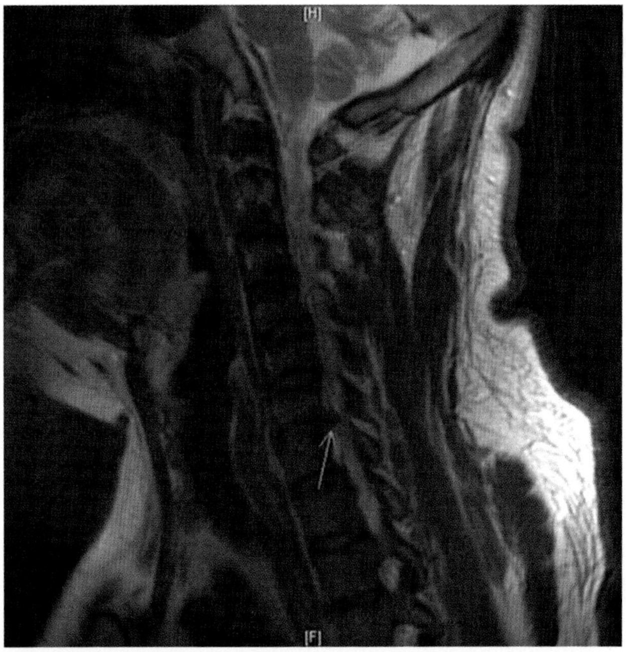

Fig. 12.2 Sagittal T2 MRI with C6–C7 disk herniation identified by *arrow*

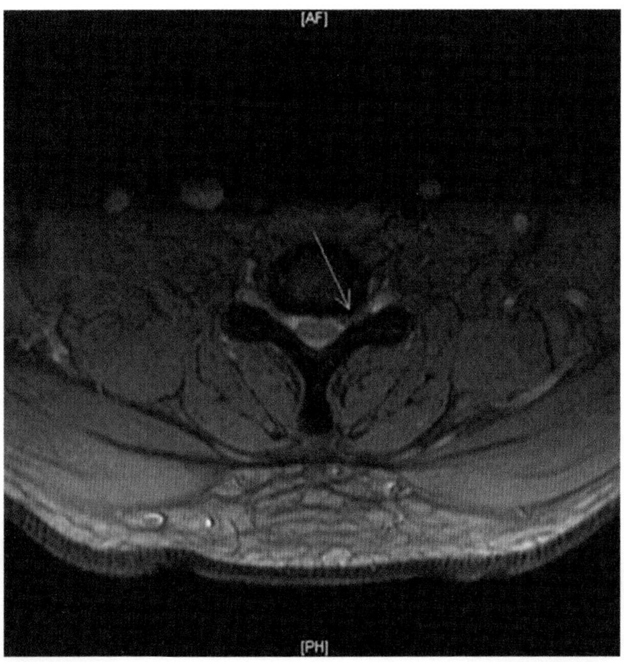

Fig. 12.3 Axial T2 MRI with leftward C6–C7 disk herniation identified by *arrow*

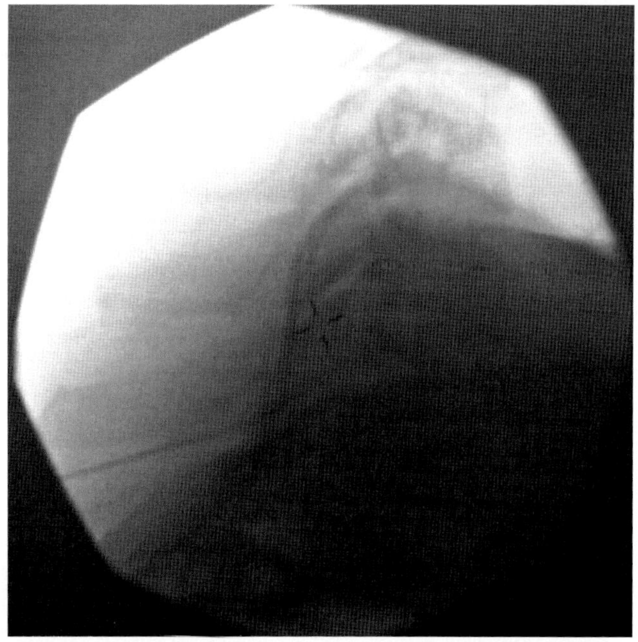

Fig. 12.4 Lateral fluoroscopic view post-contrast injection; note contrast spread in the posterior epidural space to C6 level

of resistance to saline was obtained at a depth of 7 cm. A lateral fluoroscopic view was obtained at this time, confirming appropriate needle placement in the posterior epidural space. After negative aspiration for blood or cerebrospinal fluid (CSF), 2 mL of contrast dye was injected through the needle, spreading up to the C6 level in the posterior epidural space (see Fig. 12.4). An AP fluoroscopic view was then obtained, and an additional 1 mL of contrast dye was injected, without evidence of intravascular or intrathecal spread (see Fig. 12.5). A mixture of methylprednisolone 80 mg and lidocaine 2% 1.5 mL was then injected. Immediately after injection, the patient complained of paresthesias of his upper extremities, difficulty speaking, developed profound hypotension and bradycardia, and suddenly lost consciousness. The patient was immediately turned supine on the table, mask ventilation was initiated and endotracheal intubation performed, and intravenous (IV) access was established for fluid resuscitation and administration of vasoactive medications. Approximately 60 min after the injection of lidocaine, the patient recovered consciousness and spontaneous respiration, returned to baseline hemodynamic values, and was extubated. The patient was observed for 4 h post-procedure and was discharged—accompanied by someone—in stable condition, with no new complaints and no change in his baseline neurological examination. A telephone call later that night and in the morning confirmed that he was doing fine.

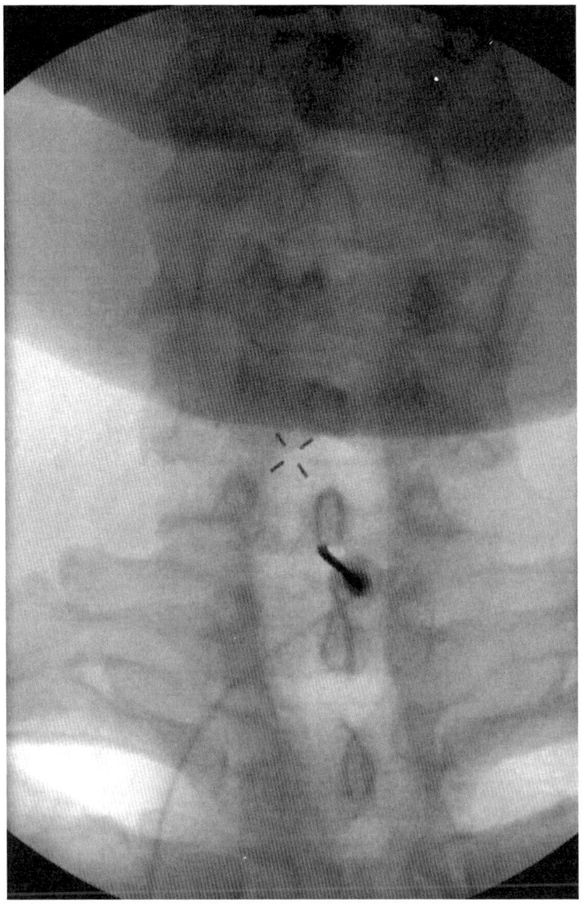

Fig. 12.5 AP fluoroscopic view post-contrast injection; note needle placement at C7-T1 interspace

12.2 Case Discussion

12.2.1 Anatomy of the Cervical Epidural Space

The boundaries of the epidural space are as follows: superiorly by the foramen magnum, inferiorly by the sacral hiatus, anteriorly by the posterior longitudinal ligament, and posteriorly by the ligamentum flavum. The diameter of the posterior epidural space is approximately 3–5 mm at the C7–T1 interspace. The ligamentum flavum is also relatively thin (and possibly discontinuous in the cervical spine) as compared to the lumbar region, making LOR more subtle in the cervical spine. Cadaver evidence has shown that the ligamentum flavum frequently fails to fuse in the midline over the cervical interspaces and that midline gaps were observed in more than 50% of specimens [1, 2]. Therefore, injection at the C7–T1 level is favored, taking into account that injected substances will likely spread over multiple interspaces in the cervical spine, so most levels can be reached from a C7–T1 epidural entry. Some practitioners favor a paramedian approach due to the possibility of incomplete fusion of the ligamentum flavum in the midline, whereas other practitioners favor a midline approach to avoid neural and vascular structures that may be located more laterally.

12.2.2 Technique for Interlaminar Cervical Epidural Steroid Injection

Typically the patient is positioned prone on the fluoroscopy table. Some practitioners perform the procedure in the sitting position; however, it may be more difficult for the patient to hold his/her head in a fixed position while sitting. After sterile prep and drape is performed, fluoroscopy is used to identify the C7–T1 interspace and optimize the angle of entry. Local infiltration is performed, and the epidural needle is introduced through the skin and subcutaneous tissue. The first structure to be encountered deep to the subcutaneous tissue is the supraspinous ligament. After passing through the supraspinous ligament, the needle will next traverse the ligamentum nuchae, a large structure that bridges the dorsal edges of the cervical spinous processes. Next, the interspinous ligament is encountered, which runs between the spinous processes. The density of this ligament is such that the needle will remain seated even when released, as compared with more superficial structures. The interspinous ligament then adjoins the ligamentum flavum, and occasionally the practitioner may sense a change in resistance at the junction between these two ligaments. Resistance will often increase once again as the needle progresses into the ligamentum flavum. (See Fig. 12.6 for an illustration of the above structures and their anatomical relationships.) A noticeable and complete LOR should occur as the needle passes through the ligamentum flavum into the epidural space. Whether using LOR to saline or air, there should be almost no resistance to injection into the epidural space. If the patient complains of a significant increase in pain or the practitioner notes a change in resistance to injection, the procedure should be halted and needle placement reassessed. The use of the hanging drop technique, whereby a non-styletted epidural needle topped with saline is advanced until the saline is pulled into the needle, has fallen out of favor due to an increased risk of dural puncture when compared with other methods. This phenomenon is best explained by the fact the epidural space may not always be in a negative pressure state, particularly in patients with spinal pathology (who are often

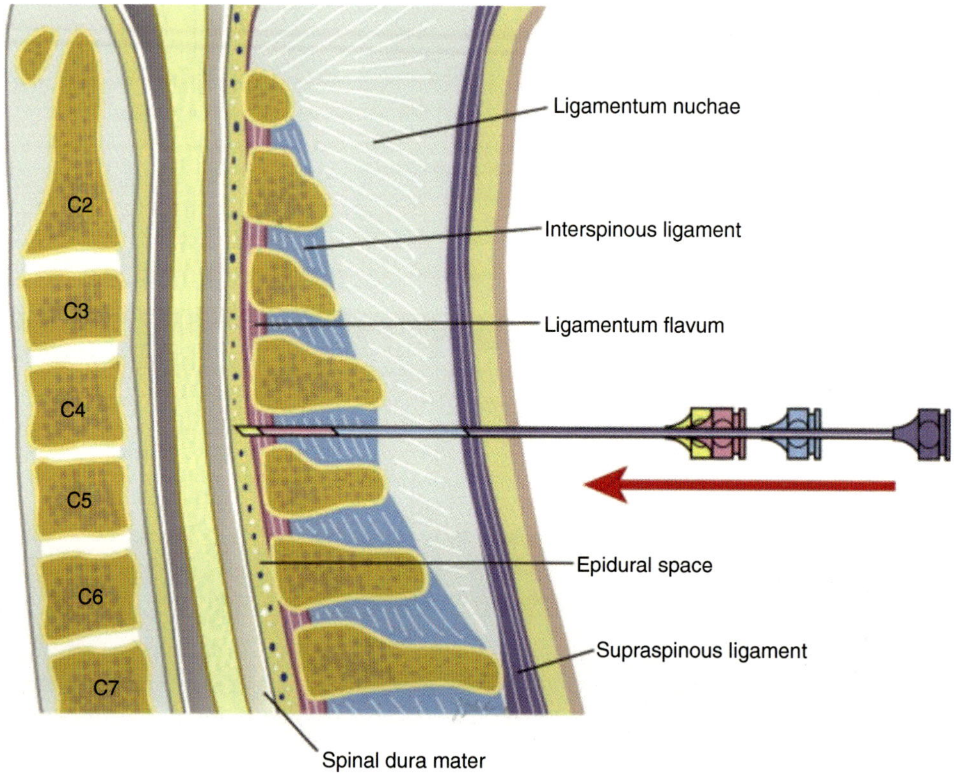

Fig. 12.6 Ligamentous anatomy of the cervical spine. Reprinted from Atlas of Interventional Pain Management, 4th Ed., Waldman SD, Cervical Epidural Block, pp. 178–187, Copyright (2015), with permission from Elsevier

presenting for ESI). If the epidural space is in a positive pressure state, no LOR will be obtained on entry into the epidural space, and the needle may be inadvertently advanced into the subarachnoid space or, worse, the spinal cord. Fluoroscopy is advocated as a safety measure among many practitioners; however, it is not a guarantee against complications. Following a negative aspiration for blood or CSF, injection of contrast should be done under live fluoroscopy. Another image may be obtained shortly after injection to verify that the location of the contrast has not changed or disappeared. Digital subtraction imaging (whereby images are produced using contrast medium by subtracting a pre-contrast image from post-contrast images) may also be useful to clarify contrast spread.

12.2.3 Potential Complications of Interlaminar Cervical Epidural Steroid Injection

1. Dural puncture +/− intrathecal injection—estimated incidence less than 1%. Failure to recognize improper needle placement may result in immediate total spinal anesthesia (if local anesthetic is injected) with associated loss of consciousness, hypotension, and apnea (see Table 12.1 for signs and symptoms of total spinal anesthesia).
   (a) Management of high spinal anesthesia—the clinician must address and manage signs or symptoms, including applying the ABCs (airway, breathing, circulation):

Table 12.1 Signs and symptoms of total or high spinal anesthesia

Numbness, tingling, or weakness in upper extremities
Difficulty speaking
Nausea/vomiting
Respiratory depression, apnea, oxygen desaturation
Profound hypotension, bradycardia
Loss of consciousness, cardiac arrest

   - Airway support including oxygen supplementation and positive pressure ventilation via mask or endotracheal tube if indicated
   - Administration of intravenous fluids and vasopressors and initiation of advanced cardiovascular life support (ACLS) protocol in the event of a cardiac arrest

   (b) Management of dural puncture—there is currently no data to support the immediate treatment of dural puncture with epidural blood patch (EBP), saline injection, or mobility restrictions. The patient should be counseled about the possibility and characteristics of a post dural puncture headache (PDPH). If a PDPH presents, many practitioners advocate aggressive fluid intake, consumption of caffeinated beverages, and/or over-the-counter or prescription analgesics. If the patient does not respond to conservative measures, an EBP could be considered.

   (c) Spinal cord injury—typically from direct needle trauma to the cord or injection of volume into the cord. Immediate reimaging and neurosurgical consultation is advised.
   (d) Arachnoiditis—a late, potential complication of intrathecal injection of steroid; often presents as an insidious, progressive motor and sensory change.
2. Additional potential complications of CESI.
   (a) Intravascular injection—presentation may vary depending on the type and volume of injectate (local anesthetic, saline, and/or steroid) and location of injection (arterial or venous).
   (b) Subdural injection—signs/symptoms in between that of epidural and intrathecal injection, with odd or unexpected levels of sensory and motor block for the dose of local anesthetic injected.
   (c) Epidural hematoma—greater risk in patients on anticoagulant or antiplatelet agents, and patients with clotting dysfunction, e.g., liver disease; often presents with significant pain at the site of injection, along with profound neurological complaints such as complete numbness, weakness, and loss of bowel or bladder continence, and is considered a surgical emergency.
   (d) Epidural abscess—greater risk in patients with active infection or an immunocompromised state, e.g., acquired immune deficiency syndrome (AIDS), cancer patients receiving chemotherapy, and patients taking TNF-alpha inhibitors; presentation similar to that of epidural hematoma with the addition of possible fevers/chills, also a surgical emergency.

12.2.4 Recommendations to Minimize Complications During CESI

1. It is important to obtain and evaluate MRI findings prior to performing CESI. Often in cases of severe disk protrusion/extrusion, there may be little to no CSF signal posterior to the spinal cord. In these cases, it may be best to avoid injection directly at the level of pathology, as the risk of dural puncture and spinal cord trauma may be higher. Additionally, if a patient has had prior spinal surgery, the presence of scar tissue or dural adhesions raises the incidence of dural puncture at that level, as well as increasing the risk of needle trauma to the spinal cord.
2. Patients should be monitored during the procedure, even if it is being done under local anesthesia. Complications are much more likely to be promptly recognized when continuous monitoring is being used, from a more mild vasovagal episode to an intrathecal injection of local anesthetic. At a minimum, pulse oximetry and NIBP should be monitored, and/or electrocardiography (ECG), particularly if sedation is being administered.
3. Optimal epidural needle entry is at C7–T1. As mentioned previously, the ligamentum flavum may be incompletely fused in the cervical spine and possibly more so at higher levels. Epidural fat that is more common at lower cervical levels may also provide a buffer between the ligamentum flavum and the dura. As evidenced by contrast spread on fluoroscopy, the limited capacitance of the cervical epidural space allows distribution of injection to multiple spinal levels (as compared with lumbar injections). To date, there is no evidence that a cervical ESI done at C7–T1 is any less efficacious for a mid-cervical radiculopathy than an injection done at a higher level. If an injection at C7–T1 fails to provide relief for spinal pathology at a considerably higher level, one might consider making an epidural entry at C7–T1 and threading an epidural catheter to the level of the pathology under fluoroscopy.
4. Both AP and lateral fluoroscopic views should be obtained prior to injection. The lateral view may be compromised by the presence of the shoulders at lower cervical levels. Options to optimize this view include asking the patient to reach toward his/her feet, taping the shoulders down toward the feet, utilizing a "swimmer's view," with one arm at the side and the other raised above the head, has been used successfully to obtain a view of the needle within the spinal canal, as well as the use of a contralateral oblique fluoroscopic view [3].
5. Sedation should be avoided unless necessary for patient comfort. When sedation is required, it should be limited to the amount needed to keep the patient comfortable but also awake and conversant. A patient under deep sedation is unable to communicate abnormal sensations that may be warning signs of improper needle placement, in addition to the fact that they may not remain deeply sedated and possibly move suddenly during the procedure due to disinhibition. There are many anecdotal accounts of patients who have had intense paresthesias and/or motor responses to contact of a needle with the spinal cord, as well as a number of cases in which general anesthesia or moderate to deep sedation appeared to block such responses [4]. Unfortunately, even in the nonsedated patient, needle entry into the cord may not result in a noticeable response [5, 6]. An awake and conversant patient still offers added safety to the procedure.
6. Many practitioners choose not to inject local anesthetic into the cervical epidural space (as opposed to saline). While it may provide some diagnostic value and possibly temporary pain relief, there is no sustained therapeutic benefit from injection of local anesthetic into the epidural space.
7. Regarding the risk of epidural abscess and hematoma, these procedures should never be performed on patients who are ill or taking anticoagulant or antiplatelet agents. These are elective procedures and should be delayed until it is safe to proceed.

8. Arachnoiditis is a known potential complication of intrathecal steroid injection. In the 2014 FDA briefing report on the safety of epidural steroid injections, particulate steroids were identified in the majority of cases of arachnoiditis that were analyzed. Some have advocated the use of non-particulate steroid to minimize this complication; however, if the practitioner is not absolutely certain about the needle placement, the procedure should be aborted and the needle repositioned.

12.3 Closed Claims from Cervical Pain Treatments

Rathmell et al. investigated injury and liability associated with cervical procedures for chronic pain between January 1, 2005, and December 31, 2008 [7]. Of course closed claims data is limited in that reported claims are only a subset of an unknown total number of incidents, but the information is valuable nonetheless. Cervical claims were specifically examined as the number of cervical procedures being performed was increasing at the time. A total of 294 chronic pain claims were reviewed, 22% of which involved cervical spinal procedures. Spinal cord damage was noted in 59% of cervical claims, compared to 11% of other chronic pain claims. In 31% of cervical cord damage cases, direct needle trauma was identified as the proximate cause. Another trend identified in the analysis was the high proportion (67%) of claims involving general anesthesia or sedation associated with cord trauma, with 25% of these patients being classified as unresponsive during the procedure. Significantly, only 19% of cervical procedure claims not associated with spinal cord injuries involved sedation. It is therefore recommended to minimize sedation needed to achieve optimal procedural conditions. Patients should remain awake, alert, and conversant, so they may communicate abnormal sensations including pain or paresthesias during needle placement. "Heavily sedated patients are unable to respond with the expected pain and paresthesias due to spinal cord irritation in the event of errant needle placement" [8].

Key Concepts

- Cervical epidural steroid injection is a safe option for managing pain related to cervical spinal pathology. There is a significant body of literature to support the generally low complication rates, with minimal permanent morbidity or mortality [8–11].
- The practitioner performing CESI must be aware of the anatomy, technical steps, and potential complications of the procedure, as well as how to diagnose and manage complications that may arise during or after the procedure.
- Continuous monitoring is essential during CESI. Resuscitation equipment and medications should be available.
- The use of fluoroscopy is encouraged to improve safety; however, it is not a guarantee against complications.
- Safety of CESI is compromised by deep sedation and should be avoided.
- It is critical to promptly recognize the signs/symptoms of an intrathecal injection of local anesthetic and support the patient as needed.

References

1. Lirk P, Kolbitsch C, Putz G, et al. Cervical and high thoracic ligamentum flavum frequently fails to fuse in the midline. Anesthesiology. 2003;99(6):1387–90.
2. Stojanovic MP, Vu TN, Caneris O, et al. The role of fluoroscopy in cervical epidural steroid injections: an analysis of contrast dispersal patterns. Spine. 2002;27(5):509–14.
3. Abbasi A, Malhotra G. The "swimmer's view" as alternative when lateral view is inadequate during interlaminar cervical epidural steroid injections. Pain Med. 2010;11:709–12.
4. Hodges SD, Castleberg RL, Miller T, et al. Cervical epidural steroid injection with intrinsic spinal cord damage. Two case reports. Spine. 1998;23:2137–42.
5. Tripathi M, Nath SS, Gupta RK. Paraplegia after intracord injection during attempted epidural steroid injection in an awake patient. Anesth Analg. 2005;101:1209–11.
6. Simon SL, Abrahams JM, Sean Grady M, et al. Intramedullary injection of contrast into the cervical spinal cord during cervical myelography: a case report. Spine. 2002;27:E274–7.
7. Rathmell JP, Michna E, Fitzgibbon DR, et al. Injury and liability associated with cervical procedures for chronic pain. Anesthesiology. 2011;114(4):918–26.
8. Johnson BA, Schellhas KP, Pollei SR. Epidurography and therapeutic epidural injections: technical considerations and experience with 5,334 cases. Am J Neuroradiol. 1999;20(4):697–705.
9. Waldman SD. Complications of cervical epidural nerve blocks with steroids: a prospective study of 790 blocks. Reg Anesth. 1989;14(3):149–51.
10. Cicala RS, Westbrook L, Angel JJ. Side effects and complications of cervical epidural steroid injections. J Pain Symptom Manag. 1989;4(2):64–6.
11. Botwin KP, Castellanos R, Rao S, et al. Complications of fluoroscopically guided interlaminar cervical epidural injections. Arch Phys Med Rehabil. 2003;84(8):627–33.

Death After Transforaminal Cervical Epidural Steroid Injection

13

Irina Khrenova and Mario De Pinto

13.1 Case Description

Fifty-eight-year-old male patient with history of right-sided neck, shoulder, and upper extremity pain along the C7 nerve root distribution. A cervical spine magnetic resonance imaging (MRI) shows degenerative disk disease at the C5–C6 and C6–C7 levels with a protruding C6–C7 disk herniation moderately impinging on the right C7 nerve root (Figs. 13.1 and 13.2). Pain has started 6 weeks earlier with no inciting event and has been getting progressively worse despite rest, use of NSAIDs, muscle relaxants, gabapentin, short-acting opioids, and physical therapy.

The patient has hypertension that is managed with beta-blockers. A focused physical examination shows mildly decreased sensation along the right C7 nerve root distribution without motor and tendon reflexes abnormalities. He reports that pain is affecting the quality of life and impairing his ability to work. He has undergone a surgical evaluation and referred to the pain clinic for a right C7 transforaminal epidural steroid injection. Risks and benefits of the procedure have been discussed with the patient and his family. The plan is to start an intravenous (IV) line and provide a small amount of sedation with fentanyl and midazolam. The injection will be performed with the patient in the supine position, under fluoroscopic guidance. A 25-gauge 2.5″ Quincke spinal needle is placed in the desired position, but aspiration is positive for blood. The needle position is adjusted, and the injection of a small amount of contrast medium reveals an appropriate flow along the right C7 nerve root with negative aspiration for blood. Two milliliters (mL) of lidocaine 2% mixed with 2 mL of a solution containing a particulate steroid (betamethasone—Celestone 6 mg/mL) are injected in 1 mL aliquots. The needle is removed, and the patient is transported back to the recovery room. Upon arrival in the recovery room, 5 min after completion of the procedure, the patient becomes agitated and confused. Vital signs show a blood pressure of 141/95, heart rate 94, respiratory rate 7 breath/min, and O_2 saturation 97% on room air. During the following 10 min, the vital signs deteriorate, and the patient becomes unresponsive. A code blue is called. He is intubated and transported to the emergency department. A brain CT scan obtained in the emergency room reveals the presence of a large hemorrhage around the

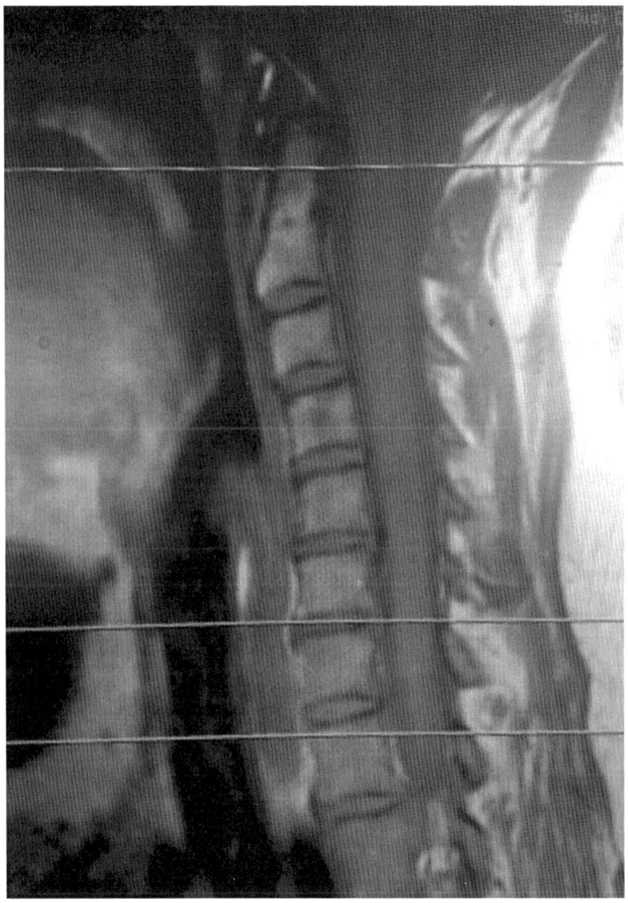

Fig. 13.1 Sagittal view of the cervical spine showing a disk herniation at the C6–C7 disk level (Courtesy of Dr. M. De Pinto)

I. Khrenova, M.D. • M. De Pinto, M.D. (✉)
Department of Anesthesiology and Perioperative Care, University of California San Francisco—UCSF, UCSF Pain Management Center, San Francisco, CA 94143-1654, USA
e-mail: Mario.DePinto@ucsf.edu

M. Anitescu et al. (eds.), *Challenging Cases and Complication Management in Pain Medicine*,
https://doi.org/10.1007/978-3-319-60072-7_13

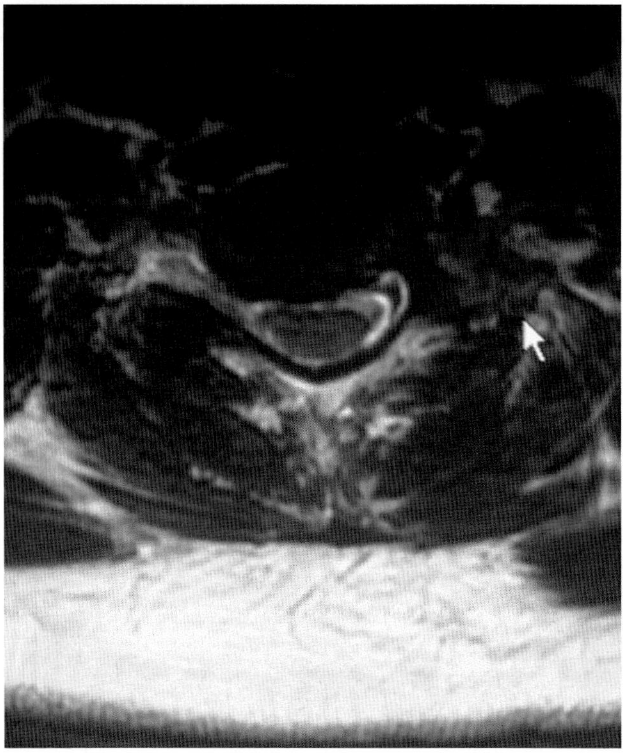

Fig. 13.2 Sagittal view of the cervical spine showing a disk herniation at the C6–C7 disk level with moderate compression of the right C7 nerve root (Courtesy of Dr. M. De Pinto)

brainstem extending through the midbrain and pons into the lateral ventricles with obstructive hydrocephalus. The gravity of the clinical condition is immediately evident and explained to the patient's family. Treatment is initiated but does not result in improvement of the clinical conditions. After consultation with the patient's wife and family, support is withdrawn 2 days after the injection. The patient expires soon afterward.

13.2 Case Discussion

13.2.1 Indications for Cervical Transforaminal Epidural Steroid Injections

Cervical transforaminal epidural steroid injections (CTESIs) are used in the management of radicular pain and may restore function in patients with cervical radiculopathies [1–3].

The main indication for CTESIs is the presence of radicular pain that:

- Persists beyond the usual natural resolution.
- Is not responsive to conservative therapy (~10–20%) [4].
- Surgery may be the only available option.
- Has no other causes (e.g., tumor, fracture, infection, etc.).

The release of nociceptive and inflammatory mediators (e.g., nitric oxide (NO), prostaglandin E2 (PGE2), interleukin 6 (IL-6), phospholipase A2) around disk herniations and areas of spondylosis can lead to chemical radiculitis and nerve root irritation. Compression of irritated nerve roots results in prolonged firing of the nerve fibers and consequent pain production [5, 6]. Moreover, dorsal root ganglions (DRG) can fire repetitively even with minimal compression and in the absence of irritation [7].

Corticosteroids suppress inflammation, limit the ectopic discharge of DRGs and injured nerve fibers, and decrease phospholipase A2 activity [5, 6]. In addition, the combination of local anesthetic and steroid has been reported to have anti-inflammatory effect on nucleus pulposus-induced nerve injuries [8]. Data in an animal model also have shown that the injection of lidocaine increases intra-radicular blood flow, thereby decreasing ischemia-like pain that may be induced by the compression of the nerve root [9].

13.2.2 Effectiveness of Cervical Transforaminal Epidural Steroid Injections

Cervical epidural steroid injections are performed as part of a conservative approach in patients with radicular pain. However, the evidence suggesting that these procedures may be effective long term is minimal and of low quality. A paper published in 2014 [10] has provided a systematic review and comprehensive analysis of the literature data available on the topic. Most of the studies published are observational and retrospective in nature, include a limited number of patients, and have some methodology flaws [1, 11–16]. No randomized, double-blind, placebo-controlled study is included in this review, even though a few of them are prospective in nature and are the ones providing the most compelling evidence of the effectiveness of CTFESIs for relief of radicular pain and avoidance of surgery [17, 18]. The authors conclude that:

- Review of the literature indicates that CTESIs help some patients with short-term relief of radicular pain but have questionable long-term benefit.
- The benefit of CTESIs appears limited in the proportion of patients who benefit (~40%), the extent to which they benefit (50% relief of radicular pain), and the duration of effect (4 weeks).
- At 3, 6, and 12 months, the proportion of patients with any degree of benefit decreases, as does the quality of the published studies.
- CTESIs carry the risk of serious and catastrophic complications, including permanent quadriplegia and death.

13.2.3 Risks and Complications of Cervical Transforaminal Epidural Steroid Injections

CTESIs have been associated with catastrophic and devastating complications. Numerous case reports have been published reporting on injuries following a CTESI that eventually led to death or permanent neurological damage including:

- Spinal cord infarction leading to death [19]
- Vertebral artery occlusion leading to death [20]
- Cerebellar and cerebral infarction leading to death [21]
- Cerebral injury and cortical blindness [22]
- Lateral spinal cord infarction [23]
- Cerebral ischemia and hippocampal atrophy [23]
- Posterior spinal cord and cerebellar infarction [23]
- Spinal cord infarction leading to quadriparesis and quadriplegia [24–26]
- Cerebellar infarction and main stem herniation [27]
- Permanent Horner's syndrome [28]

In other published case reports, the injury occurring at the time of the injection did not lead to permanent damage, and the patients made a full recovery; in some cases a long recovery time was necessary [29–36].

13.2.4 Anatomy of the Vertebral Arteries as They Relate to Cervical Transforaminal Epidural Steroid Injections

A careful review of the literature regarding risks and complications of CTESIs seems to suggest that the vertebral artery and the small radicular arteries supplying blood to the cervical spinal cord are at risk of being penetrated and injected into while performing these procedures.

Typically the vertebral arteries (VA) arise from the subclavian arteries and enter deep to the transverse process at the level of the sixth cervical vertebrae (C6) or occasionally (7.5% of cases) at the level of C7. They then proceed superiorly in the transverse foramen of each cervical vertebra. Once they have passed through the transverse foramen of C1, they travel across the posterior arch of C1 and through the suboccipital triangle before entering the foramen magnum. Inside the skull, the two vertebral arteries join to form the basilar artery at the base of the pons. The basilar artery is the main blood supply to the brainstem and connects to the circle of Willis and potentially supplies the rest of the brain if there is compromise to one of the carotid arteries [37] (Fig. 13.3).

Clinically the VA is described as having four discreet segments [38]. The first segment (V1) begins at the origin of the VA from the subclavian artery and extends to the level of the C6 transverse process. The second segment (V2) runs in the transverse foraminal column from C6 to C2. The third segment (V3) extends from the C2 transverse foramen to the foramen magnum, and the fourth segment (V4) runs from the foramen magnum to the formation of the basilar artery (Fig. 13.3).

The majority of CTESIs are performed along the V2 segment of the VA, which typically enters the C6 foramen and remains within the protection of the bony column of the cervical transverse processes throughout its length [39]. The safe target area for CTESIs, described in relation to the normal pathway of the vertebral artery, is located in the posterior aspect of the neuroforamen. To avoid cannulating the VA, interventionalists are taught to direct the needle, using an oblique view, toward the superior articular process while maintaining a posterior approach. After touching periosteum, the needle is directed slightly anteriorly and advanced medially into the neuroforamen taking care not to pass beyond the midpoint of the articular pillar in the anteroposterior (AP) view (Fig. 13.4) [40]. In a patient with normal anatomy, these guidelines should keep the needle from puncturing the exiting nerve root, vertebral artery, or dural sac (Fig. 13.5). However, studies performed on cadavers and in living subjects show that anatomical anomalies of the VA, anomalies that place an arterial segment posteriorly into the CTESI target zone, can occur in 20% of patients [41]. The VA may lie in the posterior foramen and within 2 mm of the ideal needle location in at least one location in 29% of patients. The more commonly affected levels are C3–C4, C4–C5, and C5–C6. Although possible, it is less common for the VA to be located posteriorly at the C6–C7 level (Fig. 13.6). The VA proximity to the typical target location for CTESIs correlates with the severity of foraminal stenosis

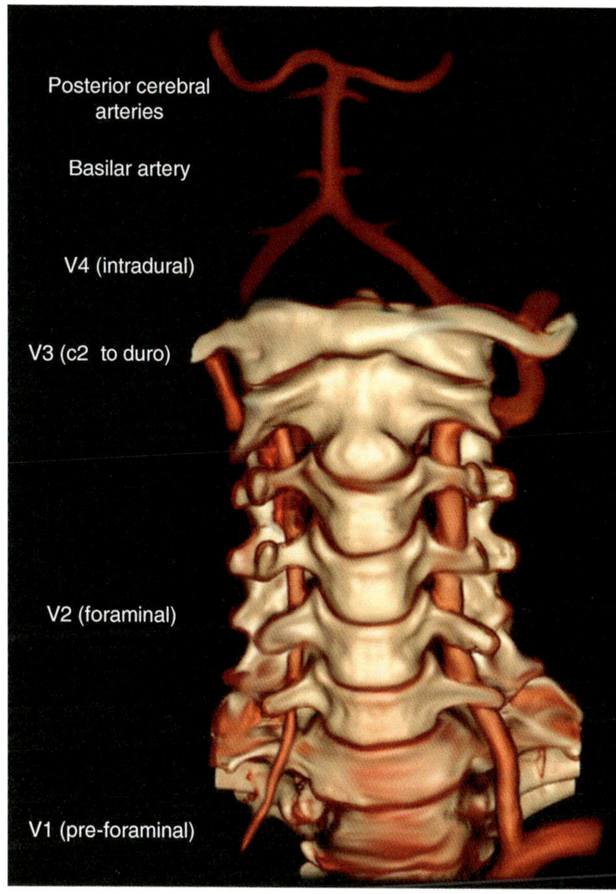

Fig. 13.3 Anatomy of the vertebral artery (Courtesy of Dr. F. Gaillord—Reprinted with permission)

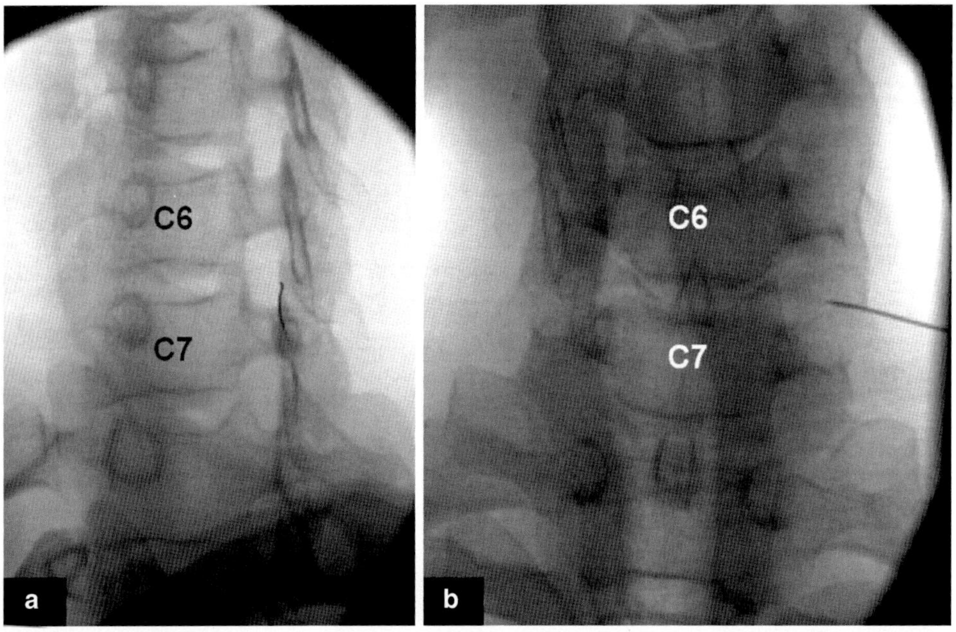

Fig. 13.4 (**a**) Needle directed toward the anterior half of the superior articular process in the most dorsal aspect of the intervertebral neuroforamen. (**b**) Tip of the needle to lie opposite the sagittal midline of the articular pillars on AP fluoroscopic view (Courtesy of the Spine Intervention Society and Dr. P. Dreyfuss—Reprinted with permission)

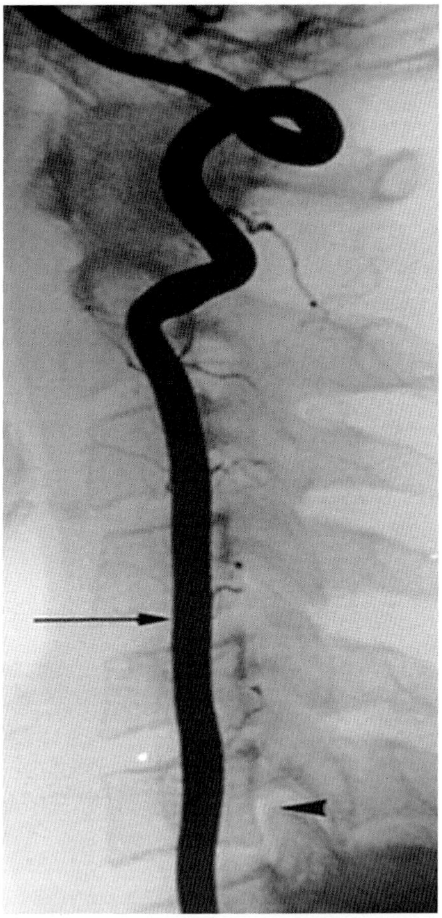

Fig. 13.5 Outline of the vertebral artery (*left arrow*) and its relationship with the cervical neuroforamen (*right arrow*) (Courtesy of Dr. J.N. Vallee—Reprinted with permission)

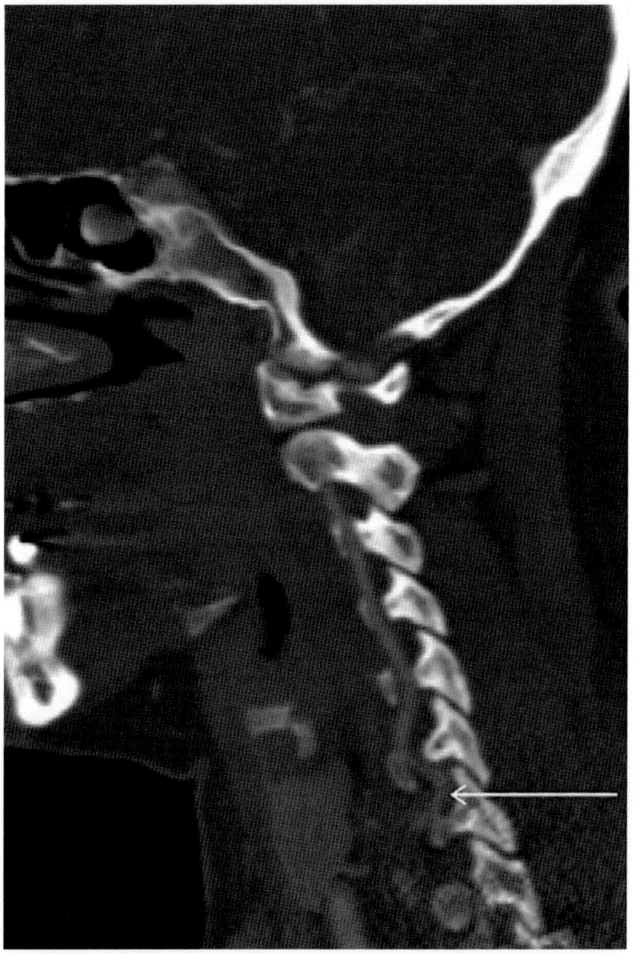

Fig. 13.6 Vertebral artery loop in the posterior foramen near the location of the needle placement for CTESIs (Courtesy of Dr. W.J. Beckworth—Reprinted with permission)

and loss of disk height. It is possible that in the case that we describe, the patient may have had such an anomaly that was not identified before the procedure was performed.

Physicians should be cognizant of this and evaluate the T2 axial MRI images to check the location of the VA before performing CTESIs [42].

13.2.5 Blood Supply to the Cervical Spinal Cord: Implications for Cervical Transforaminal Epidural Steroid Injections

Cervical spinal cord blood supply is provided by the radicular arteries. Eighty percent of the radicular arteries in the cervical region originate from the vertebral arteries, whereas the remainder originates from deep cervical, superior intercostal arteries, and the ascending cervical artery. The ascending and deep cervical arteries are formed by branches of the subclavian artery and anastomose with the vertebral artery posterior to the spinal nerve (Fig. 13.7) [43–45]. Cadaver studies show that these arteries are located within the cervical intervertebral foramina [46, 47]. They tend to enter the foramina just inferior to the exiting spinal nerve and follow a tortuous course along the inferior and anterior aspect of the spinal nerve until they penetrate the dura to join the anterior or posterior spinal artery. The arteries (vertebral, deep cervical, superior intercostals, or ascending cervical) from which the radicular arteries originate determine the depth within the intervertebral foramen at which the artery will first be encountered. Branches that arise from the vertebral artery lie over the most anteromedial aspect of the foramen, whereas those that arise from the deep cervical, superior intercostals, or ascending cervical arteries traverse the entire extent of the foramen.

The location of these arteries within the cervical intervertebral foramen in the near proximity of the area where the needle is usually placed for CTESIs may in part explain why ischemic neurologic events occur while performing these injections. Available studies support the current technique of fluoroscopic or CT-guided needle insertion into the posterior aspect of the intervertebral foramen, with the needle tip remaining over the anterior portion of the superior articular process (SAP), as the radicular arteries are most commonly located inferior and anterior to the spinal nerve roots (Fig. 13.4) [40]. However, anatomic variations in the origin and locations of these critical vessels are wide, and even with strict adherence to this technique, a properly placed needle could penetrate a radicular artery.

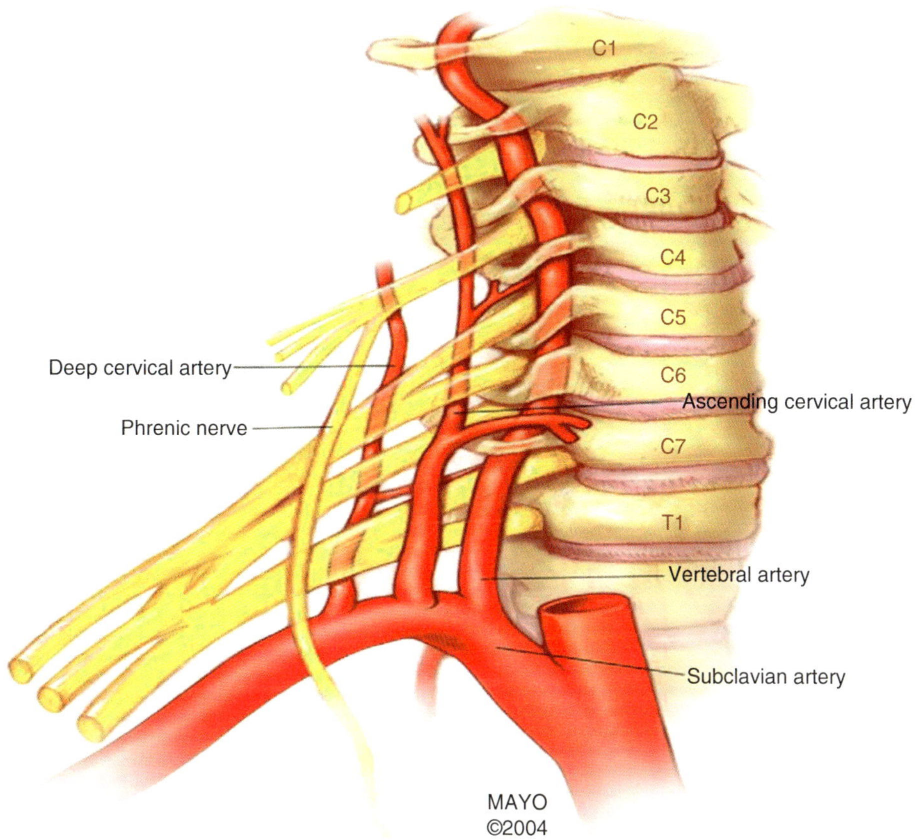

Fig. 13.7 Blood supply to the cervical spinal cord (Courtesy of Mayo Foundation for Medical Education and Research—Reprinted with permission)

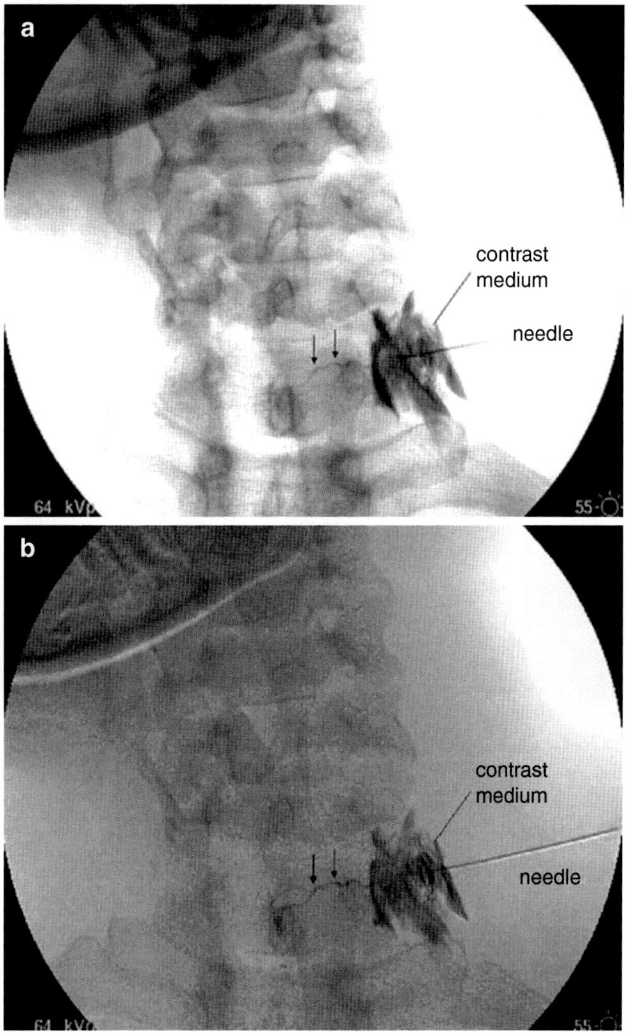

Fig. 13.8 The needle lies in the C6–C7 neuroforamen no further medially than its lateral midpoint. The *arrows* indicate the artery that was filled which passes medially to the spinal cord. (**a**) Conventional fluoroscopic exposure. (**b**) Digital subtraction angiography (Courtesy of Dr. R.M. Baker—Reprinted with permission)

Thus, intravascular needle location must be ruled out by injection of a small volume of radiographic contrast under real-time fluoroscopy with digital subtraction angiography (DSA) enhancement before a steroid solution is injected (Fig. 13.8) [48–50].

13.2.6 The Role of Steroid Solutions

The depot steroid preparations used for epidural injections contain significant amount of large particles that are a factor contributing to microvascular "sludging" and subsequent occlusion and ischemia in the event of an inadvertent intravascular injection.

The size of the particles measured is enough to occlude capillaries, metarterioles, and, in some cases, arterioles and even arteries [21].

The use of a preservative-free, non-particulate steroid solution (i.e., dexamethasone) is therefore recommended [51].

13.2.7 Can We Perform These Procedures Safely?

13.2.7.1 Procedural Factors

The complex and delicate anatomy of the cervical intervertebral foramen and the reports of possible serious and catastrophic complications while performing CTESIs raise questions about procedural factors that may help minimize such sequelae.

These procedures should be performed with fluoroscopic and/or CT guidance.

Even though radiographic confirmation of needle placement does not entirely prevent these events, confirming its correct placement by ***injecting a small amount of contrast with real-time fluoroscopy and digital subtraction angiography (DSA) may increase the chance of detecting the potential intravascular penetration of the needle and the injection of medications that can potentially cause a devastating complication.*** Many observational studies have demonstrated the value of DSA in preventing subsequent intravascular injections [52–55].

The production of a proximal neurogram (a fluoroscopic image of the target nerve root outlined by contrast medium injected into the epidural space) is another measure supposed to be protective against injecting at an inappropriate site. The theory is sound, but evidence shows that what is interpreted as a proximal neurogram may not be. In the case reported by Chung [35], what was interpreted as outlining of the epidural space was actually contrast medium spreading up along the walls of the vertebral artery.

Fitting a small-volume extension tube to the hub of the needle, rather than connecting syringes directly to it, in theory, reduces the chance of the needle tip moving during or between injections, possibly preventing its inadvertent penetration into a vessel or another inappropriate site.

Aspiration to check for blood is a traditional practice that has been assessed for validity: the evidence shows that blood seen on aspiration has 97.9% specificity but only 44.7% sensitivity for intravascular needle tip placement [26]; ***therefore, there is no guarantee that the absence of blood on aspiration means extravascular injection.***

The injection of a local anesthetic test dose is thought to protect against injection of steroid at an inappropriate site. Theoretically the effects of local anesthetics are less enduring than those of steroids. There are three case reports wherein the injection of a local anesthetic test dose resulted in symptoms and termination of procedure, preventing serious complications if the steroid had been injected [29, 35, 36].

Always inject a test dose of a short-acting local anesthetic before injecting the steroid solution.

The evidence suggests that the risk of CTESIs is increased if particulate steroids are injected. Even though it is not entirely clear that steroid particles are responsible for all the effects that can occur if inadvertently injected into the vascular system, particulate steroids were used in most of the cases involving catastrophic complications, including all of those that were fatal [19–21].

The use of a preservative-free non-particulate liquid steroid solution such as dexamethasone is recommended in therapeutic cervical TFESIs.

13.2.7.2 Other Suggestions and Recommendations

Always discuss honestly and in detail the risks and benefit of the procedure with the patient and family.

Only with all the information known about the intervention can a patient give proper informed consent and decide whether the potential risk is worth taking or not.

Do not proceed with the injection if a cervical spine MRI scan is not available.

Beckworth et al. [42] have shown that the vertebral artery may lie within 2 mm of the ideal needle location in at least one posterior neural foramen in 29% of 198 consecutive patients whose CT angiograms were studied. Severity of foraminal stenosis and disk height correlated with the proximity of the vertebral artery to the typical needle location. Therefore ideal needle placement does not guarantee protection from injury to, or injection into, the vertebral artery during CTESIs. It is recommended that physicians examine T2 axial MRI views to check the location of the vertebral artery before performing CTESIs.

Consider other approaches (i.e., interlaminar) if you have concerns after careful review of cervical MRI scan and if the patient is not willing to proceed with the transforaminal injection after risks and benefits have been fully disclosed.

However, be cognizant that the interlaminar approach is not entirely foolproof [56, 57].

Equipment for emergency resuscitation should always be available.

Avoid deep sedation.

Consider aborting the procedure in case of persistent venous runoff and/or persistent vertebral artery.

Abort the procedure immediately if there is evidence of rapid vascular runoff, especially ascending (vertebral artery) or directed medially (radicular artery) under real-time fluoroscopy and DSA.

When in doubt abort the procedure and do not inject.

Conclusions

CTESIs may provide 50% pain relief in approximately 40% of the patients with a cervical radiculitis/radiculopathy secondary to cervical spondylosis and disk herniation for a period of 4 weeks. At 3, 6, and 12 months, the proportion of patients with any degree of benefit attenuates.

The published evidence shows that CTESIs carry the risks of serious and catastrophic complications, including permanent quadriplegia and death. It does not clearly identify the causes of those complications and does not show conclusively how they can be avoided.

Each practitioner should carefully review the anatomy of the cervical spine, order images as appropriate if they are not available for review, and establish the correct indication for CTESIs.

Fluoroscopic and/or CT guidance, the use of short-acting local anesthetics (lidocaine), and non-particulate steroid preparations (dexamethasone) are strongly recommended.

When in doubt abort the procedure and do not inject.

References

1. Slipman CW, Lipetz JS, Jackson HB, Rogers DP, Vresilovic EJ. Therapeutic selective nerve root block in the nonsurgical treatment of atraumatic cervical spondylotic radicular pain: a retrospective analysis with independent clinical review. Arch Phys Med Rehabil. 2000;81(6):741–6.
2. Anderberg L, Annertz M, Persson L, Brandt L, Savelund H. Transforaminal steroid injections for the treatment of cervical radiculopathy: a prospective and randomized study. Eur J Pain. 2007;16(3):321–8.
3. Costandi SJ, Azer G, Esheaghi Y, Zeyed Y, Atalla JE, Looka ME, Mekhail NA. Cervical transforaminal epidural steroid injections: diagnostic and therapeutic value. Reg Anesth Pain Med. 2015;40(6):674–80.
4. Ellenberg MR, Honet JC, Treanor WJ. Cervical radiculopathy. Arch Phys Med Rehabil. 1994;75(3):342–52.
5. Lee HM, Weinstein JN, Meller ST, Hayashi N, Spratt KF, Gebhart GF. The role of steroids and their effects on phospholipase A2. An animal model of radiculopathy. Spine (Phila Pa 1976). 1998;23(11):1191–6.
6. Furusawa N, Baba H, Miyoshi N, Maezawa Y, Uchida K, Kokubo Y, Fukuda M. Herniation of cervical intervertebral disc: immunohistochemical examination and measurement of nitric oxide production. Spine (Phila Pa 1976). 2001;26(10):1110–6.
7. Howe JF, Loeser JD, Calvin WH. Mechanosensitivity of dorsal root ganglia and chronically injured axons: a physiological basis for the radicular pain of nerve root compression. Pain. 1977;3(1):25–41.
8. Yabuki S, Kawaguchi Y, Nordborg C, Kikuchi S, Rydevik B, Olmarker K. Effects of lidocaine on nucleus pulposus induced nerve root injury. A neurophysiologic and histologic study of the pig cauda equina. Spine (Phila Pa 1976). 1998;23(22):2383–90; discussion 2389–90.
9. Yabuki S, Kikuchi S. Nerve root infiltration and sympathetic block. An experimental study of intraradicular blood flow. Spine (Phila Pa 1976). 1995;20(8):901–6.

10. Engel A, King W, MacVicar J, Standards Division of the International Spine Intervention Society. The effectiveness and risks of fluoroscopically guided cervical transforaminal injections of steroids: a systematic review with comprehensive analysis of the published data. Pain Med. 2014;15(3):386–402.
11. Slipman C, Lipetz J, De Palma M, Jackson H. Therapeutic selective nerve root block in the nonsurgical treatment of traumatically induced cervical spondylotic radicular pain. Am J Phys Med Rehabil. 2004;83(6):446–54.
12. Lin E, Lieu V, Halevi L, Shamie A, Wang J. Cervical epidural steroid injections for symptomatic disc herniations. J Spinal Disord Tech. 2006;19(3):183–6.
13. Razzaq A, O'Brien D, Matthew B, Bartlett R, Taylor D. Efficacy and durability of fluoroscopically guided cervical nerve root blocks. Br J Neurosurg. 2007;21(4):365–9.
14. Kumar N, Gowda V. Cervical foraminal selective nerve root block: a "two-needle technique" with results. Eur Spine J. 2008;17(4):576–84.
15. Chunk JY, Yim JH, Seo HY, Kim SK, Cho KJ. The efficacy and persistence of selective nerve root blocks under fluoroscopic guidance for cervical radiculopathy. Asian Spine J. 2012;6(4):227–32.
16. Shakir A, Ma V, Mehta B. Comparison of pain score reduction using triamcinolone vs. dexamethasone in cervical transforaminal epidural steroid injections. Am J Phys Med Rehabil. 2013;92(9):768–75.
17. Kolstad F, Leviseth G, Nygaard O. Transforaminal steroid injections in the treatment of cervical radiculopathy. A prospective outcome study. Acta Neurochir (Wien). 2005;147(10):1067–70.
18. Persson L, Anderberg L. Repetitive transforaminal steroid injections in cervical radiculopathy: a prospective outcome study including 140 patients. Evid Based Spine Care J. 2012;6(4):13–20.
19. Brouwers PJ, Kottink EJ, Simon MA, Prevo RL. A cervical anterior spinal artery syndrome after diagnostic blockade of the right C6 nerve root. Pain. 2001;91(3):397–9.
20. Rozin L, Rozin R, Koehler SA, Shakir A, Ladham S, Barmada M, Dominick J, Wecht CH. Death during transforaminal epidural steroid nerve root block (C7) due to perforation of the left vertebral artery. Am J Forensic Med Pathol. 2003;24(4):351–5.
21. Tiso RL, Cutler T, Catania JA, Whalen K. Adverse central nervous system sequelae after selective transforaminal block: the role of corticosteroids. Spine J. 2004;4(4):468–74.
22. McMillan MR, Crumpton C. Cortical blindness and neurologic injury complicating a cervical transforaminal injection for cervical radiculopathy. Anesthesiology. 2009;99(2):509–11.
23. Windsor RE, Storm S, Sugar R, Nagula D. Cervical transforaminal injections: review of the literature, complications, and a suggested technique. Pain Physician. 2003;6(4):457–65.
24. Ludwig MA, Burns SP. Spinal Cord infarction following cervical transforaminal epidural injection. A case report. Spine. 2005;30(10):E266–8.
25. Muro K, O'Shaughnessy B, Ganju A. Infarction of the cervical spinal cord following multilevel transforaminal epidural steroid injection: case report and review of the literature. J Spinal Cord Med. 2007;30(4):385–8.
26. Ruppen W, Hugli R, Reuss S, Aeschbach A, Urwyler A. Neurological symptoms after cervical transforaminal injection with steroids in a patient with hypoplasia of the vertebral artery. Acta Anaesthesiol Scand. 2008;52(1):165–6.
27. Beckman WA, Mendez RJ, Paine GF, Mazzilli MA. Cerebellar herniation after cervical transforaminal epidural injection. Reg Anesth Pain Med. 2006;31(3):282–5.
28. Kaplowitz K, Lee AG. Horner syndrome following a selective cervical nerve root block. J Neuroophthalmol. 2011;3(7):54–5.
29. Karasek M, Bogduk N. Temporary neurologic deficit after cervical transforaminal injection of local anesthetic. Pain Med. 2004;5(2):202–5.
30. Wallace MA, Fukui MB, Williams RL, Ku A, Baghai P. Complications of cervical selective nerve root blocks performed with fluoroscopic guidance. Am J Roentgenol. 2007;188(5):1218–21.
31. Lee JY, Nassr A, Ponnappan RK. Epidural hematoma causing paraplegia after a fluoroscopically guided cervical nerve root injection. A case report. J Bone Joint Surg Am. 2007;89(9):2037–9.
32. Schellhas KP, Pollei SR, Johnson BA, Golden MJ, Eklund JA, Pobiel RS. Selective cervical nerve root blockade: experience with a safe and reliable technique using an anterolateral approach for needle placement. Am J Neuroradiol. 2007;28(10):1909–14.
33. Lee MH, Cha YD, Song JH, An YM, Han JU, Lee du I. Transient quadriplegia after fluoroscopic-guided selective cervical nerve root block in a patient who received cervical interbody fusion—a case report. Korean J Anesthesiol. 2010;59(Suppl):S95–8.
34. Kim W, Kim JS, Lim SC, Kim YI, Moon DE. Reversible posterior leukoencephalopathy syndrome after cervical transforaminal epidural steroid injection presenting as transient blindness. Anesth Analg. 2011;112(4):967–70.
35. Chung SG. Convulsion caused by a lidocaine test in cervical transforaminal epidural steroid injection. PM R. 2011;3(7):674–7.
36. Tofuku K, Koga H, Komiya S. Subdural spread of injected local anesthetic in a selective transforaminal nerve root block: a case report. J Med Case Rep. 2012;6(1):142.
37. Gilchrist R. Developmental and functional anatomy of the cervical spine. In: Slipman C, Derby R, editors. Interventional spine: an algorithmic approach. Philadelphia: Saunders Elsevier; 2008. p. 518–21.
38. Hong JT, Park D, Lee MJ, Kim SW, An HS. Anatomical variations of the vertebral artery segment in the lower cervical spine: analysis by three-dimensional computed tomography angiography. Spine. 2008;33(22):2422–6.
39. Bruneau M, Cornelius J, Marneffe V. Anatomical variations of the V2 segment of the vertebral artery. Neurosurgery. 2006;59(1 Suppl 1):ONS20–4.
40. Furman M, Lee T, Berkowitz L. Atlas of image-guided spinal procedures. Philadelphia: Elsevier Saunders; 2013. p. 243–9.
41. Gitkind AI, Olson TR, Downie SA. Vertebral artery anatomical variations as they relate to cervical transforaminal epidural steroid injections. Pain Med. 2014;15(7):1109–14.
42. Beckworth WJ, Sood R, Katzer AF, Wu B. Anomalous location of the vertebral artery in relation to the neural foramen. Implications for cervical transforaminal epidural steroid injections. Pain Med. 2013;14(8):1119–25.
43. Gillilan LA. The arterial blood supply of the human spinal cord. J Comp Neurol. 1958;110(1):75–103.
44. Turnbull IM, Brieg A, Hassler O. Blood supply of cervical spinal cord in man: a microangiographic study. J Neurosurg. 1966;26(6):951–65.
45. Dommisse GF. The blood supply of the spinal cord: a critical vascular zone in spinal surgery. J Bone Joint Surg Br. 1974;56(2):225–35.
46. Huntoon MA. Anatomy of the cervical intervertebral foramina: vulnerable arteries and ischemic neurologic injuries after transforaminal epidural injections. Pain. 2005;117(1–2):104–11.
47. Hoeft MA, Rathmell JP, Monsey RD, Fonda BJ. Cervical transforaminal injection and the radicular artery: variation in anatomical location within the cervical intervertebral foramina. Reg Anesth Pain Med. 2006;31(3):270–4.
48. Baker R, Dreyfuss P, Mercer S, Bogduk N. Cervical transforaminal injection of steroids into a radicular artery: a possible mechanism for spinal cord injury. Pain. 2003;103(1–2):211–5.

49. Smuck M, Fuller B, Yoder B, Huerta J. Incidence of simultaneous epidural and vascular injection during lumbosacral transforaminal and epidural injections. Spine J. 2007;7(1):79–82.
50. Kranz PG, Amrhein TJ, Gray L. Incidence of inadvertent intravascular injection during CT fluoroscopy-guided epidural steroid injections. Am J Neuroradiol. 2015;36(5):1000–7.
51. El Abd O, Amadera J, Pimentel D, Gomba L. Immediate and acute adverse effects following transforaminal epidural steroid injections with dexamethasone. Pain Physician. 2015;18(3):277–86.
52. Derby R, Lee SH, Kim BJ, Chen Y, Seo KS. Complications following cervical epidural steroid injections by expert interventionalists in 2003. Pain Physician. 2004;7(4):445–9.
53. Jasper JF. Role of digital subtraction fluoroscopic imaging in detecting intravascular injections. Pain Physician. 2003;6(3):369–72.
54. McLean JP, Sigler JD, Plastaras CT, Garvan CW, Rittenberg JD. The rate of detection of intravascular injection in cervical transforaminal epidural steroid injections with and without digital subtraction angiography. PM R. 2009;1(7):636–42.
55. Verrills P, Nowesenitz G, Barnard A. Penetration of a cervical radicular artery during a transforaminal epidural injection. Pain Med. 2010;11(2):229–31.
56. Maddela R, Wahezi SE, Sparr S, Brook A. Hemiparesis and facial sensory loss following cervical epidural steroid injection. Pain Physician. 2014;17(6):E761–7.
57. Abbasi A, Malhotra G, Malanga G, Elovic EP, Kahn S. Complications of interlaminar cervical epidural steroid injections: a review of the literature. Spine (Phila Pa 1976). 2007;32(19):2144–215.

Spinal Infarct After Lumbar Transforaminal Epidural Steroid Injection

14

Khalid M. Malik

14.1 Case Description

A 76-year-old man presented with several months history of low back pain which radiated down to his right leg, along his lateral thigh and calf in an L5 and S1 distribution. Patient's past medical history was significant for hypertension, hyperlipidemia, and osteoarthritis. His medications included valsartan, hydrochlorothiazide, diazepam, hydrocodone/acetaminophen, and pravastatin. He was not taking any nonsteroidal anti-inflammatory drugs, anticoagulants, or antiplatelet medications. His magnetic resonance imaging (MRI) revealed degenerative changes at L3–4L, L4–L5, and L5–S1 disc levels and severe right-sided L5–S1 neural foraminal stenosis. He was diagnosed with lumbar spinal stenosis and right L5/S1 radicular pain. He received two interlaminar lumbar epidural steroid injections using fluoroscopic guidance in the previous 6 months resulting in partial (60%) decrease in his pain level. For his residual right-sided radicular pain, a third injection, a right L5–S1 TF-ESI, was performed. A 5 inch, 22-gauge Quincke-type spinal needle with the tip bended was used. Foraminal placement of the needle tip was confirmed with anteroposterior, oblique, and lateral fluoroscopic views. After negative needle aspiration for blood or cerebrospinal fluid and digital subtraction angiography confirming the absence of intravascular contrast medium spread, the steroid injection was performed using 80 mg of triamcinolone acetonide in 1 cc of 1% lidocaine.

After the injection was completed, the patient instantly reported abdominal discomfort, diaphoresis, weakness of both his lower extremities, and numbness extending up to his lower abdomen. The patient was rolled from the fluoroscopy table onto the recovery bed and was observed for 2 h expecting a return of neurological dysfunction upon dissipation of the local anesthetic effect. Although he remained hemodynamically stable throughout, there was no return of neurological function in either of his lower extremities. He was transferred for further evaluation and care to the emergency department where he was noted to have complete loss of strength in both lower extremities and a loss of sensation to touch and temperature to T8-9 dermatomal level bilaterally. Reflexes were normal in his upper extremities but absent in both his lower extremities. Blood counts, chemistry panel, and coagulation studies were all within normal limits. A computed tomography (CT) angiography was performed which was negative for thoracic aortic dissection or aneurysm. An MRI of the lumbar and thoracic spine was completed 5 h after the spinal injection which showed minor increase in T2 signal intensity commencing at T7-8 level in the thoracic spinal cord. A follow-up MRI was performed at 48 h after the spinal injection which showed a hyperintense T2 signal, along with mild spinal cord expansion, in the central spinal cord from T6 to T10 level. These findings indicated spinal cord edema secondary to spinal cord infarction. The diagnosis of paraplegia from acute spinal cord infarction was consequently rendered.

The patient received a 10 mg of dexamethasone intravenous injection in the emergency department. He was subsequently transferred to the neuro-critical care unit for further treatment where he received intravenous methylprednisolone. His vital functions remained stable throughout the stay in the neuro-intensive care unit. However, he remained with flaccid paraplegia along with bowel and bladder incontinence. He was transferred to a rehabilitation facility where he remained inpatient for the next several weeks without any change in his neurological status.

14.2 Case Discussion

14.2.1 Neurological Dysfunction After Lumbar Transforaminal Epidural Steroid Injection

Etiology: Neurological dysfunction after the lumbar epidural steroid injections typically presents as inability to stand and

K.M. Malik, M.D.
Department of Anesthesiology, University of Illinois,
Chicago, IL 60612, USA
e-mail: kmalikmd@yahoo.com

M. Anitescu et al. (eds.), *Challenging Cases and Complication Management in Pain Medicine*,
https://doi.org/10.1007/978-3-319-60072-7_14

ambulate with a variable degree of weakness and numbness in one or both lower extremities. In majority of such instances, the abrupt neurological deficit is the result of local anesthetic injected into the epidural space and less commonly from its unintentional injection into the intrathecal or subdural space. In the majority of these cases, full neurological function usually returns after a variable length of time once the local anesthetic effect is dissipated. Rare but more sinister causes of postinjection neurological deficits include epidural hematoma, epidural abscess, arachnoiditis, and meningitis. In the latter uncommon scenarios, the development of neurological deficits is typically insidious and delayed and is often incomplete. These cases have characteristic findings on spinal imaging and/or CSF analysis and require specific and often urgent treatment. Abrupt and enduring flaccid paralysis after such an injection fortunately is exceedingly rare, and only few cases have been reported [1, 2]. As in this case, the presence of thoracic spinal cord edema and spinal cord expansion on the MRI imaging is consistent with thoracic spinal cord infarction. Although the exact source of spinal cord infarction in this and other analogously reported cases is not exactly clear, a vascular occlusive etiology based on the unique vascularity of the spinal cord has been suggested.

Spinal cord blood supply: Abrupt infarction of a substantial segment of spinal cord after a spinal steroid injection could be explained partially by its complex vascularity. Blood supply to the anterior two-thirds of the spinal cord emanates from a single large anterior spinal artery, which runs anteriorly along the entire length of the spinal cord. The anterior spinal artery is formed at the cervicomedullary junction by the confluence of two anterior spinal branches of the vertebral arteries. Blood supply to the posterior two-thirds of the spinal cord is by two smaller posterior spinal arteries, which run along the posterolateral aspects of the spinal cord. Radicular arteries arise bilaterally from the aorta at each vertebral level and travel along the corresponding segmental nerves into the neural foramen. The majority of these radicular arteries provide blood supply only to the concomitant nerve root, and only a limited number of larger radicular arteries, called radiculomedullary arteries, enter the dura and split into ascending and descending branches reinforcing the anterior spinal artery. The cervical spinal cord is normally supplied by three radiculomedullary arteries. However, below the level of eighth thoracic vertebra, the spinal cord is supplied only by a single large radiculomedullary artery, called the artery of Adamkiewicz. In nearly 85% of the individuals, the artery of Adamkiewicz arises on the left side between T9 and L2 vertebral segments. The origin of the artery of Adamkiewicz however is highly variable, and in a small minority of cases, it arises at lower segmental levels, and in rare instance, it may arise as low as sacral segmental level [3–5].

Proposed mechanism of spinal cord infarction after an epidural injection: The suggested mechanism of spinal cord ischemia and infarction following a spinal epidural steroid injection in this and similar cases is most plausibly either (a) direct vascular trauma and the resulting arterial spasm or (b) vascular occlusion from embolization of the injected steroids. Direct needle contact with the artery of Adamkiewicz during a lumbar transforaminal injection could perhaps cause (a) direct vascular injury and arterial spasm and/or (b) development of an intimal flap which could lead to stasis and thrombosis. The second proposed mechanism includes intra-arterial injection of the steroid suspension, causing embolization of the particulate steroids and the resulting arterial occlusion and spinal cord ischemia. Depot corticosteroid preparations routinely used for the epidural steroid injections are comprised of insoluble steroid microcrystals which aggregate to form larger particulates [6]. Methylprednisolone and triamcinolone have the largest particles which may aggregate to a fairly large size reaching up to 500 μm [7]. By comparison, an average red blood cell is only 7.5 μm in size, and the spinal medullary arterioles and arteries range from 10 to 50 μm in diameter. Even though the risk of direct contact with the artery of Adamkiewicz and consequent spinal cord ischemia and injury is highest if an injection is performed at higher lumbar or lower thoracic level, especially on the left side, an aberrant and an abnormally low origin of the artery of Adamkiewicz may explain spinal cord infarction from a lower lumbar or even sacral level epidural steroid injection.

Treatment: In the majority of the reported cases, the spinal cord injury is limited to the low to mid-thoracic levels, and the diaphragmatic and intercostal musculature innervation is spared. Hence, these patients are typically able to maintain their breathing, and the upper extremity strength is preserved. The extent of sympathectomy is also limited, and the degree of hemodynamic instability therefore is marginal. Nevertheless, this is a catastrophic complication with immense consequences for the patients and the family alike. Initially these patients are best managed in neuro-intensive care settings. The patients must maintain hemodynamic stability and should be kept well hydrated. The use of inotropic drugs may be necessary to maintain adequate perfusion of the compromised spinal cord and to limit the extent of ischemia and evolving spinal cord injury. The use of supplemental oxygen is advocated with ready availability of respiratory support in the presence of any respiratory insufficiency. The role of early high-dose parenteral steroid use and hypothermia, although disputed in the literature, may be considered [8]. Once the acute injury period is past, these patients would need protracted care in a long-term rehabilitation facility. Due to the significant psychosocial implications, psychological and social worker's help should be sought early. With possible medicolegal implications, the hospital legal, patient safety, and risk management department should be consulted early.

Prevention: Even though no evidence-based practice guidelines currently exist to prevent spinal cord infarction during epidural steroid injections, the following precautions may be taken to reduce the risk of this catastrophic outcome:

- Although the absence of blood on careful and gentle aspiration of the needle before the injection does not guarantee the absence of an intravascular injection, such a practice is prudent.
- Routine use of radiopaque contrast injection to ensure its spread along the nerve root and a lack of vascular uptake would help avoid an intravascular injection.
- The use of digital subtraction angiography (DSA) during the contrast injection is advocated to clearly delineate the lack of intravascular injection.
- The use of a blunt-tipped needle may reduce the risk of vascular trauma.
- The use of non-particulate steroids such as dexamethasone and prednisolone has been proposed [9]; however, latter practice has been considered to be less effective.
- One may precede the steroid injection with a local anesthetic and epinephrine injection [10], similar to an epidural test dose, monitoring for the signs of systemic epinephrine and local anesthetic uptake.

Key Concepts

- Epidural steroid injections may be complicated by acute onset of permanent paraplegia.
- The most likely cause of such a catastrophe is spinal ischemia and infarction.
- Spinal cord has complicated and unique blood supply which can be highly aberrant.
- Direct injury and thrombosis of major spinal cord feeding artery is possible from an injection even when performed at a low segmental level.
- Particulate steroid carries an innate risk arterial embolization and ischemia.
- Various precautions can be taken during the injection procedure to avoid vascular injury and intravascular injection.

References

1. Houten JK, Errico TJ. Paraplegia after lumbosacral nerve root block: report of three cases. Spine J. 2002;2:70–5.
2. Popescu A, Lai D, Lu A, Gardner K. Stroke following epidural injections—case report and review of literature. J Neuroimaging. 2013;23:118–21.
3. Kennedy DJ, Dreyfuss P, Aprill CN, Bogduk N. Paraplegia following image-guided transforaminal lumbar spine epidural steroid injection: two case reports. Pain Med. 2009;10:1389–94.
4. Thefenne L, Dubecq C, Zing E, et al. A rare case of paraplegia complicating a lumbar epidural infiltration. Ann Phys Rehabil Med. 2010;53:575–83.
5. Quintero N, Laffont I, Bouhmidi L, et al. Transforaminal epidural steroid injection and paraplegia: case report and bibliographic review. Ann Readapt Med Phys. 2006;49:242–7.
6. Benzon HT, Chew TL, McCarthy RJ, Benzon HA, Walega DR. Comparison of the particle sizes of different steroids and the effect of dilution: a review of the relative neurotoxicities of the steroids. Anesthesiology. 2007;106:331–8.
7. MacMahon PJ, Shelly MJ, Scholz D, Eustace SJ, Kavanagh EC. Injectable corticosteroid preparations: an embolic risk assessment by static and dynamic microscopic analysis. AJNR Am J Neuroradiol. 2011;32:1830–5.
8. Alkabie S, Boileau AJ. The role of therapeutic hypothermia after traumatic spinal cord injury—a systematic review. World Neurosurg. 2015. doi:10.1016/j.wneu.2015.09.079
9. Rathmell JR, Benzon HT, Dreyfuss P, Huntoon M, et al. Safeguards to prevent neurological complications after epidural steroid injections: consensus opinions from a Multidisciplinary Working Group and national organizations. Anesthesiology. 2015;122:974–84.
10. Smuck M, Maxwell MD, Kennedy D, Rittenberg JD, Lansberg MG, Plastaras CT. Utility of the anesthetic test dose to avoid catastrophic injury during cervical transforaminal epidural injections. Spine J. 2010;10:857–64.

Motor Weakness After Transforaminal Epidural Steroid Injection

15

John Kenny and Sheetal Kerkar DeCaria

15.1 Case Description

An 83-year-old female with a history of lumbar disc herniation at L2–L3 presents to clinic for interventional treatment of her left lumbar radicular pain. The patient has a past medical history of dementia, type II diabetes mellitus, hypertension, and cerebrovascular accident (CVA) which resulted in two-fifths right-sided weakness. She continued her aspirin 81 mg due to her CVA history but did not take any additional anticoagulants. Since her pain was primarily one-sided radicular pain and MRI showed central canal stenosis, a transforaminal epidural particulate steroid injection with lidocaine and triamcinolone was planned.

An uneventful left-sided TFESI at L2–L3 was performed in the fluoroscopy suite, and the patient was then transported to the recovery area. The AP images are seen in Figs. 15.1 and 15.2. Figure 15.2 demonstrates contrast flow along the nerve root and into the epidural space. Her vital signs remained stable, and she was responsive throughout. In the recovery area, the patient was noted to have decreased movement of her lower extremities. A thorough physical exam revealed that the patient now had two-fifths strength in bilateral lower extremities. A detailed history was challenging secondary to the patient's baseline mental status; however, the patient reported numbness in her left leg.

At this point, her differential diagnosis was broad and confounded by her preexisting right-sided weakness and dementia. The differential included weakness along her nerve root secondary to local anesthetic, nerve injury, accidental dural puncture, intrathecal injection, epidural hematoma, anterior spinal cord syndrome, and communication breakdown from dementia. The patient was admitted to the intensive care unit for frequent neurological exams, spine imaging, coagulation tests, and neurosurgical evaluation.

J. Kenny, M.D. • S.K. DeCaria, M.D. (✉)
Department of Anesthesia,
University of Chicago, Chicago, IL, USA
e-mail: SDeCaria@dacc.uchicago.edu

Given her preexisting weakness of her right lower extremity, it was unclear whether the new weakness was unilateral or bilateral. Thus, emergent MRI of the lumbar spine was conducted, which revealed normal anatomy. There was no evidence of either epidural hematoma or spinal cord ischemia. The patient's symptoms began to resolve within 2 h, and she was discharged home the following day with a diagnosis of weakness due to nerve root injection and baseline preexisting weakness in her right lower extremity.

15.2 Case Discussion

15.2.1 Complications of Transforaminal Epidural Steroid Injections

Intervertebral disc pathology is a common cause of back pain and is often treated with an epidural steroid injection. Steroid can be injected into the epidural space via the interlaminar, caudal, or transforaminal approach. Transforaminal epidural steroid injection (TFESI) is unique among the techniques in that it allows for the delivery of medication into the anterior epidural region [1]. It has been demonstrated that lower dosages of medication are effective when using the TFESI approach [2]. While the reduction of amount of medication injected decreases some risk, the transforaminal approach to the epidural space comes with its own unique risks. These include minor complications like headache and nausea or major complications such as motor weakness, nerve injury, accidental dural puncture, intrathecal injection, discitis, paraplegia, and death.

15.2.2 Anatomical Congestion in the Foramen

The epidural space is found throughout the length of the spinal canal surrounding the outermost meningeal layer, the dura mater. The superior margin is at the foramen magnum,

M. Anitescu et al. (eds.), *Challenging Cases and Complication Management in Pain Medicine*,
https://doi.org/10.1007/978-3-319-60072-7_15

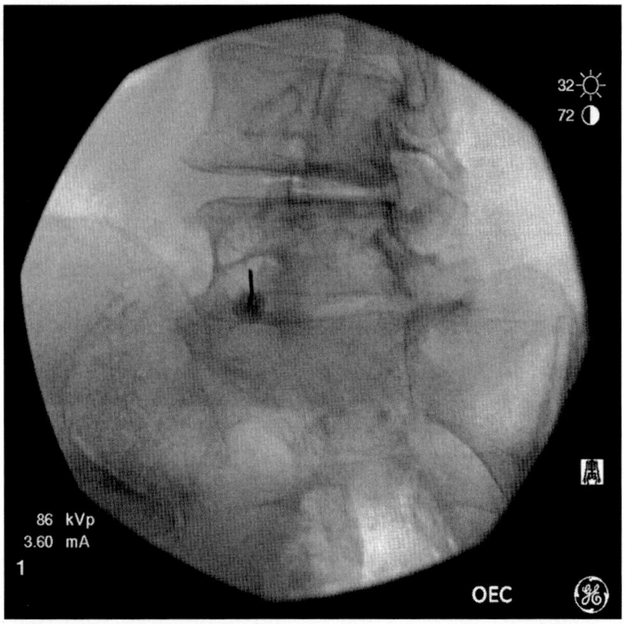

Fig. 15.1 Oblique view of transforaminal epidural steroid injection and needle placement. Image from personal library

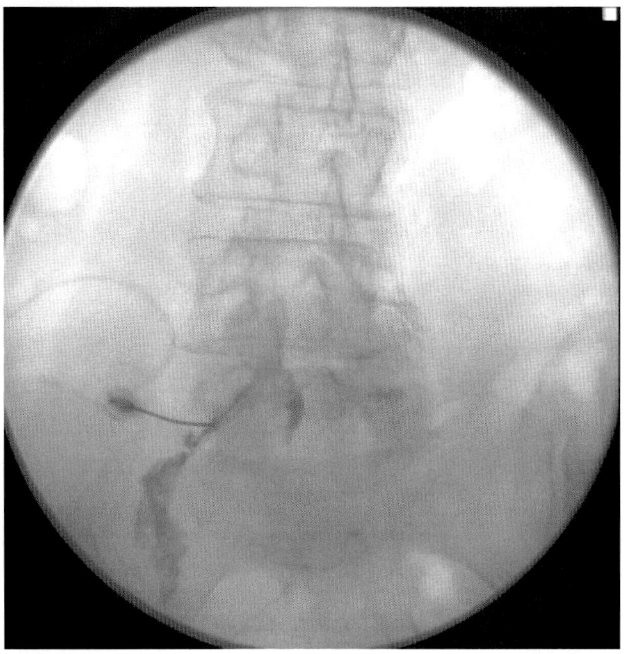

Fig. 15.2 Contrast spread in anteroposterior view showing contrast material spread primarily on the left. Image from personal library

and the sacrococcygeal membrane is the inferior extent of the space. Anteriorly the epidural space is bounded by the posterior longitudinal ligament and posteriorly by the ligamentum flavum and vertebral laminae. Part of the lateral extent is defined by the vertebral pedicles; however, the transition between the epidural space and the paravertebral space is not well defined, and there is no current consensus [3]. In 1981, Crock [4] described it as a single sagittal slice through the narrowest portion of the nerve root canal, and in 1988 Lee et al. [5] divided the foramen into three zones: lateral recess zone, midzone, and the exit zone. More recently, Gilchrist et al. have taken a more comprehensive approach, with detailed description of the anatomic boundaries moving from the medial aspect of the pedicles laterally to the psoas fascia [6].

The anterior and posterior spinal nerve roots that make up each spinal nerve exit the spinal cord cephalad to the intervertebral foramen through which they exit the spinal column. They enter the intervertebral foramen in close proximity to the inferomedial aspect of the superior vertebral pedicle [7]. As they course between the superior and inferior pedicles, the nerve roots coalesce into a single structure known as the spinal nerve. There is an enlargement of the dorsal root just proximal to the origin of the spinal nerve. This enlargement is the dorsal root ganglion (DRG) and is the location of the cell bodies of the sensory nerves [6]. The location of the DRG within the foramen can vary, though at the lumbar levels, they are most often located within the anatomic boundaries of the intervertebral foramen, directly beneath the cephalad pedicle [8, 9]. The DRG of the S1 nerve root is unique however, in that it is often located intraspinally [9].

There are multiple proposed methods of injury to the segmental arteries using the transforaminal approach. They include embolization of particulate medication, direct injury, muscle spasm, compression, intimal flaps, and arterial transection. The artery of Adamkiewicz, also known as the arteria radicularis magna, is the largest anterior segmental medullary artery. It is important as it supplies a majority of blood flow to the anterior spinal cord in the lumbar region through the anterior spinal artery. Most often the artery enters the spinal canal through the intervertebral foramen in an anterior-superior location with respect to the dural root sleeve. The vertebral level and side at which it is found is highly variable. There are conflicting data from the various anatomical studies. There is an agreement that the artery of Adamkiewicz most often occurs on the left side. However, there is a wide range of incidence in the literature, with studies concluding that the range is from 63 to 85% of the time [10, 11]. While the artery has been found as high as T5 and as low as S1, one cadaver study found the artery arose between T9 and T12 in 75% of cases [12, 13]. However, another study found that the artery arose between T12 and L3 in 84% of cases [14]. In an angiography study, the artery was found at T8–L2 in 95.4% of cases, usually from the left T11 level [15]. In one study, the artery was found between T5 and T8 in 15% of cases [13].

In addition, within the intervertebral foramen, there exist venous communications between the internal and external venous plexuses. These major venous structures are most typically found at the inferior aspect of the foramen, in a space formed by internal ligaments [16].

Apart from the spinal nerves, there are other smaller nerves traversing the intervertebral foramen. These are known as the meningeal branches of the spinal nerves, recurrent meningeal nerves, sinuvertebral nerves, or recurrent nerves of Luschka. They branch from the spinal nerve near the origin of the anterior and posterior rami and then reenter the intervertebral foramen [17]. These nerves provide innervation to the facet joints, the annulus fibrosus of the intervertebral disc, and the ligaments and periosteum of the spinal canal. They are typically found in the three o'clock position of the foramen when viewed laterally [16].

As the paired segmental nerve roots diverge from the spinal cord, they penetrate the dura as they course through the intervertebral foramen. They take with them an extension of dura and arachnoid mater, which is known as the dural sleeve. This is anatomically important when performing a TFESI as it can be the route through which medication is aberrantly delivered into the intrathecal space. The dural sleeve ends at the point when the dura becomes the epineurium of the respective spinal nerve. This extension of dura results in a potential space with a nerve surrounded by cerebrospinal fluid [18]. The widest portion of this potential space is found near the dorsal root [19]. The arachnoid mater splits from the dura and ends at about the level of the ganglion, while the dura extends slightly further laterally [19].

The incidence of dural puncture while performing TFESI is unknown. In fact, one survey involving 322 TFESIs did not identify any [20]. Because they are so rare, the most common presenting symptoms are not well defined. However, immediate signs of intrathecal injection include weakness, numbness, persistent paresthesia, respiratory depression, and unconsciousness. Intrathecal injections can also eventually lead to arachnoiditis and meningitis from chemical irritation from the injectate [19].

In contrast to intrathecal injection, subdural injection, or injection between the dura and arachnoid mater, can be difficult to diagnose. Contrast spread is irregular and different than the honeycomb appearance typically seen with epidural spread. Also, the symptoms of weakness appear more slowly than the immediate weakness seen with an intrathecal injection.

Identification of appropriate contrast spread is one of the best ways to avoid subdural injection, which can occur with proper fluoroscopic needle placement or without CSF return on aspiration. Some authors recommend live fluoroscopic injection of contrast media, which they believe that it allows the interventionalist to better identify intrathecal runoff and vascular injection. The typical intrathecal contrast image is described as flat and glasslike and is located in the central canal. This is opposed to the transforaminal epidural contrast spread, which has a honeycomb appearance at the ipsilateral side of the injection. Epidural contrast will spread along the medial wall of the pedicle and out of the foramen, extending past where the dural sleeve ends.

A complication of accidental intradiscal needle placement can be discitis. The incidence of discitis after TFESI is not well known, though there have been published case reports [21]. A study of the rate of discitis after cervical discography demonstrated the incidence to be around 0.44% [22]. The rate of discitis after accidental annulus puncture during TFESI would most likely be less than this, especially if the puncture is identified prior to injection. Some have proposed the use of prophylactic intravenous or intradiscal antibiotics to prevent discitis after disc puncture; however, the available clinical evidence currently does not support regular use of this practice [23].

Arguably, the most devastating complication of TFESI is paraplegia. There have been eight cases reported in the literature [24]. The similarities between the cases were that a particulate steroid was used, rapid onset of symptoms, and MRI evidence of distal spinal cord infarct [24]. It is commonly believed that the etiology is injection of the particulate steroid into one of the following arteries: (a) radicular artery accompanying the nerve root, (b) ascending cervical artery, (c) deep cervical artery, (d) artery of Adamkiewicz, and (e) vertebral artery (this implies faulty technique) [25]. In the cases, the immediate paraplegia was often attributed to the local anesthetic component of the injectate, and thus the diagnosis of spinal cord infarct was delayed until several hours later. The level and laterality of injection varied in the cases, though, of this small sample, it occurred more often on the left side. Of the eight reported cases, six occurred when needle entry was on the left side [24, 26–29]. One case was reported involving each of the following: T12-L1, L1-L2, L2-L3, and S1 [26, 28, 29]. Four cases were described involving L3-4 [24, 27]. As mentioned before, in all cases a particulate steroid was used. Particles in betamethasone, methylprednisolone, and triamcinolone have been shown to be larger than red blood cells [28]. It has been proposed that these particles act as emboli when injected intravascularly and occlude arterioles and meta-arterioles. Dexamethasone has no particles and has not been implicated in any cases of TFESI paraplegia [25].

Some propose using non-particulate steroids to avoid this devastating complication of TFESI. The largest opposition from this however comes from the idea that non-particulate steroids are cleared from the epidural space too quickly for them to have a sustained anti-inflammatory response. There have been limited studies to date that compare the effectiveness of non-particulate to particulate steroids in lumbar transforaminal injections. One study, recently published, examined particulate (triamcinolone) vs. non-particulate (dexamethasone) in 162 patients undergoing lumbar epidural steroid injections. The study found significantly better and more sustained relief with the particulate steroid group [30]. Other recent studies however showed equal efficacy between particulate and non-particulate steroids [31, 32].

Avoiding intra-arterial injection altogether is the best way to prevent paraplegia. Aspiration is the most frequently used method; however, the sensitivity was shown to be only 45% in one study [33]. Three of the eight reported cases of paraplegia documented a negative aspiration [24, 26, 27].Some argue that CT guidance is safest, as soft tissue structures within the foramen can be identified. CT guidance cannot, however, demonstrate arterial uptake of contrast, and there has been a report of paraplegia when the injection was performed under CT guidance [34]. Continuous fluoroscopy is the only method for identifying intra-arterial flow away from needle tip [24].

Real-time injection of contrast media or digital subtraction angiography are two commonly used methods to accomplish this, although they have not been studied specifically with regard to prevention of intra-arterial injection during TFESI [35]. Figure 15.3 is an image of the DSA study used in this particular patient demonstrating epidural, not arterial, spread.

Kennedy et al. recommend a TFESI injection protocol in which local anesthetic test dose is administered [24]. They propose that a local anesthetic solution is injected after the contrast media; then 2 min is allowed to assess for symptoms of intra-arterial injection. Only after it is determined that the patient is free from weakness, numbness, or loss of proprioception, is the corticosteroid injected. One can also consider injecting a test dose of local anesthetic with a low concentration of epinephrine prior to injection of steroid, similar to the test dose administered during epidural catheter placement.

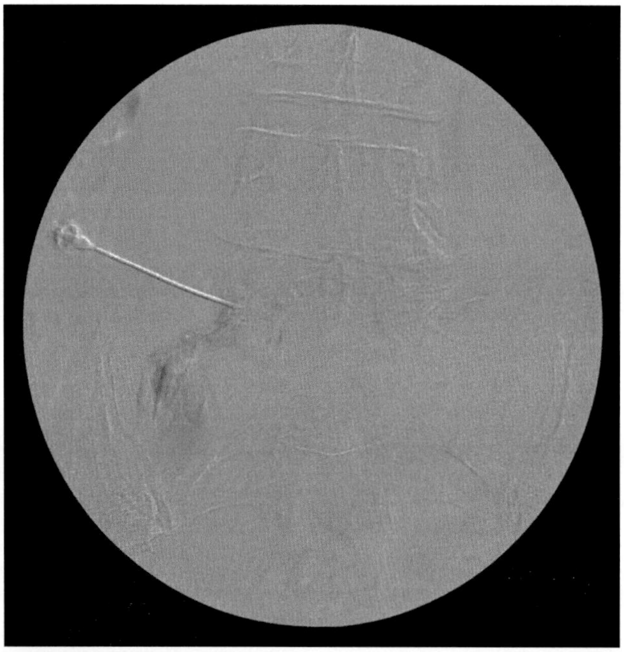

Fig. 15.3 Digital subtraction angiography study in AP view during transforaminal epidural steroid injection, showing no vascular uptake and contrast material spread primarily on the left. Image from personal library

If a patient does develop unexpected symptoms, it is imperative to initiate early neurosurgical evaluation and possible imaging. Time course is important to optimize possible recovery in the event of an epidural hematoma or abscess requiring surgical decompression. Immediate symptoms would imply an intravascular or intrathecal injection, whereas a delayed presentation may be a result of an epidural hematoma or abscess.

15.2.3 Is There an Optimal Injection Technique?

Various techniques have been developed to perform a TFESI that primarily differ in the needle tip endpoint. The subpedicular or "safe triangle" approach places the needle at the six o'clock position of the superior pedicle in the intervertebral foramen and has typically been the most commonly described approach to this injection. This technique avoids the exiting nerve root and minimizes accidental nerve injury caused by needle trauma. It has been described in detail by Bogduk [36]. The boundaries of the "safe triangle" in the AP view are a horizontal line positioned at the inferior aspect of the pedicle, a vertical line from the lateral border of the pedicles that make the intervertebral foramen, and then a line connecting the two lines. Needle placement here will result in the injectate being placed lateral and superior to the exiting spinal nerve.

TFESIs are relatively safe in the low lumbar regions. However, in the high lumbar and low thoracic regions, this approach may result in intravascular injection as this is where the segmental radiculomedullary arteries course through the foramen. The largest of these arteries, the great anterior radiculomedullary artery, also known as the artery of Adamkiewicz, is most often found in the intervertebral foramen between T9 and L2. Damage to or occlusion of this artery is especially problematic as it is responsible for the majority of blood flow to the anterior spinal cord and can cause paraplegia.

Several other approaches have been described in an effort to minimize complications via the transforaminal approach. These include the retroneural and retrodiscal approaches [37]. The needle tip target in the retroneural approach is posterior to that in the subpedicular approach. The target is at the intersection of a longitudinal line between the posterior and middle third of the intervertebral foramen and a transverse line between the upper and middle third [38]. In the retrodiscal approach, the needle will be medial to the exiting spinal nerve which differs from the other approaches. The needle will enter the intervertebral foramen just lateral to the superior articular process [39].

Each approach has its own positives and negatives. The retrodiscal approach has been said to decrease the incidence of nerve trauma; however, the epidural spread in this needle tip location may not be easily recognizable [37]. Also, there may be a lowered risk of intravascular injection in the retroneural and retrodiscal approaches as the spinal artery tends to course more anterior in the foramen. To the authors' knowledge, a comparison of the safety of these various approaches has not been formally studied as of now.

The transforaminal approach continues to be a safe technique for delivery of therapeutic drugs into the epidural space, as the incidence of major complications is low [40]. When they do occur, complications are associated with incorrect assessment of needle tip location (e.g., intraneural or intravascular). Essentials in avoiding these complications are a detailed understanding of fluoroscopic anatomy, accurate identification of appropriate contrast spread, and identification of vascular injection. Also, some authors advocate utilizing blunt-tipped needles to decrease dural puncture and reduce nerve trauma.

Although historically it was believed that the delivery of medication to the anterior epidural space resulted in superior symptomatic improvement over the caudal or interlaminar approach, more recent systematic analysis of the literature suggests otherwise [41]. Because of the unique and devastating risks that come with the transforaminal approach, patients should be selected carefully, and appropriate training and understanding of fluoroscopy imaging is essential.

According to the consensus opinions published in 2015, several measures can be undertaken to minimize risks in patients receiving transforaminal epidural steroid injections [42]. There was unanimous approval to only use non-particulate steroids for cervical transforaminal injections. They recommended initially using dexamethasone in lumbar TFESIs but acknowledge there may be times where particulate steroids are more useful. Technical considerations to improve safety include appropriate imaging-guided views, injection of contrast under real-time fluoroscopy, review of prior imaging studies, the use of sterile gloves and mask to minimize infections, the use of extension tubing, and avoidance of heavy sedation. Another consideration is digital subtraction imaging that provides the benefit of significantly increasing detection of vascular uptake of contrast medium, but the committee acknowledged it may not be readily available to all and thus did not make it a mandatory recommendation [42].

Key Points

- TFESI is a safe approach to deliver medications into the anterior epidural space.
- There are rare but devastating complications associated with TFESI which may even be life threatening.
- If intravascular injection or epidural hematoma is suspected, then early imaging and neurosurgical intervention is the best chance for functional recovery.
- The "safe triangle" approach reduces risk of nerve injury and dural puncture.
- The use of real-time injection of contrast media or digital subtraction imaging is the best way to identify accidental intravascular injection.

References

1. Karaman H, Kavak GO, Tüfek A, Yldrm ZB. The complications of transforaminal lumbar epidural steroid injections. Spine (Phila Pa 1976). 2011;36(13):E819–24.
2. Manchikanti L. Transforaminal lumbar epidural steroid injections. Pain Physician. 2000;3:374–98.
3. Westbrook JL, Renowden SA, Carrie LE. Study of the anatomy of the extradural region using magnetic resonance imaging. Br J Anaesth. 1993;71(4):495–8.
4. Crock HV. Normal and pathological anatomy of the lumbar spinal nerve root canals. J Bone Joint Surg. 1981;63-B:487–90.
5. Lee C, Rauschning W, Glenn W. Lateral lumbar spinal stenosis. Spine. 1988;13:313–20.
6. Gilchrist RV, Slipman CW, Bhagia SM. Anatomy of the intervertebral foramen. Pain Physician. 2002;5:372–8.
7. Rauschning W. Normal and pathologic anatomy of the lumbar root canals. Spine. 1987;12:1008–19.
8. Bose K, Balasubramaniam P. Nerve root canals of the lumbar spine. Spine (Phila Pa 1976). 1984;9:16–8.
9. Hasegawa T, Mikawa Y, Watanabe R, An HS. Morphometric analysis of the lumbosacral nerve roots and dorsal root ganglia by magnetic resonance imaging. Spine (Phila Pa 1976). 1996;21:1005–9.
10. Boll DT, Bulow H, Blackham KA, Aschoff AJ, Schmitz BL. MDCT angiography of the spinal vasculature and the artery of Adamkiewicz. AJR Am J Roentgenol. 2006;187:1054–60.
11. Lu J, Ebraheim N, Biyani A, Brown J, Yeasting R. Vulnerability of great medullary artery. Spine. 1996;21:1852–5.
12. Murthy NS, Maus TP, Behrns CL. Intraforaminal location of the great anterior radiculomedullary artery (artery of Adamkiewicz): a retrospective review. Pain Med. 2010;11:1756–64.
13. Lazorthes G, Gouza A. Supply routes of arterial vascularization of the spinal cord. Applications to the study of vascular myelopathies. Bull Acad Natl Med. 1970;154:34–41.
14. Biglioli P, Spirito R, Roberto M, et al. The anterior spinal artery: the main arterial supply of the human spinal cord—preliminary anatomic study. J Thorac Cardiovasc Surg. 2000;119:376–9.
15. Minatoya K, Karck M, Hagl C, et al. The impact of spinal angiography on the neurologic outcome after surgery on the descending thoracic and thoracoabdominal aorta. Ann Thorac Surg. 2002;74:S1870–2.
16. Amonoo-Kuofi HS, el-Badawi MG, Fatani JA. Ligaments associated with lumbar intervertebral foramina L1-L4. J Anat. 1988;156:177–83.
17. Drake RL, Vogl W, Mitchell AWM. Gray's anatomy for students. New York: Elsevier; 2005. p. 69–70.
18. Bogduk N. Clinical anatomy of the lumbar spine and sacrum. 4th ed; London, UK: Elsevier Health Sciences Limited; 2005. p. 123–39.
19. Goodman BS, Bayazitoglu M, Mallempati S, Noble BR, Geffen JF. Dural puncture and subdural injection: a complication of lumbar transforaminal epidural injections. Pain Physician. 2007;10:697–705.
20. Botwin KP, Gurber RD, Bouchlas CG, Torres-Ramos FM, Freeman TL, Slaten WK. Complications of fluoroscopically guided transforaminal lumbar epidural injections. Arch Phys Med Rehabil. 2000;81:1045–50.
21. Hooten WM, Mizerak A, Carns PE. Discitis after lumbar epidural corticosteroid injection: a case report and analysis of the case report literature. Pain Med. 2006;7:46–51.

22. Kapoor SG1, Huff J, Cohen SP. Systematic review of the incidence of discitis after cervical discography. Spine J. 2010;10:739–45.
23. Sharma SK1, Jones JO, Zeballos PP, Irwin SA, Martin TW. The prevention of discitis during discography. Spine J. 2009;9:936–43.
24. Kennedy DJ, Dreyfuss P, Aprill CN, Bogduk N. Paraplegia following image-guided transforaminal lumbar spine epidural steroid injection: two case reports. Pain Med. 2009;10:1389–94.
25. Benzon HT, Chew TL, McCarthy RJ, Benzon HA, Walega DR. Comparison of the particle sizes of different steroids and the effect of dilution: a review of the relative neurotoxicities of the steroids. Anesthesiology. 2007;106:331–8.
26. Houten J, Errico T. Paraplegia after lumbosacral nerve root block: report of three cases. Spine J. 2002;2:70–5.
27. Huntoon M, Martin D. Paralysis after transforaminal epidural injection and previous spinal surgery. Reg Anesth Pain Med. 2004;29:494–5.
28. Derby R, Lee S, Date E, Lee J, Lee C. Size and aggregation of corticosteroids used for epidural injections. Pain Med. 2008;4:227–34.
29. Glaser SE, Falco FM. Paraplegia following a thoracolumbar transforaminal epidural steroid injection: a case report. Pain Physician. 2005;8:309–14.
30. Kim JY, Lee JW, Lee GY, Lee E, et al. Comparative effectiveness of lumbar epidural steroid injections using particulate vs non-particulate steroid: an inter-individual comparative study. Skelet Radiol. 2016;45:169–76.
31. El-Yahchouchi C, Geske JR, Carter RE, Diehn FE, Wald JT, Murthy NS, Kaufman TJ, Thielen KR, Morris JM, Amrami KK, Maus TP. The noninferiority of the nonparticulate steroid dexamethasone and triamcinolone in lumbar transforaminal epidural steroid injections. Pain Med. 2013;14:1650–7.
32. Kennedy DJ, Plastaras C, Casey E, Visco CJ, Rittenberg JD, Conrad B, Sigler J, Dreyfuss P. Comparative effectiveness of lumbar transforaminal epidural steroid injections with particulate versus non-particulate corticosteroids for lumbar radicular pain due to intervertebral disc herniation: a prospective, randomized, double-blind trial. Pain Med. 2014;15:548–55.
33. Furman M, O'Brien E, Zgleszewski T. Incidence of intravascular penetration in transforaminal lumbosacral epidural steroid injections. Spine. 2000;25:2628–32.
34. Somayaji HS, Saifuddin A, Casey ATH, Briggs TWR. Spinal cord infarction following therapeutic computed tomography-guided left L2 nerve root injection. Spine. 2005;30:E106–8.
35. Bogduk N, Dreyfuss P, Baker R, et al. Complications of spinal diagnostic and treatment procedures. Pain Med. 2008;6:S11–34.
36. Bogduk N. Clinical anatomy of the lumbar spine and sacrum. New York: Churchill Livingstone; 1997. p. 127–44.
37. Goodman BS, Posecion LWF, Mallempati S, Bayazitoglu M. Complications and pitfalls of lumbar interlaminar and transforaminal epidural injections. Curr Rev Musculoskelet Med. 2008;1(3-4):212–22.
38. Bogduk N. Practice guidelines for spinal diagnostic and treatment procedures. ISIS. 1st ed. San Francisco: International Spine Intervention Society; 2004.
39. Jasper JF. Lumbar retrodiscal transforaminal injection. Pain Physician. 2007;10:501–10.
40. Huston CW, Slipman CW, Garmin C. Complications and side effects of cervical and lumbosacral selective nerve root injections. Arch Phys Med Rehabil. 2005;86:277–83.
41. Manchikanti L, Abdi S, Atluri S, Benyamin RM, Boswell MV, Buenaventura RM, Bryce DA, Burks PA, Caraway DL, Calodney AK, Cash KA, Christo PJ, Cohen SP, Colson J, Conn A, Cordner HJ, Coubarous S, Datta S, Deer TR, Diwan SA, FJE F, Fellows B, Geffert SC, Grider JS, Gupta S, Hameed H, Hameed M, Hansen H, Helm S II, Janata JW, Justiz R, Kaye AD, Lee M, Manchikanti KN, CD MM, Onyewu O, Parr AT, Patel VB, Racz GB, Sehgal N, Sharma M, Simopoulos TT, Singh V, Smith HS, Snook LT, Swicegood J, Vallejo R, Ward SP, Wargo BW, Zhu J, Hirsch JA. An update of comprehensive evidence-based guidelines for interventional techniques of chronic spinal pain: part II: guidance and recommendations. Pain Physician. 2013;16:S49–253.
42. Rathmell JP, Benzon HT, Dreyfuss P, Huntoon M, Wallace M, Baker R, Riew KD, Rosenquist RW, Aprill C, Rost NS, Buvanendran A, Kreiner DS, Bogduk N, Fourney DR, Fraifeld E, Horn S, Stone J, Vorenkamp K, Lawler G, Summers J, Kloth D, O'Brien D, Tutton S. Safeguards to prevent neurologic complications after epidural steroid injections: consensus opinions from a multidisciplinary working group and national organizations. Anesthesiology. 2015;122(5):974–84.

Permanent Paralysis Caused by Epidural Hematoma After Tunneled Catheter Placement

16

Alina Lazar, Johal Gurbir, and Magdalena Anitescu

16.1 Case Description

A 61-year-old male with stage IVb pancreatic cancer with intractable abdominal pain and severe opioid-induced nausea refractory to conventional therapy is scheduled to undergo placement of a tunneled epidural catheter for palliative pain management. His medical history is significant for hypertension and depression. Preoperative laboratory values, including international normalized ratio (INR) and platelet count, are within normal limits. His preoperative medication consists of metoprolol, hydrochlorothiazide, morphine, ondansetron, and fluoxetine. In the pain clinic, a wire-reinforced epidural catheter is placed without difficulty at the T8–T9 level using a paramedian approach with a 17-gauge Touhy needle after loss of resistance to saline. Upon epidural injection of 1.5% lidocaine and epinephrine, a bilateral T6–T8 sensory level is noted, and subsequently a 0.0625% bupivacaine infusion is started. After returning to the hospital room, the patient receives ketorolac 30 mg for shoulder pain from severe osteoarthritis. He is scheduled to receive this dose every 6 h for 48 h. Subcutaneous heparin, 5000 units, is administered two times per day for deep vein thrombosis prophylaxis.

On post-procedure day 1, he inadvertently receives enoxaparin, 40 mg subcutaneously, 2 h after his last scheduled dose of heparin. Three hours later, he complains of back pain and numbness from the waist down; he is unable to move his legs. Physical examination confirms sensory and motor loss below the T6 level. Magnetic resonance imaging (MRI) of the spine is emergently obtained. However, because of distortion at the site of catheter insertion (Fig. 16.1), an epidural hematoma cannot be ruled out. Repeat MRI after removal of the catheter reveals a T1 hypointense and T2 hyperintense extradural fluid collection along the posterior spinal canal from T4 to T9, consistent with epidural hemorrhage, causing spinal cord compression (Fig. 16.2). The patient undergoes emergent decompression laminectomy. Despite this intervention and extensive perioperative rehabilitation, the sensory and motor

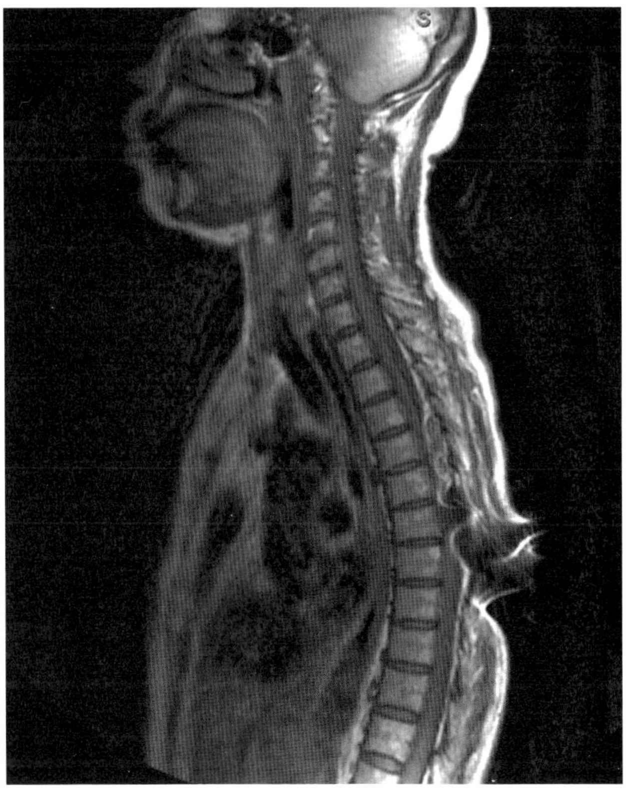

Fig. 16.1 MRI of lumbar spine with artifact due to epidural catheter. Personal library

A. Lazar (✉) • M. Anitescu, M.D., Ph.D.
Department of Anesthesia and Critical Care, University of Chicago Medical Center, 5841 S. Maryland Ave., Chicago, IL, USA
e-mail: ALazar@dacc.uchicago.edu

J. Gurbir
Prestige Pain Centers, Carteret, New Jersey, USA

M. Anitescu et al. (eds.), *Challenging Cases and Complication Management in Pain Medicine*,
https://doi.org/10.1007/978-3-319-60072-7_16

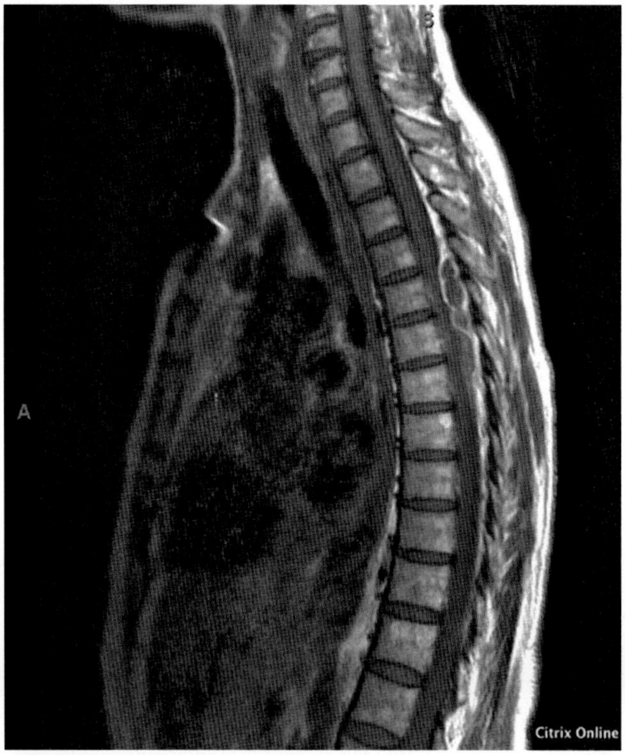

Fig. 16.2 MRI prior to decompression revealing a large extradural collection from T5 to T6 causing significant compression of the spinal cord. Personal library

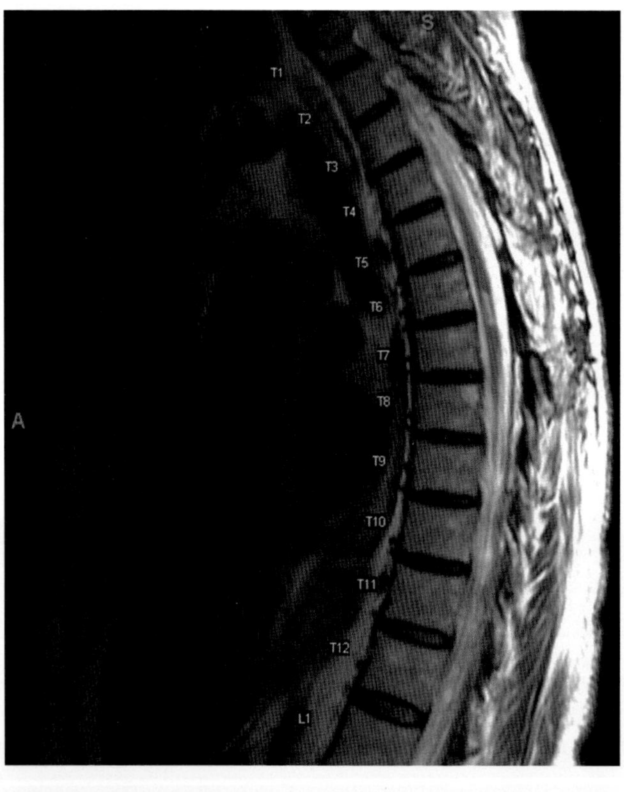

Fig. 16.3 Thoracic MRI, T2-weighted image: follow-up 3 years later reveals postoperative changes after T4–T6 laminectomy, with myelomalacia at the T6–T7 level. Personal library

loss continues. His postoperative course is complicated by postlaminectomy syndrome with ongoing back pain and muscle spasms, for which he requires chronic pain treatment with methadone, oxycodone, and a cetaminophen, combined with baclofen, gabapentin, and periodic trigger point injections. After 2 months of intense rehabilitation, his motor function recovers only minimally. He is able to walk short distances with assistance, has bladder and bowel incontinence, and a marked sensory deficit below T7. His subsequent MRI scans are consistent with stable myelomalacia (Fig. 16.3).

16.2 Case Discussion

Permanent paralysis after epidural catheter insertion is a rare but catastrophic event. Epidural hematoma is the most common cause of permanent neurological deficit after epidural block. Other common causes are epidural abscess, spinal cord infarction, traumatic injury, arachnoiditis, and local anesthetic and adjuvant toxicity. Spinal epidural hematoma has been described in autopsies since 1682 as "spinal apoplexy" and as a clinical diagnosis since 1867 [1, 2].

16.2.1 Incidence

The estimated incidence of epidural hematoma commonly cited in the literature is <1 in 150,000 epidurals and <1 in 220,000 spinal anesthetics [3]. In a recent report, using a multidimensional search strategy including analysis of the electronic medical records at a single major US institution, others have found a rate of 1:7200 [4]. In an Australian review of more than 8000 cases, in which an epidural catheter was placed by the acute pain service and managed for several days, the combined rate of epidural abscess and hematoma was 1 in 1026 [5]. In females undergoing knee arthroplasty, the risk was 1 in 3600 [6]. The incidence of epidural-related serious morbidity and mortality is higher when blocks are placed perioperatively, rather than for obstetric and pediatric populations or for chronic pain management [7]. A review of the ASA Closed Claims database revealed that spinal cord injuries were the leading cause of nerve injury claims in the 1990s [8]. Spinal epidural hematomas accounted for nearly half of the spinal cord injuries reported, and the median payment was very high. In an analysis of claims after regional anesthesia between 1980 an1999, three-fourths of patients had evidence of a preexisting or iatrogenic coagulation abnormality [9]. In an analysis of the closed claims data from 2005 to 2008, there were three cases of compressive epidural hematoma after cervical injections. The unfavorable outcomes from these interventions were more severe than adverse outcomes from all other procedural interventions for pain [10].

16.2.2 Etiology and Risk Factors

Epidural hematomas are caused by bleeding from the prominent valveless venous plexus found in the low-pressure epidural space [6]. They are more likely to be present in the thoracic spine where a prominence of the epidural venous plexus has been described. Because the thoracic vertebral canal in the mid-thoracic area is narrower than the lumbar one and contains less fatty and fibrous connective tissues, even a small hematoma can compress the spinal cord in this area. The amount of epidural fat in the posterior epidural space decreases with age and body weight, making older patients more vulnerable. Some argue that because venous pressure is generally lower than intrathecal pressure, venous bleeding should not cause acute spinal cord compression [11]. On the other hand, bleeding from an arterial source accumulates rapidly and causes neural ischemia soon after vessel trauma. Most epidural hematomas become symptomatic days after epidural needle or catheter placement, suggesting the bleeding is not arterial.

Among the causes of epidural hematomas reported in the literature are spinal surgery, trauma, spinal or epidural injection, arterial venous malformations, tumor hemorrhage, lumbar puncture, myelography, and spinal manipulation [12]. In a review of 613 cases published between 1826 and 1993, epidural hematoma was idiopathic or spontaneous in 30% of cases, related to anticoagulation in 17% and related to spinal or epidural anesthesia in 10% of cases [13].

Numerous predisposing factors for epidural hematoma have been described: patient-, technique-, and medication-related (Table 16.1). In the majority of cases, it is difficult to identify a sole cause for epidural hematoma. The interplay of various predisposing factors creates the conditions for epidural bleeding to occur. Radiographic imaging, reviewed before performing interventional spine and pain procedures, assesses for central and foraminal stenosis, disc herniations that compromise canal diameter, ligamentum flavum hypertrophy, epidural fibrosis, and previous surgical scarring that can alter the level of procedural difficulty [14].

Table 16.1 Risk factors for spinal hematoma-personal table

Patient-related risk factors	Procedure-related risk factors	Medication-related risk factors
Coagulopathy—inherited, acquired (renal or liver failure) History of major bleeding episodes from procedures	Traumatic procedure or multiple needle passes	Antithrombotics (warfarin, heparin, LMWH)
Advanced age Female gender	Presence of blood in the catheter during insertion or removal	Antiplatelets (aspirin, NSAIDs)
Spine abnormalities (ankylosing spondylitis, Paget's disease of the vertebral bones, osteoporosis, spinal stenosis, previous spine surgeries, and epidural interventions)	Type of neuraxial block (indwelling epidural catheter > single-shot epidural block > single-shot spinal block)	Selective serotonin reuptake inhibitors (SSRIs)
Hypertension		Dietary supplements (fish oil, vitamin E, gingko biloba, garlic, ginseng, magnesium)
Epidural vessel abnormalities		
Increased intra-abdominal pressure		
Coughing, straining, Valsalva maneuver		

16.3 Clinical Manifestations

The symptoms of epidural hematoma result from compression of the spinal cord or nerve roots below the affected spinal level: neck or back pain and radicular pain, followed by more or less severe, but usually progressive, paralysis. The pain is intense, constant, and knifelike and worsens with coughing, sneezing, or straining. High cervical epidural hematomas can lead to spinal shock or even death [15]. Cauda equina syndrome due to hematoma formation, a rare complication with a reported incidence of 2.7 in 100,000 epidural blocks, resulted in permanent deficit in more than two-thirds of cases [6]. Its symptoms are low back pain, altered proprioception, decreased sensation to pinprick and temperature in the lumbar and sacral distribution, voiding and defecation disturbances, and progressive loss of muscle strength.

Not all of these symptoms are present at the same time. A literature review of nonoperative and operative cases of epidural hematoma found that 16% of the cases managed conservatively suffered only backache or neck pain and another 9% of cases had mild radicular symptoms [16]. In 88% of these patients, diagnosis was based on MRI. Conversely, among the series of hematomas managed operatively, local pain or isolated radicular symptoms and signs were present in only 6% of the patients [16]. Isolated vesicorectal dysfunction also has been described [17]. In patients who are receiving local anesthetics epidurally, the most common

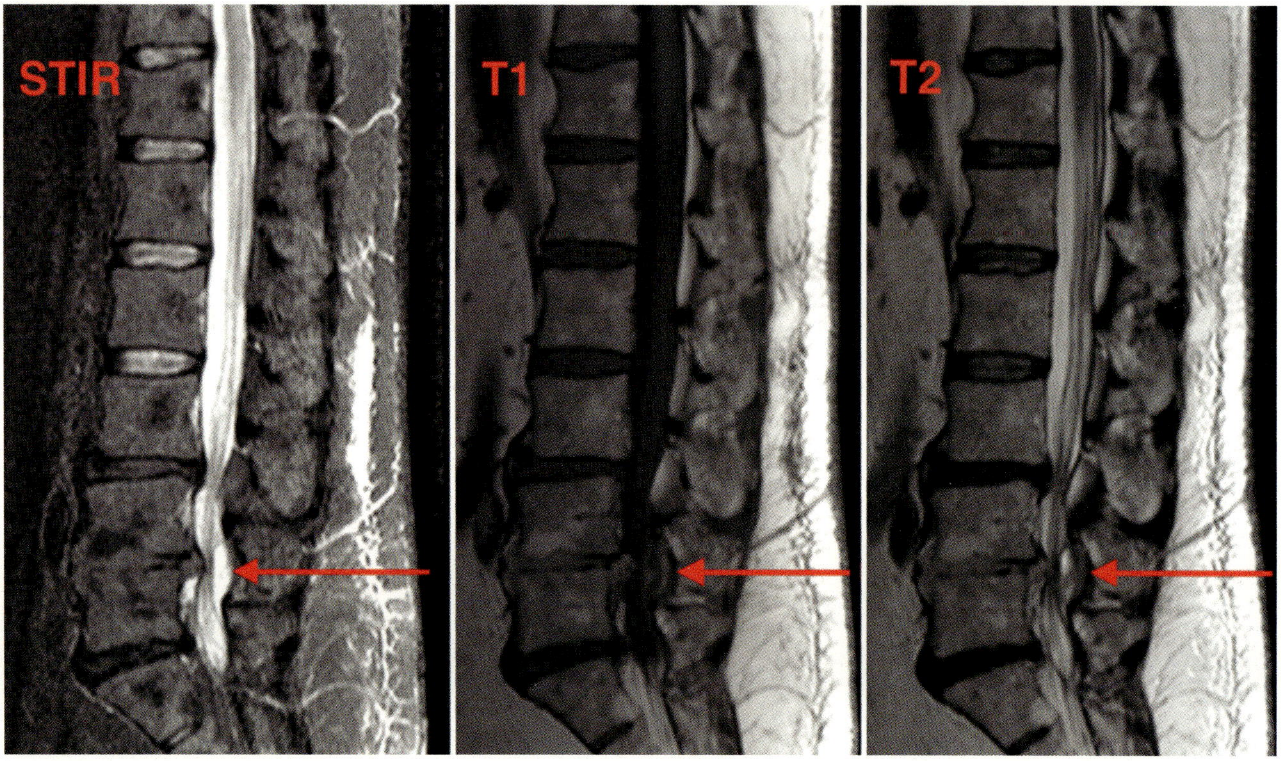

Fig. 16.4 MRI of chronic posterior epidural hematoma at L4–L5, sagittal views. Personal library

presenting symptom may be increased motor block rather than back pain [9]. The presence of postoperative numbness or weakness may be erroneously attributed to local anesthetic effect rather than spinal cord ischemia, which may delay diagnosis.

Although some symptoms manifest within 24 h, most epidural hematomas become symptomatic several days after an epidural placement. Far less frequently, symptoms are slowly progressive, chronic or relapsing, or mimic an acute intervertebral disc prolapse (Fig. 16.4).

16.3.1 Imaging

Emergent magnetic resonance imaging (MRI) or computed tomography scan (CT) when MRI is contraindicated is recommended as soon as spinal hematoma is suspected. An urgent neurosurgical consult sought to evaluate for decompressive surgery is required if an epidural hematoma is detected. On MR imaging, a hematoma appears as an isointensity on the spinal cord seen on T1-weighted images or as a heterogeneous hyperintensity with focal hypointensity on T2-weighted images [18]. In regard to CT imaging, it appears as a high-density mass in the spinal canal compressing the cord [19].

Though MRI is considered the gold standard for diagnosing an epidural hematoma, whether to leave in place or remove epidural and peripheral nerve catheters during MRI is not clear. Potential concerns encompass catheter movement, device heating, or interference with MRI scanning. Depending on the material of catheters, MRI may not be advisable to confirm diagnosis. Many catheters are wire reinforced or contain a flexometallic ring, thus making MR imaging contraindicated [20].

Newer packaging contains a label specifically identifying MRI unsafe catheters. Caregivers who screen patients for MRI compatibility may not know which catheters are unsafe. See Table 16.2 for commonly used catheters and their MRI compatibilities. Clinicians should plan in advance for the uncertainty of catheter compatibility with MRI and have alternate diagnostic strategies, such as proceeding to surgery without MRI guidance or performing computerized tomography with a myelogram [21]. Manipulation of a catheter may increase bleeding; thus, removal of a catheter is not advisable before imaging. Careful consideration must be given for each individual case.

Table 16.2 Epidural catheter types and MRI compatibility-personal table

Catheter type	MRI compatibility
Arrow International	
Flextip Plus Epidural Catheter (304V SS)	Unsafe 2
TheraCath (304 V SS)	Unsafe 2
Braun Medical	
Perifix ONE Marked Polyamide/Polyurethane Epidural Catheter	Conditional 8
Perifix FX Springwound Epidural Catheter	Unsafe 1

Information incorporated from www.mrisaftey.com
Unsafe 1: Object poses a risk or hazard to a patient or individual in the MR environment. The presence of this object is contraindicated for an MR procedure
Unsafe 2: Object is contraindicated for an MR procedure or for any individual in the MR environment. Potential risks include possible induced currents, excessive heating, as well as other potentially hazardous conditions
Conditional 8: Pertaining to an implant/device that has MRI labeled as 1.5-T and 3-T, only. In some cases, may be associated with single- and two-overlapped versions of a stent

16.3.2 Treatment

Neurologic recovery is more likely if decompressive laminectomy is performed within 8 h of symptom onset. In a retrospective case series of 61 epidural hematomas, patients who had decompressive surgery less than 8 h after onset of paraplegia had better neurologic outcomes than if surgery was performed more than 24 h after symptom onset [22]. In this series only 38% of patients had partial or good neurologic recovery, and even with prompt diagnosis and decompression, many patients had permanent neurologic deficits [22]. The final neurologic outcome depends on the time span between hematoma formation and surgical decompression, the speed with which the hematoma develops, the severity of the preoperative neurologic deficit, the size of the hematoma, and the patient's age (the older the patient the worse the prognosis) [13, 22].

Hematomas that are found incidentally, chronic stable hematomas, or hematomas with minimal symptoms that appear to be resolving have a good outcome when managed nonsurgically, provided that the patients are evaluated with regular neurologic exams and MRI (Fig. 16.4) [23]. Leakage of the hematoma through the intervertebral foramen and its spread along the epidural space may explain spontaneous recovery [16].

In patients with an acute epidural hematoma from an indwelling epidural catheter, the removal of the catheter can worsen the bleeding. When an epidural hematoma is diagnosed, anticoagulation is discontinued immediately, and reversal of anticoagulation should be considered with fresh frozen plasma, vitamin K, plasmapheresis, and dialysis. These interventions should not delay decompressive surgery.

16.3.3 Prevention

Patient selection and identification of risk factors for epidural hematoma are essential for an optimal outcome. A safety checklist includes an evaluation of the patients and family history of bleeding disorders, screening for medication and supplements known to influence coagulation status, review of radiographic images to identify anatomic challenges, and determination of the best time for (re)initiation of anticoagulation and antiplatelet therapy. Close communication with prescribing physicians is necessary. Alerts built into computerized physician order sets and computer-assisted decision support systems have proved to be effective in increasing adherence to practice guidelines and preventing inadvertent coadministration of multiple anticoagulants [24].

Various techniques have been proposed to minimize the risk of epidural hematoma. Medial insertion of needle is preferred because a lateral puncture increases the risk of injuring epidural veins. Some interventionalists advocate the use of short-beveled or blunt-type needles [25]. In a prospective study of 2376 interlaminar cervical epidural steroid injections, no significant hemorrhagic complications were discovered, regardless of the needle type [26]. The epidural catheter should not be introduced more than 3–5 cm into the epidural space.

The guidelines for the management of regional anesthesia in the presence of anticoagulation are continuously evolving. A special concern exists for patients undergoing interventional spine and pain procedures with high risk for neuraxial bleeding (Table 16.3). These patients tend to be older and more likely to have spinal abnormalities, previous epidural interventions, and renal or hepatic insufficiency. They may take several concomitant medications with antiplatelet effects including aspirin, nonsteroidal anti-inflammatory drugs (NSAIDs), and selective serotonin reuptake inhibitors (SSRIs). Interventional pain procedures involve large gauge needles and long-term indwelling catheters which increases the risk of epidural bleeding. For these patients, the 2010

Table 16.3 Pain procedures with high risk for epidural hematoma

Spinal cord stimulator trial and implant
Intrathecal catheter and pump implant
Vertebral augmentation
Epiduroscopy and epidural decompression
Tunneled epidural catheters

Personal table, based on modified from Narouze et al. [21]

American Society of Regional Anesthesia and Pain Medicine (ASRA) guidelines for regional anesthesia in patients taking anticoagulants or thromboprophylactics [3] are insufficient. Separate guidelines were created in 2015 for patients undergoing spine and pain procedures [21]. Among the major areas of difference from the 2010 guidelines are discontinuation of aspirin and NSAIDs before high-risk spine procedures, delayed reinstatement of low molecular weight heparin (LMWH) therapy after neuraxial procedures, and a more nuanced management of patients taking antidepressants. Simultaneous use of multiple agents with anticoagulant properties (e.g., NSAIDs, aspirin along with SSRIs, fish oil) increases the risk of morbidity. Consideration should be given to their discontinuation based on an assessment of risk and benefits. A summary of the ASRA 2010 and 2015 guidelines appears in Tables 16.4, 16.5, and 16.6.

Table 16.4 Guidelines for indwelling epidural catheters: antiplatelets and NSAIDs

Therapeutic class	Drug	When to stop before placement	When to restart after removal	Can be continued while catheter in place?[a]
Aspirin	Aspirin primary prophylaxis	6 days	24 h	No
	Aspirin secondary prophylaxis	Shared assessment	Shared assessment	Yes, as monotherapy (i.e., no prophylactic UFH, LMWH, NSAIDs)
PDE inhibitors	Cilostazol	2 days	24 h	No
	Dipyridamole	2 days	N/A	No
	Aspirin combinations	See aspirin	See aspirin	No
P2Y12 inhibitors	Clopidogrel	7 days	12–24 h	No
	Prasugrel	7–10 days	12–24 h	No
	Ticagrelor	5 days	12–24 h	No
GPIIb/IIIa inhibitors	Abciximab	2–5 days	8–12 h	No
	Eptifibatide	8–24 h	8–12 h	No
	Tirofiban	8–24 h	8–12 h	No
NSAIDs	Diclofenac	1 day	N/A	No
	Ketorolac	1 day	N/A	No
	Ibuprofen	1 day	N/A	No
	Etodolac	2 days	N/A	No
	Indomethacin	2 days	N/A	No
	Naproxen	4 days	N/A	No
	Meloxicam	4 days	N/A	No
	Nabumetone	6 days	N/A	No
	Oxaprozin	10 days	N/A	No
	Piroxicam	10 days	N/A	No

Personal table based on modified from Narouze et al. [21] and Horlocker et al. [3]
[a]Recommend against concurrent use of medications that affect clotting (NSAIDs, aspirin, low molecular weight heparins, and subcutaneous heparin)

Table 16.5 Guidelines for indwelling epidural catheters: anticoagulants and fibrinolytics

Therapeutic class	Drug	When to stop before placement	When to restart after removal	Can be continued while catheter in place?[d]
Thromboprophylaxis	Enoxaparin ≤40 mg/day	12 h	4 h	No
	Enoxaparin 30 mg Q12h/40 mg Q12h	12 h	4 h	No
	Fondaparinux ≤2.5 mg/day	4 days	24 h	No
	Unfractionated heparin 5000 units BID[a]	8–10 h	2 h	Yes, as monotherapy (i.e., no NSAIDs or ASA)
	Unfractionated heparin 5000 units TID[a]	8–10 h	2 h	No
	Rivaroxaban 10 mg daily	No recommendations	No recommendations	No

Table 16.5 (continued)

Therapeutic class	Drug	When to stop before placement	When to restart after removal	Can be continued while catheter in place?[d]
Therapeutic anticoagulants	Enoxaparin 1 mg/kg Q12h[b]	24 h	4 h	No
	Enoxaparin 1.5 mg/kg Q24h[c]	24 h	4 h	No
	Fondaparinux 5–10 mg/day	4 days	24 h	No
	Unfractionated heparin Intravenous	4 h	2 h	No
	Rivaroxaban 20–30 mg/day	3 days	24 h	No
	Dabigatran	5 days	24 h	No
	Apixaban	3–5 days	24 h	No
	Edoxaban	3 days	24 h	No
	Argatroban	8–10 h	2–4 h	No
	Warfarin	5 days, INR <1.5	24 h	No
Fibrinolytics	Alteplase Full-dose stroke, MI, etc	Contraindicated	Contraindicated	No
	Alteplase Intracatheter	N/A	N/A	No

Personal table based on modified from Narouze et al. [21] and Horlocker et al. [3]
[a]Check platelet count if on heparin therapy >4 days before placement
[b]For single daily dose, restart 6–8 h postoperatively and remove catheter prior to first dose
[c]For twice daily dose, start 24 h postoperatively and remove catheter prior to first dose
[d]Recommend against concurrent use of medications that affect clotting (NSAIDs, aspirin, low molecular weight heparins, and subcutaneous heparin)

Table 16.6 Guidelines for indwelling epidural catheters: herbals, vitamins, and antidepressants

Therapeutic class	Drug	When to stop before placement	When to restart after removal	Can be continued while catheter in place?[b]
Herbals	Gingko	No contraindication[a]	No contraindication	No contraindication
	Garlic	No contraindication[a]	No contraindication	No contraindication
	Ginseng	No contraindication[a]	No contraindication	No contraindication
	Omega-3 fish oil	No contraindication[a]	No contraindication	No contraindication
	Turmeric	No contraindication[a]	No contraindication	No contraindication
Vitamins	Vitamin C	N/A	N/A	No contraindication
	Vitamin E	N/A	N/A	No contraindication
Antidepressants	SSRI	N/A	N/A	No contraindication

Personal table, based on, modified from Narouze et al. [21] and Horlocker et al. [3]
[a]High-risk patients (advanced age, renal or hepatic disease, history of major bleeding from procedures) should discontinue use prior to elective procedures
[b]Recommend against concurrent use of medications that affect clotting (NSAIDs, aspirin, low molecular weight heparins, and subcutaneous heparin)

Patients having neuraxial anesthesia who have received antithrombotic drugs need more frequent neurologic evaluation—every 1–2 h for the first 6–12 h. The frequency of the checks can be decreased subsequently, if no changes in the epidural management are made (e.g., bolus administration, change in concentration). Especially in patients with multiple risk factors for epidural hematoma, the lowest effective dose of local anesthetic makes it possible to recognize motor or sensory loss promptly. Any change in neurologic status should immediately trigger clinical assessment and additional evaluation. Vigilance, prompt diagnosis, and intervention are required to optimize the neurologic outcome.

Conclusions

Although the incidence of neurological complications from hemorrhage associated with neuraxial blockade is low, the consequences can be devastating. In patients receiving antithrombotic and thrombolytic therapy, no more than one anticoagulant is given at a time. Concurrent use of anticoagulants with different mechanisms of actions and medications and supplements with the potential to impair coagulation increases the risk of hematoma. Safety mechanisms should be in place in order to prevent inadvertent administration of anticoagulants with epidural analgesia. Vigilance in monitoring is critical for early evaluation of neurological dysfunction and prompt intervention.

Key Points

- The incidence of the spinal epidural hematoma increases with age, female sex, underlying coagulopathy, difficult epidural placement, and an indwelling catheter.
- Common symptoms are rapidly progressing muscle weakness, severe localized back and radicular pain, and urinary and fecal disturbances.
- The diagnosis of spinal hematoma is confirmed with emergent magnetic resonance imaging.
- Prompt diagnosis and surgical decompression within 8 h after diagnosis are paramount for optimizing neurological outcome.
- Patients receiving anticoagulants are at increased risk for a hematoma and require close monitoring.

References

1. Plagne R. L'hématome extra-dural rachidien non traumatique (hématome épidural spontané). Thèse pour le Doctorat en Médecine (Diplôme d'Etat). Université de Clermont, Faculté mixte de Médecine et de Pharmacie; 1961.
2. Jackson R. Case of spinal apoplexy. Lancet. 1869;2:5–6.
3. Horlocker TT, Wedel DJ, Rowlingson JC, et al. Regional anesthesia in the patient receiving antithrombotic or thrombolytic therapy: American Society of Regional Anesthesia and Pain Medicine evidence-based guidelines (third edition). Reg Anesth Pain Med. 2010;35:64–101.
4. Ehrenfeld JM, Agarwal AK, Henneman JP, Sandberg WS. Estimating the incidence of suspected epidural hematoma and the hidden imaging cost of epidural catheterization. A retrospective review of 43,200 cases. Reg Anesth Pain Med. 2013;38:409–14.
5. Cameron CM, Scott DA, McDonald WM, Davies MJ. A review of neuraxial epidural morbidity: experience of more than 8,000 cases at a single teaching hospital. Anesthesiology. 2007;106:997–1002.
6. Moen V, Dahlgren N, Irestedt L. Severe neurological complications after central neuraxial blockades in Sweden 1990–1999. Anesthesiology. 2004;101:950–9.
7. Cook TM, Counsell D, Wildsmith JA. Major complications of central neuraxial block: report on the Third National Audit Project of the Royal College of Anaesthetists. Br J Anaesth. 2009;102(2):179–90.
8. Cheney FW, Domino KB, Caplan RA, Posner KL. Nerve injury associated with anesthesia: a closed claims analysis. Anesthesiology. 1999;90(4):1062–9.
9. Lee LA, Posner KL, Domino KB, Caplan RA, Cheney FW. Injuries associated with regional anesthesia in the 1980s and 1990s: a closed claims analysis. Anesthesiology. 2004;101:143–52.
10. Rathmell JP, Michna E, Fitzgibbon DR, et al. Injury and liability associated with cervical procedures for chronic pain. Anesthesiology. 2011;114:918–26.
11. Beatty RM, Winston KR. Spontaneous cervical epidural hematoma. A consideration of etiology. J Neurosurg. 1984;61:143–8.
12. Chang Chien GC, McCormick Z, Araujo M, Candido KD. The potential contributing effect of ketorolac and fluoxetine to a spinal epidural hematoma following a cervical interlaminar epidural steroid injection: a case report and narrative review. Pain Physician. 2014;17:E385–95.
13. Kreppel D, Antoniadis G, Seeling W. Spinal hematoma: a literature survey with meta-analysis of 613 patients. Neurosurg Rev. 2003;26:1–49.
14. Smith CC, Lin JL, Shokat M, Dosanjh SS, Casthely D. A report of paraparesis following spinal cord stimulator trial, implantation and revision. Pain Physician. 2010;13:357–63.
15. Adamson Bulsars DCK, Bronec PR. Spontaneous cervical epidural hematoma: case report and literature review. Surg Neurol. 2004;62:156–60.
16. Groen RJM. Non-operative treatment of spontaneous spinal epidural hematomas: a review of the literature and a comparison with operative cases. Acta Neurochir. 2004;146:103–10.
17. Kamoda H, Ishikawa T, Miyagi M, et al. Delayed postoperative epidural hematoma presenting only with vesicorectal disturbance. Case Rep Orthop. 2013;2013:1–4.
18. Narouze S, Benzon HT, Provenzano DA, et al. Interventional spine and pain procedures in patients on antiplatelet and anticoagulant medications. Guidelines from the American Society of Regional Anesthesia and Pain Medicine, the European Society of Regional Anaesthesia and Pain Therapy, the American Academy of Pain Medicine, the International Neuromodulation Society, the North American Neuromodulation Society, and the World Institute of Pain. Reg Anesth Pain Med. 2015;40:182–212.
19. Mhyre JM, Greenfield ML, Tsen LC, Polley LS. A systematic review of randomized controlled trials that evaluate strategies to avoid epidural vein cannulation during obstetric epidural catheter placement. Anesth Analg. 2009;108:1232–42.
20. Shih CK, Wang FY, Shieh CG, Huang JM, Lu IC, et al. Soft catheters reduce the risk of intravascular cannulation during epidural block—a retrospective analysis of 1117 cases in a medical center. Kaohsiung J Med Sci. 2012;28:373–6.
21. Law EM, Smith PJ, Fitt G, Hennessy OF. Non-traumatic spinal extradural haematoma: magnetic resonance findings. Australas Radiol. 1993;192:192–6.
22. Vandermeulen EP, Van Aken H, Vermylen J. Anticoagulants and spinal-epidural anesthesia. Anesth Analg. 1994;79:1165.
23. Shin JJ, Kuh SU, Cho YE. Surgical management of spontaneous spinal epidural hematoma. Eur Spine J. 2006;15:998–1004.
24. Jajosky J, Howell SM, Honaker J, et al. Improving adherence for practice guidelines for anticoagulation in patients receiving neuraxial anesthesia using an electronic order entry alert system. J Patient Saf. 2015; doi:10.1097/PTS.0000000000000219.
25. Özcan U, Şahin Ş, Gurbet A, et al. Comparison of blunt and sharp needles for transforaminal epidural steroid injections. Agri. 2012;24(2):85–9.
26. Manchikanti L, Malla Y, Wargo BW, Cash KA, Pampati V, Fellows B. A prospective evaluation of complications of 10,000 fluoroscopically directed epidural injections. Pain Physician. 2012;15:131–40.

Sheared or Break of Caudal Catheters After Epidural Steroid Injection

17

Tariq Malik

17.1 Case Report

A 54-year-old male was referred to the pain clinic for the management of post-laminectomy pain syndrome. He had a long-standing history of chronic back and left leg pain. His medical history was noncontributory. A truck driver by profession, his back pain and leg pain were affecting his work. He had no neurological deficit. MRI was positive for L4–L5 left neuroforaminal stenosis compatible with his left leg pain. He had been treated with a series of lumbar interlaminar epidural steroid injections in conjunction with physical therapy. The pain relief was short term, leading him to opt for surgical decompression. He underwent L4 laminectomy, which provided pain relief for 6 months, and then his pain returned gradually to its presurgical level. He was evaluated by the surgeon who, deeming him not a candidate for another surgery, referred him to the pain clinic for nonsurgical pain management. Evaluation revealed a man of average built, a stable gait, non-focal neurological examination, and full range of motion in the lumbar spine. There was a midline scar on his back from his previous surgery. He was scheduled for a caudal epidural steroid injection for possible relief of his pain. When he returned for the procedure, he was placed prone, and the sacral area was prepped with chlorhexidine. The caudal epidural space was accessed under fluoroscopic guidance using a 18 g R.K.™ epidural needle (Epimed, Farmer Branch, TX). The needle position was confirmed by injecting iohexol, which revealed appropriate spread of the dye. A 20 g flexible wire-reinforced R.K.® epidural catheter was threaded up until the tip of the catheter was at the L4 vertebral level. Intravascular and intrathecal placement of the catheter was excluded by injection of contrast via the catheter, which revealed spread of the dye along the left L4 nerve root. Then 60 mg of triamcinolone was injected in 4 mL of 0.0625% bupivacaine. At the completion of the procedure, the needle was removed easily, but the catheter was stuck. Tugging caused uncoiling of the catheter at which time further tugging was discontinued. Imaging revealed an intact catheter inside the epidural space with unraveling of the catheter at the subcutaneous level. Constant gentle tension under live fluoroscopic guidance showed that the catheter had slipped out without further uncoiling. This gentle constant traction under live fluoroscopic guidance continued until the entire catheter was removed. The catheter was examined, and its tip was noted to be intact. Its sheath revealed a slight shearing resulting in a small flap pointing backward. This flap could have anchored onto tissue, offering enough resistance to cause uncoiling but fortunately not enough to shear the catheter (Fig. 17.1).

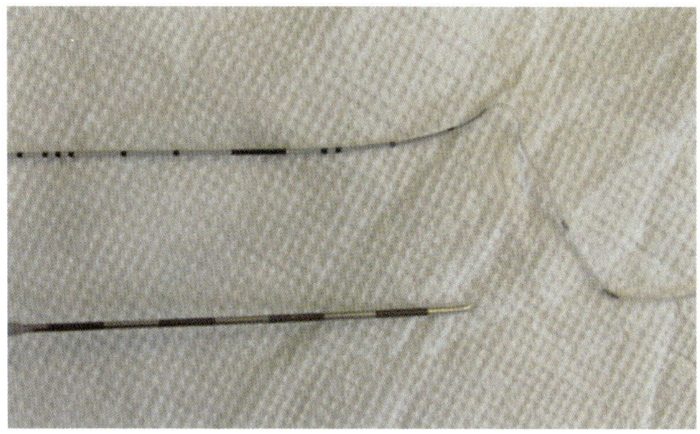

Fig. 17.1 Catheter sheared when threaded through a needle with a bent tip

17.2 Discussion

The physical and social impact of low back pain is enormous. It is one of the leading causes of disability in the past several decades [1]. Lifetime prevalence of back pain is

T. Malik, M.D.
University of Chicago Hospitals, 5841 S. Maryland Avenue, Chicago, IL 60637, USA
e-mail: tmalik@dacc.uchicago.edu

M. Anitescu et al. (eds.), *Challenging Cases and Complication Management in Pain Medicine*, https://doi.org/10.1007/978-3-319-60072-7_17

reported at 50–90% [2, 3]. The economic cost of back pain is increasing both in terms of health-care expenses and lost productivity [4]. The etiology of back and leg pain varies, but the exact etiology is needed for proper treatment. Epidural steroid injections are commonly performed procedures for the relief of back pain. Epidural injection with a catheter has seen a 127% increase in Medicare patients in the decade 2000–2011 [5]. The purpose of using a catheter is twofold: (1) scar tissue, which prevents the steroid from reaching the nerve roots, is loosened or removed by either using a chemical agent like hyaluronidase or mechanically by injecting 10–20 mL of normal saline. (2) Drug delivery is targeted by positioning the catheter tip very close to the nerve root. In some studies, the use of a catheter has been proven to be more effective than regular epidural steroid injections in relieving leg pain in patients with post-laminectomy pain syndrome [6, 7]. The caudal epidural catheter technique is safe with a low incidence of complications. The true incidence of sheared or broken epidural catheters is unknown. The first report of epidural catheter breakage was published in 1957 [8]. In one study of 250 patients, the incidence of Racz catheter shearing was 1.2% [9]. There have been a number of case reports of epidural catheters shearing, knotting, or breaking [10, 11]. These complications are attributed to patient characteristics, insertion or removal technique, catheter type, or entrapment of the catheter by tissue. Catheters vary in tensile strength and breaking point. In one in vitro study, flexible wire-reinforced epidural catheters were shown to break more easily than non-wire catheters [12]. A damaged catheter is more prone to breakage [13]. Strength variability is attributed to the different material used in making catheters. The average force required to remove an epidural catheter in a clinical setting was found to be around 130–390 g with an upper limit of 1170 g [14]. Removal force is much lower than the force that breaks a catheter, which measured around 2000 g in a laboratory setting [12]. Often other factors are at play that necessitate the use of more than average force. These factors include coiling and knotting of the catheter, which offer much higher resistance to removal. Coiling and knotting are more likely with excessive threading of catheters in the epidural space. Excessive threading also can cause looping, which damages catheter integrity. The lumbar level is most vulnerable to coiling and knotting of a catheter. In one study, the mean distance before a catheter started to coil was 10 cm at the thoracic level versus 4.5 cm at the lumbar level [15]. During insertion, the needle tip can touch the bone and bend if force is used in order to walk up the bone [9]. Bending is more likely when accessing the epidural space at the thoracic or caudal level, damaging the epidural catheter both during placement and on removal. Catheters normally break when force is used to remove them; therefore, force should not applied on insertion or removal. Once the catheter is out of the needle, it is risky to rotate or move the needle because the needle tip is bound to shear the catheter. The catheter should be withdrawn into the needle before the needle is moved in any direction if at all. No manufacturer recommends catheter withdrawal into the needle, but a modern catheter can be withdrawn carefully and without resistance [10] (Fig. 17.2).

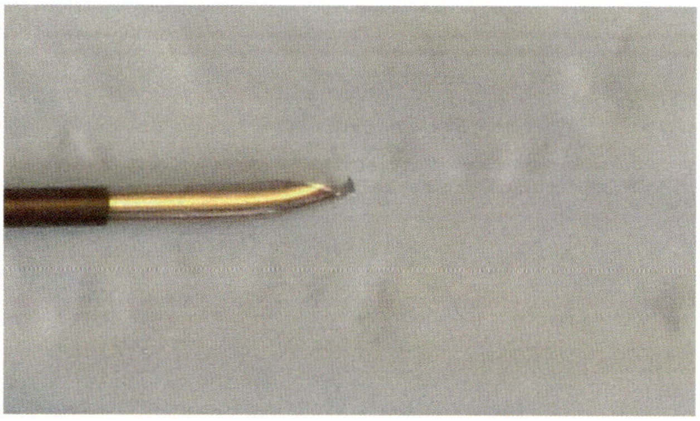

Fig. 17.2 Bent tip when needle was used to walk of the bone while looking for interlaminar space

Management of a broken catheter is controversial. As catheters are biologically inert, catheters in asymptomatic patients are not retrieved unless they are present in the intrathecal space. Catheters in the intrathecal space produce a granuloma that puts pressure on the spinal cord, necessitating surgical removal [16, 17]. Epidural catheters also produce symptoms by direct pressure effect [18], by cyst formation [19], or by excessive scar formation that affect the nerves or spinal cord. Migration of a retained catheter segment from one epidural level to another level has not been reported. Retained catheter segments in the epidural space have caused symptoms requiring surgery. Based on several case reports, some have suggested removing all epidural catheters. Patients should be informed about the broken catheter, and the final decision about how to proceed should be made after consultation with the patient irrespective of the location of the broken piece of the catheter. The exact location of the broken piece may determine the action to be taken. If a catheter is not radiopaque, an X-ray may reveal its location. Also an X-ray cannot localize exact anatomical position of the sheared catheter piece even if the catheter is radiopaque. An MRI is unsafe for visualization of a catheter with a wire because of the migration of the catheter under magnetic force or the effect of heating. An MRI, however, has been used to localize a broken wire-reinforced catheter without harm to the patient [20]. Visualization with an MRI may not be possible if a catheter is surrounded by an isodense

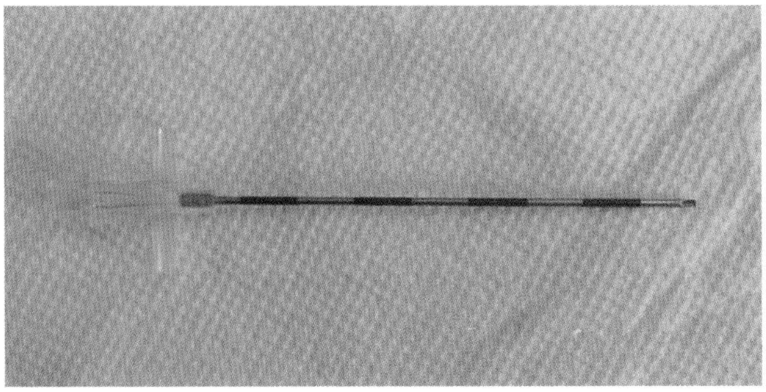

Fig. 17.3 Tuohy needle with bent tip

material. A CT without infusion is best at localizing a broken catheter and is the imaging modality of choice [21, 22]. Sheared catheters in the epidural space are not withdrawn if the patient is not symptomatic and he/she agrees to follow up observations [23]. However, it's advisable to scan the catheter in 6 months to 1 year to evaluate the catheter in case it is inciting granuloma formation that can cause any pressure effects (Fig. 17.3).

Appendix 1: Factors That Cause Catheter Breakage

1. Factory based
   (a) Bad catheter
   (b) Bad needle
2. Operator based
   (a) Inexperience
3. Technique based
   (a) Use of force on inserting needle
   (b) Forced catheter insertion
   (c) Excessive threading of catheter
   (d) Forced removal despite resistance

Appendix 2: Managing a Stuck/Broken Catheter

1. No more than moderate traction if catheter is not slipping out.
2. Put patient in a different position with varying degree of flexion if possible.
3. Leave the catheter in place (covered and taped) and try again after a few hours.
4. Use fluoroscopic guidance if catheter is radiopaque to see if catheter is slipping out when tugged.
5. If catheter breaks, inform the patient.
6. Use computed tomography to localize the catheter exactly.
7. If catheter is not intrathecal and the patient is asymptomatic, no intervention is needed if the patient agrees.
8. If patient is symptomatic, remove the catheter surgically.

References

1. US Burden of Disease Collaborators. The state of US health, 1990-2010: burden of diseases, injuries, and risk factors. JAMA. 2013;310:591–608.
2. Hoy D, Bain C, Williams G, et al. A systematic review of the global prevalence of low back pain. Arthritis Rheum. 2012;64:2028–37.
3. Juniper M, Le T, Mladsi D. The epidemiology, economic burden, and pharmacological treatment of chronic low back pain in France, Germany, Italy, Spain and the UK: a literature-based review. Expert Opin Pharmacother. 2009;10:2581–92.
4. Crow W, Willis D. Estimating cost of care for patients with acute low back pain: a retrospective review of patient records. J Am Osteopath Assoc. 2009;109:229–33.
5. Manchikanti L, Falco FJ, Singh V, et al. Utilization of interventional techniques in managing chronic pain in the Medicare population: analysis of growth patterns from 2000 to 2011. Pain Physician. 2012;15:E969–82.
6. Manchikanti L, Singh V, Cash KA, Pampati V, Datta S. A comparative effectiveness evaluation of percutaneous adhesiolysis and epidural steroid injections in managing lumbar post surgery syndrome: a randomized, equivalence controlled trial. Pain Physician. 2009;12:E355–68.
7. Manchikanti L, Singh V, Cash KA, Pampati V. Assessment of effectiveness of percutaneous adhesiolysis and caudal epidural injections in managing post lumbar surgery syndrome: 2-year follow-up of a randomized, controlled trial. J Pain Res. 2012;5:597–608.
8. Bonica JJ, Backup PH, Anderson CE, Hadfield D, Crepps WF, Monk BF. Peridural block: analysis of 3,637 cases and a review. Anesthesiology. 1957;18:723–84.
9. Talu GK, Erdine S. Complications of epidural neuroplasty: a retrospective evaluation. Neuromodulation. 2003;6:237–47.
10. Collier C. Epidural catheter breakage: a possible mechanism. Int J Obstet Anesth. 2000;9:87–93.
11. Dounas M, Peillon P, Lebonhomme JJ, et al. Difficulties in the removal and rupture of a peridural catheter. Ann Fr Anesth Reanim. 2002;21:600–2.
12. Asai T, Yamamoto K, Hirose T, Taguchi H, Shingu K. Breakage of epidural catheters: a comparison of an arrow reinforced catheter and other non-reinforced catheters. Anesth Analg. 2001;92:246–8.
13. Ates Y, Yücesoy CA, Ünlü MA, et al. The mechanical properties of intact and traumatized epidural catheters. Anesth Analg. 2000;90:393–9.
14. Boey SJ, Carrie LES. Withdrawal forces during removal of lumbar extradural catheters. Br J Anaesth. 1994;73:833–5.
15. Muneyuki M, Shirai K, Inamoto A. Roentgenographic analysis of the positions of catheters in the epidural space. Anesthesiology. 1970;33:19–24.
16. North RB, Cutchis PN, Epstein JA, Long DM. Spinal cord compression complicating subarachnoid infusion of morphine: case report and laboratory experience. Neurosurgery. 1991;29:778–84.
17. Murphy PM, Skouvaklis DE, Amadeo RJ, Haberman C, Brazier DH, Cousins MJ. Intrathecal catheter granuloma associated with isolated baclofen infusion. Anesth Analg. 2006;102:848–52.

18. Kang JH, Choi H, Kim JS, Lee MK, Park HJ. A sheared Racz catheter in cervical epidural space for thirty months: a case report. Korean J Anesthesiol. 2015;68(2):196–9.
19. Staats PS, Stinson MS, Lee RR. Lumbar stenosis complicating retained epidural catheter tip. Anesthesiology. 1995;83:1115–8.
20. Perkins WJ, Davis DH, Huntoon MA, Horlocker TT. A retained Racz catheter fragment after epidural neurolysis: implications during magnetic resonance imaging. Anesth Analg. 2003;96(6):1717–9.
21. Dam-Hieu P, Rodriguez V, De Cazes Y, Quinio B. Computed tomography images of entrapped epidural catheter. Reg Anesth Pain Med. 2002;27:517–9.
22. Moore DC, Artru AA, Kelly WA, Jenkins D. Use of computed tomography to locate a sheared epidural catheter. Anesth Analg. 1987;66:795–6.
23. Bridenbaugh PO, Wedel DJ. Complications of local anesthetic neural blockade. In: Cousins MJ, Bridenbaugh PO, editors. Neural blockade in clinical anesthesia and management of pain. Philadelphia: Lippincott-Raven; 1998. p. 639–6.

18 Epidural Abscess After Epidural Steroid Injection in a Patient on TNF-Alpha Inhibitors

Geeta Nagpal

18.1 Case Description

A 58-year-old female, who is known to the pain clinic, returns for follow-up of low back pain and radiating symptoms into her bilateral lower extremities. She has been treated for both sacroiliac (SI) joint dysfunction and lumbar radiculitis in the past. Her most recent intervention was a left SI joint injection that completely resolved her left buttock and groin pain. On presentation, she complains of her typical low back pain with radiation into the bilateral posterior thighs and into the calves. This acute exacerbation started about 3 weeks ago. She has been very dedicated to her home exercise plan, taking nonsteroidal anti-inflammatory drugs (NSAIDs) around the clock and gabapentin 600 mg TID. She saw her rheumatologist last week who prescribed a steroid taper. Her pain is relentless despite this multimodal conservative management.

On examination, she has a slow and non-antalgic gait (she uses a cane typically), full strength in the lower extremities, and reflexes and sensation are intact throughout. Review of her MRI from 2 years ago reveals the moderate spinal stenosis at the L4–L5 level with L4 on L5 spondylolisthesis. During routine inquiry for any other major changes in health or medications, she mentions that she is trying a new treatment for her rheumatoid arthritis. One month ago, her methotrexate was discontinued, and she started etanercept. She states that her functional status has improved because the pain in her hands, wrists, and shoulders is much better controlled.

Without complication, an L4–L5 epidural steroid injection is performed under fluoroscopic guidance using 80 mg depomedrol and 1 mL of 1% lidocaine. She has 100% immediate relief of her symptoms and is discharged in excellent condition.

Five days after her visit, she is taken to the Emergency Department at a local hospital because of a fall in the morning. She states she was going to the bathroom, her legs "gave out," and she fell backward and hit her head. She was down for 7 h before being able to call for assistance and did have an episode of urinary incontinence. She reports frequent falls at home but states that she is feeling weaker. She did not mention any recent injection. She denies fevers or chills but does endorse some low back pain, which seems worse than baseline. On exam, she has a temperature of 101.1, pulse of 122, blood pressure of 135/78, and respiratory rate of 16. Although she cannot walk, she has 5/5 strength on exam. She has some tenderness over the thoracic and lumbar spine to palpation. Her white blood cell count is 6.0 with a left neutrophil shift, and platelets are 50. She was admitted to the hospital with a diagnosis of lower extremity weakness and adult failure to thrive and was started on empiric antibiotic therapy. Given her fall, a computed tomography (CT) scan of the head and lumbar X-rays were ordered, which were negative for bleed or fracture, respectively. The following morning her neurologic exam reveals 4/5 strength throughout; she was unable to stand and complains of worsening back pain. An MRI (magnetic resonance imaging) of the lumbar and thoracic spine without contrast is ordered to rule out cauda equina. The MRI reveals a dorsal hyperintense lesion on T2-weighted images extending from L3 to T9. She is sent to the operating room for emergent decompression and is started on oxacillin for a methicillin-sensitive *Staphylococcus aureus* (MSSA)-positive epidural abscess. She has near full neurologic recovery with continued pain in the lower extremities.

Twelve weeks after discharge from a rehabilitation center, she returns to the pain clinic and states her left buttock and groin are starting to "act up" and asks for repeat SI joint injection.

G. Nagpal, M.D.
Department of Anesthesiology,
Northwestern University, Feinberg School of Medicine,
251 E Huron Street, Suite 5-704, Chicago, IL 60611, USA
e-mail: gnagpal@nm.org

M. Anitescu et al. (eds.), *Challenging Cases and Complication Management in Pain Medicine*,
https://doi.org/10.1007/978-3-319-60072-7_18

18.2 Case Discussion

18.2.1 TNF-Alpha Inhibitors

TNF is a naturally occurring pro-inflammatory cytokine that is pivotal in the normal inflammatory and immune responses [1]. Within the TNF family, TNF alpha and TNF beta are the most significant for signaling in the immune system [2]. TNF alpha is essential for the activation of macrophages and phagosomes, the recruitment of neutrophils, eosinophils, and macrophages, as well as the formation and maintenance of integrity of granulomas [3, 4]. TNF also stimulates synovial cells to proliferate and synthesize collagenase, which leads to the degradation of cartilage.

There are currently five TNF inhibitors approved by the US Food and Drug Administration (FDA): etanercept, infliximab, adalimumab, certolizumab pegol, and golimumab. All of these therapies inhibit TNF-alpha activity to varying degrees and by varying mechanisms, providing symptomatic and functional improvement in inflammatory conditions (Table 18.1).

Perhaps the most serious acute complication of treating patients with TNF-alpha inhibitors is the development of life-threatening infection. The risk of tuberculosis (TB) (primary infection or reactivation) is the most notorious infectious risk for TNF-alpha inhibitors. The association was noted a few years after the initial approval of infliximab in 1998 [5]. These biologics carry an FDA black box warning for physicians and patients, and current recommendations are to perform a chest X-ray and tuberculin skin test prior to and during the administration of these medications [6].

In a meta-analysis of nine randomized clinical trials of anti-TNF-alpha therapy (infliximab or adalimumab) in rheumatoid arthritis (RA), there was a reported 2.0 odds ratio for serious infection as compared to placebo [7]. This is similar to what was found with the German biologics register where the relative risk of serious infection was 2.2 for etanercept and 2.1 for infliximab compared to disease-modifying anti-rheumatic drugs (DMARDs) [8]. In an earlier study, a total of 60 charts were reviewed of patients with RA for 2 years prior to the start of anti-TNF-alpha therapy and for about 1 year during treatment. The incidence of serious infection preceding therapy was 0.008 versus 0.181 per anti-TNF-alpha treatment year [9].

Table 18.1 TNF-alpha inhibitors approved by the US Food and Drug Administration

Name of anti-TNF drug	Structure/mechanism of action
Infliximab	Chimeric (mouse/human) anti-TNF-alpha antibody
Etanercept	TNF-alpha receptor fusion protein
Adalimumab	Human TNF-alpha monoclonal anti-TNF-alpha antibody
Certolizumab pegol	Antigen-binding fragment (Fab) of human monoclonal antibody bound to polyethylene glycol
Golimumab	Human TNF-alpha monoclonal anti-TNF-alpha antibody

Analysis of the comprehensive national registry data of RA patients in the United Kingdom (UK) had differing results [10]. They compared the risk of serious infection in 8659 patients treated with anti-TNF-alpha agents with that of 2170 patients treated with traditional DMARDs. The rate of serious infection was 3.9 per 100 person-years in the DMARD cohort and 5.5 per 100 person-years in the anti-TNF-alpha group. However, after the adjustment for multiple comorbidities, sex and age, there was no significant difference in risk of infection between any of the anti-TNF-alpha cohorts and the comparison cohort.

This analysis compared the risk between the cohorts based upon an assumption of constant risk over time. This assumption has been shown to be incorrect [11]. Fu et al. analyzed the same database from the UK and found that the infection risk reaches a peak within the first month of use and then declines over the next 2 years until "stabilizing" [11]. Their analysis also suggests that patients are still at risk of developing serious infections outside of the "lag window" (the time after a patient is taken off of a drug but is still exposed to the effects of its therapy). In the case of most TNF-alpha inhibitors, this lag window is five half-lives, or 90 days.

Epidural abscess in patients on TNF-alpha inhibitors has been reported with patients on etanercept and infliximab; however, none of the reported cases were associated with epidural steroid injection [6, 12–15]. Three of the cases had no primary infection site where as one was thought secondary to a dental cleaning [12] and another from hematogenous seeding from a septic joint and cellulitis [13]. Epidural abscess is a rarely reported complication of epidural steroid injections, and the incidence remains undetermined [16]. With the paucity of reports of epidural abscess in patients on TNF-alpha inhibitors, we cannot recommend to abstain from injection therapy. However, one may consider postponing injection therapy in the setting of a patient recently starting an anti-TNF drug, as in the case of our patient.

18.2.2 Spinal Epidural Abscess

18.2.2.1 Epidemiology and Risk Factors

Spinal epidural abscess (SEA) is a surgical emergency that requires prompt diagnosis and treatment. It is generally a pyogenic infection and space-occupying lesion in the epidural space that causes neurologic sequel, including pain, paresthesias, paralysis, and even death. Bacteria can access the epidural space by direct extension from infected surroundings or, more commonly, from hematogenous seeding [17]. Abscesses can be located in the anterior or posterior space causing neurologic compromise from either direct compression or thrombosis of the vasculature. Spontaneous epidural abscess is rare, accounting for 0.2–2 cases per 10,000 hospital admissions per year [18, 19]. The incidence after central nerve block is quite varied and reported as 1:1000–1:100,000 [19]. In the literature, there is a definite prevalence for males with a male/female ratio of 1:0.56 [18].

In a meta-analysis of 915 patients with SEA, only 6% were attributed to either epidural anesthesia, injections in the epidural space, or spinal anesthesia [18]. The majority of patients will present with an identifiable source such as skin and soft tissue infections, indwelling catheters, frequent venous puncture, or spinal trauma/procedure.

Patients at increased risk of infection are more likely to develop an epidural abscess. Known risk factors for spinal epidural abscess are [18]:

1. Compromised immunity: diabetes mellitus, immunosuppressive therapy, malignancy, pregnancy, HIV infection, cirrhosis, and alcohol abuse
2. Disruption of the spinal column: degenerative disk disease, surgery, neuraxial blocks, and blunt trauma
3. Source of infection: respiratory, urinary tract, soft tissue, IV drug users, and patients with indwelling catheters

18.2.2.2 Clinical Manifestations

As with many infectious processes, the initial manifestations of a spinal epidural abscess can be vague and nonspecific, presenting as malaise and fever. The diagnosis can be a challenge as it is quite rare among patients presenting with back pain. In a retrospective review of 46 patients who were diagnosed with SEA over a 10-year period, 89% had spinal pain, 67% had fever and chills, 57% had radicular pain, 37% had bowel or bladder dysfunctions, and 80% had paralysis (paraparesis, paraplegia) [20]. In an analysis of 871 patients, 71% had back pain, 66% had fever, 24% had incontinence, and 31% had paraplegia/paraparesis [18]. The combination of severe back pain as well as fever should be regarded as an early warning of SEA.

18.2.2.3 Clinical Examination

Fever and pain on palpation or) percussion may be noted. The neurological exam can be variable as the epidural abscess progresses. The clinical exam should include muscle strength testing, sensory testing, reflexes, and rectal exam.

18.2.2.4 Laboratory Studies

The laboratory findings that are markers for severe inflammation or infection may accompany SEA; however, they are not all specific: leukocytosis, erythrocyte sedimentation rate (ESR), C-reactive protein (CPR), and thrombocytopenia. Patients presenting with an abscess will frequently have a leukocytosis [18, 20]. In a prospective study in Emergency Department patients, Davis et al. found that a treatment algorithm that incorporated risk factor assessment followed by erythrocyte sedimentation rate (ESR) and c-reactive protein (CRP) testing was highly sensitive and moderately specific for identifying patients with SEA [21]. They found the sensitivity and specificity for those with risk factors pointing toward SEA to be 100% and 67%, respectively. The mean CRP level was significantly higher in SEA patients than those with risk factor who were non-SEA. They found the rate of delayed diagnosis drops 80% after the implementation of this protocol.

While thrombocytopenia is not sensitive or specific for the diagnosis, it may be a risk factor for poor outcome [20]. The low platelet count, as seen in our patient, implies sepsis and the commencement of disseminated intravascular coagulation, thus more likely resulting in greater morbidity.

Lumbar puncture comes with significant risk, such as spread of the infection to the CSF and meninges. While it could yield information from the analysis of the CSF or even pus, radiologic imaging is preferred [19].

18.2.2.5 Radiologic Studies

The plain film yields little utility in the initial evaluation of SEA, providing useful information in about 20% of cases [19]. However, abnormalities of the end plate should not be ignored as they can point toward an associated osteomyelitis [22]. A myelogram will reliably demonstrate a space-occupying lesion, but the same risks of lumbar puncture apply. While the computed tomography (CT) scan used to be the imaging modality of choice, the MRI is now the gold standard. Some recommend a full spinal MRI in the evaluation of suspected SEA [23]. The sensitivity of MRI is 91% compared to 92% with CT myelography [18]. However, MRI can be done without intervention and in all planes without moving a patient who may have neurologic compromise. It can also detect spinal and paraspinal infections [19]. The MR images will reveal a T1 hypointense and T2 hyperintense mass in the epidural space (Figs. 18.1 and 18.2). Gadolinium enhance-

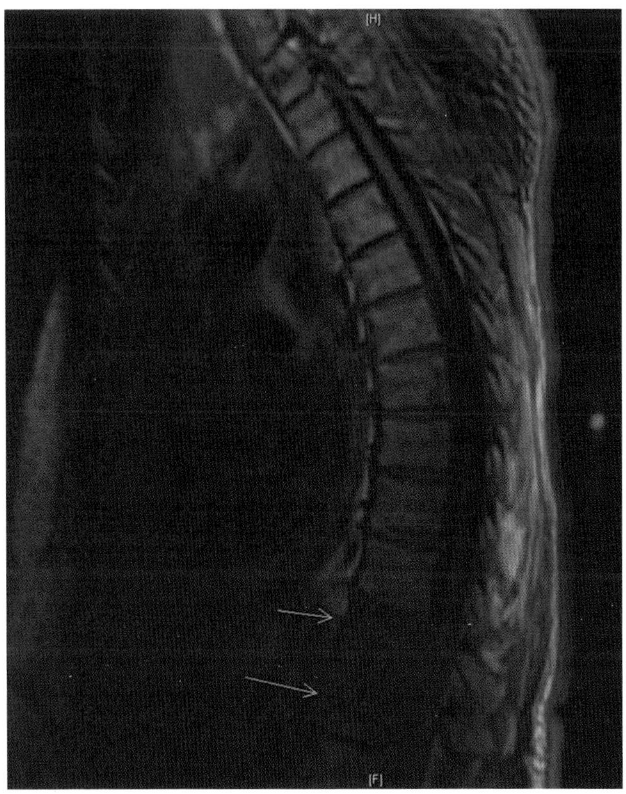

Fig. 18.1 Sagittal plane, T1-weighted image where the epidural abscess in a hypointense mass at the T11–T12 level

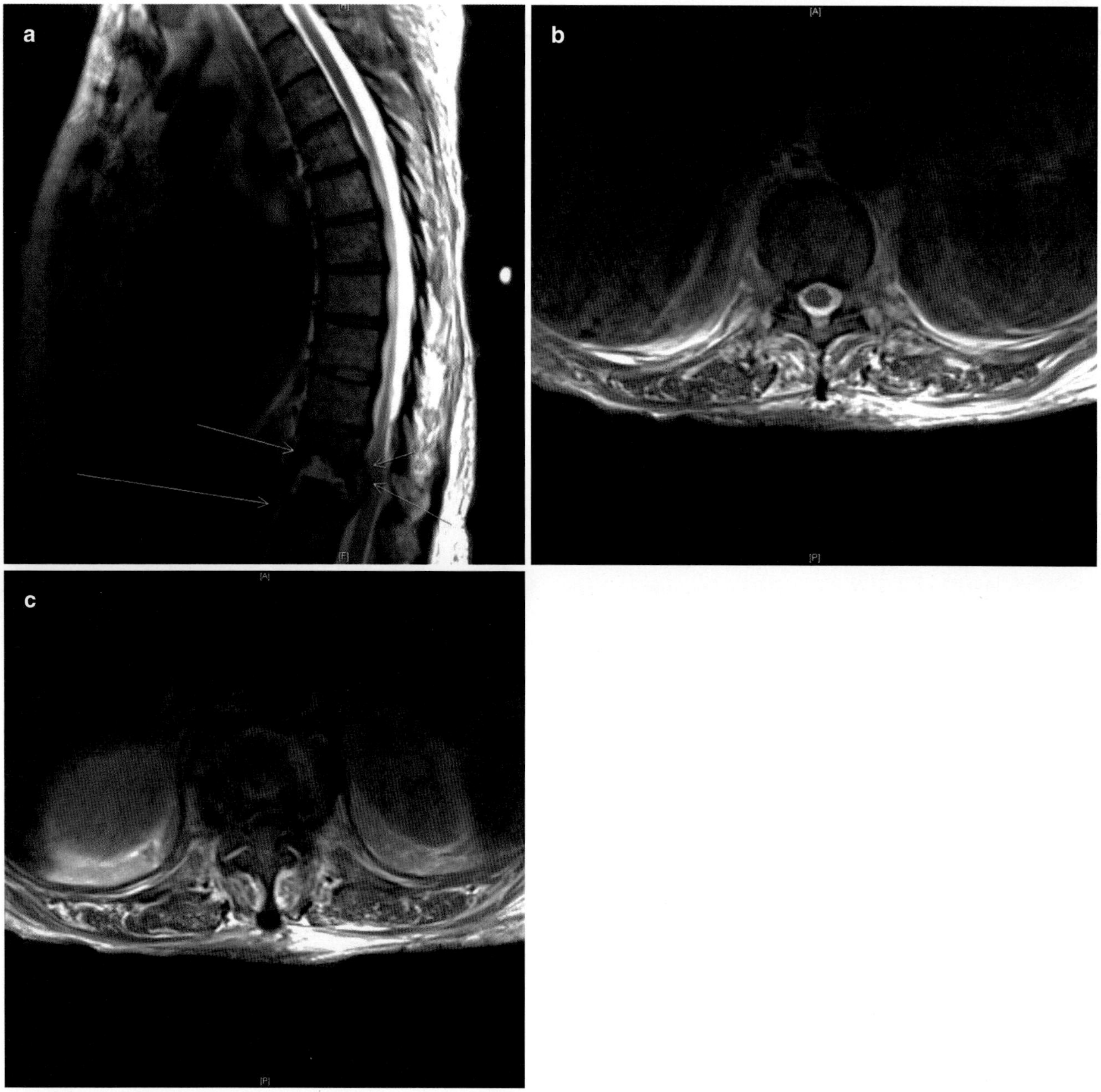

Fig. 18.2 (**a**) Sagittal plane, T2 weighted showing diskitis-osteomyelitis at T11–T12, with extension of an abscess into the epidural space circumferentially and severe canal compromise. (**b**) Axial plane, T2 weighted at the T10–T11 level where there is no evidence of epidural abscess or canal compromise. (**c**) Axial plane, T2 weighted at the T11–T12 level where the epidural abscess is causing severe canal compromise

ment increases sensitivity and gives a better differentiation between the abscess and the surrounding neurologic structures (Fig. 18.3).

18.2.2.6 Treatment

"Ubi pus, ibi evacua" (Where there is pus, there evacuate it).

SEA treatment calls for reduction in size and elimination of the causative organism, usually accomplished by a combination of aspiration, drainage, and antibiotic therapy. In a retrospective review of 128 cases of SEA, the authors found that early surgical decompression improved neurologic outcomes compared to surgical treatment delayed by medical management. In this study, over 40% of the patients that initially started with medical management failed and required a surgical intervention [24]. The conclusion of the majority of the articles in the literature is to evacuate the abscess [18].

If surgery is not feasible because of patient comorbidities, or the rare case of patient refusal, medical therapy can be

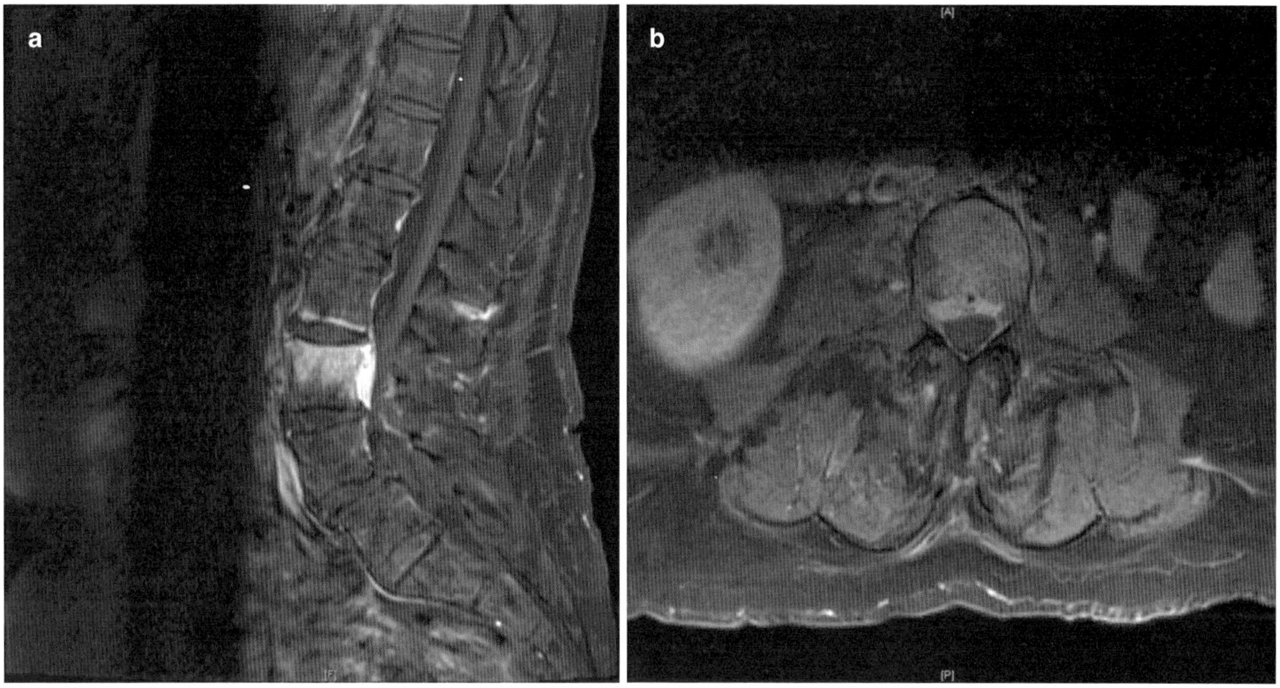

Fig. 18.3 (**a**) Sagittal post-gadolinium image with edema and enhancement within the superior two thirds of the L3 vertebral body and inferior one third of the L2 vertebral body. There is extension of enhancement into the ventral epidural space at the L3 level. (**b**) Axial post-gadolinium image with extension of abscess in the ventral epidural space

instituted. There is a case series of 38 patients that had successful outcomes with medical management only, all of which had the causative organism recovered from cultures [25]. Other studies have mixed results with either no significant difference in the medical versus surgical group or significantly worse outcome in the medical group [26, 27]. The interpretation of this data is important as successful cases are more likely to be published as case reports and those in medical groups have varying comorbidities and reasons for delaying surgery. If medical therapy is chosen, there must be intensive neurologic monitoring, follow-up imaging to confirm the regression of the abscess, and immediate surgical decompression if there is neurologic decline.

18.2.2.7 Antimicrobial Therapy

From a meta-analysis and systematic review of SEA, the most common pathogen found in either blood or tissue culture was *S. aureus* (~65%), gram-negative bacteria (8.1%), coagulase-negative *Staphylococcus* (7.5%), and *Streptococcus* species (6.8%) [18, 28]. Antibiotics should be directed against the known pathogen. If an aspirate cannot be obtained, an empiric regimen with antibiotics active against staphylococci, streptococci, and gram-negative bacilli is reasonable. A common parenteral regimen includes vancomycin, metronidazole, and either cefotaxime or ceftriaxone. If cultures return and the *S. aureus* is methicillin-sensitive, the vancomycin should be replaced with an agent that has better central nervous system (CNS) penetration, such as oxacillin, as in the case of our patient. Patients are often treated for 6–8 weeks with parenteral antimicrobial therapy. An MRI should be done if further neurologic progression is noted but is otherwise performed at 4–6 weeks post initiation of treatment.

18.2.2.8 Prognosis

Early diagnosis and treatment of SEA greatly decreased the morbidity and mortality associated with the disease. With diagnostic imaging, mycrobacterial therapy, and heightened physician awareness, the mortality rate has dropped from 34% in the 1950s to about 15% in the 1990s [18, 27]. However, the percentage of patients that achieve full neurologic recovery is less than 50% [27]. Neurologic recovery is related to the duration of neurologic deficit, only emphasizing the importance of early diagnosis. Neurologic recovery is unlikely if paralysis is present for greater than 24 h prior to surgical decompression [28].

Conclusion

Spinal epidural abscess is a medical emergency, often with a delayed diagnosis, and can be associated with catastrophic and permanent neurologic damage. While there are some small series of cases reported, it remains a rare complication of epidural steroid injections. A known risk factor for developing SEA is an immunocompromised state. While biologic response modifiers seem to carry an increased risk of infection, we cannot report on this risk in the setting of epidural steroid injections. Any immunocompromised patient, including those on TNF-alpha inhibitor therapy, should be identified prior to treatment, and the small, but possibly devastating, complications should be carefully weighed against the potential benefit of the procedure. These patients should also have a thorough understanding of the signs and symptoms of infection to help decrease the time between diagnosis and before irreversible neurological symptoms occur.

Key Concepts

- Epidural abscess of the spinal column is a rare condition that can lead to significant morbidity and mortality.
- Risk factors for epidural abscess include immunocompromised states such as diabetes mellitus, alcoholism, cancer, acquired immunodeficiency syndrome, as well as spinal procedures, surgery, and trauma.
- The signs and symptoms of SEA can be nonspecific and range from low back discomfort to sepsis. Prompt diagnosis is based on history, physical exam, and imaging techniques.
- The mainstays of treatment typically include surgical decompression and 4–6 weeks of antibiotic therapy.
- TNF-alpha inhibitors have been shown to increase likelihood of infection, but it is unknown if this is clinically significant in the setting of epidural steroid injections.

References

1. Scott L. Etanercept: a review of its use in autoimmune inflammatory diseases. Drugs. 2014;74:1379–410.
2. Doss GP, Agoramoorthy G, Chakraborty C. TNF/TNFR: drug target for autoimmune and immune-mediated inflammatory diseases. Front Biosci (Landmark Ed). 2014;19:1028–40.
3. Koo S, Marty FM, Baden L. Infectious complications associated with immunomodulating biologic agents. Hematol Oncol Clin North Am. 2010;25(1):117–38.
4. Strangfeld A, Listing J. Infection and musculoskeletal conditions: bacterial and opportunistic infections during anti-TNF therapy. Best Pract Res Clin Rheumatol. 2006;20(6):118–95.
5. Keane J, Gershon S, Wise RP, et al. Tuberculosis associated with infliximab, a tumor necrosis factor alpha-neutralizing agent. N Engl J Med. 2001;345:1098.
6. Darabi K, Jaiswal R, Hostetler S, et al. Infectious complications in patients with psoriasis and rheumatoid arthritis treated with antitumor necrosis factor agents and methotrexate. J Drugs Dermatol. 2009;8(2):175–8.
7. Bongartz T, Sutton AJ, Sweeting MJ, et al. Anti-TNF antibody therapy in rheumatoid arthritis and the risk of serious infections and malignancies: systemic review and meta-analysis of rare harmful effects in randomized control trials. JAMA. 2006;295:2275–85.
8. Listing J, Strangfeld A, Kary S, et al. Infections in patients with rheumatoid arthritis treated with biologic agents. Arthritis Rheum. 2005;52:3403.
9. Kroesen S, Widner AF, Tyndall A, Hasler P. Serious bacterial infections in patients with rheumatoid arthritis under anti-TNF-alpha therapy. Rheumatology. 2003;42(5):617–21.
10. Dixon WG, Symmons DP, Lunt M, et al. Serious infection following anti-tumor necrosis factor alpha therapy in patients with rheumatoid arthritis: lessons from interpreting data from observational studies. Arthritis Rheum. 2007;56:2896.
11. Fu B, Lunt M, Galloway J, et al. A threshold hazard model for estimating serious infection risk following anti-tumor necrosis factor therapy in rheumatoid arthritis patients. J Biopharm Stat. 2013;23:461–7.
12. Darley MD, Saad D, Haydoura S, et al. Spinal epidural abscess following minimally invasive dental examination in a rheumatoid arthritis patient receiving methotrexate, glucocorticoids, and antitumor necrosis factor therapy. J Clin Rheumatol. 2015;21(1):52–3.
13. Rose AM, Barnett J, Morris-Jones S, et al. *Staphylococcus lugdunensis* septic arthritis and epidural abscess in a patient with rheumatoid arthritis receiving anti-tumor necrosis factor therapy. Rheumatology (Oxford). 2014;53(12):2231.
14. Vasoo S, Gurnanu P, Agustin T, et al. Chest pain as presenting symptom of *Staphylococcus aureus* epidural abscess associated with anti-tumor necrosis factor therapy. J Clin Rheumatol. 2009;15(8):39608.
15. Smith AP, Musacchio MJ, O'Toole JE, et al. Spinal epidural abscess associated with infliximab treatment for psoriatic arthritis. Case report. J Neurosurg Spine. 2008;9(3):261–4.
16. Hooten WM, Kinney MO, Huntoon MA, et al. Epidural abscess and meningitis after epidural corticosteroid injection. Mayo Clin Proc. 2004;79(5):682–6.
17. Diehn FE. Imaging of spine infection. Radiol Clin North Am. 2012;50(4):777–98.
18. Reihsaus E, Waldbaur H, Seeling W. Spinal epidural abscess: a meta-analysis of 915 patients. Neurosurg Rev. 2000;232:175–204.
19. Grewel S, Hocking G, Wildsmith JAW. Epidural abscesses. Br J Anaesth. 2006;96(3):292–302.
20. Tang HJ, Lin HJ, Liu YC, et al. Spinal epidural abscess—experience with 46 patients and evaluation of prognostic factors. J Infect. 2002;45:76–81.
21. Davis D, Salazar A, Chan T, et al. Prospective evaluation of a clinical decision guideline to diagnose spinal epidural abscess in patients who present to the emergency department with spine pain. J Neurosurg Spine. 2011;14(6):765.
22. Felton B, Dao T, Gerstner B, Letarte S. Diagnosis of spinal epidural abscess by abdominal-film radiography. West J Emerg Med. 2014;15(7):885–6.
23. Tompkins M, Panuncialman I, Lucas P, et al. Spinal epidural abscess. J Emerg Med 2010; 39(3): 384–90
24. Patel A, Alton T, Bransford R, et al. Spinal epidural abscesses: risk factors, medical vs. surgical management, a retrospective review of 128 cases. Spine J. 2014;14:326–30.
25. Wheeler D, Keiser P, Rigamonti D, Keay S. Medical management of spinal epidural abscesses: case report and review. Clin Infect Dis. 1992;15:22.
26. Siddiq F, Chowfin A, Tight R, et al. Medical vs. surgical management of spinal epidural abscess. Arch Intern Med. 2004;164:2409.
27. Curry WT Jr, Hoh BL, Amin-Hanjani S, Eskandar EN. Spinal epidural abscess: clinical presentation, management, and outcome. Surg Neurol. 2005;63:364.
28. Arko L IV, Quach E, Nguyen V, Chang D, Sukul V, Kim BS. Medical and surgical management of spinal epidural abscess: a systematic review. Neurosurg Focus. 2014;37(2):E4.

Part III

Interventional Pain Procedures: Sympathetic Chain Blocks and Neurolysis

Stroke: A Complication of Stellate Ganglion Block

19

Ariana Nelson

19.1 Case Description

A 56-year-old male presented for initial evaluation at a pain clinic associated with a tertiary care center. Three months prior he suffered a work-related crush injury and now carries a diagnosis of CRPS in the distal portion of the left upper extremity. The patient reported severe pain that is burning in quality in the forearm and left hand. Pain is described as constant and exacerbated by any contact, even the touch of clothing against his skin. He noted the skin on his left hand occasionally becomes mottled, swollen, or cold compared to his other hand. Since the injury, the hair on his fingers had become increasingly longer and darker as compared to the other hand. When asked about differences in sweating, he reported that he has not noted any changes, but he avoids sweating as heat can exacerbate his pain. On physical exam his left upper extremity below the mid-forearm fit the description of the patient. He exhibited hyperalgesia and allodynia in non-dermatomal distribution. He was reluctant to participate in motor examination as he was severely limited by pain. Additionally, the left forearm was 2 °C cooler than the right upper limb. The patient had exhausted conservative measures and was scheduled for follow-up visit to undergo a SGB.

At his follow-up appointment, the patient presented appropriately NPO with a driver present to transport him home. For safety purposes, a 20 gauge IV was placed in the right hand. The patient walked to the procedure room and was positioned supine with slight neck extension to improve exposure of the stellate ganglion and move the esophagus medially underneath the trachea. Ultrasound was used to identify the carotid sheath, the longus colli muscle, and the anterior tubercle of the sixth cervical vertebrae (Chassaignac's tubercle) on the patient's left side. Using sterile technique and under direct ultrasound guidance, a needle was advanced to the plane between the posterolateral surface of the longus colli muscle and the prevertebral fascia covering the posterior aspect of the carotid sheath. The proceduralist began to inject 0.5% bupivacaine, but during injection of the initial 2 mL by the assistant, the patient swallowed, and the needle tip was no longer visualized on the ultrasound screen. Aspiration after the patient returned to a motionless state revealed a trace of blood. The needle was removed, and within seconds the patient became unresponsive to commands and completely apneic, although his eyes remained open. His heart rate decreased to 45 bpm and the systolic BP decreased to 70 mmHg. Resuscitation efforts were initiated, including mask ventilation and administration of atropine, and an endotracheal airway was placed within 2 min of onset of symptoms. One liter of normal saline was rapidly infused, and the patient was ventilated using 100% oxygen. The patient's hemodynamic parameters improved, and within 5 min the patient was following commands, and the artificial airway could be removed. When the patient had completely recovered from the event, he reported that after he swallowed during the procedure, he experienced tinnitus and what he described as "fireworks" in his eyes. He lost the ability to move any of his muscles or speak, and he could no longer take breaths. He stated he was conscious during the entire episode and could see and hear all that had taken place. During the episode, he had a profound sense of foreboding and reported that he did believe at the time that he would die. He was observed for 3 h in the clinic recovery area without further incident and then discharged home.

A. Nelson, M.D.
Department of Anesthesiology and Perioperative Care, UC Irvine School of Medicine, Irvine, CA 92697, USA
e-mail: arianamn@uci.edu

M. Anitescu et al. (eds.), *Challenging Cases and Complication Management in Pain Medicine*,
https://doi.org/10.1007/978-3-319-60072-7_19

19.2 Case Discussion

19.2.1 Complex Regional Pain Syndrome (CRPS)

Historically known as reflex sympathetic dystrophy or causalgia, CPRS is a constellation of signs and symptoms that occurs after major or minor trauma. The defining symptom is pain, but the affected region will also demonstrate abnormalities in the sensory, vasomotor, sudomotor, and motor systems.

19.2.1.1 Etiology and Pathogenesis

If the pain and associated symptoms of CRPS begin after demonstrable damage to a nerve, as evidenced by EMG or other definitive evidences, then the syndrome is categorized as CRPS type II (previously known as causalgia). If symptoms develop without an injury or after a minor trauma that results in symptoms markedly worse than expected from the injury, it is termed CRPS type I (previously known as reflex sympathetic dystrophy) [1]. Recent neurophysiological research has revealed a complex pathophysiology that results in the clinical disease state. The most significant components of the maladaptive pain state include neurogenic inflammation, cytokine release, sympathetically mediated pain, and reorganization of cortical structures in response to the constant painful stimulus, which is known as neuroplasticity [2].

19.2.1.2 Diagnostic Criteria

Although a defining characteristic of CRPS is pain, the patient must also exhibit sensory/motor and autonomic signs and symptoms to truly warrant a diagnosis of CRPS. A new set of diagnostic criteria, known as the Budapest Criteria, was recently proposed by a group of experts (Table 19.1). The criteria differ from those recommended by the International Association for the Study of Pain and have been widely adopted by clinicians and researchers alike. A diagnosis of CRPS most importantly requires a report of pain that is disproportionate to any injury incurred and that cannot be explained by any other etiologies. After these criteria have been met, the patient must also then report a symptom in three of four categories: sensory, vasomotor, sudomotor/edema, and motor/trophic. At the time of evaluation, a medical provider must also identify an objective sign on physical exam in two of four categories: sensory, vasomotor, sudomotor/edema, and motor/trophic. Of note, these are the criteria for clinical diagnosis. Diagnosis of the condition for research purposes requires that the patient report one symptom in each of the four categories and demonstrate one sign in at least two categories. These differing guidelines were established to ensure that the criteria are sufficiently sensitive for a clinical diagnosis, but adopt a better relative balance between sensitivity and specificity as is suitable for use in research studies [3].

Table 19.1 Budapest Criteria for clinical diagnosis of chronic regional pain syndrome [3]

1. Patient reports pain that is disproportionate to that which is expected given the injury		
2. Subjective symptoms (must report 3 of 4 categories)	Sensory	Hyperesthesia Allodynia
	Vasomotor	Temperature asymmetry Skin color changes Skin color asymmetry
	Sudomotor/edema	Edema Sweating changes Sweating asymmetry
	Motor/trophic	Decreased range of motion Motor dysfunction (weakness, tremor, dystonia) Trophic changes (hair, nail, skin)
3. Objective signs (must exhibit 2 of 4 categories)	Sensory	Hyperalgesia Allodynia
	Vasomotor	Temperature asymmetry Skin color changes Asymmetry
	Sudomotor/edema	Edema Sweating changes Sweating asymmetry
	Motor/trophic	Decreased range of motion Motor dysfunction (weakness, tremor, dystonia) Trophic changes (hair, nail, skin)
4. No other diagnosis better explains the signs and symptoms		

19.2.1.3 Subtypes of CRPS

The first subtype of CRPS patients have a fairly limited pain component to their syndrome and have strong vasomotor signs as the main concern. The second type is also relatively limited, respectively, in terms of pain and demonstrates neuropathic pain/sensory abnormalities as the principal feature. The third and most functionally limiting subtype is the most similar to the classic descriptions of reflex sympathetic dystrophy wherein the patients have very severe pain and are extremely limited in functional status [4].

19.2.2 Treatment

The input of multiple different therapists and use of multimodal analgesic medications are two mainstays of the treatment plan for a patient with CRPS. The concept of functional restoration has always been a foundation of treatment for patients that have CRPS. Outside of actual reduction in reported pain score, functional recovery is often considered the most critical component of interdisciplinary pain management programs for CRPS. Various types of therapy are employed, and the therapists may use multiple techniques to achieve treatment goals. Outside of these less invasive treatments, several procedures exist that often ease the pain of CRPS and may be used concomitantly with medications and therapies for optimum benefit. It has long been established that optimal treatment of neuropathic pain and CRPS is through multimodal treatment that includes behavioral and physical therapies, pharmacotherapies, injection therapy, and psychotherapy, if indicated [1, 5, 6].

19.2.2.1 Therapies

Reanimation: The concept of emphasizing physical activity in the patient, given that commonly patients with CRPS are reluctant to move or permit manipulation of their affected limb, is vital to rehabilitation. As a corollary to this, immobilization is a poor prognostic sign, and pain programs must emphasize movement in CRPS patients as even healthy individuals will develop pain symptoms after prolonged immobilization [7]. Several therapy techniques aid in achieving reanimation.

Physical therapy: PT has long been a critical component of functional restoration, but it is used in conjunction with other therapies. It is often a first-line treatment of CRPS, and concomitant sympathetic nerve blocks may be used to improve the ability of the patient to participate in physical therapy and regain function [8]. PT may be intensive and can include desensitization, aerobic physical therapy, or hydrotherapy. Often it is supplemented by cognitive behavioral therapy. This has been shown to be particularly effective in treating childhood CRPS, reducing the rate of long-term dysfunction [9].

Graded motor imagery: This is one of the therapies with very strong evidence from multiple clinical trials that support its efficacy in CRPS patients. Graded motor imagery exercises are mental in nature and consist of three different components [10]:

1. *Laterality training*: The patient is presented with a picture of a limb and will answer as quickly as possible as to the laterality and view of the limb shown in the image. These can range in difficulty, from a completely visible limb to one that is almost entirely obscured or out of frame.
2. *Explicit motor imagery*: The therapist will show the patient an image of a healthy limb executing an activity that the patient is unable to perform. The patient is encouraged to imagine performing the activity. This can be quite traumatic for patients with severe CRPS; therefore, it is recommended to start with an unaffected limb and to move from a proximal point to a more distal point on the extremity.
3. *Mirror feedback therapy*: Patient will be seated such that a mirror is at the midline of their body obstructing the view of the affected limb and reflecting a mirror image of the benign limb. The patient is then encouraged to move the healthy limb, and due to neuroplasticity the brain can better adapt to the affected limb performing the same movements without pain.

These three components used for an intensive 2-week period can reduce pain in a statistically significant manner even in patients with long-standing intractable CRPS [11].

Occupational therapy: Occupational therapists (OTs) will evaluate the patient's initial active range of motion, edema, coordination, dexterity, and ability to use the extremity during activities of daily living. This therapy may also utilize mirror visual feedback in an attempt to desensitize the patient to performing normal activities. Additionally, OTs often use a stress-loading program to improve the patient's ability to use the affected limb for activities requiring strength or contact with substances causing pain [12]. In severe cases of CRPS, e.g., subtype 3, patients may need desensitization therapy with OT in order to tolerate the touch of clothing on the affected skin surfaces. If the patient is limited in even relatively benign activities due to pain, a sympathetic nerve block may assist in enabling the patient to participate in therapy [13].

Recreational therapy: In particularly recalcitrant cases of CRPS, recreational therapy is an attractive option to engage the patient in activity to break their phobia of movement or contact. If planned appropriately, recreational therapy may incorporate the goals of the physical therapist and occupational therapist [14].

Vocational rehabilitation: This is an advanced level rehabilitation therapy in which the patient is prepared for return to work. Alternatively it is termed "work hardening." The vocational rehabilitation specialist must work closely with the patient to fully understand the physical demands of the patient's prior occupation. Although it is utilized late in the rehabilitation process, vocational rehabilitation should also be addressed early on to ensure that the final goal of return to work is constantly the focus of the patient's therapeutic process. The therapist may also work with the patient's employer in an attempt to optimize the workplace for any new limitations the patient may possess [15].

19.2.2.2 Medications

A handful of medications have been evaluated in randomized controlled trials (RCTs) specifically for use in CRPS, but the majority of medications prescribed for the disease state have only been evaluated in other neuropathic syndromes.

Anti-inflammatory Drugs

Oral corticosteroids have level 1 evidence demonstrating benefit in CRPS. However, these trials typically took place in early acute cases of the disease, at which time inflammation is a common pathophysiologic factor [16]. There are no trials regarding corticosteroid use in chronic CRPS. Other nonsteroidal anti-inflammatory medications (NSAIDs) have only been trialed in neuropathic pain and only in small clinical trials. Specific NSAIDs may be more beneficial in treating CRPS, an example of this being ketoprofen. Celecoxib, a COX-2 inhibitor, and infliximab, a tumor necrosis factor inhibitor, both have some degree of evidence demonstrating their efficacy in CRPS [17, 18].

Antiepileptic Medications

Gabapentin has shown efficacy in the treatment of neuropathies and has strong anecdotal evidence regarding its benefit in CRPS patients [19]. Carbamazepine showed considerable benefit in a randomized controlled trial when used in doses of 600 mg per day for an 8-day course in patients with CRPS [20]. Other related medications such as oxcarbazepine, phenytoin, and lamotrigine also showed some benefit in neuropathic processes but are not as widely prescribed for CRPS [1].

Antidepressants

Tricyclic antidepressants are among the most widely prescribed medications for neuropathic conditions. Although they have not been specifically studied for CRPS, multiple RCTs support their use in neuropathies, and as a consequence they are widely prescribed for CRPS [21]. Serotonin/norepinephrine reuptake inhibitors have shown some benefit in neuropathies, but none have been studied in CRPS patients. Selective serotonin reuptake inhibitors do not show analgesic benefit in any pain state, neuropathic, or otherwise [1].

N-Methyl-D-aspartate (NMDA) Receptor Antagonists

Ketamine is often prescribed for CRPS, either in oral or IV form. Currently level 4 evidence exists for its use in CRPS [22, 23], but its widespread use is limited by its abuse potential and toxicity at therapeutic doses. Ketamine has shown benefit in both oral form and after IV infusion [24].

Opioids

Opioids are not typically recommended for CRPS. Few randomized controlled trials exist, but given the neuropathic nature of CRPS, the disease state does not seem to respond to opioid therapy as reliably as patients with nociceptive pain. When considering opioid therapy for a CRPS patient, optimal choices include methadone or tramadol, due to the NMDA antagonism and serotonin/norepinephrine reuptake, respectively, of the two agents [22, 23].

Topical Analgesics/Local Anesthetics

Capsaicin cream has shown promising results when used topically in areas affected by CRPS, but given that it causes an initial burning pain prior to the desensitization of the nerve fibers, patient adherence tends to be poor. Lidocaine and clonidine are also prescribed as they have shown pain benefit in neuropathic conditions; however, they have not been studied expressly in patients with a CRPS diagnosis [18]. Similarly, although not studied in CRPS, IV lidocaine has also been shown to reduce hyperalgesia and allodynia in patients with neuropathic pain [5].

Antihypertensives

Nifedipine, a calcium channel blocker often used for cardiac disorders, has demonstrated weak evidence for utility in management of CRPS. Clonidine, which is a more common medication for pain states, is an alpha-2 adrenergic agonist and has shown no benefit in CRPS according to a systematic review [16].

Anti-osteoporotic Medications

Calcitonin, which is produced by the thyroid and is instrumental in bone growth, has been shown in several randomized controlled trials to improve pain scores in CRPS patients. However, other trials have revealed conflicting results. Bisphosphonates, another medication commonly used to treat osteoarthritis, slows bone resorption and has shown significant improvement in pain in CRPS patients. Although level 2 evidence supports the use of bisphosphonates for pain in CRPS, the effect of the drug on the symptom of osteopenia that so commonly accompanies late-stage CRPS has not been studied [1].

Intravenous Immunoglobulin

Immunoglobulin G is a human blood product component that consists of immunomodulating peptides and antibodies that act against not only exogenous antigens but also many normal human proteins. Intravenous immunoglobulin G has been shown to decrease pain scores when administered to patients with CRPS [25].

19.2.3 Stellate Ganglion Block

19.2.3.1 Anatomy

Fusion of the inferior cervical and first thoracic ganglia forms the stellate ganglion, which is only present in 80% of the population and provides sympathetic innervation to the upper extremities, head, and neck. With a pure stellate ganglion block, a majority of the sympathetic nerves of the upper extremity will be blocked, but anomalous pathways exist that bypass the ganglion. These pathways, known as Kuntz's nerves, are responsible for the incomplete nature of sympathetic blockade if a pure stellate ganglion block is performed without blockade of the second and third thoracic ganglia [26]. The stellate ganglion itself is usually 1–2.5 cm long, 1 cm wide, and 0.5 cm thick near the level of the C7 vertebrae. Although its location may vary, it is most often at the lateral border of the longus colli muscle (LCM) in the region anterior to the first rib and posterior to the vertebral vessels [27]. Therefore, the stellate ganglion is located in close proximity to various fragile soft tissue structures, which is responsible for the increasing popularity of ultrasound guidance as compared to the blind or even fluoroscopic techniques. Vulnerable soft tissues in the vicinity of the stellate ganglion include the esophagus, recurrent laryngeal nerve, pleural space, subarachnoid and epidural spaces, thyroid artery, and vertebral artery.

The vertebral artery consists of four segments. The first section stems from the subclavian artery and travels superiorly to the transverse foramen of the C6 vertebral body. At this point, the second segment begins and passes through the transverse foramina of C6–C2 vertebral bodies. The C2 level delineates the beginning of the third segment of the vertebral artery, which exits the C2 foramen and courses posteriorly to enter the dura at the foramen magnum. The fourth portion of the vertebral artery is entirely intracranial and spans from the foramen magnum to the basilar artery, where it joins the contralateral vertebral artery [28]. SGB requires needle manipulation in a position that is very near in the second segment of the vertebral artery. As this artery has wide anatomic variability, the distribution of stroke symptoms may differ for any patient that suffers an injury. However, the insult may fall into two broad categories: (1) CNS toxicity from direct injection of local anesthetic to the blood supply or (2) vertebral injury/spasm causing decreased blood flow to critical central nervous system structures.

19.2.3.2 Indications

Although SGB is most commonly performed for CRPS of the upper extremities, researchers continue to discover novel indications for the technique. Currently the procedure is performed for vascular diseases of the upper extremity, lymphatic dysfunction following mastectomy, vasomotor insufficiency due to menopause ("hot flashes"), PTSD of various etiologies, hearing loss or tinnitus, cardiac arrhythmias, postherpetic neuralgia, phantom limb pain, Bell's palsy, trigeminal neuralgia, and other neuropathic pain of the head and neck [26, 29, 30].

19.2.3.3 Procedure

Stellate ganglion blocks may be performed blind or with image guidance, either fluoroscopic or ultrasound. When using the blind approach, the proceduralist will palpate for the anterior tubercle of the transverse process of the C6 vertebrae (Chassaignac's tubercle). The sternocleidomastoid is then retracted with two fingers, which draws the internal jugular vein and the carotid artery lateral to the target, and the needle is inserted between the fingertips [26]. With fluoroscopic guidance, the procedure is similar, but the site for insertion can be more precisely determined, and the use of contrast more reliably rules out intravascular/epidural injection as compared to aspiration alone. The trachea and carotid artery are separated by the proceduralist using constant manual pressure from the

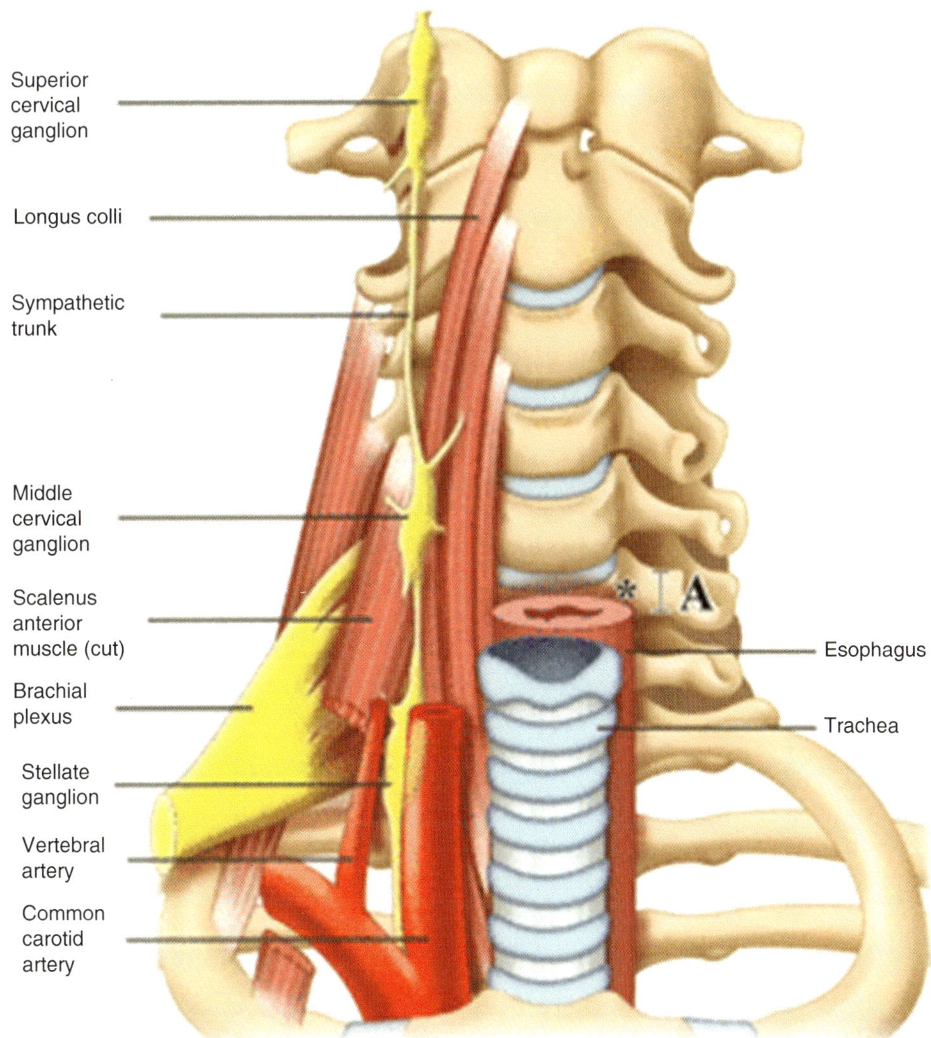

Fig. 19.1 Anatomy of the stellate ganglion. Illustration of deep tissues of the prevertebral region in the neck. "A" designates the transverse process of the C6 vertebral body (Chassaignac's tubercle). The needle insertion site for the fluoroscopic and blind technique is designated with an *asterisk*

distal portion of the first two fingers, and the needle is inserted perpendicular to the skin until it contacts the bony surface of the C6 tubercle (Fig. 19.1). The needle is then withdrawn 1–2 mm and injectate is then inserted. If the image is fluoroscopically guided, contrast may be injected prior to the local anesthetic to ensure spread along the fascial plane and absence of vascular uptake [26, 31]. Another method wherein the C7 vertebral body is targeted is exclusively performed using fluoroscopic guidance [32]. When performed using ultrasound guidance, the needle is inserted using the in-plane technique and advanced to the fascial plane between the posterolateral surface of the longus colli muscle and the prevertebral fascia on the posterior surface of the carotid artery [33]. Fragile soft tissue structures such as vasculature, the esophagus, and thyroid tissue can be identified with ultrasound and therefore carefully avoided during needle advancement (Fig. 19.2). Additionally, smaller volumes are needed to ensure targeting of the ganglion as the injectate can be directly visualized as surrounding the nerve bundle [31]. Although, in the past, volumes as high as 20 mL have been routinely injected, new data shows that 5 mL is the optimal volume, even if fluoroscopic guidance is used, to avoid side effects and ensure adequate sympathetic blockade [34].

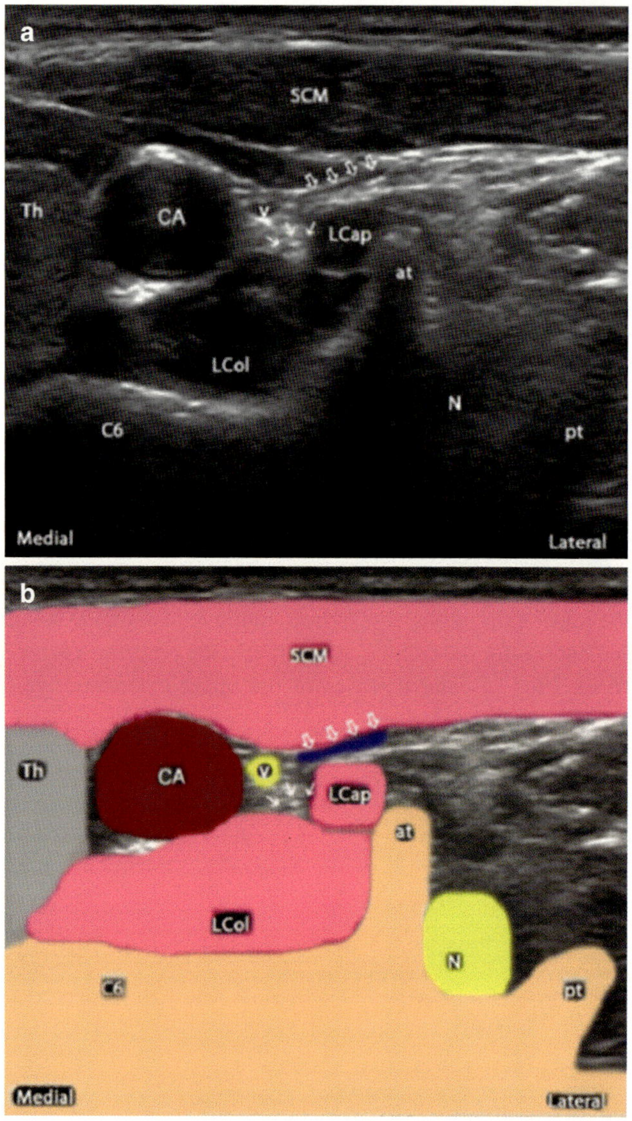

Fig. 19.2 Ultrasound short axis view at C6 level. (**a**) Ultrasound view (**b**) overlay of regional tissues. *Red*: artery. *Blue*: vein. *Pink*: muscle. *Yellow*: nerve. *Tan*: bone. *Gray*: thyroid tissue. During visualization, the physician will position the transducer in a cephalad and lateral trajectory until the sharp anterior tubercle (at) of C6 comes into view. The sternocleidomastoid muscle (SCM), thyroid (Th), vagus nerve (V), and carotid artery (CA) are posterior and medial to the target, the sympathetic chain (*three small arrows*). *White open arrows* designate the collapsed internal jugular vein. The sympathetic chain is located in the groove between the longus capitis muscle (Lcap) and the longus colli muscle (LCol). Reprinted with permission [31]

19.2.3.4 Efficacy

A successful block will result in the patient developing Horner's syndrome: miosis (pinpoint pupil), ptosis (droopy eyelid), anhidrosis (absence of sweating), scleral injection, and enophthalmos (posterior displacement of the eyelid). Patients will also experience symptoms of nasal congestion, throat "fullness," and facial flushing on the affected side. The extremity should also be tested, as the above symptoms alone do not indicate a true successful sympathetic blockade of the extremity. If the temperature of the skin on the affected hand is elevated by 1–3° as compared to pre-procedure temperature, then the block may be deemed successful [26, 31].

The efficacy of SGB in treating pain decreases as time elapses after the initial trauma or nerve insult. If symptoms have been present for greater than 16 weeks prior to the first SGB procedure, the treatment efficacy is decreased. Severity of the disease can also adversely impact results of the block in that a decrease in skin perfusion of the affected limb compared to the contralateral may portend poor relief from the block [35].

19.2.3.5 Contraindications

Contraindications to stellate ganglion block include the omnipresent contraindication triad: patient refusal, anticoagulation, and infection at the site of injection. Other contraindications specific to SGB include contralateral recurrent laryngeal nerve or phrenic nerve palsy, as bilateral blockade of these nerves causes severe respiratory consequence. For this reason, bilateral SGBs are not advised [26].

19.2.3.6 Associated Risks

A survey of 76 anesthesia departments, which represented approximately 45,000 total SGBs, revealed the incidence of

Table 19.2 Differential diagnosis of altered mental status during stellate ganglion block

Vasovagal reaction	Blockade of cardiac accelerator fibers
Intravenous injection	Intra-arterial injection
Phrenic nerve paralysis	Recurrent laryngeal nerve paralysis
Pneumothorax	Seizure
Retropharyngeal hematoma	Arterial injury

severe complication as 1.7 in 1000 procedures [36]. These data were collected at a time prior to the widespread use of ultrasound guidance for SGB, and therefore the measured risk may be elevated compared to the actual current incidence of severe complication. However, it remains prudent practice for the proceduralist to ensure immediate availability of emergency airway equipment and proximity of anticonvulsant medications and to obtain IV access on the patient prior to initiating the procedure. Presence of an assistant and monitoring of vital signs throughout the procedure, including EKG monitoring, are also strongly recommended (Table 19.2).

Common side effects of the sympathetic blockade of the stellate ganglion include hoarseness due to unilateral blockade of the recurrent laryngeal nerve, "fullness" of the throat, Horner's syndrome (described in detail above), and unilateral phrenic nerve palsy. True complications that can occur after SGB are rare but include allergic reaction, pneumothorax, intrathecal or epidural injection, and brachial plexus blockade. The most common complication is local anesthetic toxicity or seizure [36] resulting from intravascular injection of local anesthetic into cephalad vasculature [26, 27, 31, 33, 37, 38].

Retropharyngeal hematoma: This is a rare adverse event from SGB, with a reported incidence of 1:100,000. Typical symptom presentation occurs 2 h after the procedure and is more common in patients on anticoagulation or with risk factors for bleeding. Early symptoms of retropharyngeal hematoma are fairly nonspecific and most commonly include abnormal sensations and pain in the neck, head, or chest. It should be noted that in about half of cases, even these initial symptoms do not present for 2 h after the procedure. Later symptoms include hoarseness, stridor, dyspnea, and neck swelling. The three principal signs for diagnosis of an established retropharyngeal hematoma are superior mediastinal obstruction, ventral displacement of the trachea, and subcutaneous ecchymosis in the neck and anterior chest wall. These signs are significantly delayed in presentation and therefore unlikely to develop, while the patient is in the recovery area after SGB. Therefore all patients who receive a SGB should be cautioned to monitor for these indicators that a hematoma may be present, especially in those patients with risk factors for bleeding [38].

Stroke: Stroke after SGB is almost always attributed to injury to the vertebral artery. As this artery supplies the brainstem, an injury can be catastrophic. Consequence of injury to the vertebral artery often results in "vertebrobasilar syndrome" as the bilateral vertebral arteries are a major blood supply to the basilar artery, which supplies the medulla, pons, and cerebellum [28]. Although the clinical presentation can vary broadly, injury to the vertebral artery most often results in cerebellar symptoms, occipital deficits, or Wallenberg's syndrome, a constellation of symptoms including ataxia, vertigo, nystagmus, ipsilateral Horner's syndrome, dysarthria, dysmetria, and crossed sensory deficits [28, 39]. The literature also reveals several case reports of locked-in syndrome after SGB [37, 40, 41]. It is unclear how frequently stroke after SGB occurs, given that it is very likely and underreported consequence of the procedure. However, the advent of fluoroscopy and ultrasound for image guidance of SGB will certainly facilitate prevention of this adverse event.

19.2.4 Neuroablative/Neurosuppressive Techniques

A more invasive option to pursue if a stellate ganglion block is effective but provides only transient relief is pulsed radiofrequency ablation of the sympathetic chain [42]. If this is ineffective, a trial of spinal cord stimulation may be the next line of treatment, as it has been shown to decrease oral morphine equivalents consumed and overall pain scores in CRPS patients even at 1 year postimplantation [43].

Key Concepts

- There are strict criteria for a diagnosis of CRPS, termed the Budapest Criteria (Table 19.1), but the natural history of the disease varies from patient to patient.
- CRPS may be treated by conservative measures such as medications and physical therapy or invasive techniques such as stellate ganglion block (SGB) and spinal cord stimulator implantation.
- Stellate ganglion block (SGB) carries a high morbidity compared to the majority of interventional pain procedures.
- There exist a variety of indications for SGB.
- Given the delicate soft tissue structures that surround the target nerve ganglion, the block is now increasingly performed under ultrasound guidance. Although fluoroscopic-guided technique remains prevalent, the blind technique is now rarely practiced.
- Despite increased visibility of vital structures when the procedure is performed under direct ultrasound guidance, precautions should be taken such that swift resuscitation may be provided for the patient in an emergency.

References

1. Harden RN, Oaklander AL, Burton AW, Perez RS, Richardson K, Swan M, Barthel J, Costa B, Graciosa JR, Bruehl S. Complex regional pain syndrome: practical diagnostic and treatment guidelines, 4th edition. Pain Med. 2013;14(2):180–229.
2. Birklein F. Complex regional pain syndrome. J Neurol. 2005;25(2):131–8.
3. Harden RN, Bruehl S, Stanton-Hicks M, Wilson PR. Proposed new diagnostic criteria for complex regional pain syndrome. Pain Med. 2007;8(4):326–31.
4. Bruehl S, Harden RN, Galer BS, Saltz S, Backonja M, Stanton-Hicks M. Complex regional pain syndrome: are there distinct subtypes and sequential stages of the syndrome? Pain. 2002;95(1–2):119–24.
5. Scholten PM, Harden RN. Assessing and treating patients with neuropathic pain. PM R. 2015;7(11):S257–69.
6. Mailis-Gagnon A, Lakha SF, Allen MD, Deshpande A, Harden RN. Characteristics of complex regional pain syndrome in patients referred to a tertiary pain clinic by community physicians, assessed by the Budapest clinical diagnostic criteria. Pain Med. 2014;15(11):1965–74.
7. Terkelsen AJ, Bach FW, Jensen TS. Experimental forearm immobilization in humans induces cold and mechanical hyperalgesia. Anesthesiology. 2008;109:297–307.
8. Severens JL, Oerlemans HM, Weegels AJ. Cost-effectiveness analysis of adjuvant physical or occupational therapy for patients with reflex sympathetic dystrophy. Arch Phys Med Rehabil. 1999;80(9):1038–43.
9. Sherry DD, Wallace CA, Kelley C, Kidder M, Sapp L. Short- and long-term outcomes of children with complex regional pain syndrome type I treated with exercise therapy. Clin J Pain. 1999;15(3):218–23.
10. Daly AE, Bialocerkowski AE. Does evidence support physiotherapy management of adult complex regional pain syndrome type one? A systematic review. Eur J Pain. 2009;13:339–53.
11. Moseley LG. Graded motor imagery is effective for long-standing complex regional pain syndrome: a randomised controlled trial. Pain. 2004;108(1–2):192–8.
12. Watson HK, Carlson LK. Treatment of reflex sympathetic dystrophy of the hand with an active "stress loading" program. J Hand Surg Am. 1987;12A:779–85.
13. Phillips ME, Katz JA, Harden RN. The use of nerve blocks in conjunction with occupational therapy for complex regional pain syndrome type I. Am J Occup Ther. 2000;54(5):544–9.
14. Ghai B, Dureja GP. Complex regional pain syndrome: a review. J Postgrad Med. 2004;50(4):300–7.
15. Teasell R, Bombadier C. Employment related factors in chronic pain and chronic pain disability. Clin J Pain. 2001;17:S39–45.
16. Kingery WS. A critical review of controlled clinical trials for peripheral neuropathic pain and complex regional pain syndromes. Pain. 1997;73(2):123–39.
17. Huygen FJ, Niehof S, Zijlstra FJ, van Hagen PM, van Daele PL. Successful treatment of CRPS 1 with anti-TNF. J Pain Symptom Manage. 2004;27(2):101–3.
18. Pappagallo M, Rosenberg AD. Epidemiology, pathophysiology, and management of complex regional pain syndrome. Pain Pract. 2001;1(1):11–20.
19. Mellick GA, Mellicy LB, Mellick LB. Gabapentin in the management of reflex sympathetic dystrophy. J Pain Symptom Manage. 1995;10:265–6.
20. Harke H, Gretenkort P, Ladleif HU, Rahman S, Harke O. The response of neuropathic pain and pain in complex regional pain syndrome I to carbamazepine and sustained-release morphine in patients pretreated with spinal cord stimulation: a doubleblinded randomized study. Anesth Analg. 2001;92:488–95.
21. Sindrup SH, Jensen TS. Pharmacologic treatment of pain in polyneuropathy. Neurology. 2000;55:915–20.
22. Ebert B, Andersen S, Krogsgaard-Larsen P. Ketobemidone, methadone and pethidine are non-competitive N-methyl-D-aspartate (NMDA) antagonists in the rat cortex and spinal cord. Neurosci Lett. 1995;187(3):165–8.
23. Harden RN, Bruehl S. The use of opioids in treatment of chronic pain: an examination of the ongoing controversy. J Back Musculoskelet Rehabil. 1997;9(2):155–80.
24. Schwartzman RJ, Alexander GM, Grothusen JR, Paylor T, Reichenberger E, Perreault M. Outpatient intravenous ketamine for the treatment of complex regional pain syndrome: a double-blind placebo controlled. Pain. 2009;147(1–3):107–15.
25. Goebel A, Baranowski A, Maurer K, Ghai A, McCabe C, Ambler G. Intravenous immunoglobulin treatment of the complex regional pain syndrome: a randomized trial. Ann Intern Med. 2010;152:152–8.
26. Elias M. Cervical sympathetic and stellate ganglion blocks. Pain Physician. 2000;3:294–304.
27. Gofeld M, Shankar H. Peripheral and visceral sympathetic blocks. In: Benzon HT, Rathmell J, Wu C, et al., editors. Practical management of pain. 5th ed. Amsterdam: Elsevier; 2014. p. 755–9.
28. Showalter W, Esekogwu V, Newton KI, Henderson SO. Vertebral artery dissection. Acad Emerg Med. 1997;4(10):991–5.
29. McLean B. Safety and patient acceptability of stellate ganglion blockade as a treatment adjunct for combat-related post-traumatic stress disorder: a quality assurance initiative. Cureus. 2015;7(9):e320.
30. Lipov EG, Joshi JR, Sanders S. Effects of stellate-ganglion block on hot flushes and night awakenings in survivors of breast cancer: a pilot study. Lancet Oncol. 2008;9:523–32.
31. Narouze S. Ultrasound-guided stellate ganglion block. Curr Pain Meadache Rep. 2014;18(424):1–5.
32. Abdi S, Zhou Y, Patel N, Saini B, Nelson J. A new and easy technique to block the stellate ganglion. Pain Physician. 2004;7:327–31.
33. Narouze S, Vydyanathan A, Patel N. Ultrasound-guided stellate ganglion block successfully prevented esophageal puncture. Pain Physician. 2007;10(6):747–52.
34. Feigl GC, Rosmarin W, Stelzl A, Weninger B, Likar R. Comparison of different injectate volumes for stellate ganglion block: an anatomic and radiologic study. Reg Anesth Pain Med. 2007;32(3):203–8.
35. Ackerman WE, Zhang JM. Efficacy of stellate ganglion blockade for the management of type 1 complex regional pain syndrome. South Med J. 2006;99(10):1084–8.
36. Wulf H, Maier C. Complications and side effects of stellate ganglion blockade. Results of a questionnaire survey. Anaesthesist. 1992;41(3):146–51.
37. Chaturvedi A, Dash HH. Locked-in syndrome during stellate ganglion block. Indian J Anaesth. 2010;54:324–6.
38. Higa K, Hirata K, Hirota K, Nitahara K. Retropharyngeal hematoma after stellate ganglion block: analysis of 27 patients reported in the literature. Anesthesiology. 2006;105:1238–45.
39. Frisoni GB, Anzola GP. Vertebrobasilar ischemia after neck motion. Stroke. 1991;22(11):1452–60.
40. Dukes RR, Alexander LA. Transient locked-in syndrome after vascular injection during stellate ganglion block. Reg Anesth. 1993;18:378–80.
41. Tüz M, Erodlu F, Dodru H, Uygur K, Yavuz L. Transient locked-in syndrome resulting from stellate ganglion block in the treatment of patients with sudden hearing loss. Acta Anaesthesiol Scand. 2003;47:485–7.
42. Djuric V. Pulsed radiofrequency treatment of complex regional pain syndrome: a case series. Pain Res Manag. 2014;19(4):186–90.
43. Sanders RA, Moeschler SM, Gazelka HM, Lamer TJ, Wang Z, Qu W, Hoelzer BC. Patient outcomes and spinal cord stimulation: a retrospective case series evaluating patient satisfaction, pain scores, and opioid requirements. Pain Pract. 2016;16:899–904.

20 Pneumothorax After Paravertebral Block and Radiofrequency

Christina C. Moore and David M. Dickerson

20.1 Case Description

A 48-year-old female with postmastectomy pain syndrome comes to the pain clinic for relief from her chronic debilitating chest wall pain. She has had a left breast lumpectomy with adjuvant radiation therapy and takes tamoxifen. Two years after lumpectomy, microcalcifications were again found on mammogram and confirmed to be ductal carcinoma in situ on biopsy. She underwent left simple, nipple-sparing mastectomy with immediate muscle-sparing flap reconstruction.

Her postoperative course was complicated by progressive tailbone and left-sided chest pain. NSAIDs and hydrocodone/acetaminophen were prescribed by the surgical care team but offered only minimal relief. Several months after surgery, the patient was referred to the pain clinic with persistent, progressively worse, burning chest wall pain. She suffered from mood lability, sleep disturbance, and pain with pressure or touch on the left lateral and anterior chest wall. The patient described a feeling of severe tightness and pressure across her chest when she took a deep breath. Coccydynia of unknown etiology was also diagnosed. It was equally severe and limiting in function. It had begun recently without any known trauma; the patient reported that she was sitting for long periods of time in the preceding weeks.

During her pain clinic visits, she underwent a caudal epidural steroid injection with subsequent ganglion impar block and left thoracic paravertebral block at T5. The coccygeal pain improved, and the left-sided paravertebral block provided >75% pain relief, though it was limited to the painful area below the nipple line. She was prescribed pregabalin and tramadol and encouraged to continue taking bupropion for her long-standing depression. In an attempt to treat the residual chest wall pain, she returned for a T3 paravertebral block, which was again successful and without complications. Both paravertebral blocks were ultrasound guided, performed using an in-plane method and visualizing a slightly obliqued short axis of the transverse process. In both cases, a mixture of local anesthetic and dexamethasone was injected anterior to the internal intercostal membrane revealing paravertebral spread.

The patient returned for radiofrequency ablation of the left T5 intercostal nerve. A similar method was used. Using ultrasound imaging and under direct visualization of pleura, a 20 gauge, 2 inch SMK needle with a 5 mm active tip was positioned in the paravertebral area. Pulsed radiofrequency ablation was performed twice for 2 min at 42 °C after localization and sensory/motor testing of the intercostal nerve. The patient tolerated the procedure well. However, after transfer to recovery, she complained of bilateral sharp chest pain with deep inspiration. She remained hemodynamically stable and nonhypoxemic on room air. Upright chest radiographs revealed a left apical 5 mm pneumothorax (see Fig. 20.1).

Repeat chest radiograph 2.5 h later confirmed persistent, unchanged, left apical pneumothorax. At this time, the patient denied dyspnea. Oxygen saturation on room air was in the high 90s despite persistent pleuritic chest pain. She was discharged home and advised to return to the emergency department if symptoms worsened. She reported no symptoms on follow-up telephone call the next day.

One month later, the patient returned to the pain clinic. She felt relief from pain after the left-sided T5 paravertebral radiofrequency ablation. She still experienced pain at the upper portion of the breast above the nipple at the T3 level. She underwent T3 pulsed radiofrequency ablation and once again suffered pleuritic chest pain and dyspnea, even though she remained hemodynamically stable without hypoxia. Chest radiograph revealed a 4 mm apical pneumothorax, and the patient was advised to return to the hospital if symptoms worsened. She was asymptomatic on follow-up telephone calls.

C.C. Moore, M.D.
Department of Anesthesia, Medical College of Wisconsin, Milwaukee, WI, USA
e-mail: christina.gavrilos@gmail.com

D.M. Dickerson, M.D. (✉)
Department of Anesthesia and Critical Care, University of Chicago, Chicago, IL, USA
e-mail: DDickerson@dacc.uchicago.edu

M. Anitescu et al. (eds.), *Challenging Cases and Complication Management in Pain Medicine*,
https://doi.org/10.1007/978-3-319-60072-7_20

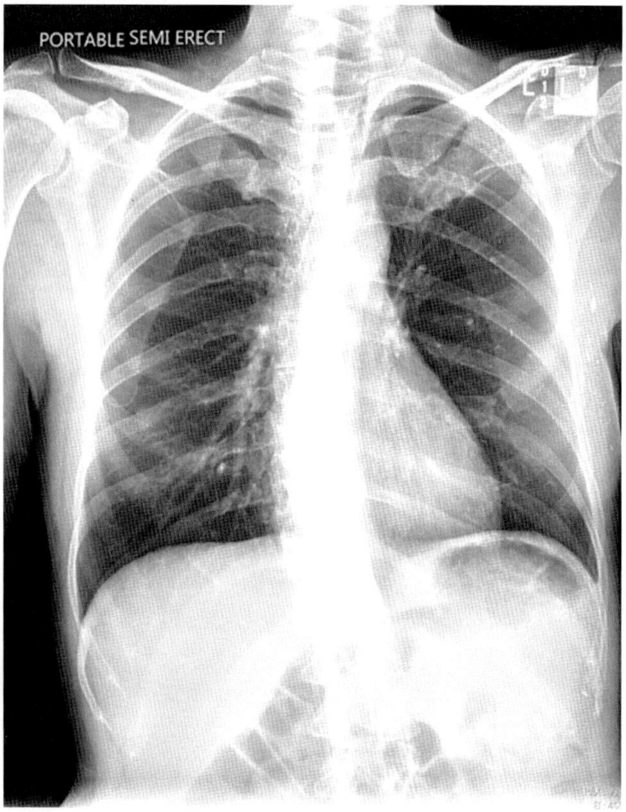

Fig. 20.1 Anteroposterior radiographic image showing left apical, 5 mm pneumothorax (Image from personal library)

Upon follow-up visit, the patient reported that the radiofrequency ablation was successful but only for several weeks. Her pain was severe and uncontrolled until initiation of transdermal buprenorphine therapy and intermittent, low-dose ketamine infusions. Her pain remains 90% relieved with this ongoing regimen. Coccydynia has not yet recurred. The decision was made not to proceed with additional paravertebral procedures because of the previous two pneumothoraces.

20.2 Case Discussion

20.2.1 Chronic Chest Wall Pain

20.2.1.1 Incidence

Fifty million people in the United States suffer from chronic pain, the direct and indirect cost of which is estimated at 80–100 billion dollars [1]. Drug therapy is inadequate for treating pain in 43% of these patients [2]. When traditional analgesic techniques are unsuccessful, interventional therapies may provide pain relief. More than 200,000 women are diagnosed with breast cancer in the United States every year, and 41% undergo surgery as part of their treatment [3]. Currently, 2.5 million women are breast cancer survivors in the United States alone. The most distressing complaint of surgically treated breast cancer survivors remains to be persistent postmastectomy pain. The estimated incidence of chronic pain after breast surgery (lumpectomy or mastectomy) is 20–30% [3, 4]. In one study, one-third of patients reported persistent postmastectomy pain on the chest wall, arm, axilla, or breast, unaffected since the surgery [3]. Chronic postsurgical chest wall pain is common after thoracic surgery as well. The incidence is 30–40% after thoracotomy, compared with 10% after other surgeries such as inguinal hernia repair or cesarean section [5, 16]. These patients experience a decrease in physical function and quality of life [6].

20.2.1.2 Pathophysiology of Post-resection Chest Wall Pain

The thoracic wall and parietal pleura are innervated by branches of the intercostal nerves originating from the anterior primary rami of T1–T12 and passing through the intervertebral foramina [7]. Surgical trauma and nerve injury modulate pain pathways with permanent synaptic neuronal changes. This neuronal plasticity is often responsible for chronic pain after surgery. Neural blockade interrupts the connection between the site of nerve trauma and the central nervous system (CNS) [8]. Denervation injury can induce neuronal dysfunction and hyperexcitation via central sensitization, disinhibition, and glial cell activation. Compounded by the possible nociceptive barrage from peripheral neuromata at the previous surgical site, the pain from mastectomy may not merely be in the chest wall itself but grossly perpetuated centrally into a debilitating, emotional experience for the patient and their family.

20.2.1.3 Treatment

Various interventional procedures target chest wall pain: thoracic paravertebral steroid injection, neuroma injection, intercostal nerve steroid injection, thoracic epidural steroid injection, dorsal root ganglion ablation, intercostal nerve neurolysis, dorsal column stimulation, and intrathecal drug delivery via implantable pump. Paravertebral block, neurolysis, and radiofrequency ablation are described below.

Paravertebral Block

A paravertebral block provides unilateral sensory and motor blockade, reduces acute postoperative pain and opioid consumption, and may reduce chronic postmastectomy chest wall pain. In a meta-analysis of 89 patients who had breast cancer surgery, paravertebral block reduced chronic pain symptoms (versus conventional analgesia) with an odds ratio of 0.37 at 6 months follow-up. Paravertebral block may decrease the risk of developing chronic pain in one in five women undergoing breast cancer surgery [8]. With paravertebral blockade, there was less motion-related and at-rest pain 12 months postoperatively [9].

Complications from paravertebral blocks are rare: a 0.5% incidence of pneumothorax, 3.8% incidence of vascular puncture, and 4.6% incidence of hypotension. In one study of 1000 paravertebral blocks, two seizures but no pneumothoraces were reported [2]. While paravertebral blockade may prevent chronic chest wall pain, the role of the block has yet to be established for chronic chest wall pain. A low-volume injection provides diagnostic information for a potential ablative therapy at the chest wall. It is thought that a steroid injectate reduces the excitability of the primary afferent neuron and its cell body in the dorsal root ganglion. More peripheral blockade via serratus anterior plane block may relieve chronic post-thoracotomy pain.

Neurolysis

Neurolytics for intractable chest wall pain from cancer are injected with the goal of destroying nerves to interrupt pain pathways. Chemical neurodestructive techniques use alcohol and phenol (carbolic acid and hydroxybenzene). Because alcohol neurolysis produces severe pain on injection, the patient is sedated during the procedure. Physical neurodestructive techniques include cryotherapy, thermocoagulation, and radiofrequency [1]. Denervation carries the risk of potential centralization of pain to cortical structures. Thus, chemical neurolysis is typically a palliative procedure.

Phenol Neurolysis

Advanced cancer pain is inadequately controlled in at least 10–15% of patients [10]. Neurolysis with phenol can improve analgesia and lessen the need for opioids and improve the quality of life [11].The ideal concentration of phenol for injection has not been established. Administration varies from 3 to 13% phenol in an aqueous solution. In a study of 42 patients with severe nonmalignant chronic pain followed 6 months after 4% phenol neurolysis, good pain relief (visual analog scale <3) was achieved in 83%.

Unfortunately, phenol neurolysis is risky, with possible devastating complications. If the phenol solution diffuses to the paravertebral gutter and through the intervertebral foramina toward the epidural space and cerebrospinal fluid (CSF), persistent paraplegia results [11].One patient underwent intervertebral injection of 10% phenol solution along the inferior border of the ribs. One hour later, the patient complained of bilateral lower extremity weakness and difficulty moving. Although IV methylprednisolone was administered and a neurosurgery consult was obtained immediately, the patient remained paraplegic for 6 months [11].

There are several ways to help mitigate complications associated with phenol neurolysis. If a glycerine-based instead of an aqueous solution is used, toxicity is 50 times lower [11]. A smaller dose of phenol may decrease the risk of paraplegia. Performing the procedure away from the spinal cord (i.e., midaxillary line injection versus paravertebral injection) can decrease risk of its entrance into the CSF [11]. In cancer metastases to the spine, adding volume can increase pressure in the epidural space, leading to symptoms of compressive myelopathy [12].

Radiofrequency Ablation

Pulsed radiofrequency ablation has gained popularity over chemical neurolysis because of fewer debilitating side effects. Its mechanism of action is thought to be the inhibition of excitatory C fibers by repetitive burst stimulation of A-delta fibers, decreased overall evoked synaptic activity, and minor structural changes in nerve tissue [13].

Case series have shown pulsed radiofrequency to be effective in spinal, groin, extremity, and facial pain [13]. In a study of 49 patients with chronic postsurgical thoracic pain, pulsed radiofrequency ablation of the intercostal nerves or dorsal root ganglia was performed. Compared to medical management, at 3 months follow-up, 53.8% with radiofrequency ablation reported 50% or greater pain relief compared to 19.9% of patients managed medically. Only 6.7% of the group with intercostal nerve pulsed radiofrequency reported pain relief greater than 50% [13]. In a case study of three patients with intercostal neuralgia, post-thoracotomy pain syndrome, or postherpetic neuralgia, respectively, ultrasound-guided pulsed radiofrequency therapy was performed at 42 °C for 120 s. Visual analog scale pain scores decreased from 7, 6, and 7 to 2, 0, and 1, respectively, and remained that way throughout the 6-month follow-up [14].

Unlike continuous thermal radiofrequency, pulsed radiofrequency does not damage tissue, although sensory or motor dysfunction may result from destruction of nervous tissue. Complications from radiofrequency ablation include pneumothorax, hemothorax, intravascular injection, and intrathecal injection. In the previously mentioned study of 49 patients with radiofrequency ablation of the dorsal root ganglion or intercostal nerves, 1 in 13 (7.6%) patients in the dorsal root ganglion group and 1 in 15 (6.7%) patients in the intercostal nerve group developed pneumothorax. Radiofrequency in the thoracic spine can damage blood supply if it affects the small radicular arteries or the artery of Adamkiewicz between T9 and L2 [13].

20.2.2 Pneumothorax

20.2.2.1 Etiology and Pathogenesis of Pneumothorax

Traumatic pneumothorax occurs when the chest wall and pleura are pierced, letting air enter the pleural space to become trapped in the thorax [15, 16].The incidence of idiopathic pneumothorax ranges from 0.11 to 2.68% according to a study of 7.5 million hospital discharge notes [16]. The rate of pneumothorax after paravertebral block is estimated at 0.5% [17]. The rate of iatrogenic pneumothorax has increased over the years, possibly because more interventional procedures are performed or methods of detection are more reliable [16]. Pneumothorax in the pain clinic can become an emergency, possibly leading to respiratory distress and cardiovascular compromise. Knowing the signs and symptoms, diagnostic modalities, and treatment options is important for the patient and provider.

20.2.2.2 Clinical Manifestations of Pneumothorax

Signs and symptoms of pneumothorax include dyspnea, tachypnea, chest pain, pleurisy, hypoxia, decreased breath sounds, hyperresonant percussion, and subcutaneous emphysema [15, 16].

Tachycardia and hypotension may signify tension pneumothorax, a condition requiring immediate intervention. Two signs of tension pneumothorax are severe respiratory distress and mediastinal shift on radiologic imaging. Some patients with pneumothorax may be asymptomatic. Patients at risk of developing pneumothorax during an interventional procedure are those with chronic obstructive pulmonary disease, primary lung cancer, older age, pleural effusion, empyema, and chronic steroid use [16].

20.2.2.3 Diagnostic Modalities for Pneumothorax

Computed tomography (CT) is the gold standard for evaluating pneumothorax; however, it is rarely the diagnostic method of choice because of high radiation exposure, cost, and transport of a possibly unstable patient [18]. CT is also infrequently available in outpatient pain clinics. Chest radiographs have been traditionally used for diagnoses, but ultrasound has recently gained popularity. Ultrasound is typically available in the pain clinic and has been shown in studies to be more sensitive than supine chest x-ray and as sensitive as CT scan in detecting traumatic pneumothorax. In a study of 28 patients, using ultrasound for diagnosis of pneumothorax had a sensitivity of 0.87 and specificity of 0.99 [17]. To detect a pneumothorax, the ultrasound is placed longitudinally on the anterior chest wall of the supine patient in search of the pleural line. In an intact lung, the pleural line is made of the visceral pleura, parietal pleura, and interpleural fluid [17]. The parietal pleura slides on the visceral pleura in a cyclic pattern corresponding to spontaneous ventilations. In pneumothorax, however, the pleural line consists only of the parietal pleura, and a collection of air is seen in the interpleural space [17]. Therefore, observing an intact pleural line, along with other ultrasonic findings, may help rule out pneumothorax.

20.2.3 Treatment of Pneumothorax

Treatment depends on both clinical assessment and diagnostic imaging. Once diagnosis has been established, management consists of either observation, aspiration, or chest tube placement [18].

20.2.3.1 Observation

For pneumothorax involving less than 20% of the hemithorax in an asymptomatic patient, observation is appropriate, as small pneumothoraces are unlikely to progresses to respiratory failure or tension pneumothorax and tend to resolve spontaneously [16, 17]. Oxygen is supplemented at a high flow rate to accelerate resorption up to fourfold [16]. Observation is either in the hospital for 24 h or at home with instructions to return to the hospital if symptoms worsen. In a study of 154 patients with pneumothorax, 91 were placed on outpatient observation, 82 of whom had spontaneous resolution without the need for treatment [17]. Repeat imaging 12–24 h after the diagnosis is appropriate. If the patient develops symptoms or imaging demonstrates worsening of the defect, aspiration or chest tube drainage is recommended.

20.2.3.2 Aspiration

To aspirate a pneumothorax, a needle or small cannula is placed into the pleural air. This method of treatment is reserved for patients without underlying lung disease who are only slightly symptomatic and with the pneumothorax involving <20% of the hemithorax volume [17]. Aspiration of an iatrogenic pneumothorax <20% in volume has an 87% success rate [17]. Undergoing aspiration as opposed to chest tube placement decreases hospitalization admissions for pneumothorax [18]. Post-aspiration, an asymptomatic patient with either resolved or unchanged imaging may be discharged with instructions to return within 48 h if symptoms worsen [17].

20.2.3.3 Chest Tube Placement

Severely symptomatic patients or patients with large pneumothoraces (more than 20% hemothorax volume) require chest tube placement and hospital admission [17]. Chest tube placement is necessary in a patient requiring mechanical ventilation, which substantially increases the risk of tension pneumothorax. Chest tubes are the most definitive way to treat a pneumothorax nonsurgically [18]. They are inserted under the axilla to prevent damage to organs. A one-way valve ensures that air escapes without reentering the chest cavity. Typically, the chest tube is left in place until either air is no longer observed or x-ray confirms re-expansion of the lung. If the air leak continues, surgery may be necessary (Table 20.1).

Table 20.1 Initial management of iatrogenic pneumothorax

Pneumothorax treatment	
Pneumothorax characteristics	Treatment
<20% and asymptomatic	Supplemental oxygen, observation, and repeat x-ray in 24 h
<20% and symptomatic	Chest tube with suction at −20 cm H_2O for 24 h
>20%	Chest tube with suction at −20 cm H_2O for 24 h

Chest tube evacuation depends on defect size, symptoms, and progression at 24 h (Adapted from Loiselle et al. [15])

Conclusion

Although procedures in the pain clinic are not risk-free, there are techniques to mitigate complication rates. Fluoroscopy-guided or ultrasound-guided blocks are correlated with lower risk of complication as opposed to their non-image-guided procedural counterparts [16, 17]. The specific therapeutic benefit of chest wall procedures must be weighed against the risk of a specific procedure in a specific patient. A low-risk, low-cost method should be utilized coupled with a vigilant system for postprocedural monitoring before discharge from the clinic. A standardized evaluation is specific to the procedure performed. With an incidence of pneumothorax of 5–10% after paravertebral or intercostal blocks, all patients having chest wall procedures should be given clear and specific postprocedural instruction for monitoring and seeking acute care.

References

1. Weksler N, Klein M, Gurevitch B, et al. Phenol neurolysis for severe chronic nonmalignant pain: is the old also obsolete? Pain Med. 2007;8(4):332–7.
2. Vila H, Liu J, Kavasmaneck D. Paravertebral block: new benefits from an old procedure. Curr Opin Anesthesiol. 2007;20:316–8.
3. Belfer I, Schreiber KL, Shaffer JR, et al. Persistent postmastectomy pain in breast cancer survivors: analysis of clinical, demographic, and psychosocial factors. J Pain. 2013;14:1185–95.
4. Peng Z, Li H, Qian X, et al. A retrospective study of chronic postsurgical pain following thoracic surgery: prevalence, risk factors, incidence of neuropathic component, and impact on quality of life. PLoS One. 2014;92:e90014.
5. Kehlet H, Jensen T, Woolf C. Persistent postsurgical pain: risk factors and prevention. Lancet. 2006;367:1618–25.
6. Enck R. Postsurgical chronic pain. Am J Hosp Palliat Care. 2010;27:301–2.
7. Gulati A, et al. A retrospective review and treatment paradigm of interventional therapies for patients suffering from intractable thoracic chest wall pain in the oncologic population. Pain Med. 2015;16:802–10.
8. Andreae M, Andreae D. Local anesthetics and regional anesthesia in preventing chronic pain after surgery. Cochrane Database Syst Rev. 2012;10:CD007105.
9. Wardhan R. Update on paravertebral blocks. Curr Opin Anesthesiol. 2015;28:588–92.
10. Sloan P. The evolving role of interventional pain management in oncology. J Support Oncol. 2004;2(6):491–500. 503
11. Gollapalli L, Muppuri R. Paraplegia after intercostal neurolysis with phenol. J Pain Res. 2014;7:665–8.
12. Kim B, No M, Han S, et al. Paraplegia following intercostal nerve neurolysis with alcohol and thoracic epidural injection in lung cancer patients. Korean J Pain. 2015;28:148–52.
13. Cohen S, Sireci A, Wu C, et al. Pulse radiofrequency of the dorsal root ganglia is superior to pharmacotherapy or pulsed radiofrequency of the intercostal nerves in the treatment of chronic postsurgical thoracic pain. Pain Physician. 2006;9:227–36.
14. Akkaya T, Ozkan D. Ultrasound-guided pulsed radiofrequency treatment of the intercostal nerve: three cases. J Anesth. 2013;27:968–9.
15. Zanogoulidis P, Kioumis I, Pitsiou G, et al. Pneumothorax: from definition to diagnosis and treatment. J Thorac Dis. 2014;6:S372–6.
16. Loiselle A, Parish J, Wilkens J, et al. Managing iatrogenic pneumothorax and chest tubes. J Hosp Med. 2013;8:402–8.
17. Park J, Young H, Su A, et al. Ultrasound-guided aspiration of the iatrogenic pneumothorax caused by paravertebral block- a case report. Korean J Pain. 2012;25:33–7.
18. Chen L, Zhang Z. Quantitative imaging in medicine and surgery. Quant Imaging Med Surg. 2015;5:618–23.

Retroperitoneal Hematoma After Celiac Plexus Block

21

Ryan Mattie and Ramana K. Naidu

21.1 Case Description

A 68-year-old gentleman with a history of hypertension, smoking tobacco abuse, and carcinoma of the head of the pancreas presented 3 weeks status post palliative gastrojejunostomy and cholecystojejunostomy with intractable mid-epigastrium pain radiating to the back. Attempts at alleviating the symptoms included the use of nonsteroidal anti-inflammatory drugs (NSAIDs); neuropathic membrane stabilizers, specifically gabapentinoids; and extended-release/long-acting opioid analgesia that proved ineffective due to altered sensorium. His oncologists stated that the patient's life expectancy was in the order of months. After a discussion regarding risks, benefits, and alternatives to intervention, the patient elected to undergo celiac plexus neurolysis under CT guidance for potential long-lasting relief from his abdominal pain and improvement in quality of life. Prior to the procedure, the patient denied any noticeable bruising or bleeding or use of any antithrombotic medications. Routine laboratory workup for his chemotherapy was negative for thrombocytopenia or coagulopathy. He had no food or liquid for 8 h in preparation for the procedure.

The patient underwent celiac plexus neurolysis using a posterior *transaortic* approach. He was placed in the prone position, the injection area was prepared with chlorhexidine, and the skin, subcutaneous tissues, and muscle were anesthetized with 1% lidocaine at a point approximately 6–7 cm from the left of the midline. A 13-cm, 20-G Quincke spinal needle was placed through the anesthetized area and directed toward the posterior aorta. With the aid of computerized tomography (CT), the needle was oriented slightly laterally to the T12–L1 interspace and carefully shifted until its tip rested in the retro-aortic space. With advancement, aortic pulsations were transmitted to the needle. The needle was advanced gradually through increased resistance until it passed through the posterior wall of the aorta. The stylet was removed, and immediately Luer-locking tubing with a three-way stopcock at the end was attached to the needle and held until a free flow of arterial blood was seen, indicating needle position within the aortic lumen. The needle was advanced in a slow constant-rate progression with the tubing demonstrating a pulsatile column of blood. The three-way stopcock was available to cease overflow during the procedure. The needle was advanced through increased resistance until a change in resistance was felt as it passed through the anterior aortic wall and confirmed under CT guidance. The pulsations had ceased, and the needle was advanced another 3 mm indicating a probable location within the substance of the celiac plexus. The stylet was removed, and after gentle aspiration, contrast medium was injected. A CT scan at the level of the needle showed contrast medium in the preaortic area and surrounding the aorta, confirming satisfactory needle placement. No contrast was observed in the retrocrural space or intravascularly.

Initially, an injection of lidocaine 1% 10 ml was injected to reduce the pain with subsequent injection of alcohol. Then after 4 min of waiting to allow neural blockade to prevent significant pain with alcohol, an injection of 15 mL of absolute alcohol was performed. The needle was flushed with a small amount of sterile saline, the stylet was replaced, and then the needle was removed. The patient was observed carefully in the recovery area for hemodynamic changes including hypotension and tachycardia for 30 min after the procedure, and no complications were noted with ambulation just prior to departure from the clinic.

Twelve hours later, the patient developed severe left-sided flank and back pain and presented to the emergency department at his local hospital. He was lethargic and pale and had thready pulses. Initial vital signs were notable for tachycardia (HR = 121 bpm) and hypotension with blood pressure of

R. Mattie, M.D.
Division of Pain Medicine Clinical Fellow, PGY-5, Department of Anesthesia and Perioperative Care, University of California at San Francisco, San Francisco, CA 94143, USA

R.K. Naidu, M.D. (✉)
Pain Physician and Anesthesiologist, Mt Tam Orthopedics, Medical Director of Pain Management for Marin General Hospital, Novato, CA 94945, USA
e-mail: ramonaidu@me.com

M. Anitescu et al. (eds.), *Challenging Cases and Complication Management in Pain Medicine*,
https://doi.org/10.1007/978-3-319-60072-7_21

82/50 mmHg. A complete blood count revealed hemoglobin of 7.3 g/dL and hematocrit of 21.6%. An emergent CT scan showed a large (10 cm × 12 cm × 8 cm) hematoma in the retrorenal space extending into the interfascial plane behind the left kidney. He was taken to the intensive care unit and treated conservatively with 2 L of normal saline for fluid resuscitation and 2 units of blood. General surgery and interventional radiology were consulted for possible interventions. Blood pressure and hemoglobin levels responded appropriately, and he remained hemodynamically stable in the ICU. Serial hematocrits and neurologic checks were performed and were stable. A repeat CT angiogram 24 h later revealed no further active bleeding or increase in the size of the hematoma, and the patient recovered well.

21.2 Case Discussion

This patient suffered a delayed retroperitoneal hematoma resulting from celiac plexus neurolysis through a posterior transaortic approach. Though it is a relatively uncommon complication of celiac plexus block, development of a retroperitoneal hematoma represents a serious condition with a risk of mortality if not treated appropriately. Potential areas at risk for bleeding during celiac plexus block, as well as retroperitoneal hematoma presentation, management, and treatment, will be discussed further.

21.2.1 Celiac Plexus Block Positioning and Techniques

In order to understand the risk of bleeding associated with a celiac plexus block, it is important to review the anatomic location of the plexus, along with the variety of approaches taken to reach the plexus itself. While the chapter on autonomic dysfunction related to these blocks focused on the nervous system, this chapter will look at the vasculature that can be impacted by these procedures. During a celiac plexus block, accurate depiction of the retroperitoneal anatomy (Fig. 21.1) and the position of the needle tip can help to avoid crucial vascular structures such as the aorta, celiac artery, superior mesenteric artery (SMA), intercostal artery, artery of Adamkiewicz, feeding spinal arteries, and renal arteries [1, 2].

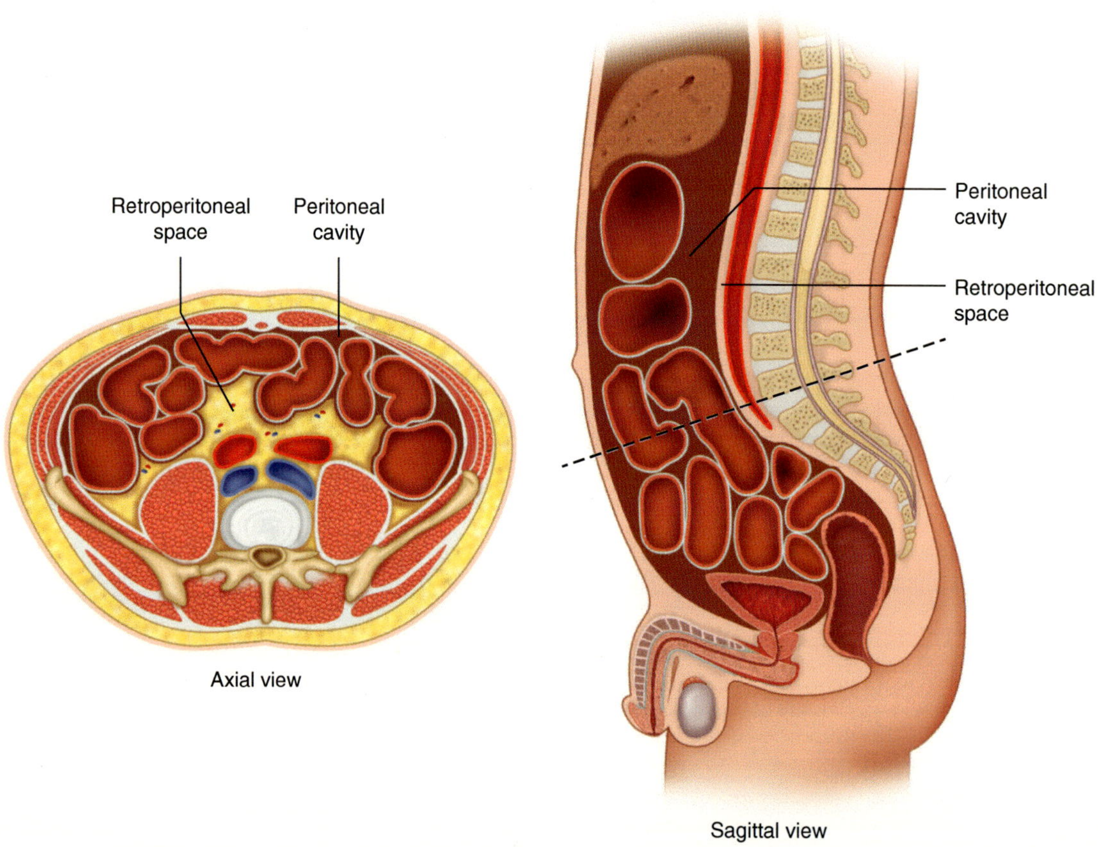

Fig. 21.1 Retroperitoneal space

The celiac plexus is located deep in the retroperitoneum, behind the stomach and omental bursa, and anterior to the crura of the diaphragm on the level of the first lumbar vertebra. It lies over the anterolateral surface of the aorta and around the origin of the celiac trunk for several centimeters, demonstrating considerable variability in size, number, and position [1–5]. The position of the celiac ganglia has been reported to be anywhere from the T12–L1 disk space to the middle of the L2 vertebral body, though prior reports indicate the most common location is at the level of T12 or L1 [1–6]. Nonetheless, the position of the celiac plexus relative to the celiac artery is more consistent than that of the vertebral column, making the celiac artery a more reliable landmark for localizing the plexus [7–9]. The right celiac ganglia are approximately 0.6 cm caudal to the celiac artery, and the left celiac ganglia are slightly more caudal at 0.9 cm [7–9].

Due to the anatomic variability of vascular structures and plexus location between patients, pre-procedure planning is essential. Prior imaging should be obtained and reviewed in detail to determine patient positioning, procedure approach, type of needle, needle entry site and path, and the site of neurolytic injection [9, 10]. Taking these steps will increase the likelihood that the neurolytic agent is delivered accurately and distributed appropriately to provide the greatest analgesic effect while reducing morbidity and mortality [9, 10].

21.2.2 Positioning

There are several positions that may be used depending on the approach and the patient's overall condition. Positioning influences the percutaneous path of the needle and is essential for a safe procedure. It is important to ensure patient comfort to minimize motion in an effort to prevent inadvertent needle puncture of nearby organs or vasculature. The positions commonly used for this procedure are prone, lateral decubitus, oblique, and supine.

The prone position is most common and permits posterior approaches [1]. Pillows are placed beneath the iliac crests to reduce lumbar lordosis. This position is not preferred in obese patients or in patients who cannot maintain a safe airway [1]. The lateral decubitus or the oblique position can be used if the prone position is not tolerated. Supine positioning is usually the most comfortable and is used with an anterior approach obviating this particular complication.

21.2.3 Retroperitoneal Hematoma

Retroperitoneal hematoma is a well-recognized but relatively rare condition, with an incidence of approximately 0.1% and possibly as high as 0.6% in patients on anticoagulation therapy [11]. The incidence, however, is increasing due to complications related to interventional and image-guided procedures [12, 13]. Despite advances in procedures and imaging, detection and treatment of retroperitoneal hematoma remain challenging [14]. Diagnosis is often delayed due to a lack of specific symptoms, and the bleeding may initially go unrecognized. A timely and accurate diagnosis is critical for survival of the patient; even if patients do not die of rapid exsanguination, they may die later on from complications of compartment syndrome [12, 15].

21.2.4 Risk Factors for the Development of Retroperitoneal Hematoma

The American Society of Regional Anesthesia and Pain Medicine (ASRA) in conjunction with the European Society of Regional Anaesthesia and Pain Therapy (ESRA), the American Academy of Pain Medicine (AAPM), the International Neuromodulation Society (INS), the North American Neuromodulation Society (NANS), and the World Institute of Pain (WIP) came up with interventional-specific guidelines on the use of antiplatelet and anticoagulant medications in 2015 [16]. The guidelines delineated in the consensus document [16] are helpful for practitioners to understand when drugs should be ceased and restarted; however, these should only serve as a guide as each case requires its own evaluation of risks versus benefits. New antithrombotic drugs are always being added to the market and may not be listed as time progresses. Celiac plexus block or neurolysis was considered an intermediate risk procedure. Patients are at higher risk if they are of old age, with history of bleeding tendency, concurrent use of antithrombotics, liver cirrhosis, or advanced hepatic or renal disease.

There are patient factors that can increase risk for bleeding complications including thrombocytopathia/thrombocytopenia (e.g., von Willebrand's disease), varices, and vascular variability, among others. Procedural factors include several passes of the needle(s) or a "traumatic entry," low-gauge (thicker diameter) needles, blunt tip needles, etc.

It is important to obtain a thorough history and physical examination in order to pick up any of these risks. Laboratory diagnostic tests are not routinely ordered, but if there are concerns from the patient's history or physical exam, such as a history of chemotherapy, bruising, bleeding gums when brushing teeth, epistaxis, etc., these should be explored with laboratory testing. Imaging is not ordered routinely prior to intervention, but often imaging is available for other reasons and should be obtained and reviewed. As with laboratory workup, if there are concerns based on the history and physical, imaging can be ordered or done in conjunction with the procedure.

21.2.5 Diagnosis of Retroperitoneal Hematoma

Patients with uncontrolled retroperitoneal bleeding rarely present with obvious cutaneous manifestations such as Grey Turner or Cullen signs. Instead they initially exhibit subtle signs of hemorrhage like relative hypotension and mild tachycardia. Confounding the picture even more is the fact that hypotension is a common side effect of celiac plexus block. Loss of sympathetic tone and dilated abdominal vasculature as a result of celiac plexus block can lead to orthostatic hypotension, a complication seen in up to 38% of patients [17, 18]. It is usually transient (1–3 days) and can be managed with intravenous hydration, but assuming a patient's hypotension is a result of the procedure when the true cause is a hematoma that delays the diagnosis, prolongs bleeding, and could potentially lead to greater morbidity or mortality [19, 20]. It is also important to consider that patients on beta-blockers may not be able to have a tachycardic response, becoming hypotensive with no change in heart rate [12].

Other signs and symptoms of retroperitoneal hematoma include abdominal pain, abdominal distention, bruising, severe back pain, flank pain, lower quadrant pain, groin discomfort, and femoral neuropathy [21]. Femoral neuropathy is often the result of bleeding after puncture of the femoral artery during coronary angiography [22]; however, retroperitoneal hematoma from other causes can lead to femoral neuropathy, and this has been infrequently reported in the literature. The most commonly reported associations are with various bleeding disorders and therapeutic anticoagulation [23], but theoretically retroperitoneal hematoma can result from any cause of bleeding into the retroperitoneal space, such as intratumoral bleeding, ruptures of a retroperitoneal organ, or aneurysm [24, 25]. Femoral neuropathy from retroperitoneal hematoma can present with severe groin and hip pain radiating to the anterior thigh and lumbar region and later on can lead to characteristic paresthesia in the anteromedial thigh and leg [23] (Table 21.1).

Imaging plays an important role in the diagnosis of retroperitoneal hematoma, providing useful information on the type, site, and extent of fluid collections. Ultrasonography is a rapid means of detecting hematoma without exposing patients to radiation, but it may not be precise enough to identify the cause. Unfortunately, ultrasound is often distorted by body habitus or underlying bowel gas, or limited by a patient's discomfort or operator skill [26, 27]. Hemodynamically stable patients with a negative diagnosis from ultrasound but a high clinical suspicion for retroperitoneal hematoma should undergo stat CT scanning [14].

CT scanning is noninvasive, rapidly obtainable, and highly sensitive for diagnosing retroperitoneal hematoma.

Table 21.1 Signs and symptoms of retroperitoneal hematoma

Retroperitoneal hematoma		
Clinical signs	CT imaging of hematoma	CT imaging of active bleeding
Hypotension Tachycardia Abdominal pain Abdominal distention Bruising Severe back pain Flank pain Lower quadrant pain Groin discomfort Femoral neuropathy	Abnormal soft tissue density Compressed adjacent normal structures	Extravasation of contrast material, which appears as a hyperattenuating pool or jet, with attenuation similar to adjacent vessels

Bleeding from arteries at high risk during a celiac plexus, such as the suprarenal aorta, the celiac axis, or the SMA, is most likely to result in an upper abdominal midline supramesocolic retroperitoneal hematoma [28, 29]. In an unenhanced CT scan, a hematoma will appear as an abnormal soft tissue density that compresses adjacent normal structures [30]. Active bleeding can be seen by extravasation of contrast material, which appears as a hyperattenuating pool or jet, with attenuation similar to adjacent vessels [31, 32]. If CT angiography shows contrast outside of the vessels, urgent treatment is required. In fact, some argue that angiography should not be performed unless an interventional radiologist is prepared to embolize, if an arterial injury is identified [33].

21.2.6 Management of Retroperitoneal Hematoma

Treatment of a retroperitoneal hematoma remains controversial, and there are no specific guidelines detailing when to use endovascular or open surgical intervention to stop the bleeding. It depends on the resources of where the patient lands. If the patient is hemodynamically stable with no evidence of active bleeding, conservative management with close monitoring, fluid resuscitation, blood transfusion, and normalization of coagulation factors is recommended. Panetta et al. have suggested that hemodynamic instability despite 4 or more units of blood transfused within 24 h, or 6 or more units transfused within 48 h, is an indication for further investigation and endovascular treatment [34].

Embolization is becoming more common as an alternative to open surgery for treating retroperitoneal hematoma and should be performed whenever arterial extravasation is seen [12]. In a retrospective analysis of 25 patients with an extraperitoneal hematoma, Farrelly et al. found transcatheter embolization to be an effective and safe procedure for treatment of bleeding extraperitoneal hematoma [35]. Several small case series have also shown successful cessation of bleeding in retroperitoneal hemorrhage with endovascular embolization [36–38]. Coils, gelatin, and polyvinyl alcohol have all been used for embolization, though a prior study commented that proximal coiling of the bleeding artery might not be sufficient in the retroperitoneum [36]. Embolic agents should be placed both proximal and distal to the bleeding site to prevent rebleeding. While there is a high technical success rate of embolization, extraperitoneal hematomas are associated with a relatively poor prognosis, with high patient mortality around the time of angiography, but this is often due to other comorbidities [35].

Though there are no guidelines detailing when to attempt open surgery to stop active retroperitoneal hematoma [35], open surgery with exploratory laparotomy is generally indicated in patients not responding to conservative treatment or when interventional endovascular embolization is not successful. Traditionally clinicians have been reluctant to operate because of the difficulty identifying or ligating bleeding vessels within the hematoma [39, 40]. As such, the procedure is typically guided by preoperative CT findings. Surgery is also indicated if a patient develops abdominal compartment syndrome as a result of a large retroperitoneal hematoma, which requires prompt decompression [41, 42]. Though surgery certainly has its place in the treatment of retroperitoneal hematoma, removal of the hematoma can also increase bleeding by removing the tamponade effect [12].

Key Points

- Retroperitoneal hematoma is a rare complication of celiac plexus block that can have severe consequences if not diagnosed quickly.
- If a patient presents with orthostatic hypotension after undergoing celiac plexus block, the possibility of hemorrhage must be ruled out before assuming that it is due to an autonomic response to the block.
- Patients may also present with back, abdominal, flank, or groin pain, but cutaneous manifestations of bruising are not likely to be present.
- Patients suspected of having a retroperitoneal hematoma should be admitted to the hospital for serial hematocrit monitoring, fluid resuscitation, and blood transfusion and will also likely need a CT scan.
- A surgical consult should be obtained as soon as possible in conjunction with interventional radiology.
- Most patients with retroperitoneal hematoma can be monitored closely and treated conservatively, but occasionally endovascular or surgical intervention is required.

References

1. Kambadakone A, Thabet A, Gervais DA, Mueller PR, Arellano RS. CT-guided celiac plexus neurolysis: a review of anatomy, indications, technique, and tips for successful treatment. Radiographics. 2011;31:1599–621.
2. Loukas M, Klaassen Z, Merbs W, Tubbs RS, Gielecki J, Zurada A. A review of the thoracic splanchnic nerves and celiac ganglia. Clin Anat. 2010;23:512–22.
3. Mercadante S, Nicosia F. Celiac plexus block: a reappraisal. Reg Anesth Pain Med. 1998;23:37–48.
4. Erdine S. Celiac ganglion block. Agri. 2005;17:14–22.
5. Rathmell JP, Gallant JM, Brown DL. Computed tomography and the anatomy of celiac plexus block. Reg Anesth Pain Med. 2000;25:411–6.
6. Zhang XM, Zhao QH, Zeng NL, et al. The celiac ganglia: anatomic study using MRI in cadavers. AJR Am J Roentgenol. 2006;186:1520–3.
7. De Cicco M, Matovic M, Balestreri L, Fracasso A, Morassut S, Testa V. Single-needle celiac plexus block: is needle tip position critical in patients with no regional anatomic distortions? Anesthesiology. 1997;87:1301–8.
8. Penman ID. Coeliac plexus neurolysis. Best Pract Res Clin Gastroenterol. 2009;23:761–6.
9. Titton RL, Lucey BC, Gervais DA, Boland GW, Mueller PR. Celiac plexus block: a palliative tool underused by radiologists. AJR Am J Roentgenol. 2002;179:633–6.
10. Wang PJ, Shang MY, Qian Z, Shao CW, Wang JH, Zhao XH. CT-guided percutaneous neurolytic celiac plexus block technique. Abdom Imaging. 2006;31:710–8.
11. Estivill Palleja X, Domingo P, Fontcuberta J, Felez J. Spontaneous retroperitoneal hemorrhage during oral anticoagulant therapy. Arch Intern Med. 1985;145:1531, 4.
12. Chan YC, Morales JP, Reidy JF, Taylor PR. Management of spontaneous and iatrogenic retroperitoneal haemorrhage: conservative management, endovascular intervention or open surgery? Int J Clin Pract. 2008;62:1604–13.
13. Lim WC, Leblanc JK. Retroperitoneal bleeding after EUS-guided FNA of a pancreatic mass. Gastrointest Endosc. 2006;63:499–500.
14. Wang F, Wang F. The diagnosis and treatment of traumatic retroperitoneal hematoma. Pak J Med Sci. 2013;29:573–6.
15. Iribarne A, Easterwood R, Yang J, Dayal R, Argenziano M. Retroperitoneal hematoma with abdominal compartment syndrome during minimally invasive mitral valve replacement. Ann Thorac Surg. 2010;89:e17–8.
16. Narouze S, Benzon HT, Provenzano DA, et al. Interventional spine and pain procedures in patients on antiplatelet and anticoagulant medications: guidelines from the American Society of Regional Anesthesia and Pain Medicine, the European Society of Regional Anaesthesia and Pain Therapy, the American Academy of Pain Medicine, The International Neuromodulation Society, the North American Neuromodulation Society, and the World Institute of Pain. Reg Anesth Pain Med. 2015;40:182–212.
17. Eisenberg E, Carr DB, Chalmers TC. Neurolytic celiac plexus block for treatment of cancer pain: a meta-analysis. Anesth Analg. 1995;80:290–5.
18. Akinci D, Akhan O. Celiac ganglia block. Eur J Radiol. 2005;55:355–61.
19. Fugere F, Lewis G. Coeliac plexus block for chronic pain syndromes. Can J Anaesth. 1993;40:954–63.
20. Haaga JR, Kori SH, Eastwood DW, Borkowski GP. Improved technique for CT-guided celiac ganglia block. AJR Am J Roentgenol. 1984;142:1201–4.
21. Murai Y, Adachi K, Yoshida Y, Takei M, Teramoto A. Retroperitoneal hematoma as a serious complication of endovascular aneurysmal coiling. J Korean Neurosurg Soc. 2010;48:88–90.

22. Farouque HM, Tremmel JA, Raissi Shabari F, et al. Risk factors for the development of retroperitoneal hematoma after percutaneous coronary intervention in the era of glycoprotein IIb/IIIa inhibitors and vascular closure devices. J Am Coll Cardiol. 2005;45:363–8.
23. Parmer SS, Carpenter JP, Fairman RM, Velazquez OC, Mitchell ME. Femoral neuropathy following retroperitoneal hemorrhage: case series and review of the literature. Ann Vasc Surg. 2006;20:536–40.
24. Daliakopoulos SI, Bairaktaris A, Papadimitriou D, Pappas P. Gigantic retroperitoneal hematoma as a complication of anticoagulation therapy with heparin in therapeutic doses: a case report. J Med Case Rep. 2008;2:162.
25. Aune S, Trippestad A. Chronic contained rupture of an abdominal aortic aneurysm complicated by infection and femoral neuropathy. Case report. Eur J Surg. 1995;161:613–4.
26. Silverstein A. Neuropathy in hemophilia. JAMA. 1964;190:554–5.
27. Merrick HW, Zeiss J, Woldenberg LS. Percutaneous decompression for femoral neuropathy secondary to heparin-induced retroperitoneal hematoma: case report and review of the literature. Am Surg. 1991;57:706–11.
28. Accola KD, Feliciano DV, Mattox KL, Burch JM, Beall AC Jr, Jordan GL Jr. Management of injuries to the superior mesenteric artery. J Trauma. 1986;26:313–9.
29. Mattox KL, Burch JM, Richardson R, Martin RR. Retroperitoneal vascular injury. Surg Clin North Am. 1990;70:635–53.
30. Lindner A, Zierz S. Images in clinical medicine. Retroperitoneal hemorrhage. N Engl J Med. 2001;344:348.
31. Scialpi M, Scaglione M, Angelelli G, et al. Emergencies in the retroperitoneum: assessment of spread of disease by helical CT. Eur J Radiol. 2004;50:74–83.
32. Murakami AM, Anderson SW, Soto JA, Kertesz JL, Ozonoff A, Rhea JT. Active extravasation of the abdomen and pelvis in trauma using 64MDCT. Emerg Radiol. 2009;16:375–82.
33. Sclafani SJ, Florence LO, Phillips TF, et al. Lumbar arterial injury: radiologic diagnosis and management. Radiology. 1987;165:709–14.
34. Panetta T, Sclafani SJ, Goldstein AS, Phillips TF, Shaftan GW. Percutaneous transcatheter embolization for massive bleeding from pelvic fractures. J Trauma. 1985;25:1021–9.
35. Farrelly C, Fidelman N, Durack JC, Hagiwara E, Kerlan RK Jr. Transcatheter arterial embolization of spontaneous life-threatening extraperitoneal hemorrhage. J Vasc Interv Radiol. 2011;22:1396–402.
36. Isokangas JM, Perala JM. Endovascular embolization of spontaneous retroperitoneal hemorrhage secondary to anticoagulant treatment. Cardiovasc Intervent Radiol. 2004;27:607–11.
37. Sharafuddin MJ, Andresen KJ, Sun S, Lang E, Stecker MS, Wibbenmeyer LA. Spontaneous extraperitoneal hemorrhage with hemodynamic collapse in patients undergoing anticoagulation: management with selective arterial embolization. J Vasc Interv Radiol. 2001;12:1231–4.
38. Pathi R, Voyvodic F, Thompson WR. Spontaneous extraperitoneal haemorrhage: computed tomography diagnosis and treatment by selective arterial embolization. Australas Radiol. 2004;48:123–8.
39. Milutinovich J, Follette WC, Scribner BH. Spontaneous retroperitoneal bleeding in patients on chronic hemodialysis. Ann Intern Med. 1977;86:189–92.
40. Pode D, Caine M. Spontaneous retroperitoneal hemorrhage. J Urol. 1992;147:311–8.
41. Dabney A, Bastani B. Enoxaparin-associated severe retroperitoneal bleeding and abdominal compartment syndrome: a report of two cases. Intensive Care Med. 2001;27:1954–7.
42. Howdieshell TR, Proctor CD, Sternberg E, Cue JI, Mondy JS, Hawkins ML. Temporary abdominal closure followed by definitive abdominal wall reconstruction of the open abdomen. Am J Surg. 2004;188:301–6.

Autonomic Insufficiency After Neurolytic Celiac Plexus Block

22

Mark J. Burish, Ryan Mattie, and Ramana K. Naidu

22.1 Case Description

A 49-year-old gentleman, with a history of chronic pancreatitis from a history of alcoholism (abstinent for 2 years) and abdominal pain, presents for a diagnostic bilateral splanchnic nerve block. The plan was to perform radiofrequency ablation if he received >50% relief from the diagnostic procedure in order to prolong the duration of relief. At the time of his procedure visit, he had lost 10 pounds over several weeks, which he attributed to decreased appetite from nausea and pain when he tried to eat. Otherwise there were no significant changes to his pain or medical history. He had no food or liquid for 8 h, except for medications with sips of water, in preparation for his procedure.

His bilateral splanchnic nerve block was uneventful. The procedure was performed in the prone position. Needle placement was at the base of the T12 vertebra, with the needle tip 3 mm anterior to the anterior border of the vertebral body. Aspiration was negative, and injection of contrast showed appropriate cephalocaudal spread confined to the plane consistent with the expected location of the splanchnic nerves. Medications used included 3 mL of 1% lidocaine into the skin and soft tissues on each side and 20 mL of injectate (10 mL per side) consisting of 17 mL of 0.2% ropivacaine, 100 mcg clonidine, and 8 mg dexamethasone. The patient also received intravenous sedation with 1.5 mg midazolam and 150 mcg fentanyl and was given 1 L of normal saline over the course of the procedure. Signs of intravascular uptake were negative including periodic re-aspiration for blood, stable blood pressure at 115/75 and pulse of 90, and lack of metallic taste or tinnitus. His pain improved from 7/10 to 1/10.

After the procedure, the patient remained on the table for 20 min and received juice and crackers in the recumbent position. His blood pressures initially were within 5 mmHg of his pre-procedure pressures. With nursing staff present, he progressed to a sitting position and then standing and stated that he felt "fine." He then ambulated 50 ft to the front of the clinic. While standing at the front desk, he verbalized that he was starting to feel flushed and light-headed. Clinic staff came to his side and then caught him as he lost consciousness for approximately 3 s. Afterward he stated that he felt "back to normal" with no confusion. He was placed in a wheelchair and brought back to the procedure room, where vital signs were BP 85/60 and HR 105. Another intravenous catheter was placed, and a second liter of normal saline was given; the patient remained in the recovery area for another 45 min. His vital signs normalized with his systolic blood pressure maintaining above 105 mmHg and HR at 91 bpm. He was warned of symptoms such as bowel or bladder incontinence or motor impairment. He was told that diarrhea was common and was told to stay hydrated. He received a follow-up phone call the following day and stated no additional episodes of light-headedness or flushing. He did have an episode of diarrhea which was unusual for him—he had no vomiting and no fevers or chills, and he and his wife ate the same food, but she did not have any diarrhea.

Our patient suffered a transient orthostatic hypotensive event in the setting of blockade of the splanchnic nerves, recent weight loss, and an 8-h fast for intravenous sedation. Transient hypotension after celiac plexus block occurs 38% of the time, with transient diarrhea occurring 44% of the time [1]. Both of these complications and adverse effects are well described in the literature and will be discussed further below.

M.J. Burish, M.D., Ph.D.
Department of Neurosurgery, University of Texas Health Science Center, Houston, TX 77030, USA

R. Mattie, M.D.
Division of Pain Medicine Clinical Fellow, PGY-5, Department of Anesthesia and Perioperative Care University of California at San Francisco, San Francisco, CA 94143, USA

R.K. Naidu, M.D. (✉)
Pain Physician and Anesthesiologist, Mt Tam Orthopedics, Medical Director of Pain Management for Marin General Hospital, Novato, CA 94945, USA
e-mail: ramonaidu@me.com

M. Anitescu et al. (eds.), *Challenging Cases and Complication Management in Pain Medicine*,
https://doi.org/10.1007/978-3-319-60072-7_22

22.2 Discussions

22.2.1 Anatomy

An explanation of the autonomic side effects of a celiac plexus block begins with a discussion of the celiac plexus, which is a prevertebral ganglion that is part of the autonomic nervous system (Fig. 22.1). Structurally, the celiac plexus is actually a distinct collection of one to five ganglia [2], each approximately 2 cm × 2 cm [3], arising immediately anterior to the aorta at the T11, T12, or L1 level [3, 4]. Relative to the celiac artery, the celiac plexus is on average 6 mm inferior on the right and 9 mm inferior on the left [5]. There is very limited data on gender differences [4] or variations in pediatric patients.

The celiac plexus receives parasympathetic innervation from the vagus nerve [6], sympathetic input from three splanchnic nerves [7, 8], and visceral sensation via both the vagus and the splanchnic nerves. In terms of the three splanchnic nerves, the first is the greater splanchnic nerve, which receives inputs from the T5–T10 levels of the sympathetic

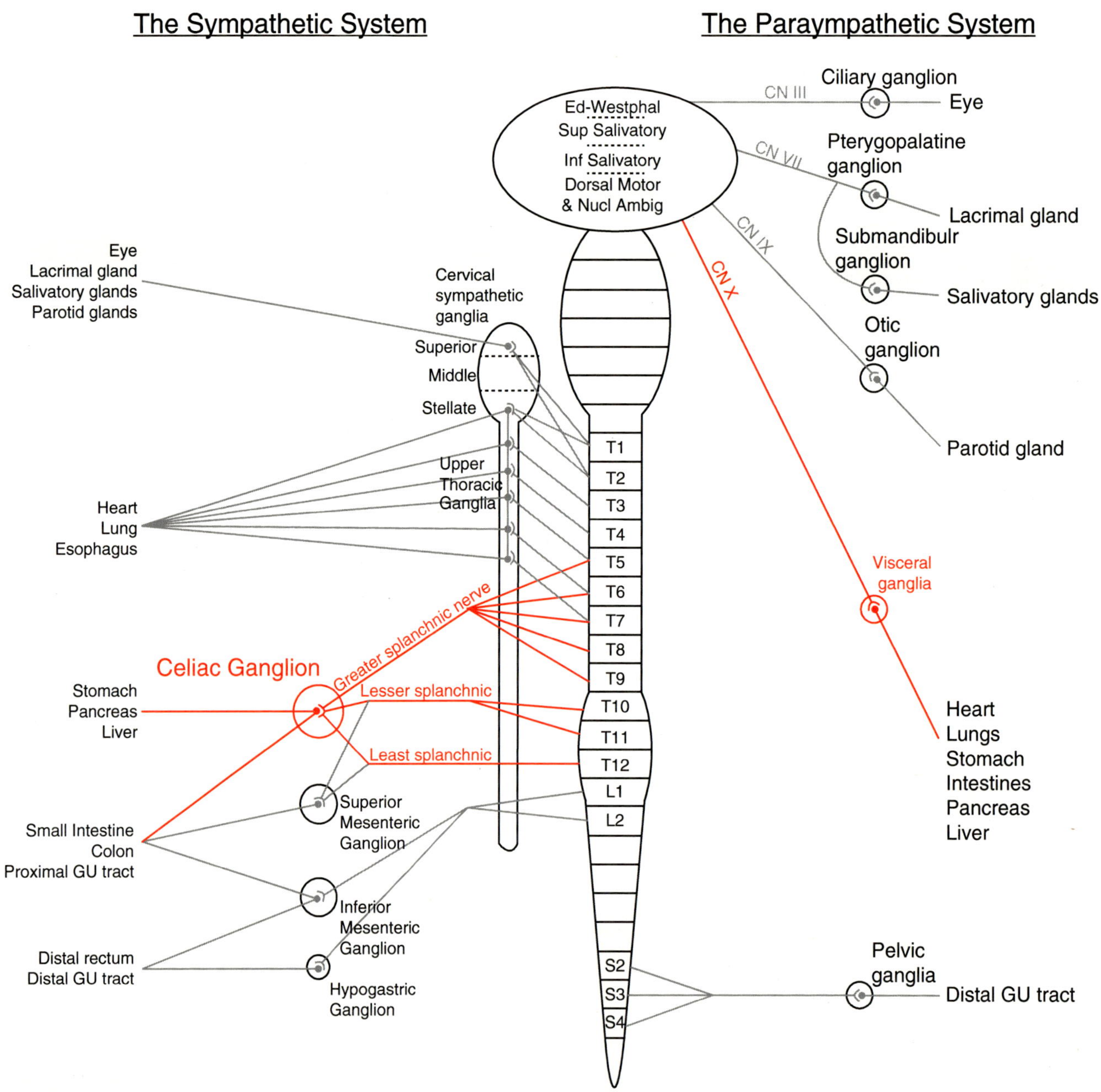

Fig. 22.1 The autonomic nervous system. *Ed-Westphal* Edinger-Westphal nucleus, *Sup Saliv* superior salivatory nucleus, *Inf Saliv* inferior salivatory nucleus, *Dorsal Motor and Nucl Ambig* dorsal motor nucleus of the vagus nerve and nucleus ambiguus. Visceral ganglia refer to ganglia located near or on the respective organs, such as the cardiac, pulmonary, celiac, myenteric, and submucosal plexuses

paravertebral chain (the T5–T10 thoracic ganglia) but may also involve T4 or T11. The second is the lesser splanchnic nerve, which receives inputs from T10–T11 but may also involve T8 and T9. The third is the least splanchnic nerve, which receives inputs from T12 but may also involve T10 and T11; the least splanchnic nerve is occasionally absent [8, 9], with its nerves presumably incorporated into the other splanchnic nerves. The most common pattern is for all three nerves to pass through the diaphragm at a single hiatus, making this a favorable location for blockade in what has been referred to as a splanchnic or retrocrural celiac block. In rare cases, however, the three nerves can go through three separate hiatuses [9]. Visceral sensation, including nociception, is derived from spinal and vagal visceral afferents that pass through the celiac ganglion; while the spinal afferents have traditionally been thought to be responsible for nociception and pass through the splanchnic nerves, some evidence suggests that vagal visceral afferents may also play a role [10].

The exact organs innervated by the celiac plexus are a matter of some debate but generally include sympathetic, parasympathetic, and visceral sensory innervation of the stomach, liver, gallbladder, bile ducts, pancreas, small intestine, ascending colon, distal esophagus, and possibly kidneys and adrenals [2, 11]. Thus, the celiac plexus is a favorable single target to provide a dense visceral sensory block of the upper abdomen, but a block at this location invariably affects autonomic nerves as well as visceral sensation.

22.2.2 Techniques

There are several approaches to the celiac plexus, and thus there is often confusion about the rationale and the risks/benefits of each technique. In performing a percutaneous needle-based procedure, the goal is simply to have the needle tip at the location or in a plane contiguous with the celiac plexus or splanchnic nerves. In some situations, an open technique can be performed in conjunction with surgeons performing a laparotomy; this allows for direct application of solution to the nerves under direct visualization. Given the central location of these nerves, multiple needle trajectories have been described.

22.2.2.1 Posterior Percutaneous Retrocrural/Splanchnic Approach

The most common trajectories currently are the posterior approaches [12]. The first posterior approach is commonly referred to as a *retrocrural celiac plexus block* and is similar in injectate spread to a *splanchnic nerve block*. The term splanchnic nerve block is often used because it specifies that these are the nerves that are blocked on their way to the celiac plexus. This block, as the name describes, is performed with the final needle position near the anterior border of the T12 or L1 vertebral body and posterior to the diaphragm; it targets the greater, lesser, and least splanchnic nerves as they all come in close proximity. This technique avoids piercing the aorta, but it does require two needles on each side of the vertebral bodies. This is also a potential target for thermal neurolysis, which can be done with radiofrequency ablation. One does not generally attempt chemical neurolysis with these blocks given the potential for nerve root neurolysis.

22.2.2.2 Posterior Percutaneous Antecrural Approach

The *antecrural* approach is, as the name implies, where the needle's final position is anterior to the crus of the diaphragm. With this technique, there are several potential locations for the needle to reside in relation to the aorta, generally a distance 10 mm anterior to the anterior border of the vertebral body. The purpose is to be in a plane where the injectate can reach the celiac plexus without diffusing into the aorta. It can lie posterior to it in the retro-aortic space or lateral to it without piercing it. This latter approach, with the needle positioned lateral and adjacent to the aorta, is often described as the *transcrural* approach. On occasion with this approach, the needle is within the aorta as noted by blood return or contrast injection revealing an aortogram; in this situation, one can proceed with the *transaortic* approach.

22.2.2.3 Posterior Percutaneous Posterior Transaortic Approach

The *transaortic approach* is performed with the needle positioned through the aorta at the T12 or L1 vertebral level until the needle is placed through and anterior to the aortic adventitia. This can be accomplished with one needle from the left side and is the preferred choice for chemical neurolysis. This particular approach is done with the provider using aortic pulsations to determine progress through the vessel. Practitioners can feel resonance through the needle, or they can attach low dead-space Luer-locking tubing with a length greater than the recorded blood pressure with conversion from mmHg to cmH_2O, and the column of blood can be seen pulsating until needle position is into the anterior aortic wall. At least another 2–4 mm of advancement is required to ensure that the needle does not remain in the intima, media, or adventitia, or any plane between; care must be taken to ensure that the needle is through the aortic wall to avoid the potential for aortic dissection during injection. The use of contrast and plunger pressure monitoring of injection can aid in reducing this complication.

In spite of the seeming danger, puncture of the aorta is actually relatively safe, and overall, major complications from celiac plexus block occur in less than 1% of patients [13]. Nonetheless, aortic dissection is one of the most concerning complications and has been reported to arise from use of the transaortic approach. Kaplan et al. described a fatal case of needle puncture in the anterior aortic intima between the superior mesenteric artery (SMA) and celiac artery causing dissection and vascular thrombosis that resulted in bowel and liver infarction [14]. Additionally, Naveira et al. reported an atheromatous aortic plaque presenting as a loss of resistance that also resulted in aortic dissection [15]. Because of the puncture of the aorta and the proximity of other vascular structures like the SMA and celiac and renal arteries, the transaortic approach is contraindicated in patients receiving anticoagulant medication and in patients with coagulopathy secondary to antiblastic chemotherapy or liver abnormalities, as they are at increased risk for retroperitoneal hemorrhage, a complication which is discussed in the previous chapter [16–18].

22.2.2.4 Posterior Percutaneous Transdiscal Approach

The posterior transdiscal approach involves passage of the needle directly through the T12–L1 or L1–L2 intervertebral disk via fluoroscopic or CT guidance. The needle is inserted 5–7 cm from the midline and directed to reach the paraaortic region at the level of the celiac trunk [19]. By traversing the intervertebral disk, this approach theoretically minimizes hazards of injury to the arteries and spinal cord, and potential damage to the liver, kidney, and pancreas as with other approaches can be avoided [20, 21]. It can also be used when the paravertebral needle path is obstructed by transverse processes or ribs or for improved access to the anterolateral wall of the aorta in patients with abnormal anatomy [16, 18, 19]. Although this procedure offers the possibility of avoiding vascular or organ trauma, it is not routinely used. There is increased risk for disk trauma that could lead to diskitis, herniation, meningeal puncture, and spinal cord puncture; this approach should be avoided in patients with degenerative disk disease in the thoracolumbar spine [16, 18, 19].

22.2.2.5 Anterior Percutaneous Approach

The celiac plexus can be approached from the ventral surface of the abdomen using CT guidance, MRI guidance, or ultrasound guidance. This approach can be more comfortable for patients who cannot lie prone with their pain or because they have a colostomy/ileostomy. In the anterior approach, the patient lies supine. The needle is inserted through the epigastrium at an entry site 1.5 cm below and 1.5 cm to the left of the xiphoid process [22]. The needle is advanced to a depth anterior to the aorta and the diaphragmatic crura between the roots of the celiac trunk and the SMA and most commonly traverses the stomach, liver, or pancreas before reaching the plexus [21, 22]. Although the anterior approach minimizes the risk of injury to the kidney and spinal cord, steps should be taken to prevent other complications [21]. It is essential to avoid major blood vessels, dilated biliary ducts, and portal hilum, and multiple punctures to the liver capsule can increase the risk of bleeding [21, 23]. Vascular structures in the neck of the pancreas must be avoided to prevent unnecessary bleeding [21]. Additionally, there have been reports of gastric perforation, pancreatic fistula, hepatic hematoma, retroperitoneal hematoma, paraplegia, and abscess with this approach [24–26]. While there is concern about contamination and potential infectious seeding, this approach, when done with a styleted and small needle (e.g., Chiba or Quincke), has been reported to be safe [5].

22.2.2.6 Endoscopic Ultrasound-Guided Approach

An endoscopic ultrasound-guided approach can be performed by endoscopists and generally is well-tolerated by patients. In a prospective randomized comparison of endoscopic ultrasound (EUS) and CT-guided celiac plexus block in 22 patients, the authors concluded that EUS-guided block provided more persistent pain relief than CT-guided block [27]. Advantages include a lack of radiation with EUS as compared to CT and costs. Challenges include visualization of deeper structures as intestinal air can impede sonographic imaging. Gastric perforation and infectious complications appear to be the most common complications associated with this approach. It can be more comfortable for patients and can also be combined with diagnostic endoscopic procedures [28, 29].

22.2.2.7 Summary of Techniques

Based on the approach, the needle may pass near the nerve roots (posterior approaches) and kidney (posterior approaches), near or through the aorta (posterior approaches), through a disk (transdiscal), or through the bowel (endoscopic and anterior approaches). Structures nearby the celiac plexus that may be affected by all the approaches include other autonomic plexuses such as the cardiothoracic, superior hypogastric, and inferior hypogastric plexuses, as well as the artery of Adamkiewicz which supplies the spinal cord. Blockade of these structures can cause additional autonomic symptoms such as hypotension, sexual dysfunction, and bowel/bladder dysfunction.

There are few reports comparing the autonomic side effects of the different approaches to celiac plexus block [18, 21, 28, 29]. The differences are also varied based on volumes and doses of drugs used as well as the drugs themselves.

In addition to local anesthetics, adjuvants such as clonidine, while off-label, are used to prolong the duration of analgesia. Symptoms of bradycardia and hypotension may be augmented with the addition of clonidine. There is insufficient data to compare the different forms of denervation, such as alcohol or phenol neurolysis, or radiofrequency ablation. There are some limited data to suggest that, when comparing the two posterior approaches, hypotension is more common with a retrocrural approach and diarrhea is more common with the anterocrural approach [30]. Celiac plexus blocks are often repeated, and hypotension and diarrhea still appear to be the most common symptoms with repeat procedures [31].

22.2.3 Adverse Effects

The autonomic side effects from a celiac plexus block are presented in Table 22.1, with the two most common side effects being transient hypotension and diarrhea. The exact incidence of hypotension is unclear: some studies have reported it in 1–3% of patients [32, 33] and others between 30 and 38% [2, 34]. It was such a well-known side effect that, in the 1940s, surgical splanchiectomy of the greater, lesser, and least splanchnic nerves was proposed as a treatment for hypertension [35]. After a celiac plexus block, autonomic symptoms usually subside within 1–3 days [36]. Risk factors include advanced age, arteriosclerosis, and hypovolemia [12, 36]. It should be noted that many patients receive sedation for the procedure and are asked not to eat or drink for several hours prior to the procedure, so many patients have some degree of hypovolemia before the block. Furthermore, patients selected for this procedure often have poor nutritional intake and have a lower threshold for compensation to insult.

Two major mechanisms have been proposed for hypotension. The first is inhibition of splanchnic vasoconstriction, which lowers blood pressure through pooling of blood in the visceral circulation [18]. Visceral vasoconstriction is a noradrenergically mediated and unopposed function of the sympathetic nervous system. While parasympathetic nerves cause vasodilation of the skin and mucosa of the face, the parasympathetic nervous system has no effect on the visceral vasculature [10]. Thus, blockade of the visceral autonomic system at the celiac ganglia inhibits vasoconstriction. In support of this mechanism, norepinephrine concentrations in all splanchnic-innervated organs are decreased after splanchnic nerve blocks [25], and in a histologic study in rats, most sympathetic nerves are not visible on mesenteric arteries and veins 2 weeks after surgical celiac ganglionectomy [37]. The second proposed mechanism is cephalad spread of the injectate, presumably involving blockade of the cardiac sympathetic nerves. In a study where contrast was injected prior to injection of bupivacaine or alcohol, cephalad spread extended to the T8–T10 levels in six of seven cases and up to T4 in one case [38]. None of these patients had hypotension.

Table 22.1 Autonomic effects of splanchnic nerve and celiac plexus block

Common side effects
Transient hypotension (1–3 days)
Transient diarrhea (1–3 days)
Uncommon side effects
Chronic diarrhea
Gastroparesis
Increased gastric acid secretion
Bowel dysfunction (most commonly in a setting of spinal artery stroke)
Bladder dysfunction (most commonly in a setting of spinal artery stroke)
Sexual dysfunction (most commonly in a setting of spinal artery stroke)
Side effects observed in animal studies
Temperature dysregulation (heat intolerance)
Altered glucose uptake
Pancreatic polypeptide release

The treatment and prevention of hypotension are done with liberal intravenous fluid administration, given the relative hypovolemia from fasting prior to sedation. Typically, patients are instructed to be nil per os (NPO) after midnight prior to their procedure. Further consideration should be given according to the American Society of Anesthesiology Preoperative Fasting Guidelines [38] which does allow patients to have clear fluids up to 2 h prior to the administration of anesthetic or sedating agents. The concern is that patients may not abide correctly (e.g., cream in the coffee), thus resulting in cancelation of procedures. In patients who are able to drink, with proper education, this allowance can mitigate the risk of post-procedural hypotension. Other preventative strategies that have previously been employed include recommending 12 h of bed rest after the procedure [21] or admitting patients for blood pressure monitoring until they are normotensive (usually overnight) [36].

The second common autonomic side effect is transient diarrhea, which is seen in 44–60% of patients and also generally lasts 1–3 days [2, 34, 39–41]. One proposed mechanism is unopposed parasympathetic activity with increased intestinal motility [21]. Of note, patients are generally able to decrease their opioid requirement after celiac plexus block [31], and opioid withdrawal effects may cause a period of temporary diarrhea, though this should correlate with the timing of the opioid down-titration.

Chronic diarrhea has been reported in less than 1% of patients [1, 39, 42], with case reports noting durations of 18 months [39, 42], 4 years [42], or even until death [43]. Some patients responded while some never fully recovered. The risk factors for chronic diarrhea have not been identified due to the paucity of cases [39]. Treatment for diarrhea includes octreotide [44], possibly in the range of 50–200 mcg total daily dose [42, 43]. Other studies have proposed the use of loperamide, the enteric mu agonist, clonidine, a high-fiber diet, and cholestyramine [39, 42].

Gastric activity appears to be affected by celiac plexus block in the form of gastroparesis and is observed in less than 1% of patients [1]. While celiac plexus blocks can be used for gastroparesis-related pain, they do not seem to help the nausea and vomiting [45]. Sympathetic innervation of the stomach also appears to function as an inhibitor of gastric acid secretion [46], and a case report has noted nausea, vomiting, increased gastric secretions, and delayed gastric emptying after a celiac plexus block [47]. One recommended treatment for celiac plexus-induced gastroparesis is cisapride 10 mg four times daily, although cisapride has been removed from many countries around the year 2000, including a voluntary recall in the United States, due to QT prolongation and risk of dysrhythmia [47].

Finally, several autonomic findings were observed in animal studies that were not seen on our review of the human literature. Temperature intolerance was seen after splanchnic nerve block in rats, which were noted to have a faster heating rate when subjected to hot temperatures, presumably from inhibition of splanchnic vasoconstriction [48]. Other digestive issues have also been noted in animals after celiac blockade, including altered glucose uptake by the liver in dogs [49] and rats [50, 51]. This hepatic glucose effect appears to be independent of steroids, as no steroids were used in these studies. Additionally, celiac plexus block caused increased pancreatic polypeptide release in response to food in dogs [52]. Theoretically these side effects could apply to humans and again warrant further study.

22.2.4 Autonomic Dysfunction and Spinal Cord Infarction from Injury to the Spinal Artery

Spinal cord infarction is one of the most feared complications of celiac plexus block; it can be associated with autonomic dysfunction. Spinal cord infarction, especially those associated with the anterior spinal artery, has been reported after celiac plexus blocks [53], and the mechanism is thought to be either direct injection into or vasospasm of a radicular artery. The common symptoms include paraplegia, loss of pain and temperature with preservation of proprioception, and bowel, bladder, and erectile dysfunction [54]. In theory, bowel, bladder, and sexual dysfunction could be independent of spinal cord damage, as the extensive spread of medication noted during some celiac plexus blocks [55, 56] could result in denervation of the lumbar and sacral autonomic nerves. However, bladder and rectal sphincter dysfunctions following celiac plexus blocks are usually seen in the setting of paraplegia [18, 53], suggesting an indirect mechanism of autonomic dysfunction through ischemia of the spinal cord. While erectile dysfunction is briefly mentioned in several papers as a side effect of celiac plexus block [18, 30, 57, 58], the correlation with myelopathic symptoms is not clear. If a patient has autonomic dysfunction along with paraplegia and sensory changes, additional diagnostic testing for spinal cord ischemia should be considered immediately.

Many morbid side effects of celiac plexus blocks have been reported, including retroperitoneal hematoma, which are discussed in Chapter 21, pericarditis [59], gastric perforation [60], pneumothorax, aortic dissection [14], aortic pseudoaneurysm [61], and retroperitoneal fibrosis after repeated blocks [62].

Key Points

- The most common autonomic symptoms of celiac denervation are transient diarrhea and orthostatic hypotension, which generally resolve over 1–3 days. Less common symptoms of celiac denervation include chronic diarrhea, gastroparesis, and other gastrointestinal issues.
- A spinal cord infarction from injury to the spinal artery is a rare but very morbid side effect of a celiac plexus block. Though not a direct effect of celiac denervation, celiac plexus blocks can indirectly cause other autonomic side effects commonly seen after spinal cord injury, such as bowel, bladder, and sexual dysfunction.
- Recommended steps to limit more common autonomic side effects:
  - If patient is having sedation, there should be an allowance of clear enteral fluids 2 h prior to procedure unless there are specific concerns about aspiration, e.g., uncontrolled gastroesophageal reflux disease, persistent nausea/vomiting, and weakened pharyngeal muscle tone.
  - Use peri-procedural liberal IV fluids if there is no contraindication. General recommendations are at least 500–1000 ml of crystalloid.
  - Monitor intra- and post-procedurally for hypotension and focal neurologic deficits (with no clear guidelines on how long patients must be monitored).
  - Educate patient and staff on more common side effects such as transient diarrhea and orthostatic hypotension.

References

1. Eisenberg E, Carr DB, Chalmers TC. Neurolytic celiac plexus block for treatment of cancer pain: a meta-analysis. Anesth Analg. 1995;80:290–5.
2. Akinci D, Akhan O. Celiac ganglia block. Eur J Radiol. 2005;55:355–61.
3. Zhang XM, Zhao QH, Zeng NL, et al. The celiac ganglia: anatomic study using MRI in cadavers. AJR Am J Roentgenol. 2006;186:1520–3.

4. Pereira GA, Lopes PT, Dos Santos AM, et al. Celiac plexus block: an anatomical study and simulation using computed tomography. Radiol Bras. 2014;47:283–7.
5. Romanelli DF, Beckmann CF, Heiss FW. Celiac plexus block: efficacy and safety of the anterior approach. AJR Am J Roentgenol. 1993;160:497–500.
6. Sisu AM, Stana LG, Petrescu CI, Motoc A. Macroscopic, mesoscopic and microscopic morphology of the gastric plexus--ontogeny of the celiac ganglion. Romanian J Morphol Embryol. 2012;53:591–6.
7. Loukas M, Klaassen Z, Merbs W, Tubbs RS, Gielecki J, Zurada A. A review of the thoracic splanchnic nerves and celiac ganglia. Clin Anat. 2010;23:512–22.
8. Yang HJ, Gil YC, Lee WJ, Kim TJ, Lee HY. Anatomy of thoracic splanchnic nerves for surgical resection. Clin Anat. 2008;21:171–7.
9. Gest TR, Hildebrandt S. The pattern of the thoracic splanchnic nerves as they pass through the diaphragm. Clin Anat. 2009;22:809–14.
10. Janig W. The integrative action of the autonomic nervous system. Cambridge: Cambridge University Press; 2006.
11. Bonica JJ. Autonomic innervation of the viscera in relation to nerve block. Anesthesiology. 1968;29:793–813.
12. Mercadante S, Nicosia F. Celiac plexus block: a reappraisal. Reg Anesth Pain Med. 1998;23:37–48.
13. Noble M, Gress FG. Techniques and results of neurolysis for chronic pancreatitis and pancreatic cancer pain. Curr Gastroenterol Rep. 2006;8:99–103.
14. Kaplan R, Schiff-Keren B, Alt E. Aortic dissection as a complication of celiac plexus block. Anesthesiology. 1995;83:632–5.
15. Naveira FA, Speight KL, Rauck RL. Atheromatous aortic plaque as a cause of resistance to needle passage during transaortic celiac plexus block. Anesth Analg. 1996;83:1327–9.
16. Titton RL, Lucey BC, Gervais DA, Boland GW, Mueller PR. Celiac plexus block: a palliative tool underused by radiologists. AJR Am J Roentgenol. 2002;179:633–6.
17. Waldman S. Atlas of interventional pain management. Philadelphia, PA: Saunders; 2015.
18. Wang PJ, Shang MY, Qian Z, Shao CW, Wang JH, Zhao XH. CT-guided percutaneous neurolytic celiac plexus block technique. Abdom Imaging. 2006;31:710–8.
19. Ina H, Kitoh T, Kobayashi M, Imai S, Ofusa Y, Goto H. New technique for the neurolytic celiac plexus block: the transintervertebral disc approach. Anesthesiology. 1996;85:212–7.
20. Jain P, Dutta A, Sood J. Coeliac plexus blockade and neurolysis: an overview. Indian J Anaesth. 2006;50:169–77.
21. Kambadakone A, Thabet A, Gervais DA, Mueller PR, Arellano RS. CT-guided celiac plexus neurolysis: a review of anatomy, indications, technique, and tips for successful treatment. Radiographics. 2011;31:1599–621.
22. Lieberman RP, Nance PN, Cuka DJ. Anterior approach to celiac plexus block during interventional biliary procedures. Radiology. 1988;167:562–4.
23. Arellano RS, Maher M, Gervais DA, Hahn PF, Mueller PR. The difficult biopsy: let's make it easier. Curr Probl Diagn Radiol. 2003;32:218–26.
24. Montero Matamala A, Vidal Lopez F, Inaraja ML. The percutaneous anterior approach to the celiac plexus using CT guidance. Pain. 1988;34:285–8.
25. Kinoshita H, Denda S, Shimoji K, Ohtake M, Shirai Y. Paraplegia following coeliac plexus block by anterior approach under direct vision. Masui. 1996;45:1244–6.
26. Navarro-Martinez J, Montes A, Comps O, Sitges-Serra A. Retroperitoneal abscess after neurolytic celiac plexus block from the anterior approach. Reg Anesth Pain Med. 2003;28:528–30.
27. Gress F, Schmitt C, Sherman S, Ikenberry S, Lehman G. A prospective randomized comparison of endoscopic ultrasound- and computed tomography-guided celiac plexus block for managing chronic pancreatitis pain. Am J Gastroenterol. 1999;94:900–5.
28. Puli SR, Reddy JB, Bechtold ML, Antillon MR, Brugge WR. EUS-guided celiac plexus neurolysis for pain due to chronic pancreatitis or pancreatic cancer pain: a meta-analysis and systematic review. Dig Dis Sci. 2009;54:2330–7.
29. Seicean A. Celiac plexus neurolysis in pancreatic cancer: the endoscopic ultrasound approach. World J Gastroenterol. 2014;20:110–7.
30. Bahn BM, Erdek MA. Celiac plexus block and neurolysis for pancreatic cancer. Curr Pain Headache Rep. 2013;17:310.
31. McGreevy K, Hurley RW, Erdek MA, Aner MM, Li S, Cohen SP. The effectiveness of repeat celiac plexus neurolysis for pancreatic cancer: a pilot study. Pain Pract. 2013;13:89–95.
32. Baghdadi S, Abbas MH, Albouz F, Ammori BJ. Systematic review of the role of thoracoscopic splanchnicectomy in palliating the pain of patients with chronic pancreatitis. Surg Endosc. 2008;22:580–8.
33. Chambers PC. Coeliac plexus block for upper abdominal cancer pain. Br J Nurs. 2003;12:838–44.
34. Carroll I. Celiac plexus block for visceral pain. Curr Pain Headache Rep. 2006;10:20–5.
35. Peet MM. Hypertension and its surgical treatment by bilateral supradiaphragmatic splanchnicectomy. Am J Surg. 1948;75:48–68.
36. Fugere F, Lewis G. Coeliac plexus block for chronic pain syndromes. Can J Anaesth. 1993;40:954–63.
37. Li M, Galligan J, Wang D, Fink G. The effects of celiac ganglionectomy on sympathetic innervation to the splanchnic organs in the rat. Auton Neurosci. 2010;154:66–73.
38. American Society of Anesthesiologists Committee. Practice guidelines for preoperative fasting and the use of pharmacologic agents to reduce the risk of pulmonary aspiration: application to healthy patients undergoing elective procedures: an updated report by the American Society of Anesthesiologists Committee on Standards and Practice Parameters. Anesthesiology. 2011;114:495–511.
39. Chan VW. Chronic diarrhea: an uncommon side effect of celiac plexus block. Anesth Analg. 1996;82:205–7.
40. Hastings RH, McKay WR. Treatment of benign chronic abdominal pain with neurolytic celiac plexus block. Anesthesiology. 1991;75:156–8.
41. Ischia S, Luzzani A, Ischia A, Faggion S. A new approach to the neurolytic block of the coeliac plexus: the transaortic technique. Pain. 1983;16:333–41.
42. Dean AP, Reed WD. Diarrhoea--an unrecognised hazard of coeliac plexus block. Aust NZ J Med. 1991;21:47–8.
43. Stafford B. More complications of coeliac plexus blockade. Aust NZ J Med. 1991;21:782–3.
44. Mercadante S. Octreotide in the treatment of diarrhoea induced by coeliac plexus block. Pain. 1995;61:345–6.
45. Lee YB, Kim WS. Celiac plexus block in a patient with upper abdominal pain caused by diabetic gastroparesis. Korean J Anesthesiol. 2014;67:S62–3.
46. Larson GM, Ahlman BH, Bombeck CT, Nyhus LM. The effect of chemical and surgical sympathectomy on gastric secretion and innervation. Scand J Gastroenterol Suppl. 1984;89:27–32.
47. Iftikhar S, Loftus EV Jr. Gastroparesis after celiac plexus block. Am J Gastroenterol. 1998;93:2223–5.
48. Kregel KC, Gisolfi CV. Circulatory responses to heat after celiac ganglionectomy or adrenal demedullation. J Appl Physiol (1985). 1989;66:1359–63.
49. Dicostanzo CA, Dardevet DP, Neal DW, et al. Role of the hepatic sympathetic nerves in the regulation of net hepatic glucose uptake and the mediation of the portal glucose signal. Am J Physiol Endocrinol Metab. 2006;290:E9–E16.

50. Fujita S, Donovan CM. Celiac-superior mesenteric ganglionectomy, but not vagotomy, suppresses the sympathoadrenal response to insulin-induced hypoglycemia. Diabetes. 2005;54:3258–64.
51. Kumakura A, Shikuma J, Ogihara N, et al. Effects of celiac superior mesenteric ganglionectomy on glucose homeostasis and hormonal changes during oral glucose tolerance testing in rats. Endocr J. 2013;60:525–31.
52. Larson GM, Sullivan HW, O'Dorisio T. Surgical sympathectomy increases pancreatic polypeptide response to food. Surgery. 1985;98:236–42.
53. Davies DD. Incidence of major complications of neurolytic coeliac plexus block. J R Soc Med. 1993;86:264–6.
54. Cheshire WP, Santos CC, Massey EW, Howard JF Jr. Spinal cord infarction: etiology and outcome. Neurology. 1996;47:321–30.
55. Garcea G, Thomasset S, Berry DP, Tordoff S. Percutaneous splanchnic nerve radiofrequency ablation for chronic abdominal pain. ANZ J Surg. 2005;75:640–4.
56. Hardy PA, Wells JC. Coeliac plexus block and cephalic spread of injectate. Ann R Coll Surg Engl. 1989;71:48–9.
57. Erdine S. Celiac ganglion block. Agri. 2005;17:14–22.
58. Rana MV, Candido KD, Raja O, Knezevic NN. Celiac plexus block in the management of chronic abdominal pain. Curr Pain Headache Rep. 2014;18:394.
59. Sayed I, Elias M. Acute chemical pericarditis following celiac plexus block--a case report. Middle East J Anaesthesiol. 1997; 14:201–6.
60. Takahashi M, Yoshida A, Ohara T, et al. Silent gastric perforation in a pancreatic cancer patient treated with neurolytic celiac plexus block. J Anesth. 2003;17:196–8.
61. Sett SS, Taylor DC. Aortic pseudoaneurysm secondary to celiac plexus block. Ann Vasc Surg. 1991;5:88–91.
62. Pateman J, Williams MP, Filshie J. Retroperitoneal fibrosis after multiple coeliac plexus blocks. Anaesthesia. 1990;45:309–10.

Aortic Dissection After Celiac Plexus Block

23

R. Lee Wagner

23.1 Case Description

A 62-year-old male was referred to the pain clinic by his oncologist for discussion of pain management options. The patient had presented 5 months earlier with a 15 lb weight loss and epigastric pain radiating through to the back. The evaluation established a diagnosis of adenocarcinoma of the head of the pancreas, and staging revealed metastases to several locations in the liver and lungs and multiple locations in the peritoneum. CT scan showed that the primary tumor mass was relatively well confined to the pancreas, with only a single localized area of enlargement of periaortic lymph nodes, and no involvement of major vessels. The patient was relatively functional, with a Karnofsky score of 80. There had been slight decrease in tumor size with three courses of gemcitabine/paclitaxel therapy, but the patient had decided against further chemotherapy because of intolerable side effects. Past medical history included hypertension and a 40-pack-year history of cigarettes.

On first presentation to the pain clinic, the patient complained of two distinct types of abdominal pain. A diffuse and vague pain throughout the abdomen, intensity 4 on a scale of 0–10, was slightly worse after meals and sometimes improved after bowel movements. A second, more intense epigastric and right upper quadrant pain, 7–8 on a scale of 0–10, has reliably worsened for 1–2 h after each meal and radiated seemingly directly through the body to the central mid back. The patient had tried hydrocodone, oxycodone, and hydromorphone with partial relief and was now taking extended-release morphine sulfate, 60 mg orally every 8 h, duloxetine, and gabapentin. This regimen provided some relief of pain but had caused unacceptable somnolence, intermittent confusion, and constipation.

On physical examination, the patient appeared intelligent and interactive but chronically ill. He was in apparent chronic distress from pain. Abdominal exam revealed normal bowel sounds, mild distention, a sense of fullness in the right upper quadrant of the abdomen without discrete palpable masses, and marked tenderness over the epigastrium. Light percussion of the central mid back was not tender, but moderate percussion was clearly tender.

A wide range of treatment options was discussed. The patient elected to proceed with a therapeutic trial of celiac plexus block with bupivacaine.

It was decided to use a two-needle, posterior, percutaneous anterocrural approach under fluoroscopic guidance [1]. With the patient prone, light IV sedation, a 22 gauge, 15 cm Chiba needle from a skin entry point just below the 12th rib, 8–10 cm lateral to the midline, was directed medially toward the L1 vertebral body. On lateral view, each needle was advanced a distance of 2–3 cm anterior to the L1 vertebral body, palpably grazing that body as the needle passed. Careful intermittent aspiration for blood was performed to avoid the aorta and vena cava. A test dose of iohexol (Omnipaque®) 300 mg/mL, 5 mL through each needle, showed good retroperitoneal spread without vascular uptake. Once in position, an injection was made of 20–30 mL 0.25% bupivacaine through each needle, in 5 mL increments.

The patient tolerated the procedure well. Within 5 min after completion of the injection, he reported a marked improvement in pain, from 7/10 preprocedure to 1/10 post-procedure. After a period of observation, he was discharged home with his caregiver wife. Over the next several days, the patient was happy with the results of the block, although pain relief was incomplete. Intensity of the epigastric pain was down to 3/10. At approximately 72 h post-procedure, however, the pain returned to its full intensity. The patient wished to proceed with a more permanent neurolytic block, as had been previously discussed at the initial clinic visit.

In an attempt to improve efficacy of epigastric pain relief, the technique was changed to a transaortic technique [2, 3]. The approach was similar to that for the first block, modified as a single needle, left-sided approach only, intentionally

R.L. Wagner, M.D.
Scripps Green Hospital, La Jolla, CA, USA
e-mail: Wagner.Lee@ScrippsHealth.org

M. Anitescu et al. (eds.), *Challenging Cases and Complication Management in Pain Medicine*,
https://doi.org/10.1007/978-3-319-60072-7_23

directed toward the posterior wall of the aorta and then advanced through the aortic wall to the anterior side, using palpation of arterial pulsation, aspiration for blood, and intermittent injection of 1–2 mL boluses of iohexol as guides. The planned injection was for 40 mL total volume of equal parts absolute alcohol and 0.5% bupivacaine, admixed, using an intermittent aspiration technique. After approximately 30 mL was injected, blood was aspirated through the needle. The needle was advanced to reposition it anterior to the aorta. When pressure was exerted on the plunger of the syringe, the patient complained of a transient unusual abdominal and lower thoracic pain, and blood was again aspirated through the needle. The pain appeared to subside within seconds. The needle was again advanced to a position likely anterior to the aorta by AP and lateral fluoroscopic view; an iohexol test dose showed good position on AP and lateral fluoroscopy, and the remaining 10 mL of alcohol/bupivacaine was injected.

The patient was observed for 4 h in the recovery room with stable vital signs, normal urination and ambulation, and a marked decrease in his preprocedure pain. He was discharged home with his wife.

Four hours post-procedure, the wife reported by telephone that the patient was experiencing diaphoresis, severe abdominal pain, and inability to move the legs. The paramedics returned the patient to the hospital with vital signs that became increasingly unstable en route. Consistent with the patient's documented wishes, advanced resuscitation was not performed, and the patient expired 30 min after arrival in the emergency room.

A coroner's autopsy was performed. The abdominal aorta had an intramural dissection of the anterior wall between outer media and adventitia layers, centered at the level of L1 and extending proximally and distally, forming a pseudoaneurysm and thrombus with occlusion of a major anterior spinal artery branch at T12 and occlusion of the celiac axis and all of the distal aortic branches. There was ischemic death of a segment of the spinal cord at T12, as well as most of the organs of the abdomen. There was moderate intraluminal plaque in the aorta.

Case discussion: (The discussion here refers to the use of celiac plexus block for relief of pain in the terminally ill cancer patient and is not the treatment of chronic benign conditions.)

Initial evaluation: Avoidance of complications can start before the initial interview, by screening for inappropriate referral. Conversation with the referring physician can clarify life expectancy and family dynamics. Life expectancy greater than 3 months may mean repeat block will be needed [4]. A life expectancy of only a few weeks may suggest insufficient benefit to the patient to match the risk and inconvenience of undergoing the procedure.

The approach strategy to celiac ganglia may be affected by tumor. For example, a celiac plexus heavily infiltrated by tumor mass may suggest a more proximal, retrocrural splanchnic approach. Prior abdominal CT scan will often be available, and reviewing abdominal imaging as part of planning the procedure is useful. At times, however, imaging may be several months old, and the patient's advanced state of disease may not warrant additional imaging.

The block is likely to help only the pain from the structures innervated by the celiac plexus [5]. In this case example, pain caused by distal colon, lung, pleura, and peritoneal metastases would not be expected to improve. Thoughtful diagnosis of specific causes of the several pain elements a patient may be experiencing is almost always valuable to the practitioner and patient.

It is also important to assess patient and family goals. The referring physician or independent patient/family research may have created unrealistic expectations. During the initial patient consultation, it is important to be supportive but modest about the benefits of celiac plexus block. There is a reasonable likelihood of significantly decreasing pain. The block cannot promise improved quality of life or prolongation of life expectancy [6]. Common possible complications should be discussed, including the possibility that the block will be ineffective.

23.2 Technical Choices

(a) Imaging: celiac plexus block was performed successfully for many decades without imaging, and that choice may still be appropriate in underdeveloped areas of the world. In developed countries, fluoroscopy, CT scan, and ultrasound are all possibilities.
(b) Approaches: posterior transcutaneous retrocrural and anterocrural (transcrural) periaortic and transaortic approaches can all be performed with either CT or fluoroscopic guidance. Anterior transcutaneous and endoscopic trans-gastric approaches can be guided with ultrasound. Discussion of success and complication rates of these various approaches is beyond the scope of this chapter, but is discussed further in other publications [1–3, 7–19]. Choice of a transaortic approach should include assessment of risk factors for aortic vascular disease (in this case, hypertension and history of smoking).
(c) Choice of medication: phenol 6–9% or ethanol 50% can be used for neurolytic block. A diagnostic block with a local anesthetic (lidocaine, bupivacaine, others) can demonstrate efficacy prior to a neurolytic block but has the disadvantage of requiring two separate procedures in a terminally ill patient.

Basic anatomy of celiac plexus and ganglia: The location of the celiac ganglia and plexus was probably first described by Galen (ca. 173 CE) and has now been more precisely described in recent anatomic dissection papers [20] and CT [21] and MRI [22] anatomic studies. Typically, both left and right celiac ganglia are approximately 2 cm in the long axis and 0.35 cm in the short axis. There is a multi-lobulated shape in approximately two thirds of ganglia, discoid in the remainder. The ganglia are thin. Both ganglia typically are between the origins of celiac trunk and superior mesenteric arteries anterior to the diaphragmatic crura and aorta and just above and medial to the adrenal glands. The left ganglion is typically slightly larger.

Histology of the aortic wall: The aorta comprises three main layers. The innermost layer is the tunica intima. This is approximately 20% of the total thickness of the aorta. Next is the tunica media, composed of smooth muscle and elastin. The outermost is the adventitia containing collagen and elastic fibers as well as blood vessels. Overall wall thickness averages 2 mm [23]. Injury to the aorta is more likely if it is diseased. In most cases, there will have been CT imaging of the abdomen somewhere in the patient's course that will have identified any aortic disease.

No clarity on relative safety of transaortic approach: It is understandable that the novice pain practitioner might reflexively conclude that intentional puncture of the aortic wall is inadvisable. However, awareness of the history of medicine and the common practice of other medical disciplines is useful. For decades before it was ever used for pain management, translumbar aortography was a common approach by radiologists, and several papers attest to its low complication rate. Szilagyi et al. reviewed the clinical course of 14,550 patients and found a very low incidence of major or fatal complications of 0.064% [24]. This makes sense when one considers that the highly elastic wall of the healthy aorta is ideally suited to immediately seal off puncture holes without sequelae. The transaortic approach was initially developed to improve efficacy of earlier techniques [2].

Diagnosis of aortic dissection: Unfortunately, arriving at the correct diagnosis may be clouded by associated clinical factors. Hypotension, a hallmark of aortic dissection, also frequently occurs with the partial sympathectomy of celiac plexus block. (See Naidu, Chap. 22.) Dissection can be associated with sudden pain; unfortunately, the initial effect of absolute alcohol on nerves can also produce increased pain, and the local anesthetic used to minimize this may also obscure this sign of aortic injury.

Mechanism of dissection unknown: Abdominal aortic dissection from all causes is rare, from iatrogenic causes rarer still, and very few of those cases have resulted in death, autopsy, and publication [25]. When an aorta is injured by needle trauma alone, a small intimal flap may be created that enlarges with the sheer force of high-pressure blood flow. A different mechanism of aortic wall injury may be the hydrodissection that occurs at either the media or intima layer of the aorta. It is this author's belief (without evidence) that the injury is primarily a mechanical one, and it is likely irrelevant whether local anesthesia, contrast media, or neurolytic agents are used.

23.3 Avoidance of Aortic Dissection

1. The usual argument of less trauma with smaller bore needle versus better tactile awareness with larger bore blunt-tipped needle may apply here. Of great interest, Ischia, the original pioneer of the transaortic technique, asserts (without supporting evidence) that "in our opinion, the possibility of aortic dissection will be greater, the smaller the needle diameter used" [10]. The present author typically uses a 22 gauge, 15 cm Chiba needle, relying primarily on fluoroscopic imaging with injection of small amounts of contrast dye, rather than tactile signs.
2. In recent years, endoscopic trans-gastric approaches with ultrasound (EUS) have been described [4, 12, 14, 16, 17]. This field is changing rapidly, and it is possible that the EUS-guided approach will continue to grow in popularity.
3. With a fluoroscopic approach, it is possible to combine radiocontrast material with the neurolytic fluid (alcohol or phenol) and use continuous fluoroscopy whenever injecting. If the needle tip were inadvertently within the wall of the aorta, a small dissection of the aortic wall may still occur, but usually an atypical dye pattern can be recognized before more than 1–2 mL of fluid is injected.
4. Avoidance of the transaortic approach altogether is another possibility. However, the interventionist should bear in mind that this complication of aortic dissection is exceedingly rare. Other approaches may cover the celiac plexus less effectively, depending on individual anatomy and pathology. There are potential complications with most other approaches as well. At this time, it is not clear that one method is safer and more reliable than another.

Treatment and prognosis of aortic dissection: It will have been valuable to clarify limits on resuscitative measures associated with this procedure with the patient and family prior to the celiac plexus block. It may be helpful that the diagnosis of aortic (or nearby artery) dissection will be made while the patient is in a hospital setting receiving the procedure and can move smoothly to intervention by vascular surgeon or interventional radiologist. Mortality for out-of-hospital, spontaneous rupture of abdominal aortic aneurysm, a different disease, was high in the past. More recent outcome data are limited, but there is at least the suggestion that recent developments in the field of endoscopic vascular repair may have decreased morbidity and mortality considerably for isolated abdominal aortic dissection, and mortality rate may be approaching 5% [26, 27].

Conclusion: Aortic dissection is only one of several risks of celiac plexus block and perhaps is the rarest. A thoughtful informed consent will strike the right balance between ensuring that there is awareness of catastrophic complications and avoiding the encumbrances of a medicolegal scenario that is burdensome to a terminally ill patient and his family.

References

1. Singler RC. An improved technique for neurolysis of the celiac plexus. Anesthesiology. 1982;56:137–41.
2. Ischia S, Luzzani A, Ischia A, et al. A new approach to the neurolytic block of the celiac plexus: the transaortic technique. Pain. 1983;16:333–41.
3. Liebermann RP, Waldman SD. Celiac plexus neurolysis with the transaortic approach. Radiology. 1990;175:274–83.
4. Le Blanc JK, Al-Haddad M, McHenry L, et al. A prospective, randomized study of EUS-guided celiac plexus neurolysis for pancreatic cancer: one injection or two? Gastrointest Endosc. 2011;74(6):1300–7.
5. Brogan SE. Interventional pain therapies. In: Fishman SM, Ballantyne JC, Rathmell JP, editors. Bonica's management of pain. 4th ed. Philadelphia: Lippincott Williams & Wilkins; 2010. p. 612.
6. Wong GY, Schroeder DR, Carns PE, et al. Effect of neurolytic celiac plexus block on pain relief, quality-of-life, and survival in patients with unresectable pancreatic cancer. A randomized controlled trial. JAMA. 2004;291:1092–9.
7. Bridenbaugh LD, Moore DC, Campbell DD. Management of upper abdominal cancer pain. JAMA. 1964;190:99–102.
8. Ischia S, Ischia A, Polati E, et al. Three posterior percutaneous celiac plexus block techniques. Anesthesiology. 1992;67:534–40.
9. Moore DC. Computed tomography eliminates paraplegia and/or death from neurolytic celiac plexus block. Reg Anesth Pain Med. 1999;24:483–4.
10. Ischia S, Polati E. Reply to Dr. Moore. Reg Anesth Pain Med. 1999;24:484–6.
11. Moore DC. The dreaded complications from neurolytic celiac plexus blocks are preventable! Reg Anesth Pain Med. 2004;29:377–8.
12. Gimeno-Garcia AZ, Elwassief A, Paquin SC, et al. Fatal complications after endoscopic ultrasound-guided celiac plexus neurolysis. Endoscopy. 2012;44:E267.
13. Kambadakone A, Thabet A, Gervais DA, et al. CT-guided celiac plexus neurolysis: a review of anatomy, indications, technique, and tips for successful treatment. Radiographics. 2011;31:1599–621.
14. Noble M, Gress FG. Techniques and results of neurolysis for chronic pancreatitis and pancreatic cancer pain. Curr Gastroenterol Rep. 2006;8:99–103.
15. Kaufman M, Singh G, Das S, et al. Efficacy of endoscopic ultrasound-guided celiac plexus block and celiac plexus block neurolysis for managing abdominal pain associated with chronic pancreatitis and pancreatic cancer. J Clin Gastroenterol. 2010;44:127–34.
16. O'Toole TM, Schmulewitz N. Complication rates of EUS-guided celiac plexus blockade and neurolysis: results of a large case series. Endoscopy. 2009;41:593–7.
17. Oh SY, Irani S, Kozarek RA. What are the current and potential future roles for endoscopic ultrasound in the treatment of pancreatic cancer? World J Gastrointest Endosc. 2016;10:319–29.
18. Poruk KE, Wolfgang CL. Palliative management of unresectable pancreas cancer. Surg Oncol Clin N Am. 2016;25:327–37.
19. Warner NS, Moeschler SM, Warner MA, et al. Bleeding complications in patients undergoing celiac plexus block. Reg Anesth Pain Med. 2016;41:488–93.
20. Loukas M, Klaasen Z, Merbs W, et al. A review of the thoracic splanchnic nerves and celiac ganglia. Clin Anat. 2010;23:512–22.
21. Wang ZJ, Webb EM, Westphalen AC, et al. Multi-detector row computed tomographic appearance of celiac ganglia. J Comput Assist Tomogr. 2010;34(3):343–7.
22. Zhang XM, Zhao QH, Zeng NL, et al. The celiac ganglia: anatomic study using MRI in cadavers. AJR Am J Roentgenol. 2006;186:1520–3.
23. Malayeri AA, Natori S, Bahrami H, et al. Relation of aortic wall thickness and distensibility to cardiovascular risk factors. Am J Cardiol. 2008;102:491–6.
24. Szilagyi DE, Smith RF, Elliott JP, et al. Translumbar aortography: a study of its safety and usefulness. Arch Surg. 1977;112:399–408.
25. Kaplan R, Schiff-Keren B, Alt E. Aortic dissection as a complication of celiac plexus block. Anesthesiology. 1995;83:632–5.
26. Trimarchi S, Tsai T, Eagle KA, et al. Acute abdominal aortic dissection: insight from the International Registry of Acute Aortic Dissection (IRAD). J Vasc Surg. 2007;46:913–9.
27. Jonker FH, Schlosser FJ, Moll FL, et al. Dissection of the abdominal aorta. Current evidence and implications for treatment strategies: a review and meta-analysis of 92 patients. J Endovasc Ther. 2009;16:71–80.

Ureteral Injury After Lumbar Sympathetic Block

24

Daniel Levin, Sophy Zheng, and Magdalena Anitescu

24.1 Case Description

A 36-year-old male presents to the emergency room with a 4-day history of persistent right-sided abdominal pain. The pain is dull and poorly localized and accompanied by nausea, malaise, and decreased appetite. In addition, he also reports new right-sided lumbar back pain that he has been treating with hydrocodone with acetaminophen. His medical history is significant for well-controlled Crohn's disease and complex regional pain syndrome (CRPS) of the left lower extremity following a motor vehicle accident 18 months earlier. For his CRPS, he was previously treated with gabapentin and sertraline but stopped a month ago as his symptoms had improved following a "pain injection." His surgical history includes small bowel resection 10 years ago and ORIF of the right femur following the MVA. Complete blood count and chemistry panel were performed by the ER and were within normal limits. An abdominal ultrasound was performed; while there was no evidence of gallbladder disease, a perirenal cystic formation was seen along with dilation of the left collecting system and proximal ureter. Computerized tomography (CT) of the abdomen revealed a 7 × 10 × 10 cm well-lineated, non-contrasted cystic lesion adjacent to the psoas muscle. The CT further demonstrated anterolateral displacement of the left kidney and a dilation of the collecting system and proximal ureter.

Given these findings, the urology service was consulted and recommended obtaining further information from the patient's pain physician regarding the "pain injection." Records obtained from the pain clinic indicate that the he had undergone a left-sided lumbar sympathetic block (LSB) with a posterior oblique approach 5 weeks ago. Upon review of the case, the pain physician revealed that the initial needle entry at L3 resulted in a urogram with dye injection (see Fig. 24.1). The needle was removed, and entry was made at L4 resulting in a successful block. The patient denied having experienced symptoms of urinary urgency, retention, and hematuria in the days immediately following the procedure.

The patient underwent anterograde pyelography which demonstrated extravasation at the upper third of the proximal ureter and concurrent formation of urinoma at the site with no passage to the distal ureter and bladder. The patient was taken to the operating room for exploration; the urinoma was drained and a ureteroureterostomy was performed; a nephrectomy was deemed unnecessary. The patient was seen 3 months later and had full resolution of his abdominal and lower back symptoms as well as full recovery from the ureteral injury.

D. Levin, M.D. • M. Anitescu, M.D., Ph.D.
Department of Anesthesia and Critical Care,
University of Chicago Medical Center,
5841 S. Maryland Ave, MC 4028, Chicago, IL, USA

S. Zheng, M.D. (✉)
Department of Anesthesia and Critical Care,
Northwestern University, Feinberg School of Medicine,
251 E. Erie St, Chicago, IL, USA
e-mail: sophy.zheng@nm.org

M. Anitescu et al. (eds.), *Challenging Cases and Complication Management in Pain Medicine*,
https://doi.org/10.1007/978-3-319-60072-7_24

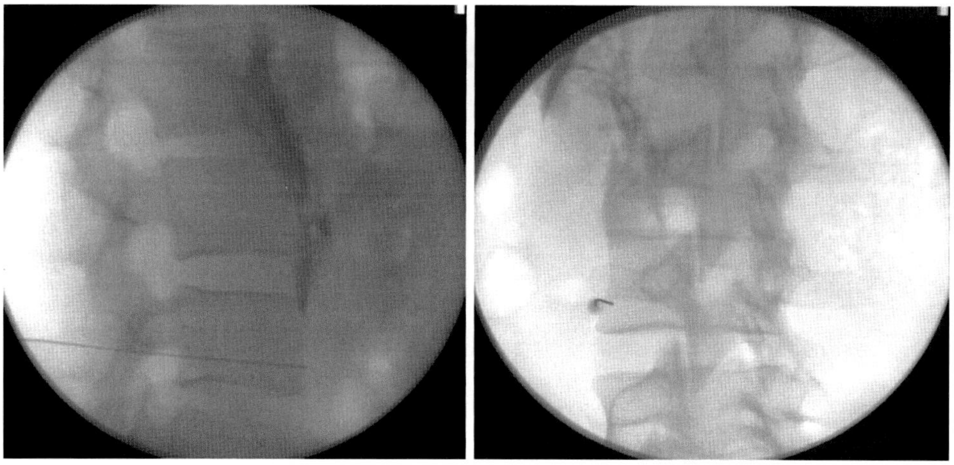

Fig. 24.1 Placement of the needle at the L3 level for a left lumbar sympathetic block shows uptake of the dye by the left kidney via ureter. Needle was removed and then positioned lower at the left L4 level; patient had excellent relief of his sympathetic mediated pain. He was cautioned regarding blood in urine but ultimately had no sequelae from the initial needle placement in the left ureter and kidney; he subsequently returned for repeat blocks that were all performed at L4 level to avoid contact with the kidney. These images are from Dr. Anitescu's personal library

24.2 Discussion

Lumbar sympathectomy was first reported by a French surgeon, Leriche. In 1920s, the first percutaneous lumbar sympathetic block was first described by Kappis and Mandl, with several subsequent variations in technique [6]. The goal of lumbar sympathetic block is to utilize local anesthetic and/or neurolytic agents to inhibit sympathetically mediated pain signal transmission at the level of the ganglion [7]. While advances in imaging techniques have increased the safety of such blocks, neither fluoroscopy nor computed tomography has precluded ureteral injury [2]. To date, there are seven case reports of such injury in the literature. Presentation of post-procedure ureteral injury is variable in both its symptoms and its time course, thereby warranting close follow-up and requiring a high index of suspicion for diagnosis.

Lumbar Sympathetic Block

1. Anatomy and physiology
   (a) The lumbar sympathetic ganglia are located in the retroperitoneum, anterolateral to the lumbar vertebral bodies at the attachment site of the psoas muscle. Variability exists in the number of ganglia as well as their location; cadaveric studies demonstrate three ganglia; however, up to five separate ganglia have been reported in the literature. The most common reported location of the ganglia is anterior to the L2/L3 intervertebral disc; as such, the ganglia can be blocked anywhere between L2 and L4 [7]. Several surrounding structures make placement of a lumbar sympathetic block precarious. These structures include the somatic lumbar plexus, the intervertebral foramen with access to the epidural space, the subarachnoid space, and the spinal cord, as well as important vascular structures including the inferior vena cava anteriorly on the right and the abdominal aorta anteromedial on the left. Smaller vascular structures, such as the lumbar arteries and veins, also are present, as are the ureters [6]. Complications may arise when such surrounding structures are compromised either by direct injury from the needle or injury secondary to injection of neurolytic agents.
2. Indications [7]
   (a) Ischemic limb pain
   (b) Complex regional pain syndrome
   (c) Post-herpetic neuralgia
   (d) Residual and phantom limb pain
   (e) Recluse spider bites [8]
   (f) Diabetic peripheral neuropathy [9]
   (g) Exercise-induced leg pain [10]
3. Techniques
   (a) Approach
      - A posterior oblique approach to the ganglia with the patient in the prone position is most commonly used. A lateral approach was also described by George Wallace in 1955 with the suggested advantage of increasing patient comfort; Wallace's approach described a patient in the lateral position with needle entrance at the apex of the "lumbar triangle" or convergence of the border of the twelfth rib, the superior border of the iliac crest, and the paravertebral musculature at L2 [11]. More recently, a transdiscal approach has been suggested with the aim of decreasing intra-psoas

injection and thus decreasing genitofemoral neuritis [12]. Approaches also vary in the number of needle placements utilized to achieve blockade. A study by Hong et al. demonstrated a significant difference in great toe temperature change with three injections (at L2, L3, and L4) as compared with single injection at L2 [13].

(b) Image guidance
- While the original technique was based solely on anatomic landmarks, complications arising secondary to the presence of local anatomic structures have led to the use of image guidance to improve safety profile. Imaging tools utilized include both ultrasound [14] and MRI [15], although fluoroscopy has been the most commonly used modality in pain management [17]. X-ray fluoroscopy is currently the primary mode of imaging among pain physicians, although computer tomography (CT) fluoroscopy may offer improved safety as it allows visualization of visceral structures not readily seen on plain radiography [16, 17].

(c) Local anesthetics and neurolytic agents
- Sympathetic blockade with local anesthetic can be diagnostic and/or therapeutic. Repeated LSBs with local anesthetic have been performed [18] to treat CRPS with success. In one study, 86% of 29 patients in a case series with CRPS following knee surgery treated with LBS with .375% bupivacaine as the injectate demonstrated partial to complete relief of knee pain for variable durations [19].
- Chemicals, thermal ablation, and radiofrequency ablation (RFA) have been used to extend the duration of the sympathetic blocking effect of LSB [20]. Phenol and alcohol are the most common chemical agents used for blockade; however, case reports of agents such as botulinum toxin [20] and clonidine [21] also exist. Studies comparing phenol ablation to thermal ablation demonstrated increased sympathectomy in the phenol group; a similar study comparing phenol ablation to RFA revealed comparable levels of sympathectomy [22]. The effects of chemical sympathectomy typically last about 3–6 months, whereas the effects of RFA last up to 1 year [23].

4. Efficacy
   (a) Ranges from 21 to 89% in the literature and is dependent on patient selection [24].
5. Complications [6]
   (a) Neuralgia
   - The incidence of neuralgia has been quoted between 6 and 40%. The most common neuralgia induced by LSB is in the genitofemoral distribution; however, symptoms affecting the lateral thigh have also been described.

   (b) Neuraxial injection
   - Subarachnoid injection, post-dural puncture headache, paraplegia, aseptic meningitis, epidural injection, and subdural injection have all been described.

   (c) Vascular complications
   - Complications arise from intravascular injection, intralymphatic injection, and bleeding secondary to puncture of vascular structures. Retroperitoneal hematoma has been reported as a complication secondary to vascular puncture in anticoagulated patients.

   (d) Other complications
   - More unusual complications also have been reported, including pneumothorax, intervertebral disc penetration, allergic reactions to injectate, inability to ejaculate in men, and ureteral and/or renal injury.

Ureteral Injury Secondary to Lumbar Sympathetic Block

1. *Mechanism*: The exact mechanism of injury is not fully understood. However, there are two predominant theories: direct injection into the ureter and migration of injectate between tissue planes to reach the ureter [3]. The latter theory is further supported by a case reported by Trigaux et al. in which CT guidance was used to confirm that the needle was placed in a location far from the ureter; ureteral injury occurred none the less, suggesting that indeed the phenol had reached the ureter by tracking through tissue planes [2]. Other sources note that penetration of the kidney, its capsule, or the ureter as seen in the case we reported does occur and may occur more commonly with the wide lateral approach [6].
2. *Presentation*: Clinical presentation of ureteral injury varies widely among the seven reported cases. One patient presented with iliac fossa pain, a second presented with nausea, and others presented with sepsis, abdominal pain, back pain, soft tissue swelling in the flank region, severe groin pain, and renal failure. This myriad of nonspecific symptoms makes diagnosis difficult. Correlation of symptoms with history of chronic pain syndrome of the lower extremity and recent treatment with LSB often helps to reach the diagnosis. However, patients have presented between 4 days and 6 months post-procedure. Image guidance during placement and confirmation of final needle placement may reduce but does not prevent these complications [1–5].
3. *Diagnosis*: The initial presenting symptoms often dictate the differential diagnosis and subsequent management. Nonetheless, in all reported cases, evidence of retroperi-

toneal fluid collection or hydronephrosis via IV urogram or abdominal ultrasound was seen on the same side as the LSB block. Further imaging included CT of the abdomen as well as more invasive urologic investigation further confirms the diagnosis [1–5].

4. *Management*: Management of ureteral injury requires consultation with urology service, and specific treatment may vary depending on the individual patient condition. Surgical intervention is frequently the mainstay of treatment [2, 4, 5]. On exploration, typical findings included urinoma, periureteral fibrosis, ureteral stricture, and hydronephrosis. Operative intervention was dependent on the degree of stricture and renal damage and included ureteral stenting, ureteral reconstruction, urinoma drainage, and, in two cases, unilateral nephrectomy. However, there was one case that reported successful nonoperative management in an 85-year-old female following percutaneous drainage under ultrasound guidance. Upon her follow-up 6 months later, her renal function had returned to baseline [3]. Two other cases report nonoperative management with follow-up studies demonstrating persistently hydronephrotic kidneys [1]. Because the literature consists only of several case reports, there is not enough data to suggest benefits of either the conservative or operative approaches, as both have been successful in varying situations. The patient's specific clinical condition and comorbidities should be taken into account in weighing the risks and benefits of surgery.
5. *Prognosis*: While no specific survey data is available, all patients in the seven cases reported in the literature attained complete resolution of symptoms; two patients had residual hydronephrosis, one had a mild elevation in creatinine (see Table 24.1), while the remainder had negative imaging, normal renal function laboratory values, or "favorable" and "unremarkable" recoveries (see Table 24.1). Notably, there is one case reported of acute kidney injury after bilateral LBS; while the patient did require a unilateral nephrectomy, follow-up at 1 year revealed no symptoms of renal failure [1–5].

Table 24.1 Case reports of ureteral injury following lumbar sympathetic block

Author	Age gender	Indication	Technique: (agent, guidance)	Time to symptoms	Presenting symptoms	Treatment	Outcomes
Fraser et al. [1]	79-year-old female	Vascular disease of foot	90% alcohol anterolateral to body of L3; X-ray guidance	4 days	RUQ pain, septicemia, DIC, GI bleed	Operative exploration, nephrectomy	Unremarkable recovery
Fraser et al. [1]	62-year-old male	Vascular disease	6.6% phenol in water; "blind" sympathectomy	2 days	Abdominal, back pain, groin swelling	Urinoma drainage with peritoneal dialysis catheter	Residual hydronephrosis, asymptomatic
Fraser et al. [1]	82-year-old female	Vascular disease of feet	6.6% phenol; "blind" sympathectomy	4 days	Severe left groin pain	Analgesia, antibiotics	Residual hydronephrosis, significant residual function
Trigaux et al. [2]	63-year-old male	Vascular disease of leg	8% glycerin phenol, CT guidance	7 days	Lumbar pain	Operative exploration, urinoma drainage, ureteral reconstruction	Favorable outcome at 8-month follow-up
Cutts et al. [3]	85-year-old female	Vascular disease, critical limb ischemia	6% phenol with niopam, X-ray guidance	17 days	Ipsilateral iliac fossa pain	Percutaneous urinoma drainage, antibiotics	Normal serum urea and creatinine 6 months later
Dirim et al. [4]	53-year-old female	Reflex sympathetic dystrophy	Unknown	3 months	Nausea	Operative exploration, urinoma drainage, ureteral reconstruction	No extravasation or obstruction on IV pyelography at 3-month follow-up
Ranjan et al. [5]	70-year-old male	Buerger's disease	Bilateral chemical sympathectomy, technique unknown	6 months	Renal failure	Hemodialysis, nephrostomy placement, urinoma drainage, ureteral reconstruction, nephrectomy	Serum creatinine 1.4–1.8 mg%, asymptomatic at 1-year follow-up

Conclusions

- Ureteral injury following lumbar sympathetic block is a rare complication and presents with a variety of symptoms making diagnosis reliant upon a history revealing recent injection as well as imaging demonstrating retroperitoneal fluid collections and sequelae of ureteral obstruction.
- All reports of ureteral damage involved chemical neurolysis; there have been no reported cases of ureteral damage following RFA of the lumbar sympathetic ganglia.
- While image guidance aids in avoiding complications of needle misplacement during LSB, it does not preclude ureteral damage; despite optimal needle placement, neurolytic agents may tract through soft tissue to cause ureteral damage.
- Management requires consultation with a urologist. Both operative and conservative interventions have demonstrated favorable outcomes, and decision making will be dictated by individual patient characteristics and specific injury seen.

References

1. Fraser I, Windle R, Smart JG, Barrie WW. Ureteric injury following chemical sympathectomy. Br J Surg. 1984;5:349.
2. Trigaux J-P, Decoene B, Beers BV. Focal necrosis of the ureter following CT-guided chemical sympathectomy. Cardiovasc Intervent Radiol. 1992;15:180–2.
3. Cutts S, Williams H, Lee J, Downing R. Lesson of the Month: ureteric injury as a complication of chemical sympathectomy. Eur J Vasc Endovasc Surg. 2000;2:212–3.
4. Dirim A, Kumsar S. Iatrogenic ureteral injury due to lumbar sympathetic block. Scand J Urol Nephrol. 2008;42(4):492–3.
5. Ranjan P, Kumar J, Chipde S. Acute renal failure due to bilateral ureteric necrosis following percutaneous chemical lumbar sympathectomy. Indian J Nephrol. 2012;22(4):292–4.
6. Middleton WJ, Chan VW. Lumbar sympathetic block: a review of complications. Tech Reg Anesth Pain Manag. 2008;2(3):137–46.
7. Abramov R. Lumbar sympathetic treatment in the management of lower limb pain. Curr Pain Headache Rep. 2014;18(4):1–5.
8. Yi X, Aubuchon J, Zeltwanger S, Kirby JP. Necrotic arachnidism and intractable pain from recluse spider bites treated with lumbar sympathetic block. Clin J Pain. 2011;27(5):457–60.
9. Cheng J, Daftari A, Zhou L. Sympathetic blocks provided sustained pain relief in a patient with refractory painful diabetic neuropathy. Case Rep Anesthesiol. 2012;1–5.
10. Gebauer A. Chronic exercise-induced leg pain in an athlete successfully treated with sympathetic block. Am J Sports Med. 2005;33(10):1575–8.
11. Wallace G. A lateral approach for lumbar sympathetic nerve block. Anesthesiology. 1955;16(2):254–60.
12. Ohno K, Oshita S. Transdiscal lumbar sympathetic block. Anesth Analg. 1997;85(6):1312–6.
13. Hong JH, Oh MJ. Comparison of multilevel with single level injection during lumbar sympathetic ganglion block: efficacy of sympatholysis and incidence of psoas muscle injection. Korean J Pain. 2010;23(2):131–6.
14. Kirvela O, Svedstrom E, Lundbom N. Ultrasonic guidance of lumbar sympathetic and celiac plexus block: a new technique. Reg Anesth. 1992;17(1):43–6.
15. König CW, Schott UG, Pereira PL, Trübenbach J, Schneider W, Claussen CD, Duda SH. MR-guided lumbar sympathicolysis. Eur Radiol. 2002;12(6):1388–93.
16. Tay VK, Fitridge R, Tie ML. Computed tomography fluoroscopy-guided chemical lumbar sympathectomy: simple, safe and effective. Australas Radiol. 2002;46(2):163–6.
17. Koizuka S, Saito S, Obata H, Tobe M, Koyama Y, Takahashi A. Anatomic analysis of computed tomography images obtained during fluoroscopic computed tomography-guided percutaneous lumbar sympathectomy. J Anesth. 2008;22(4):373–7.
18. van Eijs F, Stanton-Hicks M, Van Zundert J, Faber C, Lubenow T, Mekhail N, van Kleef M, Hoygen F. Complex regional pain syndrome. Pain Pract. 2011;11(1):70–87.
19. Cameron HU, Park YS, Krestow M. Reflex sympathetic dystrophy following total knee replacement. Contemp Orthop. 1994;29(4):279–81.
20. Choi E, Choo C, Kim H, Lee P, Nahm F. Lumbar sympathetic block with botulinum toxin type B for complex regional pain syndrome: a case study. Pain Physician. 2015;18(5):E911–6.
21. Chen L, Wong C, Huh B, Huang Y, Yang C, Yeh C, Wu C. Repeated lumbar sympathetic blockade with lidocaine and clonidine attenuates pain in complex regional pain syndrome type 1 patients—a report of two cases. Acta Anaesthesiol Taiwanica. 2006;44:113–7.
22. Haynsworth RF, Noe CE. Percutaneous lumbar sympathectomy: a comparison of radiofrequency denervation versus phenol neurolysis. Anesthesiology. 1994;74(3):455–63.
23. Jackson TP, Gaeta R. Neurolytic blocks revisited. Curr Pain Headache Rep. 2008;12(1):7–13.
24. Heindel W, Ernst S, Manshausen G. CT-guided lumbar sympathectomy: results and analysis of factors influencing the outcome. Cardiovasc Intervent Radiol. 1998;21(4):319–23.

Lower Extremity Weakness Following Neurolytic Superior Hypogastric Block

25

Jeffrey Hopcian, Bradley Silva, and Magdalena Anitescu

25.1 Case Description

A 49-year-old woman diagnosed with anorectal cancer and carcinomatosis presents with progressive pelvic pain as well as rectal tenesmus. The patient was diagnosed with cancer 2 years ago, and her prior treatments include radiation and chemotherapy with carboplatin and paclitaxel. Abdominal computed tomography (CT) reveals progressive intra-abdominal spread of malignancy. Attempts to control her pain with oral and intravenous analgesics including opioids, nonsteroidal anti-inflammatory drug (NSAID), and anticonvulsants failed to improve her pain symptoms. She underwent fluoroscopic-guided superior hypogastric plexus block. Procedural anesthesia was accomplished with local anesthetic and light sedation using 2-mg midazolam intravenous (IV) injection. The procedure was performed by a physician trainee with attending physician supervision. Needle placement was performed with direct fluoroscopic guidance using iodinated contrast agent. Diagnostic injection of 15 mL of 0.5% bupivacaine produced excellent analgesia after 3 min. Subsequently, concentrated ethanol (95%) was injected for neurolysis. Needle stylets were replaced, and needles removed (Figs. 25.1 and 25.2).

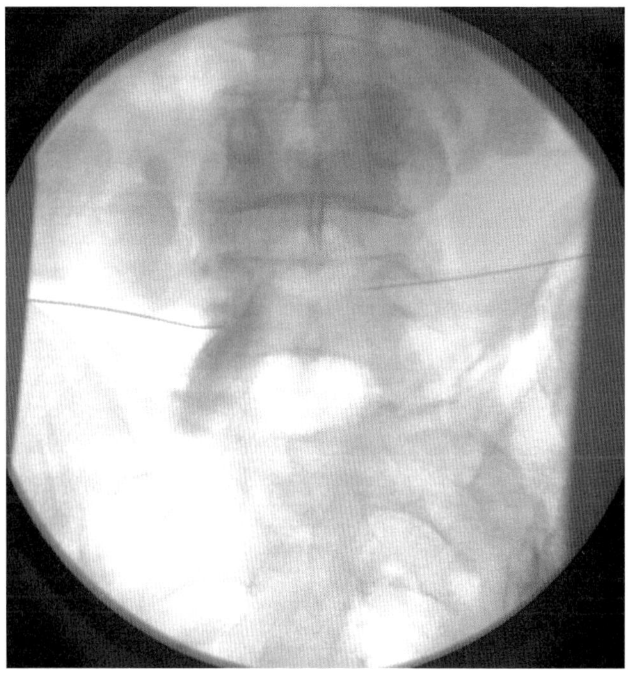

Fig. 25.1 Anteroposterior view of needle placement in the case presented. Images from Dr. Anitescu Personal Library

Following this procedure, her abdominal pain resolved completely. However, she complained of persistent weakness of hip flexion on the right side only. She was unable to tolerate magnetic resonance imaging (MRI), but a CT study with contrast did not reveal mass effect on lumbosacral nervous structures. She was discharged home with a cane for ambulation and underwent outpatient physical therapy. She experienced gradual improvement of her symptoms over the following month.

25.2 Background

The superior hypogastric plexus is formed by the coalescence of visceral afferent nerve fibers as well as autonomic fibers including lumbar sympathetic and sacral parasympathetic nerve fibers (themselves continuations of lumbar and pelvic splanchnic nerves). The superior hypogastric plexus continues as the inferior hypogastric plexus which is the source of the middle rectal plexus, the prostatic plexus, the

J. Hopcian, M.D. (✉)
University Suburban Health Center, Cleveland, OH, USA
e-mail: Jeffrey.Hopcian@UHhospitals.org

B. Silva, M.D. • M. Anitescu, M.D., Ph.D.
Department of Anesthesia and Critical Care, University of Chicago Medical Center, Chicago, IL, USA
e-mail: Bsilva1@dacc.uchospitals.org; manitescu@dacc.uhhospitals.org

M. Anitescu et al. (eds.), *Challenging Cases and Complication Management in Pain Medicine*,
https://doi.org/10.1007/978-3-319-60072-7_25

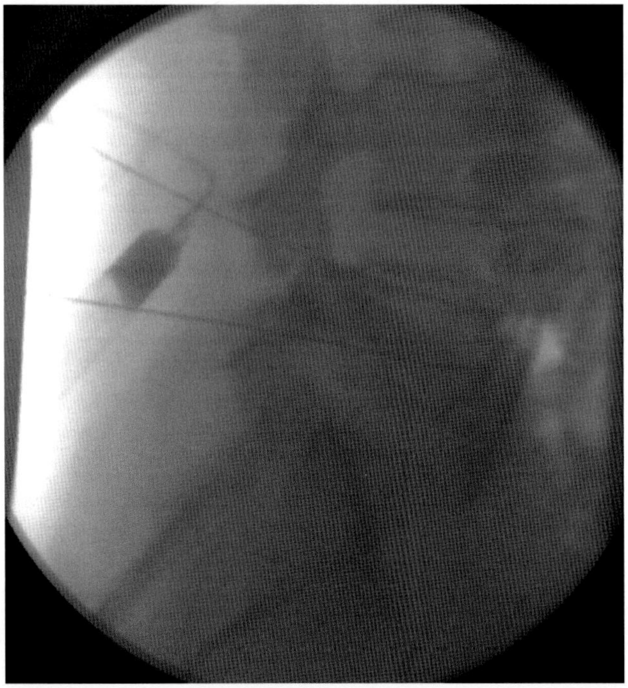

Fig. 25.2 Lateral view of the needle placement in the case presented. Images from Dr. Anitescu Personal Library

vesical plexus, and the uterovaginal plexus. The nerve fibers coalescing at the superior hypogastric plexus have many functions including transmission of nociception from the pelvic viscera [1].

Superior hypogastric plexus blockade has been performed for many years as a treatment for chronic pelvic pain. The procedure has been successfully performed via landmark techniques; however most practitioners now utilize fluoroscopic or computed tomography (CT) guidance. Commonly employed techniques include the classic bilateral, two-needle posterior approach, the single-needle medial paraspinous approach, and the single-needle transdiscal approach as well as the single-needle anterior approach. In the classic bilateral two-needle posterior approach, needle tips are advanced to the anterior margin of either S1 or the L5/S1 intervertebral disc, distal to the bifurcation of the aorta into the common iliac arteries [2, 3]. Temporary blockade for diagnostic and therapeutic purposes may be performed with any number of local anesthetic agents. Chemical neurolysis with concentrated alcohol or phenol is often performed for pain related to pelvic malignancy [3, 4].

Generally, this procedure is considered a safe method for treating severe pain with a relatively low risk of complications when performed appropriately. Expected consequences of this procedure include interruption of the sympathetic innervation distal to the inferior hypogastric nerves. Although this has not been adequately studied, disruption of autonomic function at this level may have negative consequences on bowel, bladder, and sexual function [5]. Based on neural anatomy, physiologic theory, and extrapolation from surgical data, many texts warn of bilateral hypogastric block impairing sexual function in males [6, 7]. Owing in part to lack of adequate knowledge, female sexual function has likely been overlooked on this issue [8–10]. As with any interventional spine procedure, one must be cautious to avoid inadvertent intravascular injection. Should the segmental arteries supplying the spinal cord be disrupted, permanent neurologic deficits may be encountered [11]. Local anesthetic toxicity, infection/abscess formation, hematoma formation, as well as direct needle trauma to vascular, muscular, and neural structures are also possible.

The patient that we described had weakness of her hip flexors. The major hip flexor in the body is the iliopsoas muscle. The iliopsoas is formed by the joining of the iliacus muscle with the psoas muscle. The psoas major is present in all humans and is comprised of a deep part (originating from the transverse processes of L1–L5) and a superficial part (originating from lateral portions of vertebral bodies T12–L4). It is innervated by L2–L4. In less than 50% of humans, the psoas major is joined by psoas minor which originates from the T12–T1 vertebral bodies and attaches to the iliopectineal eminence. It functions as a weak flexor of the lumbar spine [12, 13].

25.3 Case Discussion

In our case, the patient had excellent analgesia from a neurolytic superior hypogastric blockade. However, she suffered an unexpected complication of hip flexion weakness. The differential diagnosis for weakness following superior hypogastric plexus blockade includes: [2–4, 14]

1. Anesthesia or neurolysis of the spinal nerve or its rami
2. Intraneural injection and nerve trauma
3. Abscess
4. Hematoma
5. Disruption of vascular supply to spinal cord (infarction)
6. Musculoskeletal injury

1. Inadvertent anesthesia and/or neurolysis of the spinal nerves are concerns during superior hypogastric blockade. Proper needle positioning as well as use of contrast agent to visualize spread of injectate should be employed. One aims to ensure appropriate spread of injectate in a cephalad-caudad plane immediately anterior to the vertebral column without dangerous spread posterior toward the neural foramen.
2. Intraneural injection is typically characterized by severe pain felt by the patient, as well as relatively high resistance (i.e., low compliance) during the injection. This risk is

minimized by avoiding deep sedation that may blunt the patient's ability to communicate/sense severe pain. Compliance during sympathetic ganglia blocks varies depending on needle and syringe size. This element of feedback is optimized by using a standardized set of syringes and needles. In the event of damage from intraneural injection, treatment is often conservative. Outcomes are variable; pain and/or motorsensory disturbance may be self-limited or may be permanent.

3. Abscess formation is a risk of deep tissue injection, particularly in immunocompromised patients. Appropriate sterile technique and use of barrier protection (i.e., sterile gloves and masks) minimizes this risk but does not eliminate it. An abscess may form within days following an injection. Systemic illness and compressive mass effect on surrounding structures may develop as the abscess evolves. Abscess may be detected on CT imaging, ideally with IV contrast. Antibiotic treatment and possible surgical intervention may be necessary for treatment.
4. Hematoma formation is also a risk of deep tissue injection. Hematoma has a variable presentation depending on the degree of blood loss and location, but in this discussion we will focus on the direct compressive mass effect on surrounding neural structures. The risk of hematoma is minimized by ensuring pharmacologic anticoagulants, and antiplatelet agents have been discontinued appropriately prior to injection. Particular caution should be taken with newer generation anticoagulants which have limited safety data. Many herbal supplements interfere with platelet function and may alter function of concomitant anticoagulant/antiplatelet agents. Bleeding risk is increased in many pathologic states including malnourishment/vitamin deficiency, uremic platelet dysfunction, and cytopenia associated with any number of conditions including malignancy and/or chemotherapy and radiotherapy. Hematoma formation may be diagnosed via CT imaging. Depending on the underlying mechanism of hematoma formation (i.e., coagulopathy versus vascular disruption), treatment may be conservative or in some cases surgical.
5. Intravascular injection may result in systemic toxicity or disruption of vascular supply to the spinal cord. Contrast may or may not detect intravascular uptake of injectate. The use of digital subtraction angiography likely increases the sensitivity for detection of intravascular injections. The spinal cord receives vascular supply from a single anterior spinal artery supplying the anterior 2/3 of the spinal cord, as well as a pair of posterior spinal arteries supplying the posterior 1/3 of the spinal cord. Anastomoses between the spinal arteries (vasocorona) offer supply to the lateral columns of the spinal cord. The spinal arteries originate at the cervico-occipital junction and receive reinforcement from several radicular (aka segmental) arteries that include the ascending and deep cervical arteries, intercostal arteries, lumbar arteries, and lateral sacral arteries. There is a dominant segmental artery known as the artery of Adamkiewicz. Disruption of this artery has a high risk of spinal cord infarction and paralysis. Although it is typically left-sided (80% of patients) and arising from a mid- to low-thoracic intercostal artery, right-sided and/or lumbar origination of the artery of Adamkiewicz is not very uncommon. Given this variable origin, one should take care to avoid it in any thoracolumbar injection. Disruption to segmental arteries during injections is conceivable. Alcohol and phenol have been shown to induce vasospasm of segmental arteries in dogs [15]. The effects of this arterial disruption depend on many factors (i.e., significance of a given vessel's contribution to vascular supply) but may include paralysis.
6. Musculoskeletal injury during superior hypogastric block may include direct trauma from needle placement. With judicious use of local anesthetic and appropriately sized needles (22G is common), this is usually mild and self-limited. However, severe pain and muscle spasm are possible. More devastating would be chemical destruction of muscle tissue when using phenol or alcohol for neurolysis. This may occur during inadvertent intramuscular injection or unintended spreading of injectate. Following successful needle placement and chemical neurolysis, one must take care to flush needles with a nonirritating solution to remove residual neurolytic agent and reinsert stylets to avoid "backtracking" of neurolytic agent during needle removal. The relevant muscles in this case are those encountered during an oblique approach toward the anterolateral L5/S1 vertebral bodies and include the quadratus lumborum, psoas, and erector spinae (longissimus, iliocostalis, spinalis).

Review of the fluoroscopic images from the procedure reveals needle placement that is slightly cephalad and lateral to the conventional target for superior hypogastric plexus block. Appropriate needle placement is demonstrated in Figs. 25.3 and 25.4.

Although injection of contrast dye in this case does not suggest immediate threat of intravascular injection or posterior spread toward the spinal nerves, it does show spread within surrounding structures, possibly muscle tissue based on the subtle striated appearance. The patient's subsequent clinical symptom of hip flexion weakness combined with successful resolution of pain suggests a likely spread of injectate over the hypogastric plexus along with introduction of the neurolytic agent into the psoas muscle, most likely at the origin of the deep part of the psoas major.

The alternative diagnoses are less likely. The time course of the symptom onset is not consistent with abscess formation. Abscess and hematoma were not demonstrated on

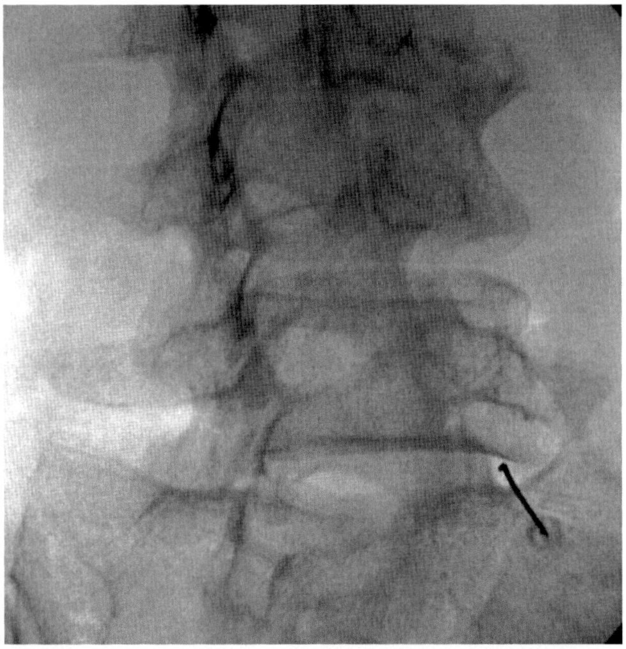

Fig. 25.3 Transdiscal approach to the superior hypogastric plexus, oblique view. Square of the L5 vertebral end plates allows easy visualization of the intervertebral disc and appropriate needle placement. Images from Dr. Anitescu Personal Library

CT imaging. Spinal cord infarction would most likely result in more widespread neurologic deficits. Although direct anesthesia or neurolysis of the spinal nerves would result in immediate deficits like those experienced by the patient above, in order to create dysfunction of hip flexion, neurolysis would have had to occur at different (i.e., higher) levels in the lumbar spine.

Importantly, this case demonstrates the importance of proper needle placement. In Figs. 25.1 and 25.2, one can appreciate placement inappropriately cephalad in both needles. In the right needle (recall right-sided weakness), needle placement is lateral to the appropriate target. This likely contributed to injury to nearby structures. Based on the patient's clinical presentation, the structures that were affected are most likely muscle fibers from the psoas major. The psoas muscle weakness may have been avoided by proper needle placement as well as proper observation of unwanted spread of injectate into nearby muscle tissue. In chemical injury to a major muscle group, outcomes vary depending on the extent of injury as well as the muscle group involved, vis-a-vis the ability of the patient to compensate for loss of muscle function with targeted physical therapy and rehabilitation. In this case, the patient's deficit

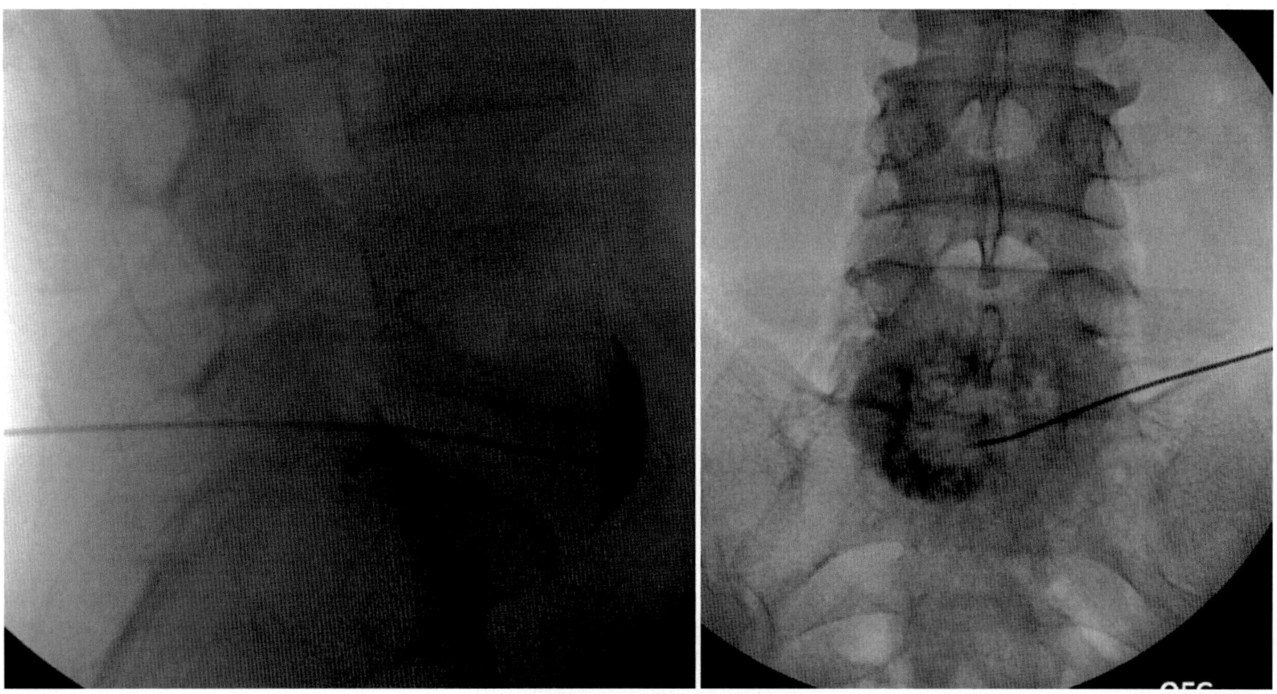

Fig. 25.4 Transdiscal approach of the superior hypogastric plexus, anteroposterior and lateral view showing appropriate spread of the dye around the plexus. Images from Dr. Anitescu Personal Library

was significant, but her functional disability was fortunately self-limited.

References

1. Snell R. The pelvis – part I: the pelvic walls. In: Snell R, editor. Clinical anatomy by regions. 9th ed. Philadelphia: Wolters Kluwer; 2012. p. 240–61.
2. Waldman SD. Hypogastric plexus block, p. 609–16. In: Waldman SD, editor. Atlas of interventional pain management. 4th ed. Philadelphia: Saunders (Elsevier); 2015. p. 602–27.
3. Plancarte R, Amescua C, Patt RB, Aldrete JA. Superior hypogastric plexus block for pelvic cancer pain. Anesthesiology. 1990;73:236–9.
4. Plancarte R, de Leon-Casasola OA, El-Helaly M, Allende S, Lema MJ. Neurolytic superior hypogastric plexus block for chronic pelvic pain associated with cancer. Reg Anesth. 1997;22:562–8.
5. Dodusek DB, Aminoff MJ. Sexual dysfunction in patients with neurologic disorders. In: Aminoff MJ, editor. Neurology and general medicine. 5th ed. London: Academic (Elsevier); 2014. p. 633–56.
6. Rastogi R, Agarwal S, Enany N, Munir MA. Sympathetic blockade. In: Smith HS, editor. Current therapy in pain. 1st ed. Philadelphia: Saunders (Elsevier); 2009. p. 612–20.
7. Byrne JR, Darling C III. Aortic surgery. In: SRT E, editor. Surgical pitfalls. 1st ed. Philadelphia: Saunders (Elsevier); 2009. p. 597–612.
8. Purves D, Augustine GJ, Fitzpatrick D, et al. Autonomic regulation of sexual function. In: Purves D, Augustine GJ, Fitzpatrick D, et al., editors. Neuroscience. 2nd ed. Sunderland: Sinauer Associates; 2001.
9. Hendren SK, O'Connor BI, Liu M, et al. Prevalence of male and female sexual dysfunction is high following surgery for rectal cancer. Ann Surg. 2005;242(2):212–23.
10. Basson R, Leiblum S, Brotto L, et al. Definitions of women's sexual dysfunction reconsidered: advocating expansion and revision. J Psychosom Obstet Gynaecol. 2003;24(4):221–9.
11. Rathmell JP, Pino CA, Ahmed S. Spinal pain and the role of neural blockade. In: Cousins MJ, editor. Neural blockade. 4th ed. Philadelphia: Wolters Kluwer; 2009. p. 1063–110.
12. Palastanga N, Field D, Soames R. Muscles flexing the hip joint. In: Palastanga N, editor. Anatomy and human movement. 1st ed. Oxford: Heinemann; 1989. p. 354–6.
13. Shoja MM. Pelvic girdle, gluteal region and thigh. In: Standring S, editor. Gray's anatomy: the anatomical basis of clinical practice. 41st ed. London: Elsevier; 2016. p. 1337–77.
14. Pollitt CI, Salota V, Leschinskiy D. Chemical neurolysis of the superior hypogastric plexus for chronic non-cancer pelvic pain. Int J Gynaecol Obstet. 2011;114:160–1.
15. Brown DL, Rorie DK. Altered reactivity of isolated segmental lumbar arteries of dogs following exposure to ethanol and phenol. Pain. 1994;56:139–43.

Discitis Following Transdiscal Approach for Superior Hypogastric Plexus Block

26

Lucia Daiana Voiculescu and Qian CeCe Chen

26.1 Case Description

A 75-year-old male was admitted with macroscopic hematuria and severe pelvic pain. He was recently diagnosed with bladder carcinoma with transmural spread to the extravesical space and rectum. The comprehensive evaluation that led to the diagnosis was prompted by patient's complaints of unexplained fatigue and pelvic pain. As part of the work-up, he underwent standard imaging, including contrast-enhanced pelvic CT and lumbar spine MRI. Pelvic lymph node involvement was visualized, but there was no evidence of metastatic spread. No suspicious lesion or significant pathology was identified at the level of the spine.

On admission he was afebrile and hemodynamically stable. Admission blood work was remarkable for microcytic anemia (Hg 9.8, Ht 30.38). The patient reported feeling "tired" and complained of diffuse pelvic pain, aggravated by bowel movements and voiding. He eventually underwent transurethral bladder fulguration to control the intravesical bleeding. An indwelling catheter was left in place for 24 h until urine cleared. Meanwhile he continued to complain of severe, intractable pain, made even worse by the bladder procedure and catheter presence. The pain was diffuse, deep, with occasional episodes of suprapubic burning and stabbing sensation. Opioid analgesics and adjuvants around the clock provided only marginal analgesia. Opioid-induced constipation resulted in increased pain and discomfort.

A pain consult was obtained for interventional pain management options. A diagnostic superior hypogastric plexus block was recommended, to be followed, if successful, by a neurolytic block. Technical difficulties in performing the classic two-needle block were anticipated by the pain specialists as recent pelvis X-rays revealed a narrow pelvis with tall iliac crests. A decision was then made to proceed with a fluoroscopically guided posteromedian transdiscal approach.

L.D. Voiculescu, M.D. (✉) • Q.C. Chen, M.D.
NYU School of Medicine, Dept. of Anesthesiology, Perioperative Care and Pain Medicine, New York, NY, USA
e-mail: Lucia.Voiculescu@nyumc.org

One gram of cefazolin was administered intravenously 30 min prior to the skin preparation.

The procedure was complicated by inadvertent vascular puncture in the targeted area, just anterior to the L5–S1 intervertebral disc. The initial intravascular placement was confirmed by both blood aspiration and contrast injection under real-time fluoroscopy. The needle was withdrawn in the disc and, after a few more attempts, was correctly repositioned. The block, performed with 8 mL 0.25% preservative-free bupivacaine, resulted in 10–12 h of good pelvic analgesia. The patient was discharged home with a recommendation to return in 1 week for the neurolytic procedure.

Over the course of the next few days, the patient continued to experience pelvic pain, worse in the rectal and suprapubic area, and noticed some low back discomfort and paraspinal muscle tension. The discomfort progressed gradually to severe, intractable lumbar pain, radiating to both hips. His sleep was interrupted by intense pain, muscle spasms, and diaphoresis. Ambulation worsened significantly due to the severity of pain and back stiffness. The patient ultimately missed his appointment for hypogastric plexus neurolysis.

One week later, the pain had progressed to unbearable levels, prompting the patient to present to the ER. On admission, he was afebrile, hemodynamically stable, and without systemic signs of infection. The severity of the symptoms following a transdiscal procedure led to a high suspicion for procedure-related pathology. Metastatic disease progression was also strongly considered in the differential diagnosis. The patient underwent an emergency lumbar MRI which revealed L5–S1 discitis. He was admitted and evaluated by a multidisciplinary team. Inflammatory markers were found to be elevated (C-reactive protein, CRP, 30 mg/dL and erythrocyte sedimentation rate, ESR, 78 mm/h). White blood cell (WBC) count was only slightly elevated. Blood was sent for bacterial (aerobic and anaerobic) cultures and Gram stain. Urinalysis and urine cultures were also ordered.

Considering patient's clinical stability, no surgical intervention was deemed immediately necessary.

M. Anitescu et al. (eds.), *Challenging Cases and Complication Management in Pain Medicine*,
https://doi.org/10.1007/978-3-319-60072-7_26

Empiric antibiotic therapy was deferred in preparation for CT-guided biopsy, to ensure optimal culture results.

While waiting to be scheduled for an image-guided aspiration biopsy, the patient became febrile. A decision was made to initiate empiric antibiotic therapy with vancomycin and cefepime. The following day, the patient underwent a successful CT-guided L5–S1 disc space aspiration. Specimens were sent for bacterial, fungal, and mycobacterial cultures. *Morganella morganii*, resistant to cefazolin, was identified in both disc biopsy and urine cultures. Specific intravenous antibiotic therapy was immediately initiated. In the interim, the patient's condition deteriorated. In addition to feeling "very ill," he complained of severe pain radiating to his legs and feet. He described dysesthesias and progressive numbness on the top and bottom of his left leg. DTRs could no longer be elicited on the left side. Gradually over a 24-h period, he developed left lower extremity weakness and foot drop.

A lumbar MRI with intravenous contrast revealed vertebral and epidural progression of the infectious process; discitis osteomyelitis at L5–S1 with probable small prevertebral abscess (1.3 × 0.7 cm) and erosive changes of the inferior L5 vertebral body; and epidural and paraspinal phlegmon spanning the L5–S1 levels and resulting in moderate spinal stenosis and severe bilateral foraminal stenosis at L5–S1. The patient was examined by neurosurgery and subsequently taken to the OR for a left L5–S1 laminotomy, evacuation of epidural infective material, and removal of an infected disk.

The patient's postoperative course showed improvement with reduction of the back pain. He regained some of the left lower extremity sensation and strength. However, he was unable to participate in physical therapy due to pelvic pain.

Intravenous antibiotics were continued for 6 weeks, followed by additional 6 weeks of oral therapy. He continued to experience severe cancer-related pain for which he was prescribed progressively higher doses of opioids. Pain control interventions, including implantable devices, were no longer deemed appropriate.

We postulate that transfer of pathogens to the intervertebral disc occurred when the bacteremic patient had an invasive, transdiscal procedure.

26.2 Case Discussion

26.2.1 Superior Hypogastric Plexus Block for Treatment of Malignant Pelvic Pain

Advanced pelvic malignancy is often associated with severe, diffuse, poorly defined visceral pain. Superior hypogastric plexus neurolysis can be used to reduce pain and minimize oral opioid therapy [1]. The superior hypogastric plexus receives, directly or via the inferior hypogastric plexus, afferent fibers that carry pain signals from all organs in the pelvis. Considering its extraperitoneal position, adjacent and anterior to the lower third of L5 vertebral body and the upper third of S1 vertebrae, neurolysis at this level is commonly utilized for the treatment of intractable pelvic cancer pain.

Due to the complexity of malignant pelvic pain, in which visceral, neuropathic, and somatic components are often involved, sympathetic plexus blocks may not always result in optimal analgesia. A recent systematic review of sympathetic blockade for visceral cancer pain management found limited data, insufficient to strongly recommend the use of superior hypogastric plexus neurolysis [2]. The authors suggested that the involvement of different pain pathways (neuropathic, somatic, and visceral) explains the inconsistent success of pelvic sympathectomy [2].

Different approaches to superior hypogastric plexus have been described in an attempt to improve the efficacy and tolerability of the block and to decrease the potential for complications (Table 26.1) [3–8]. Anatomical variability (large L5 transverse process, highly arched iliac crests), the proximity of important structures (iliac vessels, nerve roots), and possible retroperitoneal malignancy and adenopathy can create significant difficulties in needle placement. In addition, patients with severe pain or other limiting comorbidities are often unable to tolerate the prone position [7, 8].

A single needle posteromedian transdiscal approach can be used to achieve bilateral blockade with less technical difficulties. This technique, described by Turker et al. [7], is simple and can be performed with patient positioned in prone or lateral decubitus. Compared to the classic two-needle posterior approach, the transdiscal technique is easier and has less potential for complications while having the same efficacy [9]. Although no significant complications have been reported so far with any of these techniques, potential problems should always be considered.

Retroperitoneal bleeding, nerve root injury, or atherosclerotic plaque embolization from iliac arteries can occur with the posterior extradiscal needle placement. Bowel or bladder perforation can complicate the anterior approach, while discitis and disc trauma are of particular concern when transdiscal techniques are used.

26.2.2 The Intervertebral Disc: Age-Related Structural Changes

The two main components of the disc—nucleus pulposus and annulus fibrosus—are confined in the intervertebral space by the end-plate cartilage, a hyaline structure adherent

Table 26.1 Most commonly described techniques for superior hypogastric plexus block

Authors	Technique	Advantages	Disadvantages
Plancarte et al. [3]	Bilateral paramedian extradiscal approach (fluoroscopy)	Avoids risks associated with intervertebral disc and spinal canal penetration	• Technical difficulties due to anatomical variability (tall iliac crests, large L5 transverse process, L5 nerve root) • Two separate injections • Unpredictable spread in the presence of retroperitoneal adenopathy/tumor
Waldman and Wilson [4]	CT-guided paramedian single needle approach	• Avoids risk of vascular, intervertebral disc, and spinal canal penetration • Accurate needle placement	• Increased radiation exposure • Access to CT scan • Unpredictable and limited spread in the presence of retroperitoneal adenopathy/tumor
Kanazi and Frederick [5]	Single needle anterior approach (fluoroscopy, CT, or ultrasound guidance)	• Easy, simple technique • Supine position	Risk for bowel and bladder perforation or vascular injury
Erdine [6]	Single needle paramedian, transdiscal approach (fluoroscopy)	• Accurate needle placement	• Risk for disc infection, rupture, herniation • Can be painful • Unnecessary discogram
Turker [7]	Single needle posteromedian approach (fluoroscopy)	• Easy, simple • Avoids anatomical barriers • Lateral or prone position • Accurate needle placement	• Risk for infection (discitis, meningitis, epidural abscess), neural injury, postdural puncture headache

Other approaches mentioned in the literature, transvaginal and transvascular [6, 8], cannot be objectively analyzed due to scarcity of reported data

to the vertebral metaphysis, and by the anterior and posterior longitudinal ligaments. With aging all these entities undergo multiple structural changes. At birth the disc is well vascularized and contains 80–90% water. The collagen and elastin fibers are organized in very complex networks. Proteoglycans are responsible for maintaining the osmotic pressure and disc hydration, which further allows the disc to maintain height when loaded. With time the fibers become less organized and lose their strength. Proteoglycans are degraded and subsequently the osmotic pressure and water content decrease [10].

At birth, branches of the segmental arteries penetrate the annulus and provide blood supply to the entire disc. Progressively the intradiscal vascular bed contracts. In the third decade of life, the disc becomes almost avascular, maintaining only limited blood supply to the outer margin of the annulus fibrosus. The adult disc receives nutrients by diffusion through the cartilaginous end plates and from its own poor peripheral vasculature. The innervation also regresses to the disc periphery. Nociceptive and mechanosensitive fibers accompanying the blood vessels or branching from the sinuvertebral nerves are found only in the outer third of the adult annulus. Cartilaginous end plates become more frail, prone to fissures, allowing disc material to herniate into adjacent vertebrae to form Schmorl's nodes.

The disc starts to lose height and becomes more susceptible to degenerative, traumatic, and infectious processes.

26.2.3 Discitis Etiology and Pathogenesis

In adults, the infection of the intervertebral disc is most frequently the result of hematogenous spread, from a distant source (genitourinary, endocardial, respiratory, gastrointestinal, cutaneous ulcers, etc.). Infected emboli reach the well-vascularized vertebral metaphysis via arterial or retrograde venous (Batson's veins) blood flow, subsequently producing bone infarction, destruction, and osteomyelitis. From the subchondral area, the infection diffuses then into the intervertebral disc space to the avascular nucleus pulposus.

Direct hematogenous colonization of the disc occurs mostly in children, as their discs are still vascularized. Infection is often limited to the disc space [11]. The rich vascular supply allows good antibiotic penetration. Overall, in these very young patients, discitis has a better prognosis [12]. Less frequently, discitis is caused by direct iatrogenic or traumatic disc contamination. Spine surgery and intradiscal procedures are the most common iatrogenic causes of discitis. The incidence of post-discography infection varies from 1 to 4% [13].

Because discitis can be either preceded or complicated by vertebral osteomyelitis, the two conditions are frequently described as spondylodiscitis [14]. Most disc infections are bacterial, but mycobacterial and fungal etiology should be considered in specific circumstances.

Staphylococcus aureus, *Staphylococcus epidermidis*, and gram-negative *Escherichia coli* are some of the pathogens commonly isolated in the spinal infections involving the disc. Many predisposing comorbidities have been described, among them diabetes, immunocompromised states, malignancies, intravenous drug use, chronic alcoholism, previous spine surgery, infective endocarditis, etc.

26.2.4 Discitis Clinical Presentation, Diagnosis, and Treatment

26.2.4.1 Clinical Presentation

Most of the patients with discitis experience severe back pain, stiffness, muscle spasm, and tenderness to palpation. Often the onset is insidious with the pain intensifying progressively. The incidence of fever varies in different reports from 37 to 70% of patients with bacterial spondylodiscitis [15–17]. Fatigue, anorexia, and malaise can occur as the disease progresses. Sepsis is rare.

When the infection occurs as a complication of an intradiscal procedure, the symptoms become evident at 2–4 weeks after the intervention [17].

Delays in diagnosis and treatment allow infection to diffuse to the adjacent vertebral bodies, epidural space, and paraspinal muscles. Paravertebral contamination, psoas abscesses, compression fractures, and spine instability may complicate advanced stages. Depending on the site and size of the infection, different degrees of neurologic symptoms can develop. Isolated radicular pain, sensory-motor deficits, cord or cauda equina compression, or even paraplegia can complicate the course of spondylodiscitis.

26.2.4.2 Diagnosis

Although spondylodiscitis presents with non-specific symptoms, centered on progressive back or neck pain, the diagnosis should be suspected whenever fever and elevated inflammatory markers accompany the axial symptoms. Other painful spine conditions should be taken into account as part of the differential diagnosis: painful intervertebral disc disease, fractures, or vertebral metastases.

A complete clinical examination, with emphasis on neurologic and musculoskeletal aspects, can reveal axial tenderness, muscle spasms, sensory/motor deficits, or, in advances stages, spine deformities and even instability. The exam should also address the existence of a potential source of bacteremia.

Laboratory findings are remarkable for elevated erythrocyte sedimentation rate (ESR) and C-reactive protein (CRP). Leukocytosis may also be absent. Bacterial (aerobic and anaerobic) blood cultures should be sent as soon as the infection is suspected. When brucella, tuberculosis, or fungal infections are considered, specific diagnostic tests must be performed.

Essential to a correct diagnosis involves performing imaging studies as early as possible. Plain radiographs are not very reliable in the initial stages, as they tend to remain normal for many weeks, until erosions, irregularities, and bone destruction occur. With its high sensitivity (93–97%) and specificity (92.5–97%), magnetic resonance imaging (MRI) is considered the most important diagnostic tool [12, 18]. Examination with and without contrast reveals increased disc signal on T2-weighted images and post-gadolinium enhancement. The intervertebral space is narrowed and herniated disc material can be identified in the adjacent structures (end plates, spinal canal). Abscesses resulting from epidural and paravertebral spread can be identified with accuracy (Figs. 26.1, 26.2, and 26.3).

When the MRI exam is not possible, computed tomography (CT) or positron emission tomography (PET) scans should be considered. Biopsies (CT-guided or open) are performed if blood cultures fail to provide a satisfactory microbiologic diagnosis.

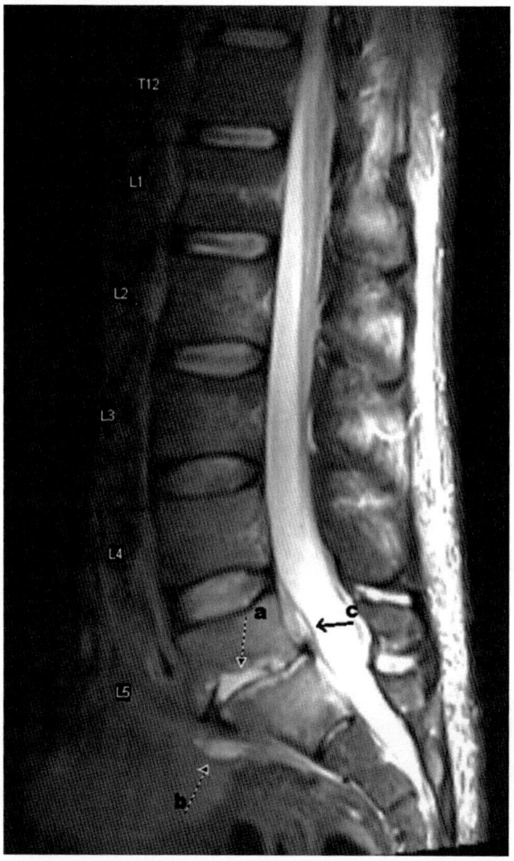

Fig. 26.1 Sagittal T2-weighted image of the lumbar spine demonstrates fluid in the L5–S1 disc space and destruction of the inferior end plate of L5 consistent with discitis and osteomyelitis (**a**). There is a small, ovoid fluid collection in the anterior paraspinal soft tissues (**b**). There is heterogeneous soft tissue in the epidural space with elevation of the posterior longitudinal ligament (**c**)

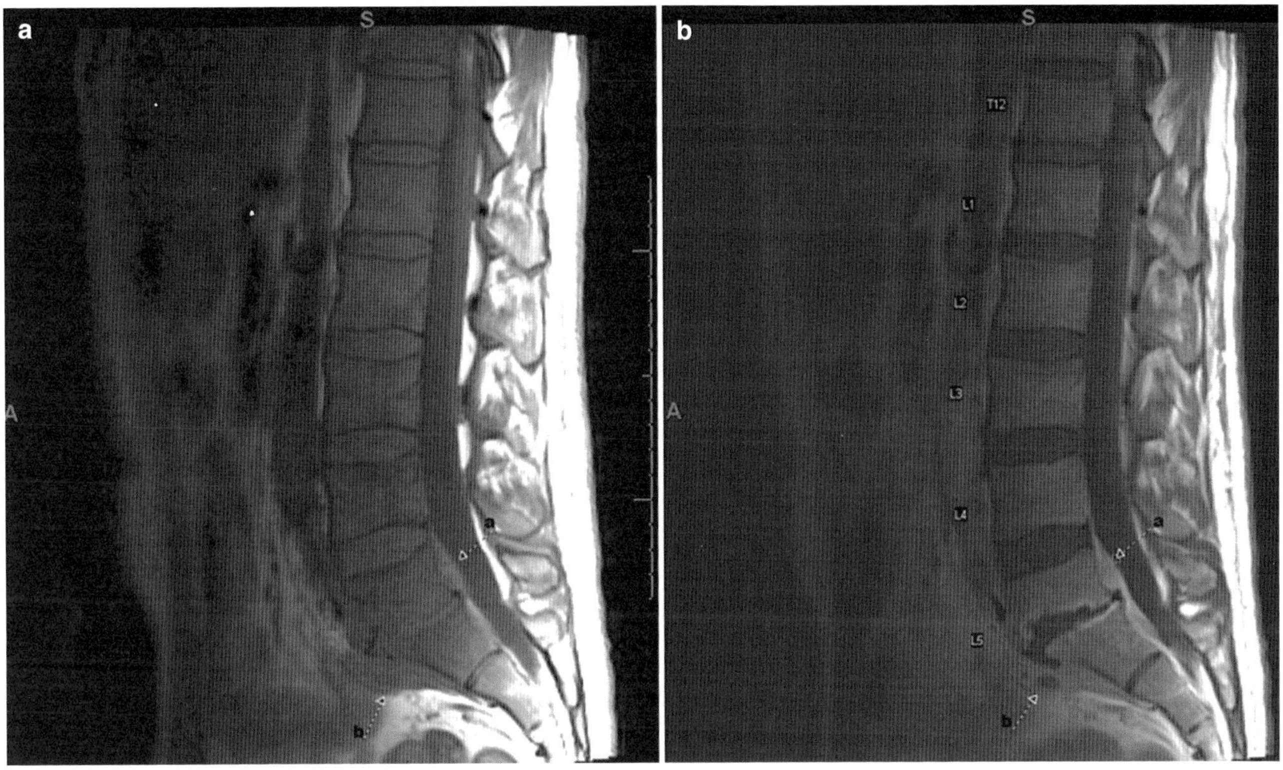

Fig. 26.2 Sagittal T1-weighted images before (**A**) and after (**B**) gadolinium administration demonstrate abnormal soft tissue in the L5–S1 disc space with enhancement after gadolinium administration consistent with discitis. There is enhancing epidural soft tissue consistent with phlegmon (**a**) and a peripherally enhancing collection in the anterior paraspinal soft tissues consistent with an abscess (**b**)

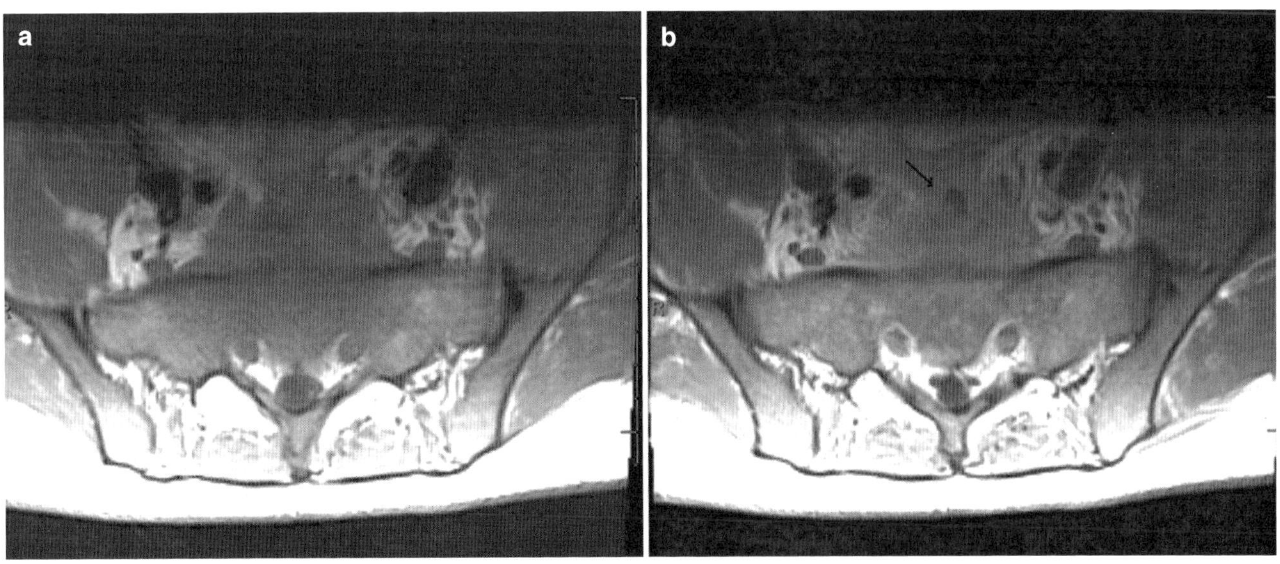

Fig. 26.3 Axial T1-weighted images before (**A**) and after (**B**) gadolinium administration demonstrate abnormal soft tissue in the anterior paraspinal soft tissues which demonstrates enhancement after gadolinium consistent with phlegmon. An ovoid area of central nonenhancement represents a small abscess (*arrow*)

26.2.4.3 Treatment

Prophylactic Management

Intravenous antibiotics are commonly administered prior to most intradiscal procedures, to minimize the risk of infection. However, animal studies have shown that not all intravenous antibiotics have equal efficacy in penetrating the intervertebral discs. The two most important factors affecting the degree of antibiotic penetration into the discs are related to the serum level of the antibiotic and the time elapsed from administration [13].

Typically a broad-spectrum antibiotic is injected intravenously 30 min prior to the disc puncture. This prophylactic measure, however, does not prevent the development of discitis if resistant bacteria from an adjacent or remote infection site are inoculated. Intradiscal procedures should be considered with caution in patients at risk for bacteremia (IV drug users, intravenous catheters, established focus of infection, etc.).

Medical Management

Management of the intervertebral space infection requires a multidisciplinary approach and long-term antibiotic therapy.

Antibiotics have been routinely used to treat discitis; however, there have been debates regarding its actual efficacy in penetrating the infected intervertebral disc.

Animal studies have shown that antibiotics, such as cefazolin when given after discitis had been diagnosed, failed to alter end-plate erosions and destructions of the discs [13]. The antibiotic therapy should be guided by microbiologic results and drug sensitivity. If sepsis or rapid neurologic deterioration develops before identifying the responsible agent, empiric antimicrobial therapy should be immediately initiated [18]. The initial intravenous antibiotic therapy is continued for 6 weeks, followed by treatment with oral antibiotics for another 6 weeks.

Symptomatic treatment is aimed at controlling pain, fever, deconditioning, and other associated symptoms. In addition, patients may be required to wear orthotic braces for external immobilization until infection is treated [19, 20].

Surgical Management

Surgery should be considered if, despite conservative treatment, infection persists or bone destruction, spinal deformity, instability, hardware failure, and intractable pain occur. Sepsis, hemodynamic instability, and compression of the thecal sac with acute neurologic compromise are indications for emergency surgical debridement or decompression [18].

Multiple surgical techniques and strategies have been described, ranging from minimally invasive techniques to complex, multistage procedures for anterior-posterior debridement and fusion [12, 20, 21]. Recent studies showed that a minimally invasive, lateral approach may be equally effective, may avoid the need to mobilize the great vessels, and may be beneficial especially for patients with severe comorbidities [19, 21].

Postoperatively, patients should finish the course of antibiotic. Systemic inflammatory markers and neurologic function are monitored, but MRI follow-ups are not routinely indicated, unless complications develop or infection persists despite appropriate therapy [18].

Key Points

- In selected patients, superior hypogastric plexus neurolysis can be successfully used to treat malignancy-related pelvic pain [1]. Different technical approaches have been described, in an attempt to improve the block efficacy and minimize the risk for complications (Table 26.1).
- Transdiscal procedures carry the risk for intervertebral disc infection, rupture, or herniation. Infected tissue can be directly inoculated by the procedural needle during the disc penetration. Discitis should be suspected when severe, intractable back pain follows a transdiscal procedure.
- Clinical manifestations of discitis are non-specific. As soon as the intervertebral disc infection is suspected, diagnostic microbiologic and imaging studies should be obtained. Antibiotic therapy should be guided by the drug sensitivity results; however, if general or neurologic deterioration occurs, emergency intravenous antibiotic and surgery should be considered.

References

1. Plancarte R, de Leon-Casasola OA, El-Helaly M, Allende S, Lema MJ. Neurolytic superior hypogastric plexus block for chronic pelvic pain associated with cancer. Reg Anesth. 1997;22(6):562–8.
2. Mercadante S, Klepstad P, Kurita GP, Sjøgren P, Giarratano A, European Palliative Care Research Collaborative (EPCRC). Sympathetic blocks for visceral cancer pain management: a systematic review and EAPC recommendations. Crit Rev Oncol Hematol. 2015;96(3):577–83.
3. Plancarte R, Amescua C, Patt RB, Aldrete JA. Superior hypogastric plexus block for pelvic cancer pain. Anesthesiology. 1990;73(2):236–9.
4. Waldman SD, Wilson WL, Kreps RD. Superior hypogastric plexus block using a single needle and computed tomography guidance: description of a modified technique. Reg Anesth. 1991;16(5):286–7.
5. Kanazi GE, Perkins FM, Thakur R, Dotson E. New technique for superior hypogastric plexus block. Reg Anesth Pain Med. 1999;24(5):473–6.
6. Erdine S, Yucel A, Celik M, Talu GK. Transdiscal approach for hypogastric plexus block. Reg Anesth Pain Med. 2003;28(4):304–8.
7. Turker G, Basagan-Mogol E, Gurbet A, Ozturk C, Uckunkaya N, Sahin S. A new technique for superior hypogastric plexus block: the posteromedian transdiscal approach. Tohoku J Exp Med. 2005;206(3):277–81.
8. Nabil D, Eissa AA. Evaluation of posteromedial transdiscal superior hypogastric block after failure of the classic approach. Clin J Pain. 2010;26(8):694–7.
9. Gamal G, Helaly M, Labib YM. Superior hypogastric block: transdiscal versus classic posterior approach in pelvic cancer pain. Clin J Pain. 2006;22(6):544–7.
10. Raj PP. Intervertebral disc: anatomy-physiology-pathophysiology-treatment. Pain Pract. 2008;8(1):18–44.
11. Duarte RM, Vaccaro AR. Spinal infection: state of the art and management algorithm. Eur Spine J. 2013;22(12):2787–99.
12. Khan IA, Vaccaro AR, Zlotolow DA. Management of vertebral diskitis and osteomyelitis. Orthopedics. 1999;22(8):758–65.
13. Osti OL, Fraser RD, Vernon-Roberts B. Discitis after discography. The role of prophylactic antibiotics. J Bone Joint Surg Br. 1990;72(2):271–4.
14. Esendagli-Yilmaz G, Uluoglu O. Pathologic basis of pyogenic, nonpyogenic, and other spondylitis and discitis. Neuroimaging Clin N Am. 2015;25(2):159–61.
15. Ramos A, Berbari E, Huddleston P. Diagnosis and treatment of Fusobacterium nucleatum discitis and vertebral osteomyelitis: case report and review of the literature. Spine (Phila Pa 1976). 2013;38(2):E120–2.

16. Kapsalaki E, Gatselis N, Stefos A, Makaritsis K, Vassiou A, Fezoulidis I, Dalekos GN. Spontaneous spondylodiscitis: presentation, risk factors, diagnosis, management, and outcome. Int J Infect Dis. 2009;13(5):564–9.
17. Cottle L, Riordan T. Infectious spondylodiscitis. J Infect. 2008;56(6):401–12.
18. Berbari EF, Kanj SS, Kowalski TJ, Darouiche RO, Widmer AF, Schmitt SK, Hendershot EF, Holtom PD, Huddleston PM 3rd, Petermann GW, Osmon DR. 2015 Infectious Disease Society of America (IDSA) clinical practice guidelines for the diagnosis and treatment of native vertebral osteomyelitis in adults. Clin Infect Dis. 2015;61(6):e26–46.
19. Madhavan K, Vanni S, Williams SK. Direct lateral retroperitoneal approach for the surgical treatment of lumbar discitis and osteomyelitis. Neurosurg Focus. 2014;37(2):E5.
20. Shiban E, Janssen I, Wostrack M, Krieg SM, Ringel F, Meyer B, Stoffel M. A retrospective study of 113 consecutive cases of surgically treated spondylodiscitis patients. A single-center experience. Acta Neurochir (Wien). 2014;156(6):1189–96.
21. Patel NB, Dodd ZH, Voorhies J, Horn EM. Minimally invasive lateral transpsoas approach for spinal discitis and osteomyelitis. J Clin Neurosci. 2015;22(11):1753–7.

Part IV

Interventional Pain Procedures: Implantable Drug Delivery System

27 Complications Related to Catheter Migration

Omar R. Qureshi and Magdalena Anitescu

27.1 Case

A 35-year-old female (height 162 cm and weight 85 kg) at 38 weeks gestation was admitted to labor and delivery for contractions. She had no significant past medical history other than an appendectomy as a child. She had a full set of prenatal labs including chemistry panel and complete blood count, all of which were within the normal range. When seen by the anesthesiologist, she requested epidural analgesia during labor.

The epidural was placed successfully using the loss of resistance technique. A 17 G Tuohy needle was used to locate the epidural space at a depth of 6 cm at the L3–L4 interspace. A 20 G epidural catheter was then threaded easily. A 3 mL test dose of lidocaine 1.5% with 1:200,000 epinephrine was given via the epidural catheter with a negative response (i.e., the heart rate and blood pressure did not change, and patient did not report any numbness or weakness in her legs). A bolus of 10 mL of 1% lidocaine was administered along with a continuous infusion of bupivacaine 0.0625% and fentanyl 2mcg/mL at a rate of 10 mL/h. The patient reported significant relief of her labor pains, and the highest level of sensory block was identified to be T9 bilaterally after testing with ice.

After 6 h of labor, the decision was made to proceed with caesarean section due to failure to progress and abnormal fetal heart tones. The patient was transported to the operating room, where she moved herself from the stretcher to the operating table. She was positioned supine with left uterine displacement. Her initial blood pressure reading was 142/81 mmHg and her heart rate recorded was 75 bpm. A surgical anesthetic dose consisting of 20 mL of 2% lidocaine with sodium bicarbonate 2 mEq and epinephrine 50 μg was administered through the epidural catheter without an aspiration test or a test dose. Within 2 min, the patient reported perioral tingling and a metallic taste in her mouth. She subsequently became drowsy and stopped responding to the anesthesiologist's commands. Her heart rate increased from 75 to 115 bpm, and her blood pressure rose from 142/81 to 165/101 mmHg. An inadvertent intravascular injection was suspected. Aspiration was performed on the epidural catheter with immediate return of bloodstained fluid.

General anesthesia was immediately induced with propofol 150 mg and succinylcholine 100 mg. Following endotracheal intubation, vecuronium was administered, and anesthesia was maintained with 2 L/min nitrous oxide and 0.75% sevoflurane. The patient's vital signs stabilized, and a 4.2 kg baby was delivered 12 min after incision. Oxytocin was then administered to assist with uterine tone. The baby had Apgar scores of 8 and 9 at 1 and 5 min, respectively. At the end of the case, neostigmine and glycopyrrolate were used to reverse neuromuscular blockade. The patient was successfully extubated and transferred to the recovery room.

In the recovery room, the patient reported that she was comfortable, and all vital signs were stable. The patient had no neurologic or cardiovascular disturbances and was subsequently discharged from the post-anesthesia recovery room to the ward.

27.2 Discussion

Epidural analgesia provides high-quality analgesia and anesthesia and has numerous applications. However, catheter migration can cause serious complications. Epidural catheter migration is a well-described entity within the field of anesthesiology. Migration of the epidural catheter even after it has been fixed to the skin has already been shown to occur.

O.R. Qureshi, M.D.
Advanced Pain Management, Stoneham, 3307 Taylor Pond Lane, Bedford, MA 01730, USA
e-mail: orqureshi@gmail.com

M. Anitescu, M.D., Ph.D. (✉)
Department of Anesthesia and Critical Care, University of Chicago Medical Center, Chicago, IL, USA
e-mail: MAnitescu@dacc.uchicago.edu

M. Anitescu et al. (eds.), *Challenging Cases and Complication Management in Pain Medicine*,
https://doi.org/10.1007/978-3-319-60072-7_27

Hazards of epidural catheter migration include intravascular, subarachnoid, or subdural injection of local anesthetic and a unilateral or failed block.

27.3 Inadvertent Intravascular Injection

Inadvertent intravascular injection of local anesthetic after catheter migration can occur in up to 0.67% of cases. Systemic toxicity of local anesthetics can occur after administration of an excessive dose, with rapid absorption and uptake, or after inadvertent intravenous injection. Because of their affinity to receptor sites in the cardiovascular and central nervous systems, local anesthetic toxicity can be exquisitely difficult to treat, and prolonged resuscitative efforts may be required [1].

Toxicity of local anesthetics typically manifests in the form of central nervous system and cardiovascular effects. Central nervous system (CNS) effects include tinnitus, disorientation, perioral numbness, and seizures. Cardiovascular toxicity displays itself as refractory hypotension, dysrhythmias, and cardiac arrest [2]. In most instances, the central nervous system effects will become apparent at lower doses than those required to produce cardiovascular toxicities due to increased susceptibility of the brain to local anesthetics. However, it is important to bear in mind that cardiovascular toxicity is more serious and difficult to treat than CNS toxicity.

Other than CNS and cardiovascular effects, local anesthetics have also been linked to other adverse events, including allergic reactions, methemoglobinemia, and bronchospasm [3].

The first signs of systemic toxicity are caused by the blockade of inhibitory pathways in the cerebral cortex. This results in disinhibition of neurons that facilitate excitatory neurons, which then leads to increased excitatory nerve activity. Many patients report symptoms such as dizziness, tinnitus, perioral numbness, or light-headedness. More objective findings consistent with local anesthetic toxicity include shivering, myoclonic jerking movements, and tremors. Eventually, tonic-clonic seizures will occur. However, this excitatory period typically leads to CNS depression, where seizure activity abates and respiratory depression and arrest may occur. Local anesthetic potency directly correlates with CNS toxicity [4].

Cardiovascular effects can be produced by all local anesthetics. With the notable exception of cocaine, all local anesthetics are cardiovascular depressants. The negative inotropic effect is dose-dependent and leads to decreased myocardial contractility and cardiac output. Dysrhythmias produced by local anesthetics can take many forms, including conduction delays (from a prolonged PR interval to third-degree heart block or asystole) and ventricular arrhythmias (ventricular ectopy, torsades de pointes, and fibrillation) (Table 27.1).

Initial low blood levels of local anesthetic typically increase most cardiac parameters, such as blood pressure, heart rate, and cardiac output. This is thought to be due to increased sympathetic tone and direct vasoconstriction.

Table 27.1 Local anesthetic systemic toxicity [28] personal table, based on, modified from Vadi MJ et al. [28]

Central nervous system toxicity	Cardiovascular toxicity
Subjective symptoms • Agitation/difficulty focusing • Auditory changes/tinnitus • Dizziness/ light-headedness • Metallic taste/tinnitus • Abrupt onset of psychiatric symptoms	Direct cardiac effects • Depression of sinus node pacemaker activity • Depression of rapid phase of depolarization in Purkinje fibers and ventricular muscle • Depression of cardiac contractility
Objective changes • Coma • Muscle tremor • Seizures • Respiratory arrest	Peripheral vascular effects • Low concentration-vascular smooth muscle vasoconstriction • High concentration-vascular smooth muscle vasodilatation

However, as the local anesthetic serum level rises, vasodilatation begins to predominate and leads to hypotension. Additionally, reduced cardiac output and dysrhythmias further worsen hypotension. This instability paves the way for cardiac arrest if not addressed immediately.

Prevention of local anesthetic toxicity is crucial due to the serious consequences of an overdose. Before any anesthetic employing local anesthetics is begun, safety equipment designed to treat emergencies, including airway equipment and resuscitative drugs, must be available. Additionally, carefully selecting the dose and concentration of local anesthetic is very important. The optimal dose is the lowest one that achieves the desired effect. Much effort has been made to develop an ideal test for detecting intravascular injection, and currently epinephrine is the most commonly used. Increases in heart rate by more than 10 bpm or systolic blood pressure by more than 15 mmHg or a decrease of 25% in the lead II T-wave amplitude are thought to be sensitive markers for intravascular injection [5]. Many problems do arise with epinephrine as a test dose, most notably in patients who are on beta-blockade therapy or those with low cardiac output states, which can delay circulation of the epinephrine. One more way of preventing intravascular injections is to use incremental dosing with frequent aspirations. Aspirating every 3–5 mL between injections and monitoring for toxicity can be instrumental in detecting intravascular injection in its earliest stages [1] (Table 27.2).

Once local anesthetic toxicity has been recognized, immediately stopping administration is of utmost importance. It is also crucial to maintain the airway and provide supplemental oxygen to the patient while assessing neurologic and cardiovascular parameters. Treatment of central nervous system toxicity is typically begun with a benzodiazepine (midazolam 0.05–0.1 mg/kg IV) to address any seizure activity. Lipid emulsion (i.e., Intralipid) is also useful in situations where cardiac toxicity is present. The current dosing guidelines recommend starting Intralipid 20% with a bolus of 1.5 mL/kg over 1 min followed by an infusion at

Table 27.2 Recognition of local anesthetic systemic toxicity [28] personal table, based on, modified from Vadi MJ et al. [28]

Recognition of severe toxicity	Immediate management	Circulatory arrest not present	Circulatory arrest present	Follow-up
• Alteration in mental status • Cardiovascular collapse • May occur some time after initial injection	• Call for help • Stop local anesthetic administration • Maintain airway • Confirm/establish IV access • Control seizures • Start IV lipid emulsion	• Conventional therapy for hypotension and arrhythmias • Continue IV lipid emulsion	• Start CPR and ACLS • Continue IV lipid emulsion • Avoid lidocaine for arrhythmia management • Consider cardiopulmonary bypass	• Admission to intensive care unit • Close monitoring until sustained recovery achieved

0.25 mL/kg/min. The bolus dose can be repeated, and the infusion rate doubled should hemodynamic instability persist [6]. Propofol is not an adequate substitute for lipid emulsion but can be used in low doses to treat seizure activity.

Dysrhythmias are managed using advanced cardiac life support modules, but providers must recognize a prolonged effort which may be required to provide enough circulation until the local anesthetic is either redistributed or metabolized. Epinephrine may aggravate some of the arrhythmias; therefore, many sources suggest vasopressin as an alternative agent [7]. The most current guidelines also recommend the use of amiodarone for local anesthetic overdose [8]. The use of lidocaine to treat dysrhythmias is controversial, with studies showing conflicting results. In instances where torsades de pointes develops, overdrive pacing may be required.

27.4 Inadvertent Intrathecal Injection

Migration of an epidural catheter into the subarachnoid space can have catastrophic consequences. While the exact cause of catheter migration into the intrathecal space remains unclear, many hypotheses have been formulated as possible explanations. Current theory suggests that exaggeration of the subatmospheric pressure in the epidural space by movement and respirations can be sufficient to propel the catheter through the dura [9]. The clinical consequences of an inadvertent large dose of local anesthetic into the intrathecal space depend on the amount administered. Symptoms can range from mild numbness in the lower extremities to unconsciousness and respiratory arrest. Spread of the local anesthetic depends on the tonicity of the solution: hypotonic solutions spread to nondependent areas, whereas hypertonic solutions will spread to the dependent areas of the spinal cord. The spread of isotonic solutions depends on the volume and concentration of the local anesthetic administered [10].

Inadvertent intrathecal administration of large doses of local anesthetic or opioids can have devastating consequences if not recognized immediately. The signs and symptoms of total spinal anesthesia result from blockade of the cervical and thoracic segments on the central nervous system as well as hypoperfusion of the medulla. Central nervous system signs can be highly variable and range from an inability to speak to unconsciousness. Often, the pupils are dilated and nonreactive due to blockade of the parasympathetic efferent fibers of the Edinger-Westphal nucleus. Cardiac signs include bradycardia due to blockade of the cardiac accelerator fibers, which have their origins from T1 to T4, as well as hypotension due to the loss of sympathetically mediated vasoconstriction. Typically, the patient's respiratory status will also be compromised from the blockade of the phrenic nerve (C3–C5). Symptoms can range from mild shortness of breath to complete apnea [10].

The most crucial first step in the management of an inadvertent intrathecal injection is early recognition and prevention of additional medication administration into the cerebrospinal fluid. Treatment is primarily supportive and revolves around maintaining a patent airway to provide adequate oxygenation and ventilation. Unconscious or apneic patients should be intubated and will need ventilator support. Hemodynamics is best maintained using a combination of volume expansion and vasopressors until the block begins to resolve.

Many methods have been established to prevent unintentional intrathecal injections. With obvious free-flowing CSF from the epidural needle or the epidural catheter, large doses of local anesthetic should not be administered. However, in many instances, the placement of an epidural catheter into the intrathecal space is not as clear. For example, if a tear is made in the dura during epidural placement, it is possible that CSF will not be seen through the Tuohy needle; however, the tear may be of sufficient size to allow for catheter passage into the intrathecal space. Careful aspiration of the catheter prior to administration of any medication is crucial and can prevent such complications [11].

The use of saline for loss of resistance can also make it difficult to identify inadvertent intrathecal placement of epidural catheters as it is unclear whether the fluid in the epidural needle is CSF or saline. Measurements of pH, temperature, glucose, and turbidity can be used to distinguish CSF from saline, but these tests are of low clinical utility because of the time necessary to obtain results [11].

Epidural test doses can also be useful in detecting intrathecal placement of a catheter. A test dose may consist of 40–60 mg of lidocaine, which would create a low-level sensory block if administered intrathecally. However, in the setting of combined spinal-epidural techniques, the test dose may be enough to create a high or total spinal when combined with the intrathecal dose administered as part of the spinal portion.

27.5 Migration into the Subdural Space

There are many cases of accidental subdural migration of epidural catheters; however, subdural drug deposition remains a poorly understood complication. The clinical presentation can be variable and is often attributed to other causes, such as an inadvertent intrathecal injection or a unilateral or patchy epidural. Most commonly, the block is disproportionate to the amount of medication injected. The motor and sympathetic fibers are typically spared. Additionally, subdural migration of an epidural catheter can lead to block failure in some instances [12].

The subdural space is a potential space between the dura mater and arachnoid mater that contains a small volume of serous fluid [13]. It extends from the cranial vault throughout the distribution of the meninges to the lower border of the second sacral vertebra. The subdural space is largest in the cervical area and narrowest in the lumbar region [14]. The subdural space extends laterally over the dorsal nerve roots and dorsal root ganglia. Because the dura mater and arachnoid mater are attached closely on the ventral root, the potential subdural space is much smaller. Therefore, injections tend to pool in the posterior segment and spare the anterior sympathetic and motor nerve roots [15].

The incidence of subdural catheter migrations is considered to be low. Most of the reported cases of subdural catheter migration have been in obstetric patients receiving neuraxial anesthesia. In one of the larger studies, Jenkins found the incidence of subdural injection to be 1 in 4200 [16]. The most common mechanism implicated is piercing of the dura but not the arachnoid, which expands the potential subdural space. Migration of epidural catheters into the subdural space is more common with prolonged catheterization. The use of a multi-holed epidural catheter can also increase the risk of subdural injections because the catheter can be placed across more than one space [17].

Several factors that can predispose a patient to subdural migration of an epidural catheter have been identified. Migration is more likely with difficult block placement, as excessive manipulations of the epidural needle can lead to a tear in the dura [18]. Additionally, patients who have had prior back surgery are at higher risk of subdural catheter migration due to altered anatomy secondary to scarring and retraction and, possibly, complete destruction of the epidural space [19]. Finally, a recent lumbar puncture increases the likelihood of subdural catheter migration due to the fact that the CSF leak distends the subdural space [20].

The presentation of a subdural block can be quite variable and depends on the spread of local anesthetic, which is a function of the highly variable anatomy of the subdural space. The block will have an onset time that is intermediate between that of an epidural and subarachnoid block. The block will typically last for 2–4 h with complete recovery [21]. The sensory level is disproportionately high for the volume of medication given and can often be patchy. Because of the limited spread to the ventral cord, subdural injections cause less hypotension and motor weakness than inadvertent intrathecal injections. In a few rare instances, permanent nerve damage can occur due to compression of the nerve roots or the radicular arteries causing ischemia [22]. There is also the potential for intracranial spread, which can cause blockade of the brainstem and periods of unconsciousness and apnea.

Diagnosis of subdural blockade can be challenging. Lubenow et al. described two major and three minor criteria that were required for the diagnosis of a subdural block. The major criteria include a negative aspiration test and unexpected extensive sensory block. The minor criteria include delayed onset by 10 min or more of the motor or sensory block, a variable motor block, or a sympathetic block disproportionate to the drug injected. Both major criteria and one minor criterion must be present for the diagnosis of subdural blockade to be made [19].

Various imaging modalities can also be used to detect subdural injections. Because the subdural compartment is considered a potential space, it is not normally seen on x-rays or computerized tomography without contrast media. A subdural injection of contrast will appear as a dense collection confined to the posterior spinal canal with primarily cranial extension. Additionally, subdural contrast media can be differentiated from subarachnoid contrast in the lateral views; the former tends to pool at the site of injection, while the latter ascends rapidly up the spinal canal [23]. Electrical stimulation of the catheter can also be used to detect subdural placement. Because the fluid injected into the subdural space can spread a large distance, there is the potential for a diffuse motor response in multiple segments [24].

Currently, there are no clear guidelines for the management of a subdural catheter. The patient should be monitored closely for high sensory levels and cardiovascular and respiratory compromise. The epidural catheter should be removed and replaced at a different level. If a subarachnoid anesthetic is planned, the anesthetist should anticipate greater cranial spread of local anesthetic because of compression of the intrathecal space from the subdural injection.

27.6 Unilateral or Patchy Anesthesia

Epidural block is a well-established and widely recognized method of providing anesthesia and analgesia. However, inadequate block may result in unsatisfactory results. Inadequate analgesia is not uncommon and can occur in 5–20% of blocks [25]. One explanation for a poor block is incorrect catheter placement. In the most common scenario, if the epidural needle is off midline, the catheter may be inserted into the lateral or anterolateral epidural space, resulting in a unilateral block. Furthermore, trabeculations in the anterior epidural space are quite common and render the potential space discontinuous. Therefore, spread of the drug to the contralateral side depends on retrograde flow around the circumference of the dural space [26].

Many authors have suggested limiting the length of catheter inserted into the epidural space as a way of reducing inadequate blockade. As greater lengths of catheter are inserted, the chances of the epidural catheter entering into the anterolateral epidural space or exiting out a neural foramen increase, resulting in a unilateral block [27]. Most current authors recommend leaving no more than 4 cm of catheter in the epidural space [25]. In cases of unilateral blockade, increasing the volume of anesthetic solution, positioning the patient with the unblocked side down, or withdrawing the catheter can promote bilateral blockade.

The amount of catheter in the epidural space is even more crucial for multi-orificed catheters. Studies have demonstrated that when a multi-holed catheter is used for epidural blockade, the more proximal holes are only 1–1.5 cm in the epidural space. Even a short outward migration of the epidural catheter can lead to an inadequate or patchy block. Therefore, when using a multi-orificed catheter, it is likely prudent to leave an additional 2–3 cm in the epidural space.

Key Points

- Epidural catheter migration is a well-described entity within the field of anesthesiology and can lead to devastating consequences. Hazards of epidural catheter migration include intravascular, subarachnoid, or subdural injection of local anesthetic and a unilateral or failed block.
- Intravascular migration can lead to local anesthetic toxicity, which typically presents with central nervous system and cardiovascular manifestations. Initial treatment consists of discontinuing the local anesthetic infusion, benzodiazepines for seizure prophylaxis, lipid emulsion, and hemodynamic support.
- Intrathecal migration can present with signs and symptoms similar to a "high" or "total" spinal. Treatment is focused on maintaining a patent airway and stable hemodynamics until the local anesthetic is metabolized.
- Subdural injections can have a variable presentation but are usually characterized by a sensory level disproportionate from the amount of medication administered. Patients should be monitored closely for high sensory levels and cardiovascular or respiratory compromise.
- A common cause of a "failed" epidural catheter is migration out of a neural foramen. Leaving no more than 4 cm of catheter in the epidural space can prevent this.

References

1. Weinberg GL. Current concepts in resuscitation of patients with local anesthetic cardiac toxicity. Reg Anesth Pain Med. 2002;27:568–75.
2. Feldman HS. Toxicity of local anesthetic agents. In: Rice SA, Fish KJ, editors. Anesthetic toxicity. New York: Raven Press; 1994.
3. Boren E, Teuber S, Naguwa S, Gershwin M. A critical review of local anesthetic sensitivity. Clin Rev Allergy Immunol. 2007;32(1):119–27.
4. Rutten AJ, Nancarrow C, Mather LE, et al. Hemodynamic and central nervous system effects of intravenous bolus doses of lidocaine, bupivacaine, and ropivacaine in sheep. Anesth Analg. 1989;69:291–9.
5. Tanaka M, Nishikawa T. A comparative study of hemodynamic and T-wave criteria for detecting intravascular injection of the test dose (epinephrine) in sevoflurane-anesthetized adult. Anesth Analg. 1999;89:32–6.
6. Picard J, Meek T. Lipid emulsion to treat overdose of local anesthetic: the gift of the glob. Anaesthesia. 2006;61:107–9.
7. Krismer AC, Hogan QH, Wenzel V, et al. The efficacy of epinephrine or vasopressin for resuscitation during epidural anesthesia. Anesth Analg. 2001;93:734–42.
8. Nolan JP, Deakin CD, Soar J, Böttiger BW, Smith G. European Resuscitation Council Guidelines for Resuscitation 2005. Section 4. Adult advanced life support. Resuscitation. 2005;67(Suppl 1):S39–86.
9. Mourisse J, Gielen MJM, Hasenbos MAWM, Haystraten FMJ. Migration of thoracic epidural catheters: three methods for evaluation of catheter position in thoracic epidural space. Anaesthesia. 1989;44:574–7.
10. Atlee JL. Total spinal anesthesia. In: Complications in anesthesia. Philadelphia: Elsevier/Saunders; 2007. p. 242–43. Print.
11. Atlee JL. Inadvertent intrathecal catheter placement. In: Complications in anesthesia. Philadelphia: Elsevier/Saunders; 2007. p. 242–43. Print.
12. Agarwal D, Mohta M, Tyagi A, Sethi AK. Subdural block and the anaesthetist. Anaesth Intensive Care. 2010;38(1):20–6.
13. Mehta M, Maher R. Injection into the extra-arachnoid subdural space. Experience in the treatment of intractable cervical pain and in the conduct of extradural (epidural) analgesia. Anaesthesia. 1977;32:760–6.
14. Romanes GJ. Cunningham's manual of practical anatomy. 14th ed. Oxford: Oxford University Press; 1986. p. 195–6.
15. Pearson RMG. A rare complication of extradural analgesia. Anaesthesia. 1984;39:460–3.
16. Jenkins JG. Some immediate serious complications of obstetric epidural analgesia and anaesthesia: a prospective study of 145,550 epidurals. Int J Obstet Anesth. 2005;14:37–42.
17. Reynolds F, Speedy HM. The subdural space: the third place to go astray. Anaesthesia. 1990;45:120–3.
18. Asato F, Nakatani K, Matayoshi Y, Katekawa Y, Chinen K. Development of subdural motor blockade. Anaesthesia. 1993;48:46–9.
19. Lubenow T, Keh-Wong E, Kristof K, Ivankovich O, Ivankovich AD. Inadvertent subdural injection: a complication of an epidural block. Anesth Analg. 1988;67:175–9.
20. Stevens RA, Stanton-Hicks MA. Subdural injection of local anesthetic: a complication of epidural anesthesia. Anesthesiology. 1985;63:323–6.
21. Collier C. Total spinal or massive subdural block. Anaesth Intensive Care. 1982;10:92–3.
22. McMenemin IM, Sissons GR, Brownridge P. Accidental subdural catheterization: radiological evidence of a possible mechanism for spinal cord damage. Br J Anaesth. 1992;69:417–9.
23. Ralph CJ, Williams MP. Subdural or epidural? Confirmation with magnetic resonance imaging. Anaesthesia. 1996;51:175–7.

24. Tsui BC, Gupta S, Emery D, Finucane B. Detection of subdural placement of epidural catheter using nerve stimulation. Can J Anaesth. 2000;47:471–3.
25. Hood DD. Obstetric anesthesia: complication and problems. In: Kirby RR, Brown DL, editors. Problems in anesthesia. Obstetric anesthesia, Hood DD (Guest ED); 1989. Vol. 3. p. 1–18.
26. Usubiaga JE, Dos Reis A, Usubiaga LE. Epidural misplacement of catheters and mechanisms of unilateral blockade. Anesthesiology. 1970;32:158–61.
27. Sanchez R, Acuna L, Rocha F. An analysis of the radiological visualization of the catheters placed in the epidural space. Br J Anaesth. 1967;39:485–9.
28. Vadi MJ, Patel N, Stiegler MP. Local anesthetic systemic toxicity after combined psoas compartment–sciatic nerve block: analysis of decision factors and diagnostic delay. Anesthesiology. 2014;120(04):987–96.

Complications Related to Intrathecal Pump Catheter Infection

28

Rena Beckerly

28.1 Case Description

A 41-year-old male presents to the emergency department with nausea, vomiting, and abdominal pain. Extensive work-up revealed a mass in his lower esophagus which was biopsied and found to be metastatic esophageal cancer. During his admission, the palliative care team was consulted and designed a pain regimen which included morphine ER 60 mg BID, fentanyl patch 300 mcq every 3 days, and morphine IR 10 mg q24 h. He reported adequate pain control (VAS 5/10) with these medications and was discharged home with plans for chemotherapy and radiation as an outpatient.

A month later, he presents to the ED with severe, intractable pain. His work-up revealed increasing tumor burden despite chemotherapy and radiation. The pain service evaluated the patient and attempted to increase his medications. However, the patient became combative, disoriented, and reported severe constipation. The pain service discussed an intrathecal pump placement with the patient and his family. The decision was made to proceed with intrathecal opiate trial. Morphine 0.1 mg single spinal dose injection produced substantial relief of his pain and no side effects. He was considered an excellent candidate for a permanent IT pump.

The patient's preoperative evaluation revealed bilateral pleural effusions and gross abdominal ascites which were stable. His labs showed neutropenia and a platelet count of 98,000. He was scheduled for his next round of chemotherapy in a week. Given the likelihood of worsening neutropenia and thrombocytopenia with chemotherapy, the patient agreed to have the intrathecal pump placed over the next few days. The next day, he was taken to the operating room for the ITP placement under general anesthesia. He tolerated the procedure well, and the infusion was started at 0.5 mg/h intrathecal. He reported excellent pain relief and a pain score of 2/10. He was discharged with seven days of cephalexin 500 mg every 6 h and detailed instructions on wound care.

Three weeks later, the patient presented to the ED with a headache, nuchal rigidity, fevers, chills, vision changes, and mental status changes. A lumbar puncture was performed in the ED which showed elevated protein (100 mg/ml), low glucose (<40 mg/dl), and **gram stain/cultures revealed staphylococcal meningitis**. Upon examining his abdominal intrathecal pump pocket, pus was expressed from the incision. The patient was quickly taken to the OR, and the IT pump was explanted. He was admitted to the intensive care unit where he was treated for sepsis and survived.

28.2 Case Discussion

28.2.1 Catheter-Related Infections

Intrathecal pumps (ITPs) have a reported infection rate of 2.5–9% [1] with the majority of infections occurring at the implantable pump pocket. While we have limited data on exact infection rates, ITPs are made of similar material as pacemakers and are placed along similar operative techniques [1]. The main differences from a pacemaker are that ITP catheter is placed intrathecally and infection of the implant may cause a life-threatening meningitis.

R. Beckerly, M.D.
University of Illinois, Chicago, IL, USA
e-mail: beckerr@uic.edu

M. Anitescu et al. (eds.), *Challenging Cases and Complication Management in Pain Medicine*,
https://doi.org/10.1007/978-3-319-60072-7_28

Fig. 28.1 Cross section of abdominal wall depicting CDC classification of surgical site infection [3]

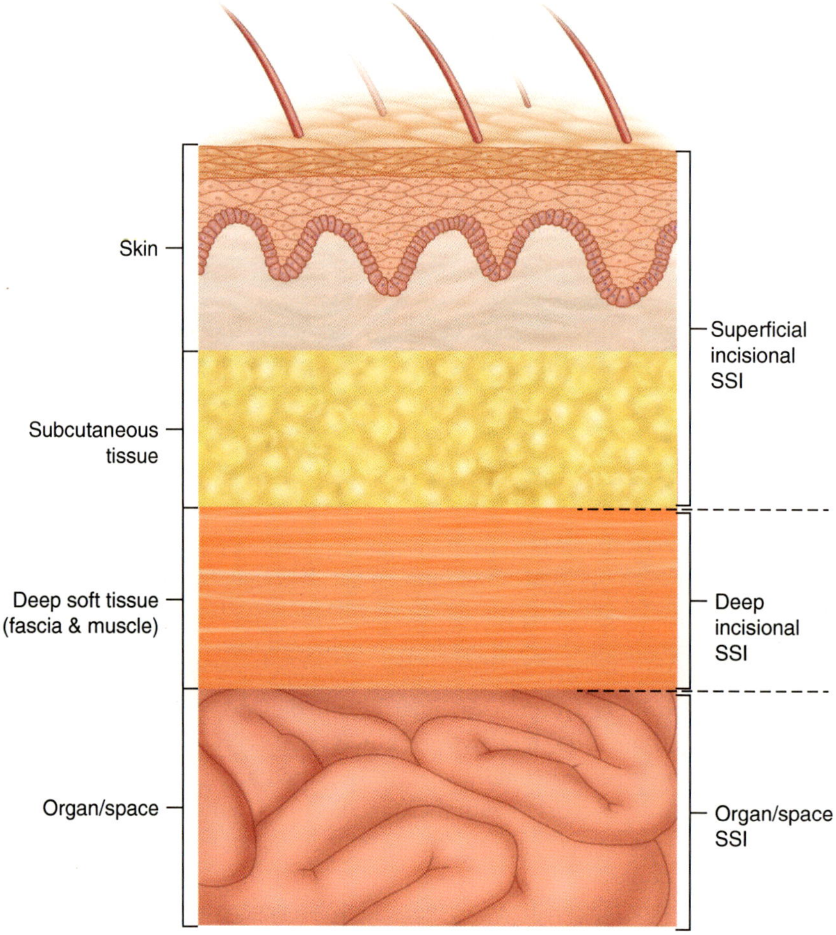

Most ITP infections present within the first 2–6 weeks after implantation. However, Deibert et al. [2] reported a case of delayed surgical site infection for 18 months after placement, where the catheter was tunneled through the abdomen, into the small bowel. The patient presented with progressively worsening tenderness at the pump pocket and mild erythema of the skin. The pump was removed with general surgery assistance. A high index of suspicion must be maintained when ITPs are implanted and monitored.

The Center for Disease Control (CDC) has classified surgical site infections (SSI) into two broad categories: incisional SSI or organ/spaces SSI [3]. The incisional SSI can be either superficial (involving the superficial layers of the skin (skin and subcutaneous tissue)) or deep incisional SSI which involve the deep soft tissue (fascia and muscles) (Fig. 28.1).

Diagnosis of surgical site infections can be very challenging but is crucial in dictating the ultimate treatment regimen. Most ITP infections present with fever, localized tenderness/pain at the site, swelling, purulent discharge, and erythema at the site. More devastating complications of CSF infections present similarly to our patient with fevers, chills, nausea/vomiting, nuchal rigidity, and headache.

A superficial incisional SSI [3] must meet several diagnostic criteria: the infection must occur within 30 days of the procedure and involve the skin or subcutaneous tissue around the incision. Additionally, the patient must present with at least one of the following criteria: purulent drainage from the incision, organisms isolated from an aseptically obtained culture of fluid or tissue from the incision, at least one sign/symptom of an infection (pain or tenderness, localized swelling, redness, or heat—and the incision is deliberately opened by a surgeon—unless the culture is negative), or diagnosis of superficial incisional SSI by a surgeon or attending physician.

Diagnostic criteria for deep incisional SSI include the following signs and symptoms: infection within 30 days of the procedure (or 1 year with an implant) and involvement of the deep soft tissue (fascia/muscle), with an infection that must be related to the procedure. Additionally, the patient must present with at least one of the following

Table 28.1 Diagnostic criteria for superficial site infections (SSI), modified from [3]

Superficial incisional surgical site infections must meet the following two criteria: • Occur within 30 days of the procedure • Involve only the skin or subcutaneous tissue around the incision Plus At least one of the following: • Purulent drainage from the incision • Organisms isolated from aseptically obtained culture of fluid or tissue from the incision • At least one of the following signs or symptoms of infection: pain or tenderness, localized swelling, redness, or heat—and the incision is deliberately opened by the surgeon—unless the culture is negative • Diagnosis of superficial SSI by surgeon or attending physician The following are not considered superficial SSI: • Stitch abscess (minimal inflammation and discharge confined to the points of suture penetration) or infected burn wounds
Deep incisional surgical site infections must meet the following three criteria: • Occur within 30 days of the procedure (*or 1 year in the case of implants*) • Are related to the procedure • Involve deep soft tissues, such as the fascia and muscles Plus At least one of the following criteria: • Purulent drainage from the incision but not from the organ/space of the surgical site • A deep incision spontaneously dehisces or is deliberately opened by a surgeon when the patient has at least one of the following: fever (>38 °), localized pain, or tenderness—unless culture is negative • An abscess or other evidence of infection involving the incision is found on direct examination or histopathologic or radiographical exam • Diagnosis of deep SSI by a surgeon or attending physician
An organ/space SSI must meet the following criterion: • Infection within 30 days after the operation procedure if no implant is left in place or within 1 year if an implant is in place *and* the infection appears to be related to the operative procedure *and* infection involves any part of the body, excluding the skin incision, fascia, or muscle layers, which is opened or manipulated during the operative procedure, *and* patient has at least one of the following: – Purulent drainage from the drain that is placed through a stab wound into the organ/space – Organisms isolated from an aseptically obtained culture of fluid or tissue in the organ/space An abscess or other evidence of infection involving the organ/space that is found on direct examination, during reoperation, or by histopathologic or radiologic

signs: purulent drainage from the incision, a spontaneously dehiscent deep incision (or is deliberately opened by a surgeon when the patient has at least one of the following signs: fever >38 °C, localized pain, or tenderness—unless the culture is negative), evidence of an abscess or other forms of infection involving the incision on direct examination or by histopathologic/radiological examination, or diagnosis of a deep incisional SSI by a surgeon or attending physician. Table 28.1 [3] includes the diagnostic criteria for superficial and deep surgical site infections.

28.3 Pathogenesis

The primary pathogens of SSI for clean procedures are *Staphylococcus aureus* and coagulase-negative staphylococci (*Staphylococcus epidermidis*) [4].

In clean-contaminated procedures, gram-negative rods and enterococci must be accounted for, in addition to skin flora. The CDC is reporting more cases of antimicrobial-resistant pathogens such as methicillin-resistant *S. aureus* (MRSA) [4] or by fungal SSI. MRSA infections are associated with higher mortality rates, longer hospital stays, and higher hospital costs compared with other infections [4]. ITPs are often classified under neurosurgical procedures where the primary infectious pathogen is *Staphylococcus aureus* [4], similar to intraventricular shunts.

The presence of these pathogens in the surgical site depends on several factors: the dose of bacterial contamination, the virulence of the pathogen, and the resistance of the host [3]:

$$\text{Risk of surgical infection} = \frac{\text{Dose of bacterial contamination} \times \text{Virulence}}{\text{Resistance of the host patient}}$$

Patients are considered to be at increased risk of SSI if the surgical site is contaminated with >1,000,000 microorganisms per gram of tissue and no foreign material is implanted (significantly lower quantities can cause a SSI if foreign material is implanted). For most patients, the source of the SSI is their native flora on skin or mucous membranes [3]. However, surgical personnel, operating room environment, instruments, or prosthetics can serve as exogenous sources of microbes.

28.3.1 Preoperative Precautions: Patient Optimization, Skin Preparation Prior to Incision, and Perioperative Antibiotics

28.3.1.1 Identification of Risk Factors for SSI

Patients with diabetes, nicotine use, chronic steroid use, malnutrition, prolonged preoperative hospital stay, preoperative colonization with *Staphylococcus aureus*, immunocompromised states (HIV, chemotherapy), and perioperative transfusion are considered to be at a higher risk for SSI (Table 28.2) [3].

Table 28.2 Selected risk factor and recommendations to prevent surgical site infections (SSI), modified from [17]

Risk factor	Recommendation	Quality of evidence
Intrinsic, patient related (preoperative)		
Unmodifiable		
Age	No formal recommendation to increase risk of SSI may be secondary to comorbidities or immune-senescence	NA
History of radiation	No formal recommendation. Prior irradiation at surgical site increases the risk of SSI, likely due to tissue damage and wound ischemia	NA
History of skin/soft infection	No formal recommendation. History of prior skin infection may be a marker for inherent in host immune function	
Modifiable		
Glucose control	Control serum blood glucose levels for all surgical patients, including patients without diabetes. For patients with diabetes, reduce glycosylated HA1c to less than 7% before surgery if possible	Category I
Obesity	Increase dosing of prophylactic antimicrobial agent for morbidly obese patients	Category I
Smoking cessation	Encourage smoking cessation within 30 days of the procedure	Category III
Immunosuppressive meds, hypoalbuminemia	No formal recommendation. Although noted risk factor does not delay surgery for use of TPN	NA
Extrinsic, procedure related (perioperative)		
Preparation of patient		
Hair removal	Do not remove unless hair will interfere with the operation. If hair removal is necessary, remove outside the OR by clipping. Do not use razor	Category II
Preoperative infections	Identify and treat infections (e.g., urinary tract infections) remote to the surgical site prior to elective surgery. Do not routinely treat colonization or contamination	Category II
Operative characteristics		
Surgical scrub (surgical team hands/forearm)	Use appropriate antiseptic agent to perform preoperative surgical scrub. For most products, scrub the hands and forearm for 2–5 min	Category I

Table 28.2 (continued)

Risk factor	Recommendation	Quality of evidence
Skin preparation	Wash and clean skin incision site. Use a dual agent skin preparation containing alcohol, unless contraindications exist	Category I
Antimicrobial prophylaxis timing	Administer only when indicated	Category I
Blood transfusions	Blood transfusions increase the risk of SSI by decreasing macrophage function. Reduce blood loss and need for blood transfusion to greatest extent possible	Category II
Duration of prophylaxis	Stop agents within 24 h after the procedure for all procedures	Category II
Surgeon skill/technique	Handle tissue carefully and eradicate dead space	Category III
Asepsis	Adhere to standard principles of OR sepsis	Category III
Operative time	No formal recommendation in most recent guidelines. Minimize as much as possible without sacrificing surgical technique and aseptic practice	Category I
Appropriate gloving	All members of the operative team should double glove and change gloves when perforation is noted	Category III
Choice of prophylactic agent	Select appropriate agents on the basis of surgical procedure, most common pathogens causing SSI for a specific procedure and published recommendations	Category I
OR characteristics		
Ventilation	Follow American Institute of Architects recommendations of proper air handling in OR	Category III
Traffic	Minimize OR traffic	Category III
Environmental surfaces	Use an EPA-approved hospital disinfectant to clean visibly soiled or contaminated surfaces and equipment	Category III
Sterilization of surgical equipment	Sterilize all surgical equipment according to published guidelines. Minimize the use of immediate-use steam sterilization	Category II

Diabetics need strict glucose control, with HbA1c less than 8 within 30 days of the trial. Nicotine use affects wound healing and should be discontinued at least 30 days prior to surgery. Patients with poor nutritional status, as exemplified by poor caloric intake, poor protein rich diets, and low albumin levels, will also increase the risk of site infections [2]. Some studies have correlated chronic steroid use (as in Crohn's patient) with an increased risk of SSI (12.5% infection in patients using steroids vs. 6.7% in patients who are not on chronic steroid use) [3]. Patients at risk for MRSA colonization should have a preoperative nasal swab and be treated appropriately in the perioperative period.

28.4 Skin Preparation Prior to Incision

Many interventions have been implemented to minimize the occurrence of SSI. Some surgeons require patients to shower with antiseptic solution to reduce the skin microbial counts prior to surgery. Two antiseptic agents are available: chlorhexidine (reduce colony counts ninefold) and povidone-iodine (reduce colony counts 1.3–1.9-fold). However, while the flora counts have been reduced, no studies have shown to reduce SSI rates [5].

Higher rates of SSI have been reported with preoperative shaving which can create cuts in the skin and can serve as foci for bacterial colonization. A study by Seropian et al. [6] reported a 5% increase in SSI in patients who had shaved prior to surgery when compared to those who did not have hair removed. Shaving immediately before the procedure was associated with a 3% SSI rate. Ultimately, any form of hair removal has been associated with increased risk of SSI. The current recommendation is the use of electrical clippers immediately prior to incision and ideally in the preoperative waiting area (prior to entering the operating room).

Many skin preparations are available in the operating room including iodophors, alcohol-containing products, and chlorhexidine gluconate. Alcohol-containing products are ideal as they are inexpensive, readily available, and rapid-acting skin antiseptic and have germicidal effects on bacteria, fungi, viruses, and spores. However, the flammability of the solution creates a hazard in the operating room. Chlorhexidine and iodophors have extensive antimicrobial activity, but chlorhexidine has shown greater reduction in hand flora when used for preoperative surgical scrub [7]. Curiously, iodophors are deactivated by blood or serum proteins, whereas chlorhexidine is not. Ideally, a 2–5 min surgical scrub is recommended. Table 28.3 [3] compares the effectiveness of different surgical scrubs.

Table 28.3 Mechanism and spectrum of activity of antiseptic agents commonly used for preoperative skin preparation and surgical scrub, modified from [3]

Agent	Alcohol	Chlorhexidine	Iodine/iodophors	Para-chloro-meta-xylenol (PCMX)	Triclosan
Mechanism of action	Denature proteins	Disrupt cell membrane	Oxidation/substitution	Disrupt cell wall	Disrupt cell wall
Gram-positive bacteria	Excellent	Excellent	Excellent	Good	Good
Gram-negative bacteria	Excellent	Good	Good	Fair except for *Pseudomonas* spp.	Good
Mycobacterium tuberculosis	Good	Poor	Good	Fair	Good
Fungi	Good	Fair	Good	Fair	Poor
Virus	Good	Good	Good	Fair	Unknown
Rapidity of action	Most rapid	Intermediate	Intermediate	Intermediate	Intermediate
Residual activity	None	Excellent	Minimal	Good	Excellent
Toxicity	Drying, volatile	Ototoxicity, keratitis	Skin absorption with possible toxicity, skin irritation	More data needed	More data needed
Uses	Skin prep, surgical scrub	Skin prep, surgical scrub	Skin prep, surgical scrub	Surgical scrub	Surgical scrub

28.5 Perioperative Antibiotics

Prophylactic antibiotics are intended to decrease the microbial burden of intraoperative contamination to a level that the host can handle. The goal is not to sterilize the tissue. In order for prophylactic antibiotics to be effective, they must be timed appropriately so that the bactericidal concentration of the drug is established in the blood and tissue prior to incision. This therapeutic level must be maintained throughout the surgery and for a few hours after the incision is closed. The choice of antibiotic is based on the classification of the surgical wound. For example, a clean wound would require a different antibiotic regimen than an anticipated clean-contaminated wound. Usually, antibiotics are indicated for surgeries where the abdomen is entered. However, if a prosthetic is to be implanted or the consequences of infection are fatal (such as with any neurosurgical operation), prophylactic antibiotics are indicated. Follett et al. [1] surveyed the literature pertaining to infections in patients undergoing ITP and found Category 1A evidence supporting antimicrobial prophylaxis.

Cephalosporins are the antibiotic class of choice as they are effective against many gram-positive and gram-negative microbes [3]. Additionally, they have proven safety and reasonable pharmacokinetics and are cost-effective. Cefazolin is the antibiotic of choice for clean and most clean-contaminated procedures. Clindamycin can be substitutes in cases of allergies. However, if the distal intestinal tract is involved, then anaerobic coverage is necessary. Vancomycin should be reserved for patients with MRSA positive preoperative, a history of surgical site infection, a prolonged hospitalization, or living in a nursing home. The 2013 American Society of Health-System Pharmacists (ASHP) [4], in conjunction with the Surgical Infection Society, recommends cefazolin for either elective craniotomy, CSF shunting procedures, or IT pump implantation. Vancomycin and clindamycin are recommended as alternatives. This represents Class A recommendation (level I–III evidence) for elective craniotomy and CSF shunting procedures. However, it is Class C recommendation (based on expert opinion) for IT pump implantation [4].

The dose and timing of the antibiotics are critical for maximized effect. Based on Surgical Site Infection Guidelines, cefazolin would be administered within 30 min of incision [2]. However, the ASHP report [4] recommends preoperative antibiotic dosing 1 h prior to incision. Other agents such as fluoroquinolones and vancomycin should be administered within 120 min of incision [4]. The therapeutic level of the antibiotics must exceed that necessary for a targeted pathogen in vitro and must be maintained for prolonged surgery; therefore, repeat doses may be required every 3–4 h. Larger doses are required for obese patients as obesity is a risk factor for surgical site infections [4].

The current guidelines for preoperative antibiotics are weight based. Cefazolin should be given 60 min prior to incision at a dose of 2 (or 3) grams intravenously for patients weighing less (or more) than 120 kg. The antibiotic should be re-dosed after 4 h. Re-dosing of antibiotics is necessary if the duration of the procedure exceeds two half-lives of the drug [4]. If the patient has an allergy to cefazolin, clindamycin 900 mg should be administered 60 min prior to incision and re-dosed in 6 h. Vancomycin 15 mg/kg should be administered 2 h prior to incision in patients with a history of SSI, prolonged hospitalization within 1 year, nursing home resident, or MRSA positive (Table 28.4) [3, 4].

New recommendations are provided for the shortened postoperative course of antimicrobials including a single dose or continuation for less than 24 h. However, these recommendations are controversial, and infection disease experts may need to be consulted. Table 28.4 reviews the recommended doses and re-dosing intervals for commonly used antimicrobials for surgical prophylaxis [4].

28.6 Intraoperative Precautions

A laminar flow, restricted access operating room should be used to implant ITPs. It is not acceptable to do this procedure in any other setting, including the pain office [8]. Operating room air can be contaminated with microbial laden dust, lint, skin squames, and respiratory drops. The level of contamination is directly related to the number of people moving around within the room [9]. Every effort should be made to minimize movement into and out of the operating room. Ventilation within the operating rooms must be in compliance with current standards.

Excellent surgical technique is critical to minimizing surgical site infections. Techniques such as maintaining effective hemostasis while preserving tissue perfusion, maintaining normothermia, gentle tissue handling, avoiding hallow viscus, removing devitalized (necrotic/charred) tissue, using drains/suture material appropriately, eliminating dead space, and appropriate wound care are essential [3]. Category II evidence exists for use of aseptic surgical techniques (2–5 min skin prep, double gloving, minimal-touch technique) [1]. High-volume irrigation has been shown to reduce the risk of SSI [10]. Special attention should be paid to wound closure to promote adequate healing and prevention of dehiscence [8]. Postoperative abdominal binder may allow for tissue compression and reduce the risk of postoperative fluid collection or seroma.

Table 28.4 Recommended dose and re-dosing intervals for commonly used antimicrobials for surgical prophylaxis, modified from [4]

Recommended dose			Half-life in adults with normal renal function, hours	Recommended re-dosing interval (from initiation of preoperative dose) h[c]
Antimicrobial	Adults[a]	Pediatrics[b]		
Ampicillin-sulbactam	3 g (ampicillin 2 g/ sulbactam 1 g)	50 mg/kg of ampicillin component	0.8–1.3	2
Ampicillin	2 g	50 mg/kg	1–1.9	2
Aztreonam	2 g	30 mg/kg	1.3–2.4	4
Cefazolin	2 g, 3 g for weight > 120 kg	30 mg/kg	1.2–2.2	4
Cefuroxime	1.5 g	50 mg/kg	1–2	4
Cefotaxime	1 g	50 mg/kg	0.9–1.7	3
Cefoxitin	2 g	40 mg/kg	0.7–1.1	2
Ceftriaxone	2 g	50–75 mg/kg	5.4–10.9	NA
Cefotetan	2 g	40 mg/kg	2.8–4.6	6
Ciprofloxacin	400 mg	10 mg/kg	2–4	NA
Clindamycin	900 mg	10 mg/kg	2–4	6
Ertapenen	1 g	15 mg/kg	3–5	NA
Fluconazole	400 mg	6 mg/kg	30	NA
Gentamicin[d]	5 mg/kg based on dosing weight(single dose)	2.5 mg/kg based on dosing weight	2–3	NA
Levofloxacin	500 mg[e]	10 mg/kg	6–8	NA
Metronidazole	500 mg	15 g/kg; neonates weighing <1200 g should receive single dose 7.5 mg/kg	6–8	NA
Moxifloxacin	400 mg	10 mg/kg	8–15	NA
Piperacillin-tazobactam	3.375	Infants 2–9 months: 80 mg/kg piperacillin component Children >9 months and <40 kg: 100 mg/kg of piperacillin component	0.7–1.2	2
Vancomycin	15 mg/kg	15 mg/kg	4–8	NA
Oral antibiotics for colorectal surgery prophylaxis (used in conjunction with a mechanical bowel preparation)				
Erythromycin base	1 g	20 mg/kg	0.8–3	NA
Metronidazole	1 g	15 mg/kg	6–10	NA
Neomycin	1 g	15 mg/kg	2–3 (3% absorbed under normal gastrointestinal conditions)	NA

[a]Adult studies obtained from studies cited. When doses cited differ, the value is based on expert opinion
[b]Maximum pediatric dose should not exceed adult dose
[c]For antimicrobials with short half-life (e.g., cefazolin), before long procedures, re-dosing in the operating room is recommended at two times the half-life of the agent in patients with normal renal function
[d]In general, the use of gentamycin for surgical prophylaxis should be limited to single dose given preoperatively, based on patient's ideal body weight. If the body weight is more than 20% ideal body weight (IDB), then the dose can be calculated using the dosing weight (DW) and the formula: DW = IBW + 0.4 × (actual weight–IBW)
[e]Although the use of fluoroquinolones was associated with tendon rupture/tendonitis in all ages, they are considered generally safe

28.7 Postoperative Treatment

The majority of SSI are superficial and require local wound care, a course of antibiotics, and close monitoring. The dressings should be removed under sterile conditions, and the wound should be evaluated. Culture and sensitivities should be sent prior to wound exploration. It may be helpful to consult infectious disease or wound care for further management. However, deep incisional/organ space infections are more serious and may require inpatient admission. The wound should be explored in the operating room, and the entire ITP must be removed along with the catheter. Cultures, gram stain, and sensitivities should be sent prior to antibiotic administration in the operating room. Additionally, the ITP catheter tip should be sent for cultures, gram stain, and sensitivity. Copious irrigation of the wound is required, and a surgical Penrose drain may help minimize seroma or abscess formation [11]. Infectious disease consultation and wound care assistance are strongly recommended. Antibiotic regimen usually involves vancomycin or meropenem depending on culture and sensitivities. Luckily, the incidence of catheter-related infections with subsequent CSF infection/meningitis is exceedingly rare and would require immediate explanation of the ITP system.

In 2014, Malheiro et al. [12] performed a retrospective analysis of 145 patients (216 pumps—some required revisions) with ITP for either spasticity or analgesia. They reported at 8.71% infection rate (19/216 pumps). Sixteen of the nineteen pumps infected were originally placed for spasticity, while three were placed for analgesia. It is possible that patients requiring baclofen pumps are more susceptible to infections as they may be bedridden and harbor more infections (chronic UTIs or compression ulcers, etc.). More than half the patients (10/19) presented with early infection defined as less than 3 months. The majority of the infections involved the pump reservoir site (14/19) and presented with a median time for occurrence of 3.2 months. Ten of the patients presented with a wound exudate. Common pathogens included MRSA, coagulase-negative staphylococci, and *Pseudomonas aeruginosa*. Ten of the patients were treated with local wound care, while eight required explantation of the entire system.

There were five cases of meningitis reported (2.3%) with the median time to meningitis development of 2.2 months. In all cases, the entire ITP system was removed, and cultures were sent from the catheter tip, pump, and blood. All five patients had positive tip and pump pocket cultures, but only two had positive blood cultures (*S. capitis*, *E. coli*, and *P. mirabilis*). Only one patient had positive CSF cultures (*S. epidermidis*). One patient died from meningitis and sepsis. The other four patients recovered without residual deficits for 1 year. The choice of antibiotics depended on sensitivities and involved vancomycin for 7–21 days along with meropenem or cefepime. Seventy-five percent of the patients were followed for over 12 months after the diagnosed infection.

There are a few case reports of ITP salvage techniques despite meningitis. Zed et al. [13] reported a case of a 19-year-old male with severe spasticity requiring a baclofen ITP. One month later, he presented with fevers/irritability and diagnosed with *S. epidermidis* meningitis (sensitive to vancomycin) per CSF culture and gram stain. He was immediately started on vancomycin 500 mg IV every 12 h without significant improvement of his symptoms. CSF levels of vancomycin IV were not detectable despite doubling the dose of vancomycin. Given the severity of his spasticity and fear of baclofen withdrawal syndrome, every effort was made to salvage the ITP. Baclofen withdrawal syndrome can present with high fever, altered mental status, exaggerated rebound spasticity, and muscle rigidity. Advanced cases can result in rhabdomyolysis, multisystem organ failure, and death. The decision was made to infuse a mixture of vancomycin and baclofen through the ITP.

The team conducted an in vitro analysis for physical compatibility of vancomycin and baclofen. An 18 cc mix of vancomycin 90 mg, baclofen 3330 μg, and 9.5 mL NS (final concentration of vancomycin 5 mg/mL and baclofen 185 μg/mL) set to infuse at 1 mL per 24 h was started. The patient became afebrile 3 days later. Additionally, Dr. Zed's group reported CSF vancomycin concentrations 40 times more than the minimal inhibitory concentration for the organisms with intrathecal infusion of the drug. Bennett et al. [14] reported a similar case report of an 18-year-old male with cerebral palsy who received a baclofen pump, complicated by staphylococcal meningitis. Despite several different intravenous antibiotics, his symptoms persisted until vancomycin 50 mg/mL at a continuous infusion of 5 mg/day was administered through the intrathecal catheter via the ITP. The patient's fever decreased after 2 days of treatment. While these case reports had successful treatment plans, there is limited data to support ITP salvage techniques in the setting of meningitis.

ITP infections may occur years after implantation and involve medication refills where there is direct skin trauma/introduction of contaminated refill. Strict antiseptic technique is required with all pump manipulation. Malheiro et al. [11] reported challenges in quantifying infection rates related to pump refills.

In 2013, Engle et al. [15] conducted a retrospective review of infection rates associated with ITP and spinal cord stimulator systems at MD Anderson in Texas. Of the 142 implants, 83 were ITPs, and 80% of the patients had cancer. They calculated an overall infection rate of 2.4% with ITP, all the infections occurring at the pocket/pump reservoir site. Overall, they reported an infection rate of 3.3% in noncancer patients and 2.7% rate for cancer patients. These rates were similar to other tertiary care facilities with similar volumes (1.7–4.5%). They concluded that cancer did *not* increase the risk of infections. Additionally, they did find an association with prolonged operative time and infection risk (215 ± 93 min vs. 132 ± 52 min—mean duration 83 min longer). They concluded that there is no increased risk of infections in cancer patients, as previously believed.

Overall, there are limited evidence-based data to help clinicians reduce infection rates for ITP procedures. Provenzano et al. [16] conducted a 15-question survey on perioperative infection control practices related to defined CDC, NICE, and SCIP evidence-based infection control (preoperative, intraoperative, postoperative stages) for spinal cord stimulator implant. Five hundred six physicians responded to the survey and revealed low compliance rates for CDC, NICE, and SCIP infection control practice recommendations. Only four of the fifteen questions revealed >80% compliance. The study revealed gaps in knowledge for perioperative infection control and identified areas of improvement: weight-based antibiotic dosing, hair removal strategies, double gloving, surgical dressing, skin antiseptic agents, and postoperative antibiotic continuation.

Key Concepts

- Patient selection and optimization are critical in minimizing the risk of surgical site infections. Patients with diabetes, nicotine use, chronic steroid use, malnutrition, prolonged preoperative hospital stay, preoperative colonization with *Staphylococcus aureus*, immunocompromised states (HIV, chemotherapy), and perioperative transfusion are considered to be at a higher risk for SSI. Patients should be optimized, as best as possible, prior to surgery. Additionally, they should be informed that they are at an increased risk for an infection.
- Strict sterile surgical techniques can minimize infection rates. Chlorhexidine surgical skin prep (2–5 min), double gloving, minimal touch technique, minimizing operative time, preoperative electrical clipper removal, and limiting traffic through the operating room can reduce infection rates. Special attention must be paid to wound irrigation, strict hemostasis, removal of charred/necrosed tissue, and use of wound occlusive dressing.
- Category IA evidence exists for preoperative antibiotics in ITP placement, as the consequences of an infection can be life-threatening. Weight-based antibiotic administration with cefazolin, clindamycin, or vancomycin within 60–120 min of incision is strongly recommended.
- Patients must be educated on appropriate wound care, especially if they are at an increased risk of wound infection. Additionally, they must be informed of the signs and symptoms of an infection: fever, chills, neck rigidity, and pain at incision sites. Wound occlusive dressings should be changed after 24–48 h (under sterile technique- sterile gloves/gauze). Usually, patients are sent home with 5–7 days of antibiotics and close postoperative follow-up. Consider an abdominal binder to minimize space for seroma/fluid collection.
- If a superficial infection occurs, the incision should be evaluated under sterile conditions. Wound culture and sensitivity should be sent. The wound should be cleaned and redressed under sterile conditions. Close patient monitoring is essential, and infectious disease consultation may be helpful.
- If a deep infection is suspected, the ITP may need to be removed. CBC, ESR, CRP, and blood cultures should be sent. The operating room should be notified, and the wound should be explored in the operating room. If the infection truly involves the deep structures, then the entire ITP needs to be removed and the patient admitted for intravenous antibiotics/observation. Wound culture, gram stain, and sensitivities should be obtained prior to intraoperative antibiotics. Additionally, ITP catheter tip should be sent for culture, gram stain, and sensitivity. Infectious disease, neurosurgical, or wound care consultations may be required. Additionally, MRI may be necessary depending on the patient's symptoms. The patient should be monitored closely for signs of meningitis or epidural abscess.

References

1. Follett K, Boortz-Marx R, Drake J. Prevention and management of intrathecal drug delivery and spinal cord stimulation system infections. Anesthesiology. 2004;100:1582–94.
2. Deibert C, Gandhoke G, Forsythe R, Moossy J. Surgical site infection 18 months following intrathecal pump placement secondary to an asymptomatic bowel injury. Pain Pract. 2015;15(7):E69–71.
3. Mangram AJ, Horan TC, Pearson ML, Silver LC, Jarvis WR. Guideline for prevention of surgical site infection, 1999. The hospital Infection Control Practices Advisory Committee. National Center for Infection Diseases. Centers for Disease Control and Prevention. Public Health Service. U.S department of health and Human Service. 1999.
4. Bratzler DW, Dellinger EP, Olsen KM, Perl TM, Auwaerter PG, Bolon MK, Fish DN, Napolitano LM, Sawyer RG, Slain D, Steinber JP, Weinstein RA. Clinical practice guidelines for antimicrobial prophylaxis in surgery. Am J Health-Syst Pharm. 2013;70:1995–283.
5. Garabaldi RA. Prevention of intraoperative wound contamination with chlorhexidine shower and scrub. J Hosp Infect. 1988;11:5–9.
6. Seropian R, Reynold BM. Wound infections after preoperative depilatory versus razor preparation. Am J Surg. 1971;121:251–4.
7. Darouiche RO, Wall MW, Itani KMF, Otterson MF, Webb AL, Carrick MM, Miller HJ, Awad SS, Crosby CT, Mosier MC, Alsharif A, Berger DH. Chlorhexidine-alcohol versus povidone-iodine for surgical-site antisepsis. N Engl J Med. 2010;362:18–26.
8. Deer TR, Mekhail N, Provenzano D, Pope J, Krames E, Thomson S, Raso L, Burton A, De Andres J, Buchser E, Buvanendran A, Liem L, Kumar K, Rizvi S, Feler C, Abejon D, Anderson J, Eldabe S, Kim P, Leong M, Hayek S, McDowell G, Poree L, Brooks E, McJunkin T, Lynch P, Kapural L, Foreman RD, Caraway D, Alo K, Narouze S, Levy RM, North R. The appropriate use of neurostimulation: avoidance and treatment of complications of neurostimulation therapies for the treatment for chronic pain. Neuromodulation. 2014;17:571–98.
9. Ayliffe GA. Role of the environment of the operating suite in surgical wound infection. Rev Infect Dis. 1991;213:1189–91.
10. Dipaola CP, Saravannja DD, Boriani L, et al. Postoperative infection treatment score for the spine (PITSS): construction and validation of a predictive model to define need for single versus multiple irrigation and debridement for spinal surgical site infection. Spine J. 2012;12:218–30.
11. Prager J, Deer T, Levy R, Bruel B, Buchser E, Caraway D, Cousins M, Jacobs M, McGlothen G, Rauck R, Staats P, Steans L. Best practices for intrathecal drug delivery for pain. Neuromodulation. 2014;17:354–72.
12. Malheiro L, Gomes A, Barbosa P, Santos L, Sarmento A. Infectious complications of intrathecal drug administration systems for spasticity and chronic pain: 145 patients from a tertiary care center. Neuromodulation. 2015;18:421–7.
13. Zed PJ, Stiver HG, Devonshire V, Jewesson PJ, Marra F. Continuous intrathecal pump infusion of baclofen with antibiotic

drugs for treatment of pump-associated meningitis. J Neurosurg. 2000;92(2):347–9.
14. Bennett MI, Tai YMA, Symonds JM. Staphylococcal meningitis following synchromed intrathecal pump implant: a case report. Pain. 1994;56:243–4.
15. Engle M, Vinh B, Harun N, Koyyalagunta D. Infectious complications related to intrathecal drug delivery system and spinal cord stimulator system implantation at a comprehensive cancer pain center. Pain Med. 2013;16:251–7.
16. Provenzano DA, Deer T, Phelps AL, Drennen ZC, Thomson S, Hayek SM, Narouze S, Rana MV, Watson TW, Buvanendran A. An interventional survey to understand infection control practices of spinal cord stimulation. Neuromodulation. 2016;19:71–84.
17. Anderson DJ, Kaye KS, Classen D, Arias KM, Podgorny K, Burstin H, Calfee DP, Coffin SE, Dubberke ER, Fraser V, Gerding DN, Griffin FA, Gross P, Klompas M, Lo E, Marschall J, Mermel LA, Nicolle L, Pegues DA, Per TM, Saint S, Salgado CD, Weinstein RA, Wise R, Yokoe DS. Strategies to prevent surgical site infections in acute care hospitals. Infect Control Hosp Epidemiol. 2008;29(suppl 1):S51–S61.

Intrathecal Pump Malfunction: Flipped, Expired, Stalled, and Malfunctioned Valves and Rotors Leading to Under- and Over-Infusion

29

Kristen Noon, Lawrence R. Poree, Kenneth Ike, and R. Carter W. Jones III

29.1 Case Description

A 55-year-old female with a past medical history of chronic low back pain secondary to failed back surgery syndrome treated for 4 years with intrathecal drug delivery on a stable dose of morphine 15 mg/ml, baclofen 600 µg/ml, bupivacaine 20 mg/ml, clonidine 225 µg/ml, and fentanyl 400 µg/ml delivered at a dose of morphine 6.5 mg/day with a personal therapy manager (PTM) dose of morphine 0.65 mg q3 h lock out via Medtronic SynchroMed® II intrathecal pump (ITP) presented to the emergency department (ED) 4 h after she heard a "double beep" alarm coming from her pump. The patient also noted an acute increase in diffuse back pain. The patient called a company representative who advised her that the alarm was likely due to ITP failure and that she should proceed directly to the ED. In the ED, she rated her back pain as "10/10" and described clinical symptoms of weakness and feeling "miserable." The patient denied fever, chills, nausea, vomiting, abdominal pain, seizures, or paresthesias. She also denied any recent falls or trauma.

On physical exam, her vital signs were stable except for a respiratory rate of 24. She appeared visibly uncomfortable. Her pupils were 5–6 mm bilaterally and reactive to light. Her mucous membranes were noted to be very dry and tacky without clear lesions or exudate. Her intrathecal pump was easily palpated in the left abdomen and was non-tender to palpation, and the overlying skin was clean, dry, and intact. Her lumbar spine was tender to palpation without focal findings. Her neurologic and psychiatric exam were normal, including normal mentation, speech, gait, affect, and behavior. While in the ED, IV hydration was initiated along with pain control and anxiolysis with IV hydromorphone, clonidine, and lorazepam. The on-call pain physician was contacted by the ED and arrived soon thereafter.

The last ITP interrogation and refill 1 month prior revealed no alarms and no discrepancies in predicted and actual fluid volume remaining in the pump reservoir. Her next refill was not due for another 2 weeks, and no changes were made to her medications or pump at the refill visit. When the ITP was interrogated in the ED, it was found to be in "safe mode" and delivering a trivial amount of medication at the pump's minimal rate. The ITP was reprogrammed at doses identical to those from the last refill and was confirmed to be functioning properly after reprogramming. The pain physician advised the ED to monitor the patient for a short time prior to discharging her home. The pain physician also advised the patient to call immediately and to return to the ED if she were to hear the critical alarm again or sense any change in pain control or mental status. The patient was discharged home 2 h later.

Five hours later, the patient returned to the ED complaining of increasing back pain. She noted that she initially felt better when her pump was reprogrammed but then developed the same severe back pain that she felt before the reprogramming. Interrogation of the ITP revealed that it was again in "safe mode" and had effectively ceased delivery of medication.

The patient was subsequently admitted to the hospital and started on morphine IR 30 mg po q 3 h prn pain, baclofen 20 mg po tid, and clonidine 0.1 mg po bid due to concern for acute withdrawal from intrathecal medications. Over the next 24 h, the patient complained of anxiety and itching in her upper and lower extremities.

K. Noon, M.D. • R.C.W. Jones III, M.D., Ph.D (✉)
Department of Anesthesiology, Center for Pain Medicine, University of California San Diego, San Diego, CA, USA
e-mail: c0jones@ucsd.edu

L.R. Poree, M.D., M.P.H., Ph.D.
Department of Anesthesia and Perioperative Care, Division of Pain Medicine, University of California San Francisco, San Francisco, CA, USA
e-mail: Lawrence.Poree@ucsf.edu

K. Ike, M.D.
Department of Anesthesiology, Stanford University School of Medicine, Stanford, CA, USA
e-mail: kennethikemd@gmail.com

M. Anitescu et al. (eds.), *Challenging Cases and Complication Management in Pain Medicine*,
https://doi.org/10.1007/978-3-319-60072-7_29

Her vital signs remained stable, and she did not develop acute neurologic compromise. On the second day after admission, her ITP was explanted, and a new Medtronic SynchroMed II pump was implanted using the previous IT catheter. The medications from the previous ITP were put into the new ITP, and the pump was reprogrammed with the original settings. Oral baclofen, morphine, and clonidine were stopped in the immediate postoperative period as the ITP was now functional. The patient was monitored for 24 h and subsequently discharged home with excellent pain relief.

29.2 Case Discussion

This case brings to light several important points regarding the management of intrathecal pump stall. First, this patient heard a "double beep" alarm indicating ITP failure. For Medtronic intrathecal pumps, a pump failure alarm sounds differently than a normal, non-emergent alarm. Traditionally, the pump failure alarm will sound every hour but can be programmed to sound as often as every 10 min if desired by the physician. The patient should be counseled to remain vigilant regarding an alarming pump. Patients should be instructed to contact their device representative as well as their pain physician in the event of an ITP alarm.

Second, this patient's Medtronic SynchroMed II intrathecal pump was in "safe mode" when it was interrogated by her pain physician. This means that the pump sensed that there could be an internal problem with delivering the correct dose of intrathecal medication. In "safe mode," a Medtronic SynchroMed II pump will significantly reduce the drug delivered to just 0.006 ml/day to avoid overdose.

Third, this patient experienced a second pump stall within hours of reprogramming her pump after its initial stall. The pain physician in this case wisely informed the patient to continue monitoring for alarms or a significant increase in her back pain after she was initially discharged from the ED. Reprogramming a stalled intrathecal pump does not prevent subsequent pump stalls if a systematic problem has occurred with the delivery system.

Fourth, if an intrathecal pump has stalled, it is important to treat the patient with oral or intravenous medications to avoid acute withdrawal from intrathecal medications. In the aforementioned case, the patient was receiving significant doses of intrathecal baclofen, clonidine, bupivacaine, morphine, and fentanyl. Withdrawal from intrathecal baclofen and clonidine can be life threatening, and the patient must be monitored for the development of severe cardiovascular and neurologic sequelae. It should be noted that oral baclofen is poorly absorbed and that in the setting of acute withdrawal from intrathecal baclofen, cardiovascular collapse may still occur in spite of supplemental baclofen. If immediate repair of the intrathecal pump is not possible, one may consider a single shot bolus of intrathecal baclofen or initiation of an intravenous propofol infusion in a monitored setting (i.e., intensive care unit, ICU) as an alternative to immediate surgical repair of the dysfunctional intrathecal delivery system. Similarly, withdrawal from intrathecal clonidine can present as malignant hypertension and require ICU monitoring and management with systemic antihypertensive medications to prevent severe sequelae. These issues are dealt with elsewhere in this book.

Withdrawal from intrathecal opioids, while distressing to the patient, is rarely fatal, and there is no known withdrawal syndrome associated with acute cessation of intrathecal local anesthetics such as bupivacaine. More information regarding intrathecal withdrawal syndromes can be found in the chapter in this book entitled, "Intrathecal Medication Withdrawal."

Finally, compounding several intrathecal medications including "off-label" medications has been shown to cause a statistically higher incidence of motor stalls in Medtronic SynchroMed II intrathecal pumps [1]. The only FDA-approved intrathecal analgesic medications are morphine, ziconotide, and baclofen. Corrosive agents in drug formulations can permeate through the internal pump tubing and initiate corrosion of internal components in this particular pump model. Damage can also occur as a result of a leak in the pump tubing, resulting in direct exposure of internal pump components to corrosive agents from the drug solution.

29.3 Pump Flip

In rare cases, intrathecal pumps have been reported to "flip" or rotate within the surgical pocket. Pump flip can occur either spontaneously or through patient manipulation of the pump. Pump flip can present as inability to access the reservoir fill port when a needle is inserted into the skin. Whenever possible, it is advisable to anchor the intrathecal pump to the underlying fascia rather than adipose tissue to reduce the

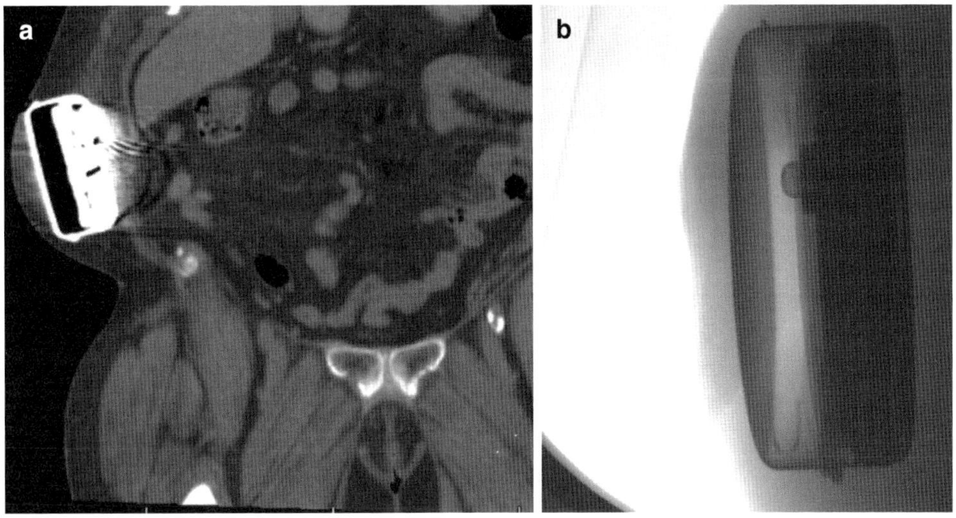

Fig. 29.1 Pump flip. CT image of a complete flipped pump. (**a**) The CT was performed after a failed pump refill with needle unable to identify the reservoir entry; fluoroscopic image performed in the pain clinic showed reservoir closer to skin consistent with pump flip. (**b**) Images from Dr. Anitescu's personal library

possibility of pump flip. Pump orientation can be readily detected using imaging with either fluoroscopy or ultrasound, where inappropriate device orientation can be easily recognized. If the pump cannot easily be returned to its normal position with external manipulation and CSF cannot be aspirated from the side port, surgical revision should be considered as soon as possible as a pump flip can also cause occlusion of the catheter and lead to an under-infusion state (Fig. 29.1).

29.4 Expired Pump

All programmable intrathecal pumps can stop functioning properly due to a natural, expected decline in battery function if the pump continues to run past the lifespan of the battery. Medtronic and Prometra pumps utilize batteries to drive function of their respective devices. The Codman pump utilizes a battery-free design that depends solely on pressured gas to promote flow.

There are currently no commercially available rechargeable battery-operated intrathecal pumps. Most battery-powered pumps have a life span of 3–9 years, primarily dependent upon how intensively the pump is used (i.e., rate of delivery). In a study by Flückiger et al., the average time to pump replacement due to battery exhaustion was 55 months [2]. Battery exhaustion was the most common indication for exchange or revision of an intrathecal pump in this study. After this point in time, the pump will be expected to stop functioning properly. Surgical replacement is usually scheduled several months before anticipated battery failure and alerts, and alarms are generated well in advance of this date to inform the patient and medical practitioner that replacement is necessary.

Perhaps less-known complications are the ones related to catheters. In majority of cases, the commercially available intrathecal drug delivery systems (IDDS) offer lifetime warranty for their products, meaning that upon placement of an intrathecal catheter, unless it breaks through trauma, develops granuloma via high opioid concentration, or migrates out of the intrathecal space, the device ensures stable and continued delivery of medication to treat patients' pain. However, it is unclear if those implants maintain their original properties during the years. In many situations, a malfunction of an intrathecal catheter may be encountered during an intrathecal reservoir change and requires changing the entire IDDS. During this operation, defective (friable, broken, punctured) catheters can be encountered although clinical reports are sparse. Special attention should be taken with replacement of intrathecal catheters that have been implanted more than 10 years as coating of the catheter may sheer from its body; in those situations, catheters become friable and can easily break, sometimes with irretrievable pieces in the intrathecal space or abdominal wall (Fig. 29.2). Multidisciplinary collaboration with neurosurgeons and/or plastic surgeons may be needed in these situations to ensure complete explant of the system. In very rare cases when risks outweigh the benefits, catheter parts may be left in place (e.g., abdominal wall) with careful monitoring of the patient.

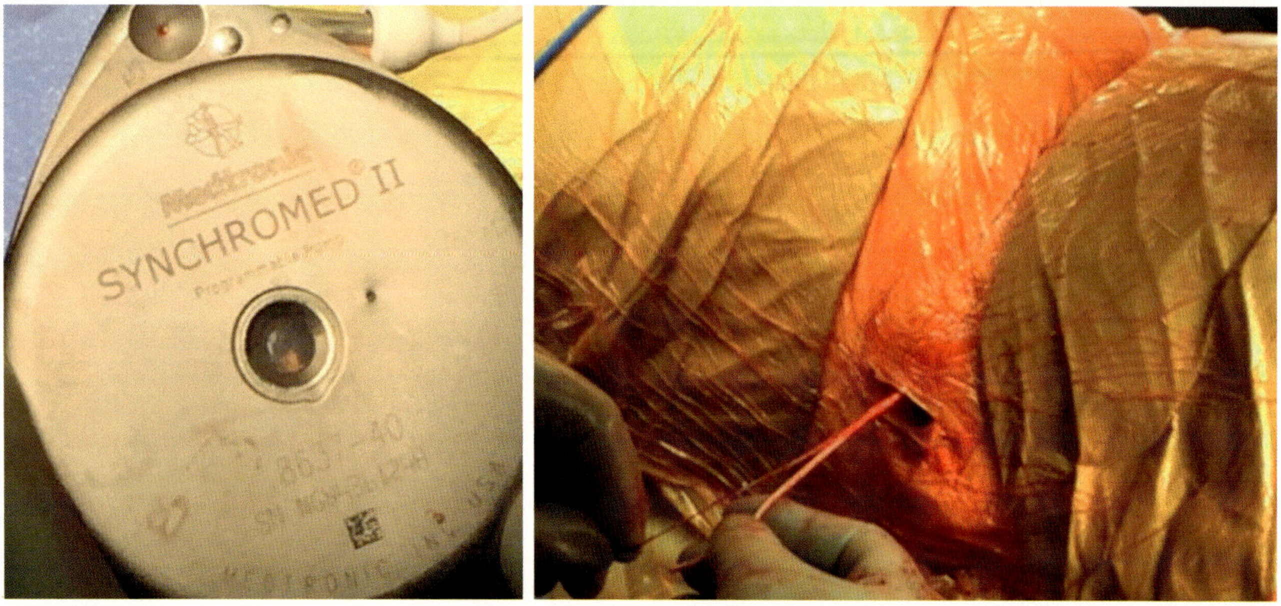

Fig. 29.2 Intrathecal pump malfunction. The original IDDS was placed 10 years ago, with replacement after 6 years. During the second replacement occurring after sudden pump stop, the catheter was unable to produce CSF upon aspiration. A complete revision of the system showed a significantly damaged catheter whose coating sheered from the catheter body. The catheter was friable but was easily removed from the intrathecal space. The picture shows the finding of the catheter during removal surgery. The entire system was removed but was not replaced with a new system as patient was weaned off intrathecal opioids during the period before surgery and tolerated it well with minimal pain and side effects

29.5 Pump Stall

There are several potential causes of mechanical failure of intrathecal pumps. In the retrospective study by Flückiger et al. [2] of 100 patients in Switzerland with implanted intrathecal pumps, the annual rate for complications requiring surgical intervention was 10.5%, with 35% of complications being pump-related and the remaining-catheter related. Pump complications included pump defect, battery exhaustion, pump repositioning, and infection.

In June 2013, a class I recall was issued for the Medtronic SynchroMed® II and SynchroMed® EL Implantable Drug Infusion Pumps [3]. This recall mentioned a potential for electrical shorting within the pump that could present as a motor stall and potentially lead to loss of or reduction in therapy. Another set of case reports by Rigoli et al. discussed two patients with symptoms of acute baclofen withdrawal with supposedly functional pumps in place [4]. In these two cases, each patient had pump reservoirs that were near empty when withdrawal symptoms presented. These cases brought attention to the concept that intrathecal drug delivery may be unreliable in some pump systems at low reservoir volumes.

Combining multiple drugs to elicit their synergistic effects at lower drug doses is common in intrathecal pump management [5]. Drug polytherapy is recommended as second-line therapy in the consensus treatment guidelines [6]. Despite these recommendations, intrathecal pumps may stall when several medications, especially "off-label" medications, are compounded for intrathecal therapy. Morphine, baclofen, and ziconotide as sole agents are the only FDA-approved intrathecal medications. None of the drugs that are FDA approved for IT administration are approved for mixing with any other drug. In clinical practice, other "off-label" medications, such as local anesthetics, opioids other than morphine, and clonidine, are routinely used in intrathecal therapy.

Combinations of intrathecal medications can contribute to internal corrosion within some intrathecal pumps. Information published by Medtronic indicates that corrosive agents (e.g., chloride ion, sulfate ion) originating from drug formulations may be to blame [1]. This report notes that some unapproved drug formations show chloride permeation rates orders of magnitude higher than those for approved drugs. Other postulated causes of internal corrosion may be due to antimicrobial and antioxidant preservatives (e.g., sodium metabisulfite), drug additives to maintain solubility, drug formulations with a pH ≤ 3, and hydrophobic drugs (e.g., fentanyl, bupivacaine).

A case report by Sgouros et al. discussed the sequela of the stall of an intrathecal pump filled with baclofen [7]. When the pump restarted after the stall, the patient received a large bolus of baclofen. The patient subsequently was unable to move her legs and later lapsed into a coma requiring intubation and ventilation. After 17 h, the patient awoke gradually from the coma with no new neurological deficits. The pump was subsequently explanted and underwent forensic examination by the manufacturer who identified no technical problems with the device.

Although a spontaneous pump stall is possible with any system at any time due to structural dysfunction (e.g., mechanical failure), these instances are very uncommon due to the high reliability of available systems. The most common time for a pump to stall is during an MRI when the mechanism for drug delivery relies upon magnetic components, as it does with the Medtronic ITP. In this instance, the pump will stop due to the magnetic field of the MRI scanner and should resume spontaneously after the patient is removed from the MRI and associated magnetic field [8]. Permanent stall, although unlikely, is possible, which is why a pump should be interrogated approximately 20 min after an MRI to determine whether the pump has resumed normal function. The event log should show messages indicating that a motor stall and subsequent motor recovery have occurred. If a recovery has not occurred or alarms have not been triggered, the patient is at risk for a withdrawal syndrome related to cessation of intrathecal therapy, especially baclofen. In this instance, it is recommended to wait another 20 min and interrogate the pump again to address delays in event logging due to electromagnetic interference from the MRI. The pump manufacturer representative should be contacted if the pump has not restarted, and appropriate care should be taken to prevent the development of withdrawal symptoms.

There have recently been case reports of stalls involving the Medtronic SynchroMed® II ITP [9–11]. We have experienced similar events at both of our institutions (University of California, San Diego, and University of California, San Francisco); characteristics of intrathecal therapy of these cases are presented in Table 29.1. All of the cases involved off-label therapy, either use of non-FDA-approved intrathecal medications (e.g., hydromorphone, meperidine, fentanyl), or polyanalgesic therapy with compounded medications. The cause of these motor stalls was identified in one case as corrosion of the internal gears (see Fig. 29.3) but is unknown in the other cases where the devices are still in the process of being analyzed by the manufacturer.

Table 29.1 Characteristics of five recent ITP stalls at two institutions

Patient	Age of pump (year of placement)	Intrathecal therapy	Use of PTM	Outcome
1	6 years (2010)	Clonidine, morphine, bupivacaine	Yes	ITP replaced
2	2 years (2013)	Meperidine	Yes	ITP replaced
3	3 years (2012)	Morphine, bupivacaine, baclofen	Yes	ITP replaced
4	5 years (2010)	Hydromorphone	Yes	ITP replaced
5	4 years (2011)	Morphine, baclofen, bupivacaine, clonidine, fentanyl	Yes	ITP replaced
6	2 years (2012)	Hydromorphone, fentanyl	Yes	ITP replaced

These cases of ITP motor stalls may certainly be related to the use of off-label medications and compounding causing corrosion of internal gears. Importantly, ITP motor stalls have been reported using FDA-approved medications as well. We also propose that a potential contributing factor to some instances of ITP stall pertains to the use of a patient therapy manager (PTM) device or "flex dosing." These modes introduce a variable, unpredictable demand on the device's battery that is not accounted for when calculating the device's "elective replacement indicator"—a time 90 days prior to the end of service life for the ITP—thus depleting the battery before its anticipated life span and potentially leading to motor stall and damage to internal components. Regardless of the cause, these cases highlight the complexity of all ITPs and the potential for their malfunction.

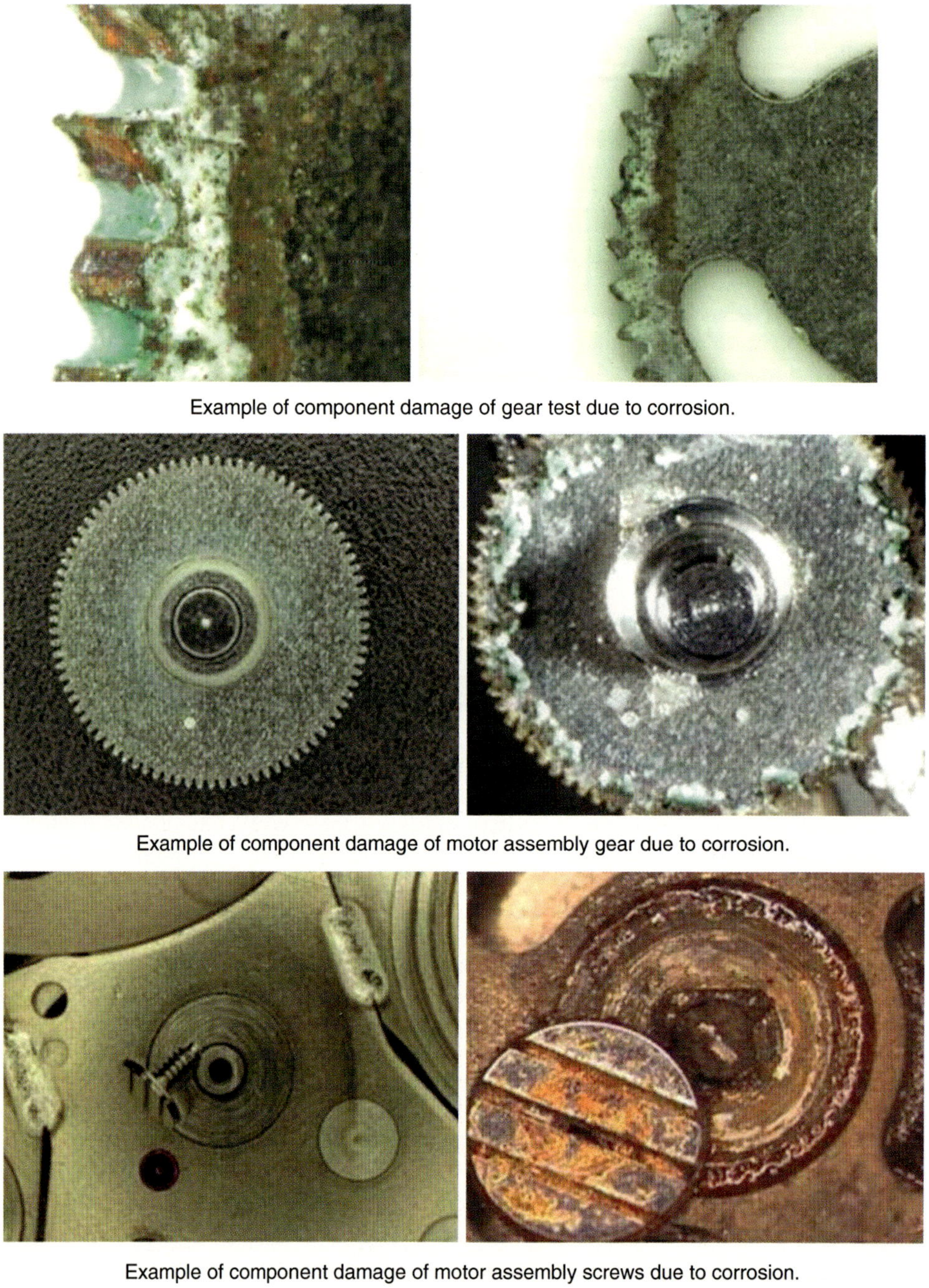
Example of component damage of gear test due to corrosion.
Example of component damage of motor assembly gear due to corrosion.
Example of component damage of motor assembly screws due to corrosion.

Fig. 29.3 Example of corrosion of internal gears of SynchroMed intrathecal pump. Reproduced with permission from Medtronic

29.6 Over-Infusion: Valve Malfunction

The Prometra intrathecal pump utilizes a valve mechanism to control drug delivery. When the Prometra pump is exposed to an MRI environment, both the inlet and outlet valves open, leading to an emptying of the drug reservoir and catheter contents into the patient. To avoid this potentially lethal complication, the drug reservoir must be emptied and the pump programmed to a rate of 0.0 mg/day. The new model Prometra II has a third shut-off valve that closes in an MRI environment, preventing the release of the contents of the pump. The Prometra does, however, require the contents of the pump to be removed after the MRI in order to reset the shut-off valve.

29.7 Over-Infusion: Side Access Port Injection

The side access port for the intrathecal catheter on an intrathecal pump can inadvertently be accessed and injected into, leading to over-infusion. The intrathecal pumps from Medtronic and Prometra both have access ports that are accessed by specific needles found in their respective side access port kits. However, if the side access port kit is used for a pump refill, an accidental injection of the catheter refill port instead of the reservoir port is possible. This error can lead to a potentially lethal overdose of intrathecal medication. Side access port injection can be avoided by determining the proper position of the pump's refill port in relation to the catheter access port and using the proper kit for refilling. In both the Prometra and Medtronic pumps, the refill port is located centrally, while the catheter access ports are located peripherally.

29.8 Over-Infusion: Chronic Pump Malfunction

Chronic over-infusion can be detected by volume discrepancies >14% expected during an intrathecal pump refill. The Medtronic registry reports that the occurrence of chronic over-infusion is <0.16% with their devices. The exact mechanism for over-infusion is still under investigation but may be related to a malfunction of the internal pumping mechanism. Clinical presentation of this will be dependent on the drug being infused but may include sedation, confusion, and respiratory depression. Patients may also present in a state of withdrawal or under-infusion if the contents of the pump are emptied prior to the pump refill alarm date. Thus, it is recommended that volume discrepancies between the actual and expected reservoir volumes be recorded, and if the discrepancy is greater than 2 ml over the course of several refills, a pump replacement should be considered.

Key Concepts

- Intrathecal pump stall can cause potentially life-threatening consequences such as acute drug withdrawal.
- Patients with a stalled ITP should be provided with oral or intravenous medications and be monitored until intrathecal therapy can be restored.
- Compounding intrathecal medications, especially "off-label" medications, can lead to pump stall due to internal pump corrosion.
- Most intrathecal pumps should be expected to stop functioning when exposed to a strong magnetic field, as occurs during an MRI. The pump should return to normal function spontaneously after removal from the magnetic field. Identification of device manufacturer should be determined before any MRI scan so appropriate precautions can be taken. Moreover, intrathecal pumps should be interrogated after an MRI to confirm proper functioning.
- Pump flip can occur when an intrathecal pump is not well secured to underlying fascia.
- Pump flip can present as inability to fill pump through the reservoir fill port when a needle is inserted into the skin.
- Intrathecal pumps have an expected battery life of 4–7 years.
- Pumps need to be replaced in anticipation of battery failure, or withdrawal symptoms may present when a pump expires.

References

1. Medtronic Inc. Increased risk of motor stall and loss of or change in therapy with unapproved drug formulations. 2012;1–2.
2. Flückiger B, Knecht H, Grossmann S, Felleiter P. Device-related complications of long-term intrathecal drug therapy via implanted pumps. Spinal Cord. 2008;46:639–43.
3. FDA. FDA—Medtronic SynchroMed II and SynchroMed EL implantable drug infusion pumps—feed through failure. 2016;1–3.
4. Rigoli G, Terrini G, Cordioli Z. Intrathecal baclofen withdrawal syndrome caused by low residual volume in the pump reservoir: a report of 2 cases. Arch Phys Med Rehabil. 2004;85:2064–6.
5. Jones RCW, Moeller-Bertram T, Wallace MS. Safety and efficacy of intrathecal drug delivery for pain. Pain Manag. 2012;2:55–61.
6. Deer TR, et al. Polyanalgesic consensus conference 2012: recommendations for the management of pain by intrathecal (intraspinal) drug delivery: report of an interdisciplinary expert panel. Neuromodulation. 2012;15:436–66.
7. Sgouros S, Charalambides C, Matsota P, Tsangaris I, Kostopanagiotou G. Malfunction of SynchroMed II baclofen pump delivers a near-lethal baclofen overdose. Pediatr Neurosurg. 2010;46:62–5.
8. Medtronic Inc. Medtronic MRI guidelines. 2016;1–4.
9. Riordan J, Murphy P. Intrathecal pump: an abrupt intermittent pump failure. Neuromodulation. 2015;18:433–5.
10. Galica R, et al. Sudden intrathecal drug delivery device motor stalls. Reg Anesth Pain Med. 2016;41:135–9.
11. Buvanendran A, Lubenow TR. Vigilance to medical device failures. Reg Anesth Pain Med. 2016;41:125–6.

30 Seroma or Hygroma Formation After Implantation of an Intrathecal Drug Delivery System or a Spinal Cord Stimulator

Dalia Elmofty

30.1 Case Description

A 53-year-old female complained of pelvic pain associated with urinary frequency and urgency for the past 6 months. A work-up by her gynecologist revealed stage IV metastatic ovarian cancer. She underwent neoadjuvant chemotherapy to reduce the size of the tumor followed by a laparotomy and tumor debulking. The procedure included a total hysterectomy, bilateral salpingo-oophorectomy, and omentectomy. In the months after surgery, severe, constant, lower abdominal pain was not controlled by escalating doses of oral opioids. Computed tomographic scan revealed extensive spread of cancer in the abdominal and pelvic cavity. Surgery, chemotherapy, and radiation were no longer an option. Because of the lack of efficacy of oral opioids, the patient was referred to the pain clinic for an infusion trial of intrathecal medication. An intrathecal infusion of hydromorphone resulted in adequate relief. Subsequently she received an intrathecal implant for drug delivery (SynchroMed® II drug pump, Medtronic, Minneapolis, MN). One week after the implant, the patient experienced severe upper back pain over the surgical incision. On physical examination in the emergency room, no sensory or motor deficit was found in the lower extremity. On her upper and lower back, a "golf ball"-like area of swelling was noted over the midline incision at the insertion site of the intrathecal catheter. The wound was healing, and no erythema or discharge was noted. The patient denied having fever, chills, or a positional headache. The differential diagnosis included the possibility of a seroma, hygroma, or abscess formation. Laboratory tests were ordered, and a C-reactive protein test and white blood cell count were normal. The patient was discharged home with a pressure dressing over the swelling and an abdominal binder and was advised to return to the emergency room if she experienced fevers or positional headaches. During a follow-up visit in the pain clinic, the swelling had increased from "golf ball" to "tennis ball" size. The patient was unable to sleep on her back because of the discomfort. An ultrasound confirmed fluid collection. Under an aseptic technique, the fluid was aspirated and sent for beta-2 transferrin, gram stain, and culture. Beta-2 transferrin was negative, and gram stain showed a moderate amount of white blood cells (mononuclear cells) with no organisms. Culture revealed no growth. A pressure dressing and abdominal binder were reapplied. The swelling subsided over 4 weeks. The most likely diagnosis was a seroma formation at the surgical incision site.

30.2 Case Discussion

Intrathecal drug delivery systems and spinal cord stimulators are devices that have brought pain relief to patients suffering chronic pain. Although the implantation technique is considered safe and reversible, mechanical and biological complications have been reported (Table 30.1) [1]. Seromas and hygromas are biological complications.

Table 30.1 Mechanical and biological complications derived from implantable devices [1]

Mechanical	Biological
Electrode fracture or migration for SCS	Infection
Catheter fracture or migration for ITDDS	Bleeding
Battery failure for SCS or ITDDS	Nerve injury
Programming or pump-fill errors for ITDDS	Seroma
	Hygroma

SCS spinal cord stimulation, *ITDDS* intrathecal drug delivery system

D. Elmofty, M.D.
Department of Anesthesia and Critical Care, University of Chicago, 5841 S. Maryland Ave., M.C. 4028, Chicago, IL 60637, USA
e-mail: DElmofty@dacc.uchicago.edu

M. Anitescu et al. (eds.), *Challenging Cases and Complication Management in Pain Medicine*,
https://doi.org/10.1007/978-3-319-60072-7_30

30.3 Etiology and Pathogenesis

A seroma is a postoperative fluid collection resulting from an accumulation of serous fluid on the skin's surface (Figs. 30.1 and 30.2). When it develops at the site of a surgical incision, it contributes to poor wound healing. The etiology of seroma formation is multifactorial; lymphatic disruptions, shearing between tissue surfaces, mediators of inflammation, and the creation of surgical dead space have been implicated [2]. Macrophages and polymorphonuclear leucocytes along with the release of histamines and prostaglandins result in vasodilatation of blood vessels and formation of interstitial fluid [2]. The fluid, known as serum, can be clear or yellowish in color.

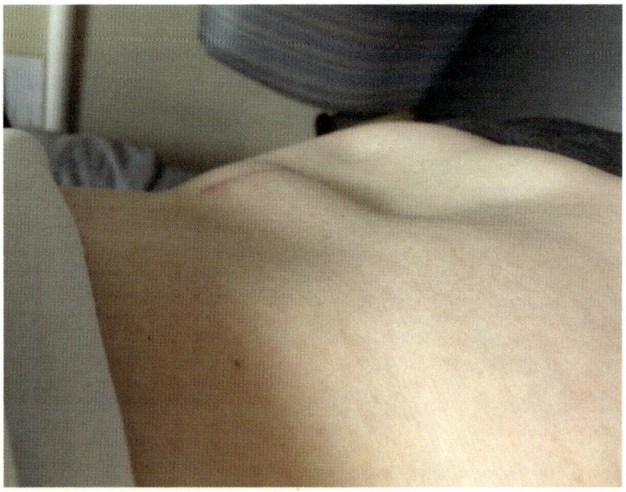

Fig. 30.1 Seroma formation along midline incision following implantation of an intrathecal drug delivery system. It developed around the incision used for placement of the intrathecal portion of the system. Image from Dr. Elmofty personal library

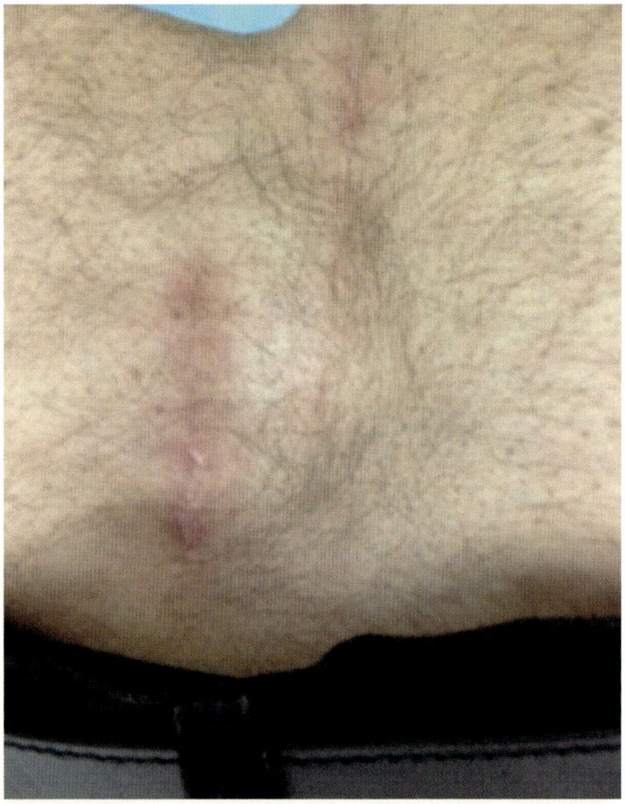

Fig. 30.2 Seroma formation along midline incision following implantation of an intrathecal drug delivery system. The patient denies positional headaches and placement of an abdominal binder has significantly reduced the size of the seroma. Image from Dr. Anitescu personal library

A hygroma is a subcutaneous collection of cerebrospinal fluid (CSF). CSF leaks when the dura is injured, for example, from an introducer during placement of an intrathecal catheter. The needle is larger than the catheter inserted, thus creating an incomplete tissue seal around the intrathecal catheter. CSF can flow from the intrathecal space down the catheter and may collect anywhere along the catheter, including the pump pocket.

30.4 Risk Factors

Certain factors increase the risk for developing a seroma or hygroma after a surgical procedure. Seromas can form after extensive surgical dissection and disruption of tissue planes. A history of seroma formation after a surgical procedure is another risk factor. Cancer patients with low protein levels or lymphedema are prone to seroma formation.

Hygromas may develop in patients with low protein levels or after improper surgical techniques or failure to place a purse-string silk suture around a Tuohy needle before removal.

30.5 Clinical Manifestations of Seroma and Hygroma

The most common symptom with a seroma is inflammation or swelling over the surgical incision from the presence of serous fluid under the skin. In many cases, a seroma will appear like a swollen lump or a large cyst. It may be tender or sore on palpation. A seroma can persist for up to 2 months. The subcutaneous fluid expands to break down the surgical scar and to discharge a clear fluid from the incision. A discharge that becomes discolored, hemorrhagic, or foul smelling indicates a possible infection or abscess. In rare cases, a seroma may calcify.

Patients with a hygroma first experience a headache. The headache is severe, involving the front or back of the head with occasional radiation to the neck and shoulders and possible neck stiffness. The headache is exacerbated by movement, sitting or standing, and relieved to a certain degree by lying down. It can be associated with nausea, vomiting, pain in arms and legs, hearing loss, tinnitus, vertigo, and dizziness. A hygroma usually resolves spontaneously within 1–2 weeks. Persistent CSF leakage can lead to meningitis, epidural abscess, and pseudomeningocele. If the leakage does not resolve spontaneously, the site of the leakage should be identified and repaired.

Table 30.2 Differential diagnosis of postsurgical fluid collection over surgical incision

Differential diagnosis	Clinical presentation	Diagnostic testing	Management
Seroma	Subcutaneous fluid collection, tender or sore on palpation, no fever or chills	Rule out infection, CBC, gram stain, and culture	*Conservative*: compressive dressing *Invasive*: aseptic aspiration, surgical excision of the bursal cavity
Hygroma	Subcutaneous fluid collection, spinal headache	Aseptic aspiration and beta-2 transferrin assay	*Conservative*: hydration, caffeinated beverages, bed rest, compressive dressing *Invasive*: surgical repair or dural patch
Abscess	Subcutaneous fluid collection, tender or sore on palpation with erythema, fever, or chills	CBC, gram stain and culture, MRI	*Conservative*: antibiotics *Invasive*: incision and drainage

30.6 Diagnostic Methods

The differential diagnosis of a fluid collection following intrathecal drug delivery systems and spinal cord stimulator implantations includes seroma, hygroma, or infection (Table 30.2). The diagnosis can be determined by the clinical presentation, appearance of the wound, and laboratory tests such as white blood cell count, C-reactive protein, erythrocyte sedimentation rate, and microbiology testing. The beta-2 transferrin assay is a highly sensitive and specific test for the presence of CSF [3]. Beta-2 transferrin is a protein found in CSF, perilymph, and the aqueous/vitreous humors of the eye [4]. It was first described in 1979 as a marker for confirming CSF leak [5]. If CFS leakage is suspected, percutaneous needle aspiration and fluid analysis may be indicated. Extreme caution and an aseptic technique are mandatory to prevent introducing bacterial contaminants. Magnetic resonance imaging also can show fluid collection. An axial T2 or sagittal T2 image can reveal a high-signal fluid collection located near the site of catheter placement to indicate a CSF leak and hygroma formation.

30.7 Prevention

Patients at high risk for a seroma may require a surgical drainage system [6]. Compression garments can be considered to help the skin and tissue heal faster. By reducing swelling and bruising after surgery, the garments may reduce the risk of a seroma. The risk of seroma formation also can be reduced by good surgical techniques. The size of the pocket for an intrathecal catheter should not be excessively large but matched to the size of the generator or intrathecal pump to be implanted. Eliminating excessive use of electrocautery or an electrosurgical scalpel has been recommended to reduce the risk [7].

Prophylactic compressive dressings or garments also can reduce the risk of hygroma formation. Small lumbar incisions promote faster healing and reduce the incidence of leakage around an intrathecal catheter. A purse-string silk suture through the lumbodorsal fascia and around the intrathecal catheter is recommended to reduce the likelihood of a CSF leak [8]. The purse-string suture is placed before the Tuohy needle is removed and then tightened around the catheter after the needle is removed.

30.8 Treatment

30.8.1 Conservative

Treatment for seroma is uncommon. Though bothersome, seromas are rarely serious if infection and spinal fluid leak are ruled out. The seroma can be left to heal on its own as the body reabsorbs the fluid that fills the cavity. An abdominal binder or pressure dressing can be helpful.

Conservative treatment for headaches from hygromas includes hydration, caffeinated beverages, bed rest, and application of a pressure dressing.

30.8.2 Invasive

In some instances wherein the size of a seroma becomes bigger than normal, aseptic drainage is performed to decrease pressure on the skin. Repeated drainage, however, may increase the risk of infection. Diluted tetracycline or doxycycline has been injected into the pocket of a seroma to prevent further fluid accumulation [9]. In some cases, seromas may require surgical excision of the bursal cavity. Surgical revision and a dural patch may be needed if a hygroma results from significant CSF flow or is associated with neurological symptoms [10].

Key Concepts

- Seroma and hygroma formations are biological complications associated with implantable devices such as intrathecal drug delivery systems or spinal cord stimulators.
- Physicians should anticipate and treat such complications.
- The diagnosis can be determined by symptoms, appearance of the wound, and laboratory tests. The beta-2 transferrin assay is a highly sensitive and specific test to confirm the presence of CSF collection.
- The treatment of seroma and hygroma is mainly self-limiting in nature. Close observation is recommended to prevent infection or, in the case of hygroma, neurological compromise from ongoing CSF leak.

References

1. Abejon D, Arango S, Riquelme I, Del Saz J. Neuromodulation techniques, complications, and troubleshooting. Tech Reg Anesth Pain Manage. 2014;18:49–57.
2. Bullocks J, Basu B, Hsu P, Singer R. Prevention of hematomas and seromas. Semin Plast Surg. 2006;20(4):233–40.
3. Bleier BS, Debnath I, O'Conell BP, et al. Preliminary study on the stability of beta-2 transferrin in extracorporeal cerebrospinal fluid. Otolarnygol Head Neck Surg. 2010;144(1):101–3.
4. Warnecke A, Averbeck T, Wurster U, et al. Diagnostic relevance of beta-2-transferrin for detection of cerebrospinal fluid fistulas. Arch Otolaryngol Head Neck Surg. 2004;130:1178–84.
5. Meurman OH, Irjala K, Suonpaa J, Laurent B. A new method for identification of cerebrospinal fluid leakage. Acta Otolaryngol. 1979;21(3):259–64.
6. Bercial ME, Sabino Neto MS, Calil JA, Rossetto LA, Ferreira LM. Suction drains, quilting sutures, and fibrin sealant in the prevention of seroma formation in abdominoplasty: which is the best strategy? Aesthet Plast Surg. 2012;36:370–3.
7. Chrintz H, Vibits H, Cordts TO, Harreby JS, Waaddagaard P, Larsen SO. Need for surgical wound dressing. Br J Surg. 1989; 76:204–5.
8. Kulkarni AV, Drake JM, Lamberti-Pasculli M. Cerebrospinal fluid shunt infection. A prospective study of risk factors. J Neurosurg. 2001;94:195–201.
9. Sterns L, Boortz-Marx R, Du Pen S, et al. Intrathecal drug delivery for the management of cancer pain. A multidisciplinary consensus of best clinical practices. J Support Oncol. 2005;3:399–408.
10. Pancal SJ, Gonzalez JA. Intrathecal pumps. Tech Reg Anesth Pain Manage. 2000;4(3):137–42.

31 Complications of Intrathecal Polypharmacy, Medication Side Effects, and Overdose

Rena Beckerly

31.1 Case Description

A 60-year-old male presented to the emergency department with hemoptysis, shortness of breath, and pleuritic chest pain. Extensive work-up revealed a thoracic mass consistent with small cell carcinoma with diffuse metastasis to his bones. During his admission, the palliative care team was consulted and composed a pain regimen which included morphine ER 60 mg BID, fentanyl patch 300mcq every 3 days, and morphine IR 10 mg every 2–4 h. He reported adequate pain relief (VAS 4/10) and was scheduled to undergo chemotherapy as an outpatient.

Two weeks later, he presented to the emergency department with severe, intractable chest pain. His work-up revealed worsening thoracic tumor burden despite chemotherapy. The pain service evaluated the patient and increased his medications. However, the patient subsequently experienced worsening shortness of breath and mental status changes. The pain service discussed an intrathecal pump with the patient and his family. The decision was made to proceed with an intrathecal opiate trial with morphine 0.1 mg single-dose injection. The patient reported excellent pain relief without side effects.

The patient's preoperative evaluation revealed bilateral pleural effusions and post-obstructive pneumonia. His laboratory values revealed neutropenia and platelet count of 90 K. He was scheduled for another round of chemotherapy in one week. Given the likelihood of worsening neutropenia and thrombocytopenia with chemotherapy, the patient agreed to have the IDDS placed as soon as possible. He was taken to the operating room the next day and had the IDDS placed under light sedation, given his tenuous pulmonary status. He tolerated the procedure well and had morphine 0.3 mg/h started. He reported excellent pain relief (VAS 2/10) without respiratory depression or mental status change.

R. Beckerly, M.D.
University of Illinois, Chicago, IL, USA
e-mail: beckerr@uic.edu

Two weeks later, the patient presented to the emergency department again with worsening shortness of breath. The pain service was consulted, and the decision was made to reduce his morphine dose (0.2 mg/h) and add bupivacaine intrathecally for improved analgesia. While the patient reported improved analgesia and improved ventilation, his blood pressure was lowered by the bupivacaine, and his antihypertensives were discontinued. A month later, the patient had worsening pain, and his IDDS medications were changed to hydromorphone/bupivacaine without improvement. Fentanyl offered minimal improvement. Ziconotide was attempted, but the patient suffered severe mental status changes. He expired shortly after.

31.2 Discussion

31.2.1 Principle Behind Intrathecal Drug Delivery Systems

Since 1981, more than 300,000 [1] intrathecal drug delivery systems (IDDS) have been implanted for the management of intractable chronic pain or spasticity. While previously utilized for cancer pain, the most common current indication for IDDS is failed back surgical syndrome [2]. IDDS allow medications to be delivered close to the spinal cord and access opiate receptors directly. Oral, intravenous, or transdermal medications attempt to access these same receptors but have to undergo first-pass metabolism and distribution. This requires larger doses of medications and often leads to side effects. Other theories suggest an increase of adenosine release into the CSF with opioid infusion through IDDS [3]. Other mediators such as nitric oxide, serotonin, and catecholamines may be involved.

Our understanding of CSF flow mechanisms comes from studies on immobilized animals and drugs other than morphine or ziconotide. Anesthetized pigs were treated with intrathecal infusions of baclofen and bupivacaine which

M. Anitescu et al. (eds.), *Challenging Cases and Complication Management in Pain Medicine*,
https://doi.org/10.1007/978-3-319-60072-7_31

showed limited distribution of the drugs in the CSF after 8 h [4]. CSF flow may be different in humans as it is replaced at least three times per day at a rate of 0.3–0.4 mL/min. This would imply more diffuse medication distribution especially in an active person.

Smith et al. [5] performed a critical study that showed IDDS medication delivery to be superior to comprehensive medical management. Patients were randomized to either IDDS drug trial with medical management or interventions (use of medications, nerve blocks, radiation, etc.). The IDDS group had better results in regard to fatigue, level of consciousness, and quality of life for the patient and caregiver. They also noted a potential for improved survival with IDDS (although not statistically significant). The authors concluded that IDDS should be the standard of care for patients suffering from cancer.

31.2.2 IDDS Trial Options

IDDS trials can be performed in several different ways including single-shot spinal injection, intermittent boluses, continuous spinal catheter, or epidural catheter infusion. Additionally, there is a lot of variability in the location of injection, duration of the trial, location of the trial (inpatient or outpatient), and how success is defined. Deer et al. [6] performed a large prospective, multicenter trial looking at trialing techniques and outcomes at 6 and 12 months. One hundred sixty-six patients had IDDS trial in different locations: outpatient procedure in a hospital (16%), inpatient procedure in a hospital (72%), or in an ambulatory surgery center (12%). Trialing methodologies were continuous epidural infusion (53%), continuous intrathecal infusion (25%), single intrathecal bolus injection (14%), and multiple intrathecal bolus injections (8%). The majority of patients (81.1%) were trialed with morphine only. The mean duration of the trial was 3.5 ± 5.4 days. One hundred fifty-four patients (93%) had successful trials, and 136 received implants (82%). Analysis of collected data revealed no statistically significant associations between most factors and IDDS trialing success. The only category that had a statistically significant association with trial success was the type of pain (mechanical and mixed pain responded better to opiate trial than neuropathic pain). The authors concluded that there were no statistically significant advantages to any trial technique or venue for IDDS trial.

Interestingly, there was a difference in outcomes in patient who received monotherapy (usually opioid) versus polypharmacy (two or more agents) during the trial. There was an 11% reduction in the success rate when polyanalgesia was not used. This was statistically evident in patients who had neuropathic or mixed pain syndromes. The study showed that opioids, when used as sole agents, may not be adequate to treat complex neuropathic or mixed pain syndromes properly. This observation may even be more significant in treatments extending longer than 1 year, because a significant number of patients develop tolerance to opioids.

31.2.3 IDDS Medications

The FDA has approved preservative-free morphine, baclofen, and ziconotide for intrathecal administration. Unfortunately, monotherapy with morphine proved ineffective for many patients, and a survey of practicing physicians revealed off-label use of adjunctive therapies in the intrathecal space. In 2000, a Cochrane Review of the literature was performed, and an expert panel reviewed existing safety data on different medications. The following algorithm [8] was composed (Fig. 31.1) after the panel reconvened in 2003 and 2007. Intrathecal morphine was previously thought to be first line in 2000 [7], but in 2003 [8], hydromorphone was included as a first-line agent. If one of the first-line agents does not work, the panel recommends trying the other. If the maximal doses of both agents do not provide adequate pain relief, adjuncts can be considered (line 2). However, if the patient has neuropathic pain, either monotherapy with morphine or hydromorphone can be considered, or an adjunct can be added (line 2). Bupivacaine may cause less hypotension than clonidine. If these changes do not offer relief, a third line of therapy is initiated (opioid, clonidine, and bupivacaine). If morphine and hydromorphone fail to provide analgesia or have significant side effects, fentanyl or sufentanil can be added (line 4). Other analgesics such as methadone, midazolam, neostigmine, adenosine, ketorolac, oxymorphone, NMDA antagonist (ketamine), ropivacaine, meperidine, gabapentin, buprenorphine, and octreotide may have a role in intrathecal therapy [8].

The 2012 Polyanalgesic Consensus on medications used for intrathecal drug delivery systems also differentiates between optimal treatments for neuropathic and nociceptive pain [9] (Figs. 31.2 and 31.3).

31.2.4 Local Anesthetics

Local anesthetics have been used in the intrathecal space since the 1880s. Usually, local anesthetic is added to the intrathecal infusion when the patient reports neuropathic symptoms such as burning or electrical-type pain. Several studies have shown improved pain control when local anesthetic is added to an opiate infusion, due to their synergistic effects and potential opiate-sparing effect. Bupivacaine is stable in the infusion system, compatible with other drugs, and safe in animal models. Tetracaine is neurotoxic at high doses. Ropivacaine has not been thoroughly studied, but a prospective, crossover, double-blinded, randomized study by Dahm et al. [10] did not show any benefit to intrathecal ropivacaine use with respect

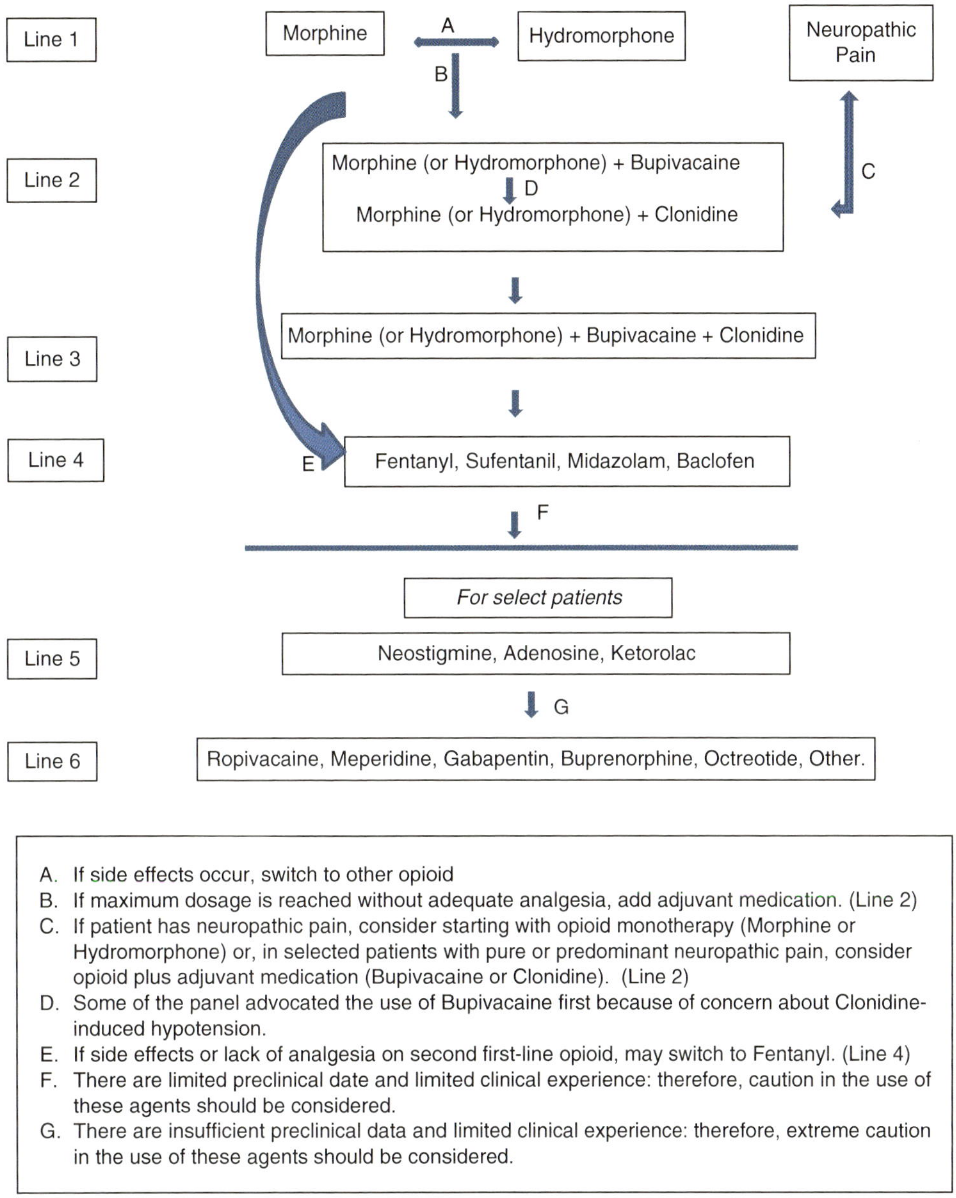

Fig. 31.1 2003 Polyanalgesic Consensus recommendations [7]

to improved analgesia, urinary retention, paresthesia, and paresis with gait impairment.

31.2.5 Ziconotide

Ziconotide is made from snail venom and works as a selective N-type voltage calcium channel blocker. It is highly hydrophilic and may require several days to demonstrate efficacy (mean time to onset is 3–9.5 days). Staats et al. [11] compared the efficacy of ziconotide with normal saline in a double-blinded, multicenter, prospective, randomized control trial in cancer and AIDS patients. They were able to show improved analgesia, quality of life, and overall satisfaction. They reported side effects of dizziness, nausea, somnolence, vomiting, postural hypotension, and fever at doses >0.1mcg/h. It is unclear if ziconotide is more powerful as a monotherapy or in combination with adjuncts. Based on the results of Staats' study, the FDA approved ziconotide for intrathecal use.

31.2.6 Opioids

Fentanyl can be considered for intrathecal infusion when morphine and hydromorphone have failed to offer analgesia or their side effects are prohibitive. Several small studies have shown the effectiveness of fentanyl in controlling pain. Mironer et al. [12] noted improved pain control with combination of fentanyl and bupivacaine when compared to fentanyl alone. No side effects were noted in either group.

Methadone has also been studied in the intrathecal space and may offer a unique advantage in that it possesses both opiate and NMDA receptor activity. Several studies have studied the efficacy of intrathecal methadone in cancer and

Fig. 31.2 2012 Polyanalgesic algorithm for optimal intrathecal treatment of neuropathic pain [9]

Line 1	Morphine	Ziconotide	Morphine and Bupivacaine
Line 2	Hydromorphone	Hydromorphone + Bupivacaine or Hydromorphone + Clonidine	Morphine + Clonidine
Line 3	Clonidine	Ziconotide + Opioid Fentanyl alone	Fentanyl + Bupivacaine Or Fentanyl + Clonidine
Line 4	Opioid + Clonidine + Bupivacaine	Bupivacaine + Clonidine	
Line 5	Baclofen		

Line 1: Morphine and ziconotide are approved by the US FDA for IT therapy and are recommended as first-line therapy for neuropathic pain. The combination of Morphine and Bupivacaine is recommended for neuropathic pain on the basis of clinical use and apparent safety.
Line 2: Hydromorphone, alone or in combination with Bupivacaine or Clonidine, is recommended. Alternatively, the combination of Morphine and Clonidine may be used.
Line 3: Third-line recommendations for neuropathic pain include Clonidine,Ziconotide plus an opioid, and Fentanyl alone or in combination with Bupivacaine or Clonidine.
Line4: The combination of Bupivacaine and Clonidine (with or without an opioid drug) is recommended.
Line 5: Baclofen is recommended on the basis of safety, although reports of efficacy are limited.

Fig. 31.3 Polyanalgesic algorithm for optimal intrathecal treatment of nociceptive pain [20]

Line 1	Morphine	Hydromorphone	Ziconotide	Fentanyl
Line 2	Morphine + Bupivacaine	Ziconotide + Opioid	Hydromorphone + Bupivacaine	Fentanyl + Bupivacaine
Line 3	Opioid (Morphine, Hydromorphone, or Fentanyl) + Clonidine			Sufentanil
Line 4	Opioid + Clonidine + Bupivacaine		Sufentanil + Bupivacaine or Clonidine	
Line 5	Sufentanil + Bupivacaine or Clonidine			

Line 1: Morphine and Ziconotide are approved by the US FDA for IT therapy and are recommended as first-line therapy for nociceptive pain. Hydromorphone is recommended on the basis of widespread clinical use and apparent safety. Fentanyl has been upgraded to first-line use by the consensus conference.
Line 2: Bupivacaine in combination with Morphine, Hydromorphone, or Fentanyl is recommended. Alternatively, the combination of Ziconotide and an opioid can be employed.
Line 3: Recommendations include clonidine plus an opioid (i.e. Morphine, Hydromorphone, or Fentanyl) or Sufentanil monotherapy.
Line 4: The triple combination of an opioid, Clonidine, and Bupivacaine is recommended. An alternate recommendation is Sufentanil in combination with either Bupivacaine or Clonidine.
Line 5: The triple combination of Sufentanil, Bupivacaine, and Clonidine is suggested.

noncancer patients. Patients received 5–60 mg/day for 3 days to 37 months. Methadone treatment consistently reduced pain and offered improved quality of life. However, patients reported vision changes and somnolence. The safety profile has yet to be clarified, and some animal studies indicate NMDA receptor drugs are linked to spinal cord injury [13].

31.2.7 Clonidine and Tizanidine

Clonidine is an alpha-2 adrenergic agonist which blocks nerve signal transmission of noxious sensory stimuli at the presynaptic and postsynaptic nerve terminals at the spinal cord level. Clonidine does not work at the opiate receptors and offers synergism when administered with opiates. Clonidine can be administered orally, transdermally, intravenously, epidurally, and intrathecally for treatment of a variety of pain syndromes. Clonidine is the only FDA-approved nonopioid intraspinal analgesic (although specified for epidural administration).

Hassenbusch et al. [14] performed a prospective open-labeled analysis of clonidine for cancer and noncancer pain. Thirty-one patients were treated with clonidine 144–1200 mcg per day with 22 patients reporting improvement in pain at 1 year. Once an effective dose was achieved, the patient rarely developed tolerance to the medication. They noted side effects of somnolence, hypotension, impotence, and urinary retention which limited dose escalation in a subset of patients. Ackerman et al. [15] showed limited improvement in pain control when clonidine is used as an adjunct. Additionally, they reported numerous side effects of hypotension, sedation, and pruritus. Tizanidine, traditionally used as a muscle relaxant, has a similar structure to clonidine as an alpha 2-adrenergic agonist. Tizanidine has similar potency to clonidine when administered intrathecally. A comparative dog study [16] showed similar efficacy of both agents, but tizanidine had fewer adverse effects of bradycardia and hypotension.

31.2.8 Octreotide

Octreotide is a growth hormone analogue which may play a role in alleviating chronic pain when administered intrathecally. Deer et al. [17] performed a randomized, prospective, double-blinded study which did not show a statistically significant improvement in pain. However, no side effects were noted, and the dose of the medication may have been inadequate.

31.2.9 Gabapentin

Gabapentin's role in treating neuropathic pain has been established. Intrathecal gabapentin has been studied in humans without side effects. The drug reduced mechanical allodynia, diminished hyperalgesia, and reduced neuropathic pain in rats as a mononeuropathy. It is more effective and potent when given intrathecally [18]. Gabapentin may be efficacious as monotherapy or an adjunct.

31.2.10 Complications of IDDS

In 2006, a cluster of three deaths were noted within 1 day of IDDS implant (nine cases were later identified). This was thought to be opiate related and prompted a review of mortality related to IDDS. Coffey et al. [19] performed a study looking at mortality associated with IDDS relaive to spinal cord stimulation implantation (a similar procedure) and lumbar discectomy. They utilized epidemiological methods along with the Medtronic device registration data from Social Security Death Master File and UnitedHealthcare population database to examine demographic/comorbidity data. This analysis revealed an intrathecal mortality rate of 0.088% at 3 days after implantation, 0.39% at 1 month, and 3.89% at 1 year (all higher than SCS implantation or lumbar discectomy in community hospitals). They attributed the excess mortality to intrathecal opioid therapy. Upon review of these sentinel cases, respiratory arrest was either the cause or contributed to patient death. No device malfunction was noted. They concluded that patients with noncancer pain treated with IDDS opiate therapy had increased mortality rates when compared to patients treated with other therapies. Given these findings, they identified physician practices that increased patient mortality.

In 2013, Prager et al. [20] composed the "Best Practices for Intrathecal Drug Delivery for Pain" article. The goal of this expert panel was to identify best practices and provide guidance for clinicians to ensure safety and pain control with IDDS. While device-related issues such as catheter complications or surgical site infections occur, the main safety issues involve inadequate patient monitoring, inflammatory mass, wound healing, dosing errors, pump refills, and interactions with systemic medications. Thus, many of these complications were preventable with clinician education. They identified three areas of focus: patient selection and trialing, safety and monitoring, and patient and device management.

31.3 Patient Selection and Trialing

Patient selection is critical to the success of an IDDS. There are a myriad of chronic pain states that may be treated with an IDDS. The expert panel noted that patients with headache, fibromyalgia, atypical facial pain, noncancer head-neck pain, and borderline personality disorder had poor responses to IDDS. Additionally, patients who cannot partner with the physician in management of the IDDS should not be implanted. Comorbidities such as sleep apnea, restricted cardiac or lung capacity, venous insufficiency, obesity, metabolic syndrome, hypertension, diabetes, and immunosuppression placed patients at an increased risk for complications. These patients need to be optimized and understand they are at increased risk. Patients with spinal stenosis may also benefit from IDDS if the catheter is placed above the conus medullaris, and the patient has stable neurologic signs. Litigation is not a contraindication to IDDS placement, but the clinician should be on alert for secondary gain [20]. Absolute contraindications include active drug use, coagulopathy, and obstruction of CSF flow. Patient on chronic anticoagulation may be candidates for IDDS but will need guidance for anticoagulation management. Any patient with psychiatric comorbidities will need a psychological evaluation prior to IDDS trial.

As discussed earlier, there are no specific guidelines for intrathecal trialing, but the panel did strongly encourage intrathecal trialing prior to implantation. There was discussion of bypassing the trial in cancer patients with severe pain who could not tolerate the side effects of systemic opiates.

The panel noted that single-dose trials were acceptable for ziconotide but not ideal for opiates. Overnight observation is recommended for opiate trials. Patients with OSA are encouraged to continue treatment throughout the trial. Pain relief and functional capacity improvement need to be assessed in determining the success of the trial.

31.4 Safety and Monitoring

The patient must be able to understand and comply with the management of the IDDS. At each visit, the clinician must review an active medication list, including over-the-counter medication. Additionally, the patient must be asked about drug and alcohol use in addition to routine urine drug screens to monitor compliance. Patients should be asked about their pain, functional capacity at home, changes in their pain perception, and new neurological symptoms.

As indicated by Coffey's [19] study, respiratory depression is the primary safety concern with IDDS. The ASA classifies respiratory depression in the context of neuraxial opioid administration as reduced respiratory rate (<10–12 breaths per minute), reduced oxygen saturation (<90–92%), hypercapnia/hypercarbia (arterial CO2 > 50 mm HG), or clinical signs of drowsiness, sedation, periodic apnea, or cyanosis. Many cases of respiratory depression can be prevented by a pretrial urine toxicity screen and full disclosure of other central nervous system depressants. Coffey et al. [19] noted the patients with fatal respiratory depression after IDDS were taking between one and nine concomitant drugs including sedatives, hypnotics, oral and transdermal opioids, antidepressants, tranquilizers, and antihistamines.

Dosing of the IDDS can be very challenging as there is a great variability in patient response to intrathecal opiates. Conversion of oral, intravenous, and transdermal opiates to intrathecal doses is inconsistent. Additionally, there is no safe ceiling dose, and the consequences of inappropriate doses/titration can be fatal. The goal is to find the lowest efficacious dose to provide the most pain relief and least side effects. Other factors that can affect analgesic levels include catheter tip location, CSF flow, and stenosis. The panel recommends reducing systemic opiate consumption by at least one half when complete cessation is not possible. The recommended initial dose of morphine is 0.1–0.5 mg/day and can be escalated based on side effects (ideally <20% of the total daily dose). More conservative increases should be considered with patients on patient-controlled analgesic devices to minimize the risk of overdose. Side effects of intrathecal morphine include delayed respiratory depression (due to the lipophilicity, rostral spread, and greater CSF diffusion), urinary retention, pruritus, nausea/vomiting, and constipation which can all be medically managed.

Close monitoring is critical, especially when initiating or reinitiating opiate therapy. As little as a week, interruption of opiate treatment can deem a patient relatively naive to opiate therapy. Vital signs should be monitored every 4 h or continuously in high-risk patients similar to our case vignette (pulmonary cripples or OSA patients). Opiate reversal agents should be readily available. Patients and their families must be educated on the side effects prior to discharge.

Preservative-free ziconotide must be titrated slowly as well. As ziconotide is highly hydrophilic, it may take several days to take effect (3–9.5 days). The panel recommends a dose of <0.5 mcg/24 h and an incremental increase of <0.5 mcg/24 h weekly. A broad range of side effects have been reported including headaches, fever, asthenia, pain, nausea/vomiting, diarrhea, anorexia, dizziness, somnolence, confusion, ataxia, abnormal gait, memory problems, hypertonia, anxiety, speech disorders, aphasia, nystagmus, abnormal vision, psychosis, hallucinations, urinary retention, and dysesthesia. Patients are at an increased risk of falls as ziconotide can cause gait imbalance and ataxia. Given the multiple CNS effects, any patient with underlying psychiatric illness should be evaluated prior to initiating ziconotide. The CNS symptoms resolve upon discontinuation of the medication. No withdrawal symptoms have been noted with discontinuation of ziconotide.

31.4.1 Neuroendocrine Dysfunction

Long-term opiate therapy (systemic or intrathecal) may cause disturbances in neuroendocrine function and affect the hypothalamic-pituitary-adrenal/gonadal axis. Fifteen percent of patient treated with opiates develop central hypocorticism, and a similar percentage develops growth hormone deficiency. Additionally, opiate-treated patients may have slightly higher body fat and higher LDL cholesterol. Close follow-up with an endocrinologist is warranted.

31.4.2 Inflammatory Mass/Granuloma

Inflammatory masses are noninfectious reactions that usually occur at the tip of IDDS catheter and can cause neurological problems if they compress the spinal cord. One theory involves an inflammatory reaction to certain opiates which recruit lymphocytes and result in severe buildup of fibrous tissue [21]. Morphine is believed to be the primary trigger, with hydromorphone, baclofen, and fentanyl as less common culprits. Higher concentrations of injectate have been linked to the development of inflammatory masses. An expert panel recommended concentration of morphine and hydromorphone of <30 mg/mL. The use of adjuncts may reduce the opiate requirement and decrease the risk of inflammatory masses. Deer [21] obtained MRI on 208 consecutive patients and reported a 3% incidence of granuloma without neurological deficits. Hypervigilance is required, and patient should have routine history and neurological exams to ensure intact function.

The manufacturer reports an incidence of granuloma to be 0.49%, but the incidence is likely higher. Four hundred forty-eight cases of inflammatory masses have been reported between 1990 and 2007 with symptoms of inadequate pain relief (33.5%), pain (32.6%), and neurological dysfunction (17.4%) [22]. Higher concentrations of morphine and higher daily doses were associated with increased risk of granuloma formation. If an inflammatory mass is suspected, prompt evaluation is needed with a detailed history and physical exam, a T1-weighted MRI with gadolinium (with thin slices in the vicinity of the catheter tip), and a scout film prior to MRI. Keep in mind the magnetic field of the MRI temporarily suspends drug infusion and the IDDS will have to be interrogated after the MRI is complete. CT side port myelogram may also be helpful if MRI is contraindicated.

If neurological symptoms exist, the catheter must be explanted. However, in the absence of symptoms, the inflammatory mass may shrink with decreasing or discontinuing the opiate. Another option is to withdraw the catheter 2 cm from the mass which may stall the masses growth. Otherwise, the opiate should be removed from the IDDS and replaced with normal saline until the mass disappears.

31.5 Patient and Device Management

31.5.1 Managing Pump and Catheter-Related Complications

Mechanical pump malfunction is rare and has declined with each updated model of IDDS. One documented source of pump failure is corrosion from off-label compound use which can cause pump stalls. The Medtronic SynchroMed II pump has an overall failure rate of 2.4% at 78 months with morphine, baclofen, or ziconotide [1]. The rate increases to 7% when off-label medications are used. The device was designed with a 7-year hard shutoff.

Catheters are the most delicate component of the IDDS and may suffer damage or dislocation which can result in microfracture, leaks, disconnection, breakage, kinks, migration, occlusion, fibroma, or inflammatory mass. Patients with active lifestyles including excessive bending and twisted should be educated about the risk of catheter damage and dislodgement. Symptoms of catheter issues may be subtle, and patients usually complain of inadequate analgesia or withdrawal symptoms. Prager et al. [20] recommended a treatment algorithm for inadequate analgesia. See Fig. 31.4.

If a catheter issue is suspected, a simple plain X-ray may help identify the location of the catheter tip on anteroposterior and lateral films. Catheter fractures are likely to occur where the catheter enters the intraspinal ligament or in the pump pocket. If the pump has a catheter access port, the medication may be withdrawn. If 2–3 cc is readily aspirated, then the catheter is patent. However, if there is difficulty aspirating, then the tip may be partially occluded. A hole in the catheter will allow for CSF aspiration but not easily. Once the catheter medication is removed, contrast dye can be injected into the access port, and the catheter can be evaluated. *Never* inject dye into the access port if you cannot withdraw 1–2 cc first. This would give the patient a bolus of the medication and potentially cause respiratory depression or significant side effects [20]. Nuclear medicine evaluation using radiolabeled indium may also be utilized to evaluate a suspect catheter.

31.5.2 Pump Refill

Pocket fill can occur if the injectate (intended for the pump) is accidentally placed subcutaneously. Three hundred fifty-one accidents were reported between 1996 and 2010 (1/10,000 refills according to the manufacturer) [20] which resulted in eight deaths and 270 interventions for serious or life-threatening injury. No consequences occurred in 58 patients. Such accidents will cause overdosing either immediately or in several hours. Underdosing will be apparent within days to weeks as the pump is empty and the patient will develop symptoms of withdrawl. Patients may sometimes notice a fluid collection around the pump site or complain of a burning or stinging sensation. However, they may not have any symptoms at all. Care must be taken to aspirate the medication frequently from the pump during a refill to ensure that the needle is still in the pump. Any volume discrepancy should be investigated, and the patient should be admitted for observation if a pocket fill is suspected. Overall, patient should be observed for 30 min after a pump refill. Prager et al. [20] composed a morphine intrathecal/epidural overdose emergency procedure. Please see Fig. 31.5 [20].

Key Points

- The FDA has approved preservative-free morphine, baclofen, and ziconotide for IDDS.
- Intrathecal morphine has inconsistently provided pain relief for cancer and noncancer patient. Clinicians have supplement infusions with adjuncts to improve pain control. An advisory panel convened and composed an algorithm to assist clinicians in managing pain when certain medications fail to control chronic pain. Please see Figs. 31.1, 31.2, and 31.3.
- While many medications have promising data in animal models and some human subjects, more studies are required to fully elucidate their efficacy and safety in managing chronic pain.

Fig. 31.4 Conceptual framework for diagnosing and managing inadequate analgesia [20]

History:

- If original presenting pain condition has worsened: neurologic changes?
- If new pain: what is quality, intensity, location?
- Do medication adjustments improve or not improve pain?
- In what dermatome is catheter tip located?
- History of pump regarding accuracy of medication remaining?

Physical:

- Neurological exam at presumed catheter tip location and at pain location: evaluate gait, balance, and sensory changes.
- Mental status: Is patient sedated? Cognitively intact? Agitated? Having hallucinations?

Pump:

- Can CSF be withdrawn through the catheter access port?
- Is a bolus dose effective?
- Is bolus painful?
- Are there any volume discrepancies?

Drug:

- Is the medication in the pump?
- Is refill medication as ordered?
- Have medications been administered within the stability specifications?
- Consider possibility of diversion of pump medications.

Radiologic work-up:

- Catheter tip location: has the location shifted? Catheter location to be used to determine location for thin slice study: see below
- Is there pain with the contrast injection
- Imaging study in reservoir vs. catheter
- T1 MRI with gadolinium (thin slice) or CT myelogram to rule out inflammatory mass
- Consider MRI/CT to evaluate new pain location and dermatome level if granuloma workup Is negative
- Does pump rotor work (movement can be visualized with CT)

- A cluster of patients died within 24 h of IDDS implant which triggered an evaluation of mortality associated with IDDS. Coffey et al. cited respiratory arrest related to opiate infusion as the culprit.
- Prager et al. composed the "Best Practices for Intrathecal Drug Delivery for Pain" in 2013 which systematically identifies areas of improvement in patient care.
  - Patients need medical optimization prior to IDDS trial/implant. Some patients require psychological testing.
  - Systemic opiates need to be weaned completely or at least reduced by 50% prior to an IDDS trial. Hypervigilance is essential in patient with PCAs and IDDS.
  - Respiratory depression is the primary safety concern with IDDS. A thorough review of the patient's medication list is essential. Every effort should be made to minimize the consumption of CNS depressant medications in combination with IDDS.
  - Overnight observation for intrathecal opiate trials is recommended. No particular trial technique or venue is suggested.
  - Oral or transdermal drug conversion to intrathecal doses can be very challenging as patients respond very differently to varying doses. The panel recommends starting at a low dose and escalating slowly (<20% of the daily dose at a time) with monitoring.
  - Ziconotide must be titrated slowly to minimized CNS side effects.
  - At each visit, clinicians should evaluate changes in the patient's pain, functional capacity, and neurological function. A thorough history and physical exam are critical to rule out inflammatory masses/granulomas. If a granuloma is suspected, prompt evaluation with an MRI is indicated.
  - Catheters are the most fragile component of the IDDS and may occlude, break, disconnect, migrate, or leak. Care must be taken to aspirate from the pump access port prior to injecting contrast as this will give the patient a bolus of intrathecal medication.
  - Pocket fill occurs in 1/10,000 pump refills and may cause immediate or delayed respiratory depression. If pocket fill is suspected or there is any volume discrepancy associated with at pump refill, the patient should be admitted for observation.

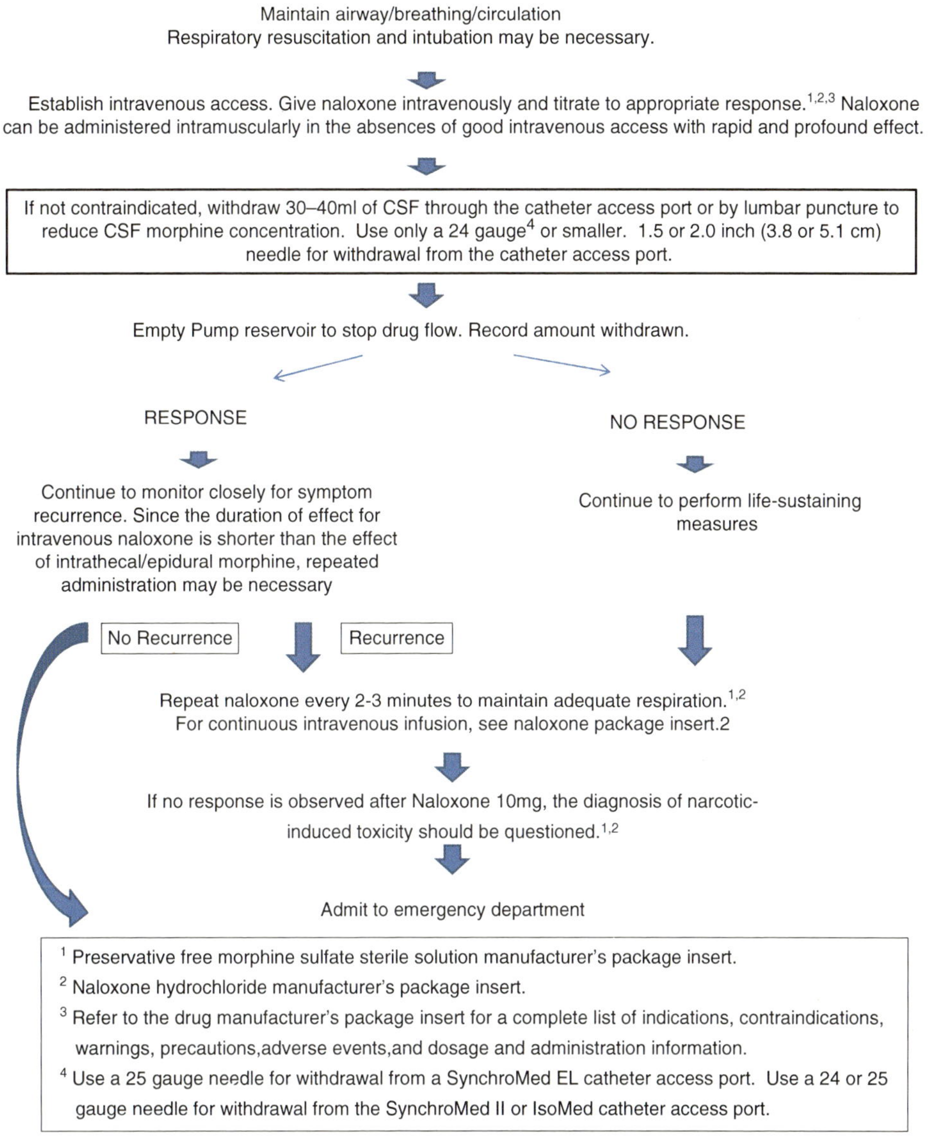

Fig. 31.5 Morphine intrathecal/epidural overdose emergency procedure. CSF, cerebrospinal fluid

References

1. Medtronic marketing data. Minneapolis, MN: Medtronic; 2013.
2. Hayek SM, Deer TR, Pope JE, Panchal SJ, Patel V. Intrathecal therapy for cancer and non-cancer pain. Pain Physician. 2011;14:219–48.
3. Eisenach JC, Hood DD, Curry R. Intrathecal but not intravenous opioids release adenosine from the spinal cord. Pain. 2004;5:64–8.
4. Bernards CM. Cerebrospinal fluid and spinal cord distribution of baclofen and bupivacaine during slow intrathecal infusion in pigs. Anesthesiology. 2006;105:169–78.
5. Smith TJ, Staats PS, Deer T. Randomized clinical trial of an implantable drug delivery system compared with comprehensive medical management for refractory cancer pain: impact on pain, drug-related toxicity, and survival. J Clin Oncol. 2002;18:4040–9.
6. Deer T, Chapple I, Classen A, Javery K, Stoker V, Tonder L, Burchiel K. Intrathecal drug delivery for treatment of chronic low back pain: report from the national outcomes registry for low back pain. Pain Med. 2004;5:6–13.
7. Bennett G, Burchiel K, Buchser E, Classen A, Deer T, DuPen S, Ferrante M, Hassenbusch S, Lou L, Maeyaert J, Penn R, Portenoy R, Rauck R, Serafini M, Willis D, Yaksh T. Clinical guidelines for intraspinal infusion: a report of an expert panel. PolyAnalgesic consensus conference 2000. J Pain Symptom Manag. 2000;20:S37–43.
8. Hassenbusch SJ, Portenoy RK, Cousins M, Buchser E, Deer TR, DuPen SL, Eisenach J, Follett KA, Hildebrand KR, Krames ES, Levy RM, Palmer PP, Rathmel JP, Rauck RL, Staats PS, Stearns L, Willis KD. Polyanalgesic consensus conference 2003: an update on the management of pain by intraspinal drug delivery-report of an expert panel. J Pain Symptom Manag. 2004;27(6):540–63.
9. Deer TR, Levy R, Prager J, Buchser E, Burton A, Caraway D, Cousins M, DeAndres J, Sudhir D, Erdek M, Grigsby E, Hutoon M, Jacobs M, Kim P, Kumar K, Leong M, Liem L, McDowell GC, Panchal S, Rauck R, Saulino M, Sitzman BT, Staats P, Staton-Hicks M, Stears L, Wallace M, Willis KD, Witt W, Yaksh T, Mekhail N. Polyanalgesic consensus conference-2012: recommendations to reduce morbidity and mortality in intrathecal drug delivery in the treatment of chronic pain. Neuromodulation. 2012;15:467–82.
10. Dahm P, Lundborg C, Janson M, Olegard C, Nitescu P. Comparison of 0.5% intrathecal bupivacaine with 0.5% intrathecal ropivacaine

in the treatment of refractory cancer and noncancer pain conditions: results from a prospective, crossover, double-blind, randomized study. Reg Anesth Med. 2000;25:480–7.

11. Staats P, Yearwood T, Charapata SG, Presley RW, Wallace MS, Byas-Smith M, Fisher R, Bryce DA, Mangieri EA, Luther RR, May M, McGuire D, Ellis D. Intrathecal ziconotide in the treatment of refractory pain in patients with cancer or AIDS: a randomized controlled trial. JAMA. 2004;291:63–70.
12. Mironer YE, Grumman S. Experience with alternative solutions in intrathecal treatment of chronic nonmalignant pain. Pain Digest. 1999;9:299–302.
13. Mironer YE, Tollison CD. Methadone in the intrathecal treatment of chronic nonmalignant pain resistant to other neuro- axial agents: the first experience. Neuromodulation. 2001;4:25–31.
14. Hassenbusch SJ, Gunes S, Wachsman S, Willis D. Intrathecal clonidine in the treatment of intractable pain: a phase I/II study. Pain Med. 2002;3:85–91.
15. Ackerman LL, Follett KA, Rosenquist RW. Long-term outcomes during treatment of chronic pain with intrathecal clonidine or clonidine/opioid combinations. J Pain Symptom Manag. 2003;26:668–77.
16. Kroin JS, McCarthy RJ, Penn RD, Lubenow TJ, Ivankovich AD. Intrathecal clonidine and tizanidine in conscious dogs: comparison of analgesic and hemodynamic effects. Anesth Analg. 1996;82:627–35.
17. Deer TR, Penn R, Kim CK, Bowman RG, Norris M, Stewart CD, Garten TG, Tolentino W, Khan Y. The use of continuous intrathecal infusion of octreotide in patients with chronic pain of noncancer origin: an evaluation of efficacy in a prospective double blind fashion. Neuromodulation. 2006;8:284–9.
18. Wallin J, Cui JG, Yakhnitsa V, Schechtmann G, Meyerson B, Linderoth B. Gabapentin and pregabalin suppress tactile allodynia and potentiate spinal cord stimulation in a model of neuropathy. Eur J Pain. 2002;6:261–72.
19. Coffey RJ, Owens ML, Broste SK, Dubois MY, Ferrante FM, Schultz DM, Stearns LJ, Turner MS. Mortality associated with implantation and management of intrathecal opioid drug infusion systems to treat non-cancer pain. Anesthesiology. 2009;111:881–91.
20. Prager J, Deer T, Levy R, Bruel B, Buchser E, Caraway D, Cousins M, Jacobs M, McGlothen G, Rauck R, Staats P, Steans L. Best practices for intrathecal drug delivery for pain. Neuromodulation. 2014;17:354–72.
21. Deer T. A prospective analysis of intrathecal granuloma in chronic pain patients: a review of the literature and report of a surveillance study. Pain Physician. 2004;7:225–8.
22. Yaksh TL, Horais KA, Tozier NA. Chronically infused intrathecal morphine in dogs. Anesthesiology. 2003;99:174–87.

32 Intrathecal Medication Withdrawal

Kristen Noon, Mark Wallace, and Timothy Furnish

32.1 Case Description

The patient is a 52-year-old female with a history of post-laminectomy pain syndrome. She has had a 40 mL Medtronic intrathecal drug delivery system device implanted 5 years ago that is nearing the estimated replacement interval known as "end of life." The patient had stable pain control over the past few years. Her past medical history is significant for diabetes mellitus type 2, hypertension, and COPD. The pump solution (hydromorphone 3 mg/mL, bupivacaine 8 mg/mL, ziconotide 11 mcg/mL, and fentanyl 100 mcg/mL) is delivering 1.5 mg per day of hydromorphone (main analgesic) as a simple continuous infusion. A Personal Therapy Manager (PTM) bolus of 0.15 mg can also be delivered as needed with a lockout interval of 4 h. The total daily hydromorphone dose range is 1.5–2.4 mg depending on PTM usage. In addition to the intrathecal analgesics, patient's oral medications include gabapentin 900 mg three times per day and cyclobenzaprine 10 mg zero to two times per day as needed.

The patient underwent a routine pump refill and interrogation. As the intrathecal device readout suggested hardware "end of life," a side port aspiration took place also during her visit. The side port was accessed in order to test catheter integrity in preparation for pump replacement scheduled in a few months. Per chart review, the catheter side port revealed free flow of cerebrospinal fluid (CSF). After the visit, the patient noticed increased pain and nausea starting the next morning following her pump refill. This progressed to diarrhea and irritability over the course of the day. She initially attributed this to a viral illness as her husband recently recovered from a cold. The symptoms worsened by day two, and she presented to the emergency room for evaluation.

K. Noon, M.D. • M. Wallace, M.D. • T. Furnish, M.D. (✉)
Department of Anesthesiology, University of California, San Diego, La Jolla, CA, USA
e-mail: tfurnish@ucsd.edu

In the emergency room, the patient presented with diaphoresis, tachycardia, hypertension, and complaints of diarrhea, nausea, and pain. Her vital signs were HR 107, BP 152/93, RR 24, and temp 36.9C, and her pain score was 7/10 (baseline score of 5/10). Pupils were dilated at 6 mm, equal and reactive to light. The pump pocket site was non-tender, without erythema or swelling.

Interrogation of the pump showed no error messages and the pump was correctly programed with the documented refill drugs and infusion rates. In the emergency room, the refill port was easily accessed, and 39 mL of medication was withdrawn and then replaced into the pump reservoir. This volume was consistent with expected reservoir volume. Next, the pump side port was accessed, but aspiration failed to produce free flow of cerebrospinal fluid.

The patient's symptoms of opioid withdrawal were treated with intravenous and oral opioids. The pump reservoir was emptied and a sample of the contents was sent for mass spectroscopy evaluation. The reservoir was filled with saline and run for 30 h to clear the internal tubing and catheter of residual drug. The patient was then taken to the fluoroscopy suite and the side port was accessed again. Contrast was injected under continuous fluoroscopy in both an AP and lateral projection. No filling of the intrathecal space was visualized. Contrast extravasation into the pump pocket was seen. The patient was scheduled for operative exploration of the pump pocket. Upon opening the pocket in the operating room, the catheter was connected to the pump but appeared partially severed just medial to the side port suggestive of needle trauma.

32.2 Case Discussion

This case demonstrates the complex clinical presentation of withdrawal from intrathecal medications. The first step is to correctly diagnose the patient with drug withdrawal based on clinical signs and symptoms. Initially, withdrawal from

M. Anitescu et al. (eds.), *Challenging Cases and Complication Management in Pain Medicine*,
https://doi.org/10.1007/978-3-319-60072-7_32

intrathecal opioids or baclofen may present with constitutional or gastrointestinal symptoms that can be misconstrued and delay correct diagnosis. In this case, the patient presented with many symptoms consistent with opioid withdrawal including increased pain, gastrointestinal upset, diaphoresis, pupillary dilation, and autonomic hyperactivity including tachycardia and hypertension.

An excellent history of the pump placement/analysis and intrathecal drug delivery therapy is necessary to discern if any recent changes to the pump, medications, or catheter have occurred. This patient had a recent pump refill with side port aspiration, and her pump was nearing the end of its battery life. A pump refill can lead to such complications such as a pocket fill, pump programming error, or drug mixing error. In this case, the skin overlying the pump did not appear edematous lowering the likelihood of pocket fill although not all pocket fills present in this manner. There was also no overlying erythema or tenderness at the site to suggest an acute infection or inflammatory process. Interrogating the intrathecal pump again can easily recognize a pump programming error. Internal programing consistent with the charted drugs and doses rules out a simple programing error. A drug mixing error could also occur. Confirmation of this is accomplished by mass spectroscopy analysis of the pump reservoir contents. Unfortunately, results from such tests may take several days, thus limiting the clinical utility. The catheter can become damaged during a refill or side port aspiration by the needle, as occurred in the case above. Finally, after 4–7 years, an intrathecal battery can fail leading to intrathecal pump stall and subsequent acute withdrawal symptoms (Fig. 32.1).

32.3 Intrathecal Withdrawal

There are only three drugs that are FDA approved for intrathecal delivery: morphine, baclofen, and ziconotide. There is no recognized withdrawal syndrome associated with ziconotide. Withdrawal from intrathecally administered opioids presents in a similar fashion as other routes of opioid administration; however, the time course may differ. The sudden halting of intrathecal baclofen administration can result in a severe withdrawal syndrome that may be much worse than seen with halting oral administration. Intrathecal baclofen withdrawal could potentially be life-threatening. In addition to these three FDA-approved drugs, there are a number of other agents that have been routinely used off-label in intrathecal pumps. These medications include the opioids hydromorphone, sufentanil, and fentanyl as well as adjuvant analgesics bupivacaine and clonidine. There is no withdrawal from bupivacaine. Clonidine withdrawal presents as hypertension and tachycardia and can be severe.

32.4 Drug Mixing Error

Any new symptoms, including signs of withdrawal, which occur shortly after a pump refill, should raise concern for a possible drug mixing error. This risk is potentially higher in patients whose intrathecal medication is compounded. Patients on simple regimens of morphine or baclofen at standard premixed concentrations do not require compounding but could have the wrong drug placed into their pump. Compounding of intrathecal medications is the added step of a pharmacist producing a special formulation of multiple drugs and/or nonstandard concentrations for a single patient. Many physicians will mix multiple drugs together for infusion intrathecally, thus requiring a compounding pharmacy. Additionally, those patients who require nonstandard drug concentrations also must have the drugs produced by a compounding pharmacist. Errors in mixing these compounded solutions could result in either overdose or underdose and withdrawal.

When a drug mixing error is suspected as a potential cause of intrathecal withdrawal, the first step is to replace the reservoir volume of drug with a new mixture.

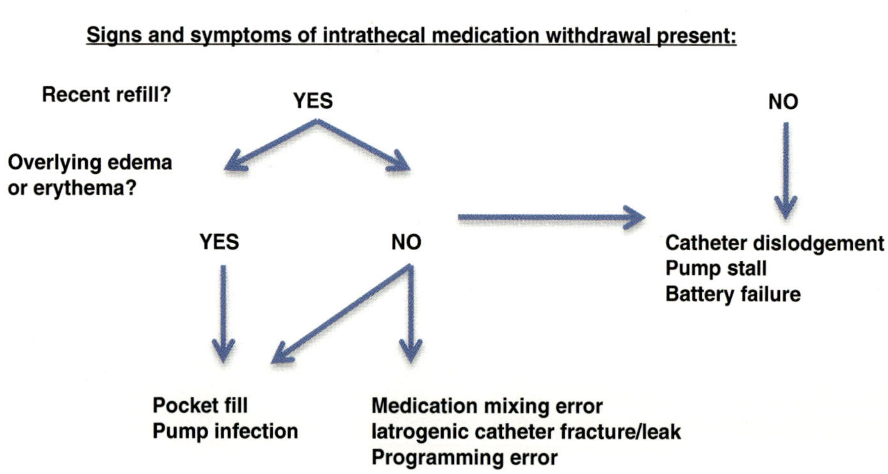

Fig. 32.1 Clinical decision tree to assess etiology of symptoms of intrathecal medication withdrawal

After removing the previous solution, it may be worth sending a sample for analysis by mass spectroscopy to determine the drugs and concentrations present in the solution. This may not always be feasible though as this is often a costly test that may take several days to receive results. Replacing the drug in the pump reservoir does not remove and replace the volume of drug in the internal tubing of the pump. As a result, it will take time for the new medication to be pumped through the tubing and catheter into to the cerebrospinal fluid. However, drug diffusion and mixing between the reservoir and catheter will rapidly equilibrate the concentration resulting in a near-normal drug dose delivery.

32.5 Pocket Fill

A "pocket fill" is the inadvertent injection of medication into the pocket or space surrounding the intrathecal pump, instead of into the pump reservoir. A pocket fill can occur if the needle is not inserted through the refill port septum until it has reached the needle stop at the back wall of the reservoir. Tactile feedback is paramount to a correctly performed refill. Without this feedback, a clinician may not realize that the needle is incorrectly positioned [1]. Properly placed needles can also inadvertently be withdrawn from the reservoir after correct placement and before drug is injected. In either case, the injected medication would either be delivered into the subcutaneous tissue around the pump pocket or within the pump pocket instead of the pump reservoir [1].

Patients with a pocket fill can show symptoms of either an overdose or underdose. An overdose usually presents quickly in a matter of minutes to hours [1]. Low-concentration intrathecal drugs are more likely to result in underdose instead of overdose. For instance, 20 mL of baclofen 500 mcg/mL injected into a pump pocket would result in systemic delivery of only 10 mg of baclofen. Similarly, 20 mL of morphine 0.5 mg/mL would result in a systemic dose of morphine of just 10 mg. An underdose can become clinically significant if a pocket fill goes unrecognized and the pump empties sooner than anticipated [1]. This interruption of therapy usually presents in several days to weeks [1]. An underdose may also present as an escalation of the primary pain complaint or withdrawal symptoms related to the pump medications [1]. However, if high concentrations of drug are used, symptoms of overdose usually occur rapidly. For instance, 40 mL of morphine 20 mg/mL would result in a systemic dose of 800 mg, which can be lethal if appropriate life support measures are not in place.

In data collected from May 1996 to September 2010, Medtronic received 351 reports worldwide related to occurrence of pocket fills with their intrathecal infusion pumps [1]. Assuming pumps are refilled six times per year on average, the reported rate of occurrence per refill opportunity is about 0.01% although the actual occurrence rate is likely higher due to underreporting [1]. Of the reported events, there have been 8 deaths, 270 events requiring medical intervention, and 58 events not requiring medical intervention [1]. There were 15 events in which the patient severity was unknown [1].

If a pocket fill occurs and is recognized, the pump pocket should be accessed with a large bore needle and attempts made to remove as much of the contents as possible. If available, ultrasound can be used to identify the fluid pocket to aspirate. The patient should be monitored for signs and symptoms of medication overdose in an appropriate facility for a reasonable amount of time or until symptoms have resolved. If a pocket fill is suspected, it may be useful to empty the pump reservoir completely and compare the volume removed to the expected volume. A discrepancy may indicate that a pocket fill has occurred [1]. Swelling at the injection site or patient report of an unusual sensation during drug injection such as pressure, stinging, or burning may also indicate the presence of a pocket fill although their absence do not rule out the occurrence of a pocket fill [1].

32.6 Pump Stall

Although a spontaneous pump stall is possible, the most common time for a pump to stall is during an MRI. Medtronic intrathecal drug delivery systems are driven by a peristaltic rotor. The rotor will stop due to the magnetic fields of the MRI scanner [2]. The pump should restart spontaneously after MRI has ended, but a permanent stall is possible. There are other pumps on the market with different mechanisms less susceptible to an MRI-related pump stall, but the number in service is substantially smaller than for the Medtronic systems [2]. Medtronic recommends that a pump should be interrogated after an MRI to determine whether the pump has resumed function [2]. The event log should show messages indicating that a motor stall and subsequent motor recovery have occurred [2]. If a recovery has not occurred, the patient is at risk for a withdrawal syndrome related to intrathecal medications, especially baclofen [2]. If a stall is identified, wait another 20 min and interrogate the pump again to address delays in event logging due to electromagnetic interference from the MRI [2]. The device representative should be contacted if the pump has not restarted at this point, and care should be taken to prevent withdrawal symptoms [2]. More information regarding pump stall can be found in the chapter entitled, "Intrathecal Pump Malfunction: Stall, Flip, Expired."

32.7 Pump Programming Error

Errors in intrathecal pump programming can occur which could result in either overdose or underdose. This may be due to incorrectly programming the concentration of the medications placed into the pump. Programming errors can also occur when entering the daily infusion dose of medication to be delivered. Changes from the previous pump settings will result in a warning if the programmed dose to be delivered is either higher or lower. Rechecking the intended settings and comparing them to doses and concentrations recorded in the patient's chart will quickly determine if this is a potential cause of withdrawal.

32.8 Catheter Fracture/Leak

Catheter fracture or leak may occur due to trauma. Trauma can occur with pulling or sheering of the catheter, repetitive motion damage, pump flip in the pocket, or needle trauma to the catheter during refill or side port aspiration. Such damage may present clinically as worsening of the primary pain complaint, cerebrospinal fluid leak including symptoms of low-pressure CSF headache, or withdrawal from intrathecal pump medications. Medtronic followed intrathecal catheters from 2003 to 2014 via a registry. Of the 7154 catheters followed in the registry, 161 catheters showed evidence of a break or a cut [3].

The first step in assessing for a catheter complication is to aspirate the side port of the intrathecal pump. If CSF can be freely aspirated, then contrast may be injected under fluoroscopy. Never inject through the side port if CSF cannot be freely aspirated. To do so may result in bolus intrathecal administration of residual drug in the catheter. Tracing contrast injected through the catheter from the pump into the intrathecal space may identify a leak of contrast or failure to deliver contrast to the subarachnoid space [4] (Fig. 32.2).

If CSF cannot be aspirated via the side port, the pump reservoir should be emptied of drug and filled with saline. The catheter must then be cleared of residual drug at the current infusion rate in order to prevent inadvertent bolus injection of drug before injection of any contrast [4]. After fluoroscopic evaluation of the contrast injection, a CT myelogram (Fig. 32.3) can be performed to help identify the location of a leak (Fig. 32.4), verify intrathecal contrast spread, or identify the formation of a granuloma at the catheter tip [4].

32.9 Catheter Dislodgement

Catheter migration is the most common catheter-related complication. Like catheter fracture, catheter dislodgement can present clinically as withdrawal from intrathecal pump medications. Most often, dislodgement occurs due to the

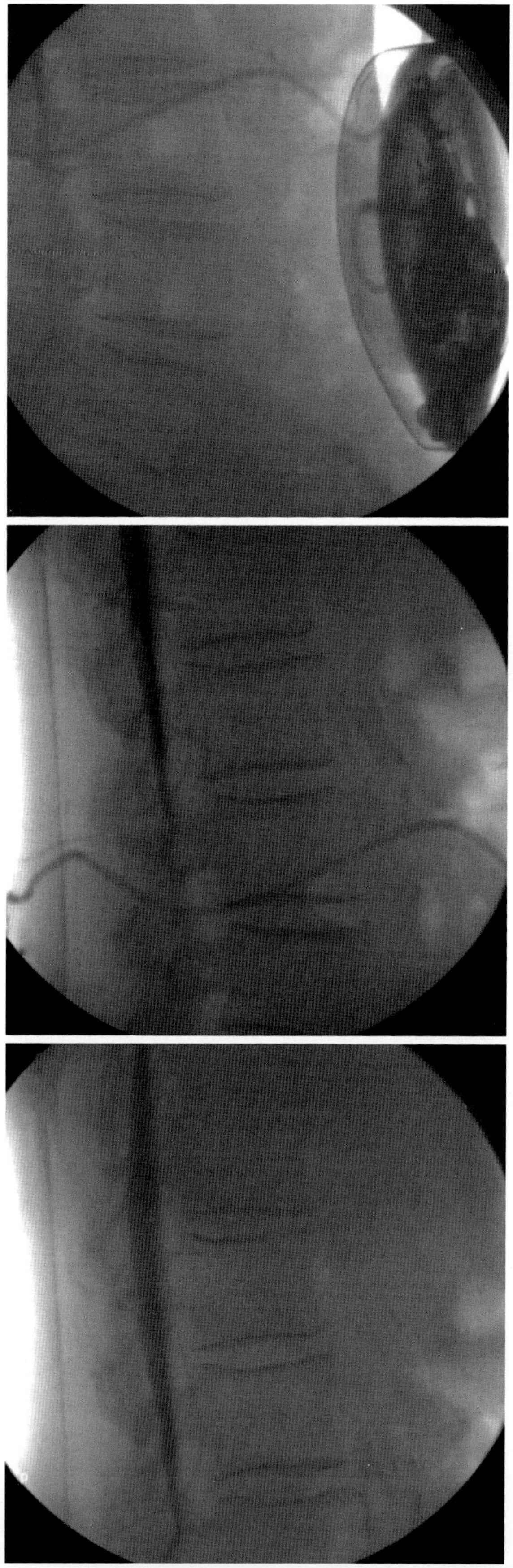

Fig. 32.2 Lateral fluoroscopic view of normal contrast dye study showing dye spread from intrathecal pump to catheter to intrathecal space

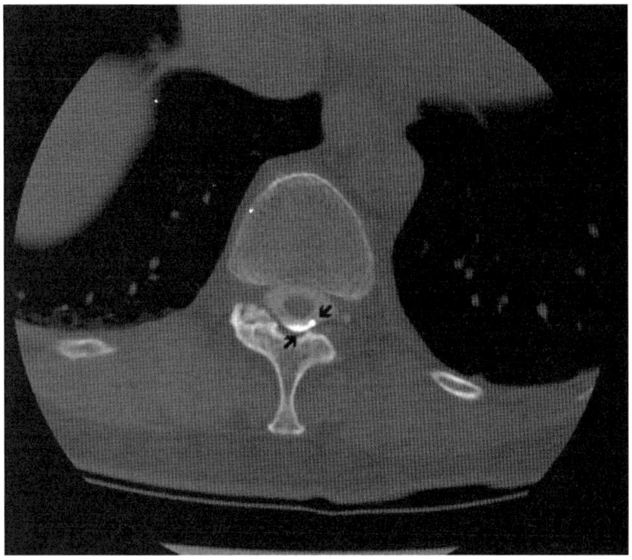

Fig. 32.3 CT myelogram showing normal extravasation of contrast from tip of intrathecal catheter into intrathecal space

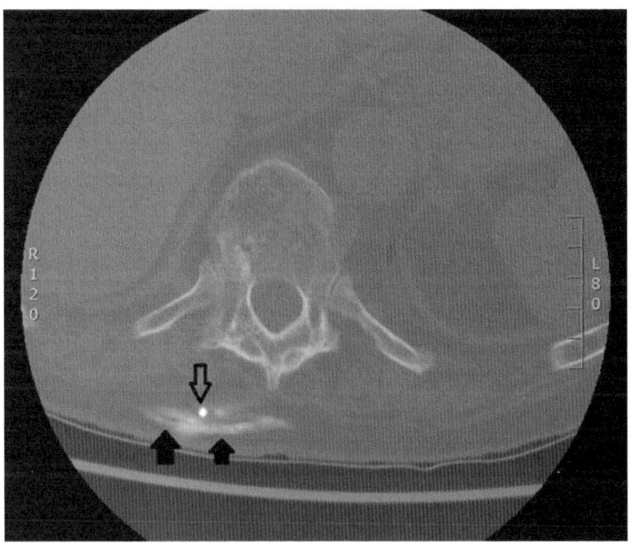

Fig. 32.4 CT myelogram showing extravasation of contrast (dark arrows) from fractured intrathecal catheter (empty arrow) into subcutaneous space

failure to adequately anchor the intrathecal catheter to underlying fascia [5]. In Medtronic's study of their one-piece catheter system, 209 patients were followed at 22 centers after implant. Catheter dislodgment/migration sufficient to interrupt drug delivery occurred in 12 cases, 10 of which were interpreted as procedure-related complications. In 6 of the 10, the catheter had not been anchored at implant. Overall, 206 of 222 implanted catheters were anchored, 6 of 222 or 2.9% of which became dislodged or migrated. In contrast, migration occurred in 6 of 13 or 46.2% of catheters that were not anchored [5]. In Medtronic's multiyear pump registry, 7154 catheters were followed and 225 of them became dislodged [3].

Assessment of catheter dislodgement is the same as for catheter fracture or leak. A side port aspiration and then dye study is necessary to determine the location and patency of the catheter.

32.10 Opioid Withdrawal Syndrome and Treatment

Opioid withdrawal, while uncomfortable and distressing to the patient, is generally not considered dangerous. Often patients will experience a rebound in their underlying pain. Common symptoms often include rhinorrhea, yawning, sweating, lacrimation, piloerection, tremors, hot and cold flashes, restlessness, vomiting, abdominal cramps, and anxiety [6]. These symptoms may be assessed using the Objective Opiate Withdrawal Scale (OOWS), which assigns points based on whether symptoms are present during a 10 min observation period [6].

Withdrawal symptoms are often managed with oral opioids as well as nonopioid adjunct agents such as clonidine, NSAIDS, loperamide, or antihistamines. Clonidine (0.1 mg PO BID) is especially useful in relieving autonomic symptoms related to opioid withdrawal. In starting oral opioids to treat intrathecal withdrawal, one should be careful to not attempt a direct conversion of the intrathecal opioid dose to an oral equivalent. Rather, it would be more judicious to start the patient on a much lower dose of oral short- and/or long-acting opioid and then titrate to effect.

Opioid withdrawal can present not only with the abrupt cessation of intrathecal opioid treatment but also when switching from one type of intrathecal opioid to another. Severe withdrawal symptoms have been observed upon switching from hydrophilic opioids such as morphine and hydromorphone to the lipophilic opioid fentanyl. This may be due to the differences in CSF spread of lipophilic versus hydrophilic drugs. Instead of an abrupt switch, it is recommended to taper intrathecal morphine while concurrently titrating fentanyl over the course of days to weeks. This may help to avoid unpleasant opioid withdrawal symptoms.

32.11 Baclofen Withdrawal Syndrome and Treatment

Baclofen withdrawal is potentially life-threatening and must be treated as a medical emergency. There have been many reported complications resulting from baclofen withdrawal including seizures [7], hallucinations [7], psychosis [8, 9], visual disturbances [8], dyskinesia [9], increased spasms [10], and hyperthermia [10]. Symptoms may progress to severe hyperthermia, rhabdomyolysis, and hypotension along with organ system failure [11]. Symptoms of central nervous system hyperexcitability may occur because chronic intrathecal baclofen infusions downregulate GABA-B receptor sensitivity [12, 13].

Sudden withdrawal of baclofen may be associated with rebound excitation neuraxially that may not be overcome by administration of small doses of oral or intrathecal baclofen or other GABA agonists [12, 14].

All patients who receive intrathecal baclofen (ITB) are at risk of underdose, or withdrawal and care should be taken to educate staff, patients, and families on the signs and symptoms of baclofen withdrawal [15]. Treatment of intrathecal baclofen withdrawal may require observation and management in a hospital setting depending on the severity and intrathecal dose [15].

The first-line treatment for intrathecal baclofen withdrawal is to restart the intrathecal pump as soon as possible [15]. If this is not immediately possible, start treatment with GABAergic agonist drugs such as oral baclofen. Additionally oral or intravenous benzodiazepines may be used [15]. Some literature has reported on the use of dantrolene and cyproheptadine as adjuncts to ITB withdrawal, but evidence is limited and consists mostly of case reports and case series.

In one published case report, dantrolene was used successfully in the care of a patient exhibiting intrathecal baclofen withdrawal resistant to oral baclofen [16]. Dantrolene has no known GABAergic effect. The clinical improvement was likely due to disassociation of the excitation-contraction coupling effect of dantrolene and suppression of the thermogenesis effect of repeated muscle contraction [16].

In a small case series, the potent serotonin antagonist cyproheptadine was used in the treatment of acute intrathecal baclofen withdrawal [17]. The rationale for treatment with cyproheptadine centers on the idea that ITB withdrawal is actually a form of serotonin syndrome. Serotonin syndrome is thought to arise from a long-term inhibition of serotonin release in the brainstem via GABA-B receptors with chronic ITB administration. When ITB stops abruptly, excessive serotonin can be released leading to serotonin syndrome [17]. Coinciding with this theory is the observation that ITB withdrawal syndrome tends to be more severe for those patients treated with ITB for several years [17]. In this small case series, cyproheptadine provided immediate relief from pruritus and a dramatic drop in fever, pulse, and temperature that appeared to depend directly on the timing of the medication [17]. In this study, 8 mg of oral cyproheptadine was given every 6 h for severe ITB withdrawal [17]. The study authors recommend starting cyproheptadine within 48 h of suspected ITB withdrawal to attenuate symptoms [17].

The initial presentation of acute opioid and baclofen withdrawal may appear similar [18]. Withdrawal of opioids or baclofen can both cause agitation, anxiety, muscle aches, nausea, and vomiting [18]. For those with both drugs infusing via an intrathecal pump, the differential must include consideration of both withdrawal syndromes [18].

32.12 Clonidine Withdrawal Syndrome and Treatment

Withdrawal from intrathecal clonidine, like baclofen, can be serious and even fatal. Clonidine withdrawal can present with acute hypertensive crisis and associated cardiac sequela. A published case report discusses an instance of stress-induced cardiomyopathy after acute intrathecal clonidine withdrawal in a 47-year-old man with low back pain. In this case, the patient was treated with clonidine for many years via intrathecal pump (550 mcg/24 h) [19]. The patient exhibited dangerously elevated blood pressures, chest pain, tachycardia, and dyspnea with pulmonary edema that eventually resolved over 3 days with repeated IV clonidine boluses and infusion, glyceryl trinitrate infusion, positive pressure ventilation, and intravenous benzodiazepines [19].

Patients with symptoms of clonidine withdrawal should be admitted to a high level of care unit within an intensive care unit where intravenous clonidine and other supportive therapies can be initiated for hemodynamic control. One should consider testing cardiac enzymes, EKG, and echocardiography in these patients. It is not known if there is any specific intrathecal clonidine dose threshold above which severe withdrawal symptoms can present.

Key Concepts

- Errors may occur in medication mixing, filling an intrathecal pump (pocket fill), or while programming an intrathecal pump which may lead to symptoms of underdose or overdose of intrathecal medications.
- MRI is an expected cause of temporary intrathecal pump stall although permanent pump stall is possible. Pumps should be interrogated after MRI to confirm that pump has begun working again.
- Catheter fractures and dislodgement are common causes of pump malfunction and may present as worsening pain symptoms, CSF leak, or withdrawal syndromes.
- Catheter dislodgment and migration is the most common catheter-related complication and is most likely due to poor anchoring to underlying fascia.
- Side port aspiration, catheter contrast dye studies, and CT myelograms can be utilized to work up catheter-related complications.
- Do NOT inject through the side port if CSF cannot be freely aspirated first.
- Opioid withdrawal is unpleasant but generally not considered dangerous. Patients should be treated symptomatically with clonidine, NSAIDS, antidiarrheals, or antihistamines.
- Baclofen withdrawal is potentially life-threatening and requires quick diagnosis and treatment. Intrathecal baclofen at previously therapeutic dose should be resumed as soon as possible. Oral or IV GABAergic medications

such as baclofen or benzodiazepines should be started if it is not possible to restart intrathecal baclofen.

- Clonidine withdrawal is potentially fatal and may present as hypertensive crisis with cardiac sequelae. Patient should be admitted to the intensive care unit for blood pressure control with intravenous clonidine. Clinicians should also consider performing a thorough cardiac workup such as cardiac enzymes, EKG, and echocardiogram.

References

1. https://professional.medtronic.com/wcm/groups/mdtcom_sg/@mdt/@neuro/documents/documents/hcp-pocket-refill.pdf
2. https://professional.medtronic.com/pt/neuro/itb/fpi/mri-guidelines/index.htm?fgm=mri:refillkit#.VlaMXHarTIU
3. https://professional.medtronic.com/ppr/intrathecal-drug-delivery-systems/index.htm#.VlaARHarTIU
4. Furnish TJ, Wallace MS. Intrathecal drug delivery: patient selection, trialing, and implantation. In: Benzon HT, editor. Practical management of pain. 5th ed. Philadelphia: Elsevier; 2014. p. 953–65.
5. Follett K, Naumann C. A prospective study of catheter- related complications of intrathecal drug delivery systems. J Pain Symptom Manag. 2000;19(3):209–15.
6. Benzon H. Essentials of pain medicine. 3rd ed. St. Louis: Elsevier/Saunders; 2011.
7. Terrence CF, Fromm GH. Complications of baclofen withdrawal. Arch Neurol. 1981;38:588–9.
8. Rivas DA, Chancellor MB, Hill K, Freedman MK. Neurological manifestations of baclofen withdrawal. J Urol. 1993;150:1903–5.
9. Kirubakaran V, Mayfield D, Rengarchary S. Dyskinesia and psychosis in a patient following baclofen withdrawal. Am J Psychiatry. 1984;141:692–3.
10. Mandac BR, Hurvitz EA, Nelson VS. Hyperthermia associated with baclofen withdrawal and increased spasticity. Arch Phys Med Rehabil. 1993;74:96–7.
11. Green LB, Nelson VS. Death after acute withdrawal of intrathecal baclofen: case report and literature review. Arch Phys Med Rehabil. 1999;80:1600–4.
12. Coffey RJ, Edgar TS, Francisco GE, Graziani V, Meythaler JM, Ridgely PM, Sadiq SA, Turner MS. Abrupt withdrawal from intrathecal baclofen: recognition and management of a potentially life-threatening syndrome. Arch Phys Med Rehabil. 2002;83:735–41.
13. Kroin JS, Bianchi GD, Penn RD. Intrathecal baclofen down-regulates GABA-B receptors in the rat substantia gelatinosa. J Neurosurg. 1993;79:544–9.
14. Samson-Fang L, Gooch C. Intrathecal baclofen withdrawal simulating neuroleptic malignant syndrome in child with cerebral palsy. Dev Med Child Neurol. 2000;42:561–5.
15. https://professional.medtronic.com/itbrc/troubleshooting/index.htm#.VlaIGnarTIU
16. Khorasani A, Peruzzi WT. Dantrolene treatment for abrupt intrathecal baclofen withdrawal. Anesth Analg. 1995;80:1054–6.
17. Meythaler JM, Roper JF, Brunner RC. Cyproheptadine for intrathecal baclofen withdrawal. Arch Phys Med Rehabil. 2003;84(5):638–42.
18. Zheng K, Brodsky J. Spinal surgery and abrupt intrathecal baclofen withdrawal. AA Case Rep. 2015;5(9):160–1.
19. Lee HM, Ruffoo V, Graudins A. Intrathecal clonidine pump failure causing acute withdrawal syndrome with 'stress-induced' cardiomyopathy. J Med Toxicol. 2016;12(1):134–8. Epub ahead of print

33 Polypharmacy: Neuraxial Anesthesia and Anticoagulation

Randall W. Knoebel and David M. Dickerson

33.1 Case Presentation

A 78-year-old male with history of type 2 diabetes mellitus, chronic renal insufficiency, coronary artery disease, hypertension, and hyperlipidemia presents for right upper lobectomy for adenocarcinoma via thoracotomy. Of note, the patient's cardiac history was significant for coronary artery bypass grafting 24 years prior. He underwent subsequent coronary stenting 4 years prior to presenting for surgery and had remained on antiplatelet therapy since his percutaneous coronary intervention. As advised by the preoperative clinic, the patient was instructed to stop clopidogrel 7 days in advance of surgery and continue with 81 mg aspirin. An epidural was placed preoperatively in the 7th thoracic spinal interspace with minimal difficulty. After an uneventful surgery, the epidural was initiated prior to emergence with a solution containing 0.0625% bupivacaine and 2 μg/mL fentanyl. Postoperative day one, the patient was without pain and stable from a cardiopulmonary standpoint. The thoracic surgical service progress notes detailed restarting clopidogrel. The medication was ordered and administered that morning although an epidural catheter remained in situ. The administration was detected shortly thereafter by the acute pain service during rounds.

Hematology was consulted for recommendations for management, and radiology was notified of potential impending urgent MRI. After a multidisciplinary discussion, it was decided that all heparin products and clopidogrel should be held until epidural removal 5–7 days post clopidogrel exposure. This plan would result in a 7-day dwell time. Neurological checks were performed every 2 h for the 24 h following clopidogrel administration. The patient remained neurologically intact and without back pain. The epidural catheter was removed postoperative day 7, and the patient remained without issue. Of note, the epidural provided significant pain relief throughout the postoperative course, and the patient was discharged home shortly thereafter.

Analysis of the factors that led to clopidogrel administration in the setting of an epidural revealed best practice alerts had been overridden by the primary service's house staff in ordering clopidogrel, pharmacy had verified the clopidogrel despite the alert and presence of active epidural medications on the patient's profile, lastly no direct communication between the primary service, pain service, and pharmacy occurred prior to overriding the alerts and medication ordering and administration.

33.2 Case Discussion

A spinal hematoma may form after a spontaneous bleed or trauma induced by neuraxial procedures. The epidural space is at particular risk from the rich epidural venous plexus, which has a high propensity for bleeding [1]. Excessive bleeding into the epidural space is a concern because the fixed anatomy surrounding the spinal cord may lead to compression, ischemia, nerve trauma, or paralysis. By comparison a bleed into the intrathecal space is less devastating with dilution by the cerebrospinal fluid [1]. The true incidence of epidural hematoma after epidural anesthesia is unknown, but it is estimated to be between 1:150,000 and 1:190,000. With spinal anesthesia, the incidence is 1:220,000 [2]. The incidence increases to 33:100,000 for epidural anesthesia and 1:100,000 for spinal anesthesia when combined with antithrombotics after surgery [2]. There are several risk factors for a hematoma after epidural/spinal anesthesia: advanced age, anatomic abnormalities of the spinal cord or vertebral column, vascular abnormalities, alcohol abuse, chronic renal

R.W. Knoebel, Pharm.D., B.C.O.P. (✉)
Department of Pharmacy, University of Chicago Medicine, Chicago, IL, USA
e-mail: Randall.Knoebel@uchospitals.edu

D.M. Dickerson, M.D.
Department of Anesthesia and Critical Care, University of Chicago, Chicago, IL, USA
e-mail: DDickerson@dacc.uchicago.edu

M. Anitescu et al. (eds.), *Challenging Cases and Complication Management in Pain Medicine*,
https://doi.org/10.1007/978-3-319-60072-7_33

insufficiency, difficult or traumatic needle placement, underlying coagulopathy, and administration of antithrombotic or antiplatelet agents [3]. Given the numerous risk factors—many non-modifiable—clinicians performing neuraxial procedures must maintain a high level of suspicion for symptoms of epidural hematoma after needle placement or catheter removal. Some symptoms are low back pain, sensory and motor loss, bowel and bladder dysfunction, and paraplegia. If symptoms develop, imaging is obtained to ensure rapid diagnosis. Delay in emergency decompressive laminectomy with hematoma evacuation may be catastrophic.

Although the direct interaction between epidural analgesics and blood thinning agents is benign, their concurrent presence on a patient's medication record is a surrogate for a suboptimal clinical scenario. The issues associated with such coadministration may be prevented or reduced through a standardized workflow that incorporates current guidelines, multidisciplinary, closed-loop communication and care coordination, and information technology driven by the electronic health record. This chapter examines the risk of various antithrombotic therapies during regional anesthesia and illustrates management strategies.

33.3 A Boom of Antithrombotic Agents

Since 2010, two novel classes of oral anticoagulants have been developed: the direct thrombin inhibitors and the direct factor Xa inhibitors. Similarly, a number of new antiplatelet inhibitors for the treatment of acute coronary syndrome have also recently entered the marketplace. The prevention of cardiovascular and cerebrovascular events through therapeutic anticoagulation has never been stress-free for patients. Inadequate, excessive, or even appropriate therapeutic anticoagulation carries risk.

It is currently estimated that approximately 250,000 patients in North America will interrupt oral anticoagulant therapy each year with an expected rise in years to come [4]. Although this situation is common, there is surprisingly little evidence to guide therapeutic recommendations because epidural hematoma is a rare phenomenon. Neuraxial procedures are frequently performed for perioperative and labor anesthesia and analgesia and for the amelioration of chronic pain. As the variety and quantity of available oral anticoagulants and antiplatelet agents increase, the potential for inadvertently inappropriate neuraxial intervention may similarly augment. The American Society of Regional Anesthesia and Pain Medicine (ASRA) first formulated guidelines to assist the anesthesia provider in caring for patients on anticoagulation. The guidelines were initially published in 1998 with the most recent update in 2010 [2]. In 2015, guidelines were published for patients receiving interventional pain procedures. Awareness and prevention through a system-based approach may prevent neuraxial hematoma and the associated catastrophic effects.

33.4 Perioperative Assessment

The perioperative management of patients receiving antithrombotic therapy, whether anticoagulant or antiplatelet, is guided by an assessment of the patient's risk for thromboembolic events considered against the risk for perioperative bleeding. These issues will determine whether antithrombotic therapy can be safely withheld around the time of surgery or a procedure or whether bridging therapy is considered [5].

33.5 Thromboembolic Risk Assessment

Thrombosis after temporary interruption in therapy is highly individualized and depends on the indication for anticoagulation. The CHEST guidelines offer a comprehensive source of information for patients with atrial fibrillation, venous thromboembolism, and heart valves. Table 33.1 is a suggested approach adapted from the CHEST guidelines; however, a patient's characteristics may modify the risk stratification. The potential risk of thrombus formation from a specific surgery or procedure also must be considered. Neurologic and vascular surgical procedures are associated with a greater risk for stroke in patients with atrial fibrillation than other types of procedures (e.g., urologic or orthopedic surgery) [6].

33.6 Bleeding Risk Assessment

The assessment of bleeding risk requires assessment of patient- and procedure-specific characteristics. The extensive venous plexus of the epidural space is vulnerable to trauma from needle puncture, advancement of spinal cord stimulator leads, or epidural and intrathecal catheters. The fragility and caliber of these vessels increase with age and various physiologic or pathologic states. The anatomic narrowing of the spinal canal from a myriad of conditions may lower the threshold for neurologic compression and injury with spinal bleeding. Table 33.2, adapted from the ASRA 2015 guidelines for pain procedures, provides a risk assessment based on type of pain procedure.

33.7 Discontinuing Anticoagulation or Antiplatelet Treatment

Concurrent use of coagulation-altering medications may increase the risk of bleeding without altering coagulation studies. Catheters are placed and removed at the nadir of

Table 33.1 Proposed risk stratification strategy for perioperative thromboembolism [4]

	Indication for anticoagulation therapy		
Risk stratum for thrombotic events	Mechanical heart valves	Atrial fibrillation	Venous thromboembolism
High risk >10% annual risk for thromboembolism	Any mitral valve prosthesis Any caged-ball or tilting disc aortic valve prosthesis Recent (within 6 months) stroke or TIA	CHADS2 score of 5 of 6 Recent (within 3 months) stroke or TIA	Recent (within 3 months) VTE Severe thrombophilia
Moderate risk 5–10% annual risk for thromboembolism	Bileaflet aortic valve prosthesis and ≥1 of the following risk factors: atrial fibrillation, prior stroke or TIA, hypertension, diabetes, CHF, age > 75 years	Rheumatic valvular heart disease CHADS2 score of 3 or 4	VTE within the past 3–12 months Recurrent VTE Active cancer (treated within 6 months or palliative) Nonsevere thrombophilia
Low risk <5% annual risk for thromboembolism	Bileaflet aortic valve prosthesis without atrial fibrillation and no other risk factors for stroke	CHADS2 score of 0–2	VTE > 12 months previous and no other risk factors

CHF congestive heart failure, *TIA* transient ischemic attack, *VTE* venous thromboembolism
The CHADS2 score is calculated by the cumulative score of CHF (1 point), hypertension (1 point), age > 75 years (1 point), diabetes mellitus (1 point), and previous stroke or TIA (2 points)
Severe thrombophilias include deficiencies in protein C, protein S, antithrombin, antiphospholipid antibodies, or multiple abnormalities
Nonsevere thrombophilias include heterozygosity for factor V Leiden or prothrombin G20210A

Table 33.2 Pain procedure classification according to the potential risk for serious bleed [1]

High-risk procedures	Intermediate-risk procedures[a]	Low-risk procedures[a]
Spinal cord stimulation trial and implant Intrathecal catheter and pump implant Vertebral augmentation Epiduroscopy and epidural decompression	Interlaminar ESIs (C, T, L, S) Transforaminal ESIs (C,T, L, S) Facet MBNB and RFA (C, T, L) Paravertebral block (C, T, L) Intradiscal procedures (C, T, L) Sympathetic blocks (stellate, thoracic, splanchnic, celiac, lumbar, hypogastric) Peripheral nerve stimulation trial and implant Pocket revision and IPG/ITP replacement	Peripheral nerve blocks Peripheral joints and musculoskeletal injections Trigger point injections including piriformis injections Sacroiliac joint injections and sacral lateral branch blocks

C cervical, *L* lumbar, *MBNB* medial branch nerve block, *RFA* radiofrequency ablation, *S* sacral, *T* thoracic, *IPG* internal pulse generator, *ITP* intrathecal pump
[a]Patients with high risk for bleeding undergoing low- or intermediate-risk procedures should be treated as intermediate or high risk, respectively. Patients with high risk for bleeding may include old age, history of bleeding tendency, concurrent uses of other anticoagulants/antiplatelets, liver cirrhosis or advanced liver disease, and advanced renal disease

anticoagulant activity. Additional anticoagulants should not be given immediately after catheter removal. Before initiating neuraxial anesthesia, the patient's medication list should identify the presence of anticoagulant or antiplatelet therapy. Common anticoagulants encountered in the surgical setting include antiplatelet medications, oral anticoagulants, unfractionated heparin, low molecular weight heparin, serotonin reuptake inhibitors, and herbal preparations.

Table 33.3 reviews pharmacokinetics and laboratory indices that reflect degree of anticoagulation. The pharmacokinetic parameters dictate the amount of cessation time before catheter placement and resumption after catheter removal. Although aspirin has a half-life of 30–40 min, its effects last well beyond the time of five half-lives because it irreversibly binds to platelets. When necessary aspirin is to be discontinued for 5–7 days before high-risk procedures. Table 33.3d (antiplatelet therapies) and Table 33.3e–f (anticoagulant therapies) recommended duration of discontinuation for antithrombotic agents before, during, and after catheter placement or removal. These times apply to patients with normal organ function; in patients with renal or hepatic dysfunction, older age, or low body weight, time to achieving normal clotting function can be delayed, making prediction difficult. In these patients, bleeding risk is assessed via thrombin time for dabigatran and via anti-Xa for factor Xa inhibitors. Normal values almost certainly exclude oral anticoagulant activity [7]. For patients on antiplatelet agents, quantitative laboratory data are helpful in risk assessment: a VerifyNow P2Y12 assay for clopidogrel, prasugrel, ticagrelor, and an Ultegra rapid platelet function assay-ASA for patients on aspirin therapy [8]. Consultation with a pharmacist and hematologist is valuable to determine the impact of drug clearance while estimating the degree of coagulation dysfunction.

33.8 Guidelines and Consensus

The first step for safe epidural management is to develop a consensus and standard methods for neuraxial procedures in the anticoagulated patient. This standard can be adopted from currently existing guidelines summarized in this chapter. Patients on anticoagulation should not receive neuraxial procedures unless duration of discontinued medications is suitable. Venous thromboembolism prophylaxis should be explicitly agreed upon preoperatively by medical, surgical, and anesthesia providers. If low-dose unfractionated heparin and serial compression device therapy is deemed insufficient for risk reduction, neuraxial techniques should be timed for effective pre- and post-procedural treatment or, ultimately, avoided altogether. In our case, a significant challenge was encountered in management and was best resolved through timely multidisciplinary care. When a patient with a neuraxial catheter in situ needs anticoagulation or inappropriately receives a dose of anticoagulant, a standard workflow is necessary to minimize risk.

Leaders from anesthesia, surgery, pharmacy, cardiology, neurology, neurosurgery, and hematology should identify a standardized method for anticoagulation in the patient with a neuraxial catheter. For elective cases, patients with coagulopathy or on anticoagulants should be evaluated in the preoperative anesthesia clinic or, if a preoperative clinic is not available, identified by the surgeon at the time of selection as a surgical candidate. At this time, a comprehensive medication reconciliation is conducted to identify and characterize the antiplatelet or anticoagulant regimen as well as the clinic managing this therapy. The cessation of such therapy may require clinical decision making about risk and benefit and may require bridging therapies meant to minimize risk. Therapy is guided by the physician or clinic managing the medical issue, and the mechanism for obtaining this plan should be agreed upon by the multidisciplinary working group [1]. The standardized workflow creates a plan, and accepted guidelines are referenced during coordinated communication between clinicians who may not be within the same institution.

Within the electronic record, electronic best practice alerts create safety nets for both the prescribing

Table 33.3 Medications appropriate while indwelling catheter in place

a **Low-dose aspirin & q12h low-dose heparin**

Therapeutic class	Drug	When to stop Before placement *Minimum time between last dose and procedure*	When to restart After Removal *Minimum time between last dose and catheter removal*
Aspirin	Aspirin < 100 mg	No time restriction	No time restriction
Thromboprophylaxis	Unfractionated Heparin (UFH), Subcutaneous Prophylactic Dose (5,000 units q 12h)[a]	8 h[b]	2 h[b]

Note: Antiplatelet agents, INCLUDING aspirin/NSAIDS, should not be used concurrently with anticoagulants while epidural catheter in-place

[a]*Check platelet count if on heparin therapy >4 days before placement; consider checking platelet count if date of removal is after >4 days of heparin therapy*

[b] *The 2015 ASRA guidelines for elective pain procedures differs from the 2010 regional anesthesia guidelines in its recommendation for subcutaneous prophylactic heparin cessation prior to catheter placement and removal. The 2015 authors note that the ASRA 2010 guidelines for regional anesthesia consider low-dose, twice daily subcutaneous dosing of heparin not to be a contraindication to catheter placement or removal. When possible 8 h should be given for maximal risk reduction. However, the decision to place or remove a catheter within this timeframe during low-dose, twice daily dosing remains low risk assuming other risks factors for spinal hematoma are not present.*

b **Herbals, vitamins & antidepressants**

Therapeutic class	Drug or supplement	When to stop Before placement *Minimum time between last dose and procedure*	When to restart After removal *Minimum time between last dose and catheter removal*	Ok to administer while catheter in place?
Herbals	Gingko	No contraindication	No contraindication	No contraindication
	Garlic	No contraindication	No contraindication	
	Ginseng	No contraindication	No contraindication	
	Omega-3 fish oil	No contraindication	No contraindication	
	Tumeric	No contraindication	No contraindication	
Vitamins	Vitamin C	N/A	N/A	
	Vitamin E	N/A	N/A	
Antidepressants	SSRI	N/A	N/A	

Table 33.3 (continued)

c Medications to be avoided while indwelling catheter in place

Aspirin & NSAIDS

Therapeutic class	Drug generic (Trade)	When to stop Before placement *Minimum time between last dose and procedure*	Ok to administer While catheter in Place?
Aspirin	Aspirin > 100 mg/day	7 days	Avoid while catheter is in place
NSAIDs	Diclofenac (Voltaren®)	1 day ($t\frac{1}{2}$ = 2 h)	
	Ketorolac (Toradol®)	1 day ($t\frac{1}{2}$ = 6 h)	
	Ibuprofen (Motrin®)	1 day ($t\frac{1}{2}$ = 4 h)	
	Etodolac (Lodine®)	2 days ($t\frac{1}{2}$ = 8 h)	
	Indomethacin (Indocin®)	2 days ($t\frac{1}{2}$ = 10 h)	
	Naproxen (Aleve®)	4 days ($t\frac{1}{2}$ = 17 h)	
	Meloxicam (Mobic®)	4 days ($t\frac{1}{2}$ = 20 h)	
	Nabumetone (Relafen®)	6 days ($t\frac{1}{2}$ = 30 h)	
	Oxaprozin (Daypro®)	10 days ($t\frac{1}{2}$ = 60 h)	
	Piroxicam (Feldane®)	10 days ($t\frac{1}{2}$ = 50 h)	

Note: obstetrics and perioperative risk benefit may differ from that of elective pain management procedures as ASRA 2015 does not discuss the specific risk:benefit for perioperative or obstetric care.

The above agents can be administered 1 h after catheter removal assuming other risks factors for spinal hematoma are not present.

d Antiplatelet agents

Drug generic (Trade)	When to stop Before placement *Minimum time between last dose and procedure*	When to restart After removal *Minimum time between last dose and catheter removal*	Antithrombotic indices for assessing adequate cessation	Ok to administer while catheter in place?
PDE Inhibitors				Avoid while catheter is in place
Cilostazol (Pletal®)	2 days	24 h	N/A	
Dipyridamole (Persantine®)	2 days	N/A	N/A	
Aspirin combinations (Aggrenox®)	7 days	4 h	N/A	
P2Y12 Inhibitors				
Clopidogrel (Plavix®)	7 days	12–24 h	VerifyNow P2Y12 assay	
Prasugrel (Effient®)	7–10 days	12–24 h	VerifyNow P2Y12 assay	
Ticagrelor (Brilinta®)	5 days	12–24 h	VerifyNow P2Y12 assay	
GPIIb/IIIa Inhibitors				
Abciximab (Reopro®)	2–5 days	8–12 h	N/A	
Eptifibatide (Integrilin®)	8–24 h (longer in renal impairment)	8–12 h	N/A	
Tirofiban (Aggrastat®)	8–24 h (longer in renal impairment)	8–12 h	N/A	

Table 33.3 (continued)

e **Anticoagulants: prophylactic dose**

Drug generic (Trade)	When to stop Before placement *Minimum time between last dose and procedure*	When to restart After removal *Minimum time between last dose and catheter removal*	Antithrombotic indices for assessing adequate cessation	Ok to administer while catheter in place?
Enoxaparin (Lovenox®)[a]	12 h (longer in renal impairment)	4 h	Anti-Xa assay	Avoid while catheter is in place
Dalteparin (Fragmin®)	12 h (longer in renal impairment)	4 h	Anti-Xa assay	
Fondaparinux (Arixtra®) 2.5 mg q 24 h	2 days (CrCrl > 80 mL/min) 3 days (CrCrl 30–80 mL/min) 4 days (CrCl <30 mL/min)	6–8 h	Anti-Xa assay	
Rivaroxaban (Xarelto®) 10 mg q 24 h	2 days (CrCrl 60–90 mL/min) 3 days (CrCrl 30–59 mL/min) 4 days (CrCrl 15–29 mL/min)	6 h	Anti-Xa assay (Rivaroxaban)	
Unfractionated Heparin 7,500 units q 8 h[a]	8–10 h	2 h	aPTT	
Unfractionated Heparin 5,000 units q 8 h[a]	8–10 h	2 h	aPTT	

[a] Check platelet count if on heparin therapy >4 days before placement

f **Anticoagulants: therapeutic dose**

Drug generic (Trade)	When to stop Before placement *Minimum time between last dose and procedure*	When to restart After removal *Minimum time between last dose and catheter removal*	Antithrombotic indices for assessing adequate cessation	Ok to administer while catheter in place?
Enoxaparin (Lovenox®), therapeutic dose 1–1.5 mg/kg q 24 h OR 1 mg/kg q 12 h	24 h (longer in renal impairment)	4 h	Anti-Xa assay	Avoid while catheter is in place
Fondaparinux (Arixtra®) 5–10 mg q 24 h	2 days (CrCrl > 80 mL/min) 3 days (CrCrl 30–80 mL/min) 4 days (CrCl <30 mL/min)	24 h	Anti-Xa assay	
Unfractionated Heparin, Intravenous	4 h aPTT < 40 s	2 h	aPTT	
Rivaroxaban (Xarelto®) 15–20 mg q 24 h	2 days (CrCrl ≥ 60 mL/min) 3 days (CrCrl 30–59 mL/min) 4 days (CrCrl 15–29 mL/min)	24 h	Anti-Xa assay (Rivaroxaban), PT	
Dabigatran (Pradaxa®)	2 days (CrCrl ≥ 50 mL/min) 3–5 days (CrCrl < 50 mL/min) (longer in renal impairment)	24 h	TT, aPTT	
Apixaban (Eliquis®)	3 days (CrCl ≥ 50 mL/min) 4 days (CrCrl < 50 mL/min)	24 h	Anti-Xa assay	
Endoxaban (Savaysa®)	3 days (CrCrl ≥ 50 mL/min) No specific recommendations for renal dose adjustments.	24 h	Anti-Xa assay	
Argatroban IV continuous infusion	8–10 h, aPTT < 40 s (longer in renal or liver impairment)	4 h	DTI or aPTT	
Bivalirudin (Angiomax) IV continuous infusion	8–10 h, aPTT < 40 s (longer in renal or liver impairment)	4 h	DTI or aPTT	
Warfarin (Coumadin®)	5 days, INR <1.5	24 h	PT/INR	

g **Fibrinolytics**

Drug	When to stop Before placement *Minimum time between last dose and procedure*	When to restart After removal *Minimum time between last dose and catheter removal*	Antithrombotic indices for assessing adequate cessation	Ok to administer while catheter in place?
Alteplase (full dose stroke, MI, etc)	Contraindicated	Contraindicated, if administered 48 h recommended	Fibrinogen	No

A 1 mg dose of Alteplace for treatment of an occluded intravascular catheter may be given without restrictions on neuraxial catheter placement or removal physician and verifying pharmacist in cases of concomitant antithrombotic therapy before an epidural. Practice guidelines are not widely appreciated outside of the anesthesiology community and can vary with altered pharmacodynamics. Therefore, computerized physician order entry systems afford a unique opportunity to improve adherence with evidence-based practice guidelines. One such method leverages an electronic clinical decision support system that alerts providers when an epidural solution is being ordered for a patient receiving a prohibited anticoagulant [9]. In one study, in the 3 months before implementation of the warning system, 213 epidurals were placed with 26 order conflicts. In the 3 months after the alerts were established, 237 epidurals were placed with only 11 order conflicts. Of potential conflicts after the warning system, most were situations in which the epidural had already been removed, but the epidural solution order had not been discontinued [9]. The best practice alerts use the following logic incorporating look-back functionality.

For the following classes of medications: aspirin, P2Y12 inhibitors, GPIIb/IIIa inhibitors, NSAIDs, thromboprophylaxis, therapeutic anticoagulants, and fibrinolytics, a best practice alert will fire:

1. If the medication was ordered within the last 5 days before an epidural order is written
2. If an active epidural order is on the medication administration record

Language appears about the risks associated with concurrent anticoagulation. A link to the guidelines assists in optimizing patient care and safety surrounding the use of regional anesthesia with antiplatelets and anticoagulants.

Within our institution, the acute pain service (APS) is responsible for epidural placement, management, and removal. In a situation necessitating emergent epidural catheter removal (i.e., postoperative, myocardial infarction, or cerebrovascular accident), a physician from the APS is available 24 h a day for recommendations for timing of anticoagulant or antiplatelet after catheter removal.

Conclusion

Epidural hematoma for epidural anesthesia, while rare, can be a potentially devastating event. Concomitant use of antithrombotics can increase this complication. It is vital that the patient's medication regimen is evaluated before placement or removal of an epidural catheter. Guidelines exist for the safe use of antiplatelet and anticoagulant medications in patients undergoing interventional spine and pain procedures.

References

1. Norouze S, Benzon HT, Provenzano DA, et al. Interventional spine and pain procedures in patients on antiplatelet and anticoagulant medications: guidelines from the American Society of Reginal Anesthesia and Pain Medicine, the European Society of Regional Anesthesia and Pain Therapy, the American Academy of Pain Medicine, the International Neuromodulation Society, the North American Neuromodulation Society, and the World Institute of Pain. Reg Anesth Pain Med. 2015;40:182–212.
2. Horlocker TT, Wedel DJ, Rowlingson JC, et al. Regional anesthesia in the patient receiving antithrombotic or thrombolytic therapy: American Society of regional anesthesia and pain medicine evidence-based guidelines (third edition). Reg Anesth Pain Med. 2010;35:64–101.
3. Kreppel D, Antoniadis G, Seeling W. Spinal hematoma: a literature survey with meta-analysis of 613 patients. Neurosurg Rev. 2003;26:1–49.
4. Douketis JD, Spyropoulos AC, Spencer FA, et al. Perioperative management of anticoagulant therapy: antithrombotic therapy and prevention of thrombosis, 9th ed: American college of chest physicians evidence-based clinical practice guidelines. Chest. 2012;141(Suppl 2):e326S–50S.
5. Ortel TL. Perioperative management of patient on chronic antithrombotic therpay. Hematology. 2012;120:529–35.
6. Kaatz S, Douketis JD, Zhou H, Gage BF, White RH. Risk of stroke after surgery in patients with and without chronic atrial fibrillation. J Thromb Haemost. 2010;8(5):884–90.
7. Tran H, Joseph J, Young L, et al. New oral anticoagulants: a practical guide on prescription, laboratory testing and peri-procedural/bleeding management. Australasian society of thrombosis and haemostasis. Intern Med J. 2014;44:525–36.
8. Gurbel PA, Bliden KP, Butler K, et al. Response to ticagrelor in clopidogrel nonresponders and responders and effect of switching therapies the RESPOND Study. Circulation. 2010;121:1188–99.
9. Gupta RK. Using an electronic clinical decision support system to reduce the risk of epidural hematoma. Am J Ther. 2014;21:327–30.

34 Intrathecal Drug Delivery System Infections (Meningitis, Encephalitis, Pump Pocket Contaminants)

Benjamin R. Beal

34.1 Case Description

A 19-year-old 56 kg male with a history of cerebral palsy and bilateral lower extremity spasticity that was refractory to pharmacological therapy was referred to our clinic for consideration of intrathecal baclofen therapy.

After a successful trial of 50 mcg intrathecal baclofen administered as a single shot, a programmable IDDS was implanted. Intravenous cefazolin 1000 mg was administered prior to incision as per routine prophylaxis. The patient was discharged on postoperative day 5 on an intrathecal dose of baclofen 45 mcg/day.

On postoperative day 21, the patient was seen in the outpatient clinic for routine follow-up and wound evaluation. Physical examination revealed mild warmth and erythema over the pump pocket incision as well as a 1 cm area over the incision that appeared to have mild tissue breakdown and dermal thinning. There was no evidence or history of purulence or fluid draining from the wound, and there was no history of fevers or headache. The patient's wound was cleansed with chlorhexidine, and he was sent home on an empiric 10-day course of cefazolin.

On postoperative day 33, the patient was again seen in clinic for routine follow-up and wound evaluation. There appeared to be an improvement in the previously noted erythema and warmth over the pocket incision, but there continued to be an area of poor wound healing. The decision was made to observe the wound, and the patient was discharged home.

On postoperative day 57, the patient was admitted to the hospital after returning from a 10-day family road trip to Mexico with a 3-day history of worsening fever and headaches. Physical examination revealed nuchal rigidity, a positive Brudzinski's sign, and a 2 cm erosion over the pump pocket with active purulence. A lumbar puncture was performed at the L3–L4 level in the emergency department and revealed an opening pressure of 32 cm H_2O and was turbid in appearance. The working diagnosis at this time was an IT pump pocket infection with an associated bacterial meningitis. Empiric antibiotic therapy with vancomycin and ceftriaxone was started. The CBC revealed a leukocytosis with a neutrophil predominance. The CSF revealed an elevated protein count, low glucose, and a white blood cell count of 2100 cells/mm^3 with a neutrophil predominance.

The patient was then taken to the OR for explant of the IDDS without any complications.

The pump pocket cultures, CSF cultures, and IT catheter tip cultures all grew out *Staph epidermidis*, so ceftriaxone was discontinued, and the patient continued to be treated with IV vancomycin. The patient was also started on oral baclofen at 15 mg po bid in order to prevent acute baclofen withdrawal.

On postoperative day (POD) #2, the patient was noted to have a gradually increasing tachycardia as well as increasing spasticity and irritability, and he reported feeling itchy. At this point there was concern for acute baclofen withdrawal, and the oral baclofen dose was gradually up-titrated to 30 mg po tid with resolution of symptoms.

By POD #4, the patient appeared to have responded well to the IV antibiotic regimen, and his initial symptoms that were consistent with bacterial meningitis had resolved. Additionally, the oral baclofen dose of 30 mg po tid continued to prevent the recurrence of acute baclofen withdrawal.

On POD #7, the patient was discharged home, and home health services were coordinated in order to administer the full 14-day course of antibiotic therapy. Upon follow-up, the patient had responded to the antibiotic therapy and had full resolution of symptoms. He continued to have bilateral lower extremity spasticity that was similar to the spasticity prior to the IDDS implant, and a discussion to reimplant the IDDS was ongoing.

B.R. Beal, M.D.
Department of Pain Medicine, UCSD Medical Center, San Diego, CA 92103, USA
e-mail: bbeal@ucsd.edu

M. Anitescu et al. (eds.), *Challenging Cases and Complication Management in Pain Medicine*,
https://doi.org/10.1007/978-3-319-60072-7_34

34.2 Case Discussion

34.2.1 Bacterial Meningitis Associated with an Intrathecal Drug Delivery System

Bacterial meningitis associated with an IDDS is perhaps the most feared complication related to this type of therapy. The reported incidence of infection of IDDS and spinal cord stimulator devices combined ranges from 2 to 8% [1]. While the most common postoperative infection associated with these devices is surgical site infections (SSIs), if not identified and treated early, these may develop into infections involving the central nervous system resulting in prolonged courses of intravenous antibiotic therapy.

34.3 Etiology and Pathogenesis

Intrathecal drug delivery system infections tend to occur early after device implantation and primarily involve the pump pocket. Additionally, the primary pathogens identified are skin floras, namely, *Staphylococcus epidermidis*, which presumably are present on either the patient or the operating room staff at the time of implantation [2]. Perioperative attention to proper sterile surgical technique, skin antisepsis, and antibiotic selection are three measures that are essential in preventing IDDS-associated infections [3]. In patients who develop IDDS-associated meningitis, one study showed that in all cases there was a concomitant pocket and tract infection at the time of diagnosis or prior to the diagnosis of meningitis [4]. This suggests that once a pump pocket infection is identified, explanting the IDDS is most often the proper course of action.

Risk factors that are associated with surgical site infections include leukopenia associated with the cancer or cancer therapy, diabetes mellitus, debilitated status, poor hygiene, poor nutritional status, smoking, and corticosteroid use [2, 5] (Fig. 34.1).

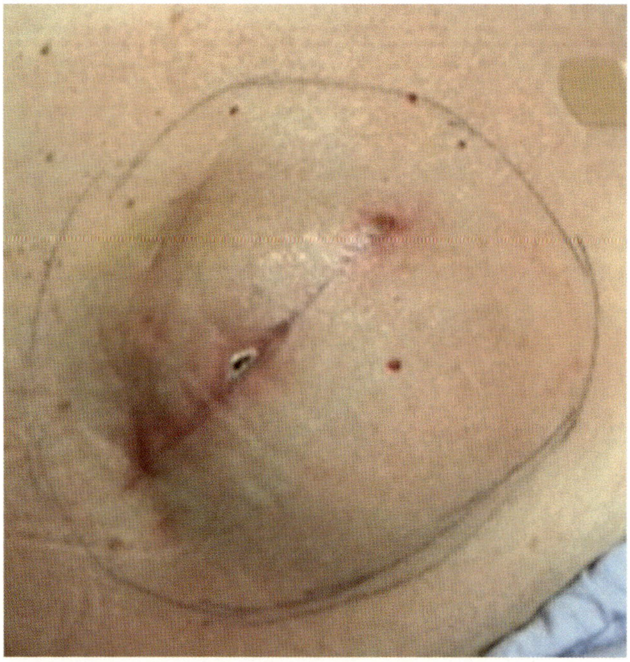

Fig. 34.1 Early would infection, localized to the intrathecal pump pocket with small dehiscence and purulent drainage 2 weeks after initial placement. Image from Dr. Malik personal library

34.4 Clinical Manifestation of IDDS Infections

1. *Classification of surgical site infections (SSIs).* The CDC classifies SSIs as either incisional, which is subdivided into those involving only the skin or subcutaneous tissue or those involving deeper soft tissues, or organ/space. Organ/space SSIs involve any part of the surgical anatomy other than the body wall layers [6]:
   (a) *Superficial incisional SSI.* This infection occurs within 30 days after the operation and involves only the skin or subcutaneous tissue. Classical signs of infection must be present on exam such as localized tenderness, swelling, warmth, or erythema. Purulent drainage from the incisional site may also be present [6].
   (b) *Deep incisional SSI.* This infection occurs within 30 days after the operation or within 1 year if implant is in place and the infection appears to be related to the operation and infection involves deep soft tissues. It will manifest as purulent drainage from the deep incisional layers, as spontaneous dehiscence of a wound in a patient with classical signs of infection on examination in the presence of a fever, or as an abscess or other signs of a deep infection noted on examination, during reoperation, or on radiologic examination [6].
   (c) *Organ/space SSI.* This infection occurs within 30 days after the operation or within 1 year if implant is in place and the infection appears to be related to the operation. The infection must involve any part of the organs or spaces that were manipulated during an operation. Finally, there must be present either purulent drainage from a drain in the organ space, an organism isolated from tissue or fluid in the organ/space, or evidence of infection involving the organ/space seen during reoperation or on radiographic examination [6].

2. *Bacterial meningitis*. Bacterial meningitis can present with the classic triad of fever, nuchal rigidity, and altered mental status. However, a recent study found the prevalence of this classical presentation to be low, but almost all patients (95%) presented with at least two of four symptoms of headache, fever, nuchal rigidity, and altered mental status [7]. Other neurologic findings such as seizures, papilledema, and cranial nerve abnormalities can be present as well but typically present later in the course of the disease [7, 8].
3. *Bacterial encephalitis*. It presents in a similar fashion as bacterial meningitis. Focal neurological deficits and seizures may be more prominent with encephalitis when compared to meningitis [9]. The most common pathogens resulting in encephalitis are viruses, but when the pathogen is bacterial in nature, meningeal signs are typically more prominent than the ones in viral encephalitic component, and as a whole it is typically referred to as meningoencephalitis [9].

34.5 Specific Diagnostic Methods

1. *Blood samples*. Once there is suspicion for IDDS-associated infection, blood samples should be sent for a complete blood cell count, which should demonstrate a polymorphonuclear leukocytosis (PMN) with a left shift. Blood samples should also be sent for gram stain and culture. Ideally, blood cultures are sent prior to the initiation of antibiotic therapy in order to have a higher success at identifying the pathogen [10]. Serum electrolytes should be evaluated in order to obtain renal function and serum glucose.
2. *Tissue cultures*. In cases that have an open and draining wound, fluid and wound samples should be sent for gram stain and culture. Ideally these samples would be sent prior to initiation of antibiotic therapy in order to have the highest likelihood of identifying the infectious pathogen.
3. *Cerebrospinal fluid (CSF) samples*. Lumbar puncture (LP) should be performed once there is suspicion for bacterial meningitis or encephalitis. The opening pressure is usually elevated in the 20–50 cm H_2O range and may be turbid in appearance due to increased white blood cells (WBC) and bacteria [10]. The WBC will have a PMN predominance, and CSF studies for glucose and protein will show a low glucose concentration and elevated protein concentration. CSF samples should also be sent for gram stain and culture. The likelihood that the gram stain will identify the pathogen depends on the bacteria responsible and ranges between 33 and 90%. This likelihood drops by about 20% in patients who receive antibiotic therapy prior to obtaining CSF [10].

   Patients presenting with focal neurologic deficits (cranial nerve abnormalities) or severe impairment of consciousness should first undergo a cranial computed tomography (CT) scan of the brain prior to LP in order to identify patients at risk for brain herniation after LP [10, 11].
4. *Radiographic studies*:
   (a) *CT scan*. CT scan of the pump pocket would be of little benefit due to metal artifact seen on the image. Sometimes, in associated cellulitis, fat strained can be present (Fig. 34.2) A contrast-enhanced cranial CT scan may reveal changes consistent with bacterial meningitis or encephalitis but is not necessary for establishing a diagnosis. These changes would be

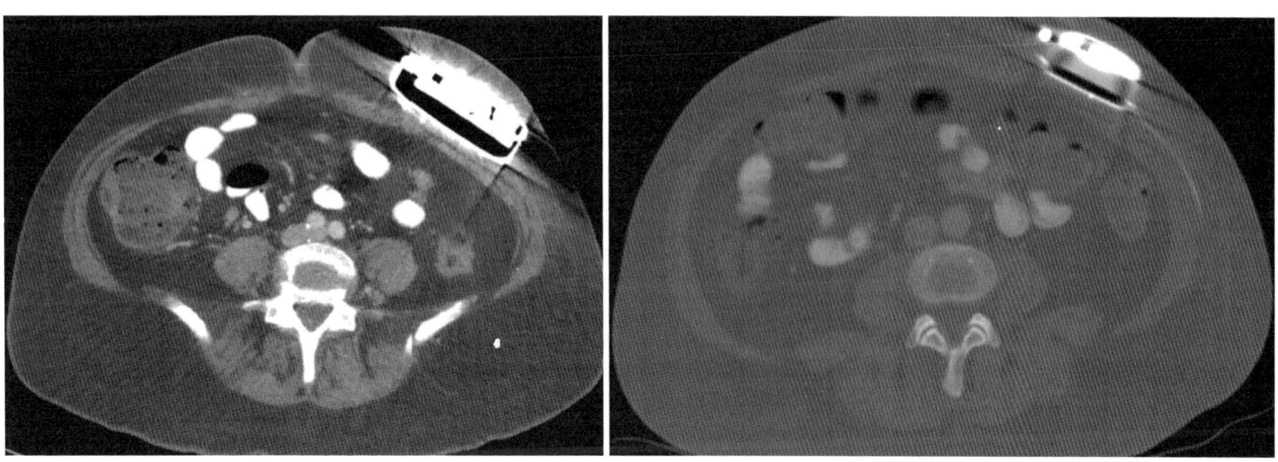

Fig. 34.2 Patient with delayed infection at the pump pocket. Despite significant artifact, both images show fat stranding consistent with cellulitis. The concern was tracking of the fat stranding toward the spine in image 2. The images are taken 6 months apart. First episode of cellulitis was treated with intravenous antibiotics and temporarily resolved the symptoms; pump was eventually explanted. Image from Dr. Anitescu personal library

noted as diffuse enhancement of the subarachnoid space as well as dural enhancement [12]. However, a cranial CT scan is most useful in detecting contraindications to lumbar puncture [11].

(b) *Magnetic resonance imaging (MRI).* Cranial MRI is more useful in identifying meningeal enhancement that is consistent with meningitis; however, it is again not necessary establishing a diagnosis and is a non-specific finding seen in other disorders involving the central nervous system [12]. MRI is also useful in identifying soft tissue changes consistent with surgical site infection as well as identifying an epidural abscess that might be associated with the infection [13].

(c) *Ultrasound.* Ultrasound has no utility in diagnosing bacterial meningitis. However, it can be used to identify fluid-filled pockets associated with soft tissue infections [14].

34.6 Prevention of IDDS Infections

The primary pathogens identified from surgical site infections are skin floras which presumably are present on either the patient or the operating room staff at the time of implantation [2, 15]. Appropriate preventative measures should be taken in the perioperative period in order to decrease the likelihood of infection. Surgical hand preparation with alcohol-based solution, povidone-iodine, or chlorhexidine gluconate is perhaps the most important measure to prevent SSI [15]. Proper selection and administration of preoperative prophylactic antibiotics as well as postponing elective surgery when there is evidence of a remote infection (urinary tract infection, pneumonia, etc.) have also been shown to decrease the incidence of SSI [15]. Intraoperatively, appropriate antisepsis of the patient's skin in conjunction with a wide prep and sterile drapes over the patient as well as over the C-arm should be used. Surgical technique should include adequate hemostasis, minimizing tissue trauma and surgical time, vigorous antibiotic wound irrigation, and proper tissue approximation during wound closure [3]. Postoperatively, occlusive dressings should remain on for 48 h, and the surgical wounds should be inspected within the first 7–10 days after implantation [3, 15].

34.7 Treatments for IDDS Infections

1. *Superficial surgical site infections.* Patients should be evaluated within 7–10 days after implantation. If there is erythema or edema beyond that which is expected postoperatively, additional follow-up and reevaluation are necessary. If, however, there is concern for a superficial surgical site infection, such as cellulitis, one should consider incision and drainage of the wound in and/or appropriate selection and administration of oral antibiotics that would cover the most likely organism (Table 34.1) [3, 16, 17].
2. *Deep surgical site infections.* When there is an IDDS-related pump pocket infection or deep tissue infection, the patient should be hospitalized and scheduled for urgent IDDS removal [4]. A 2015 study evaluated patients with infectious complications associated with IDDS in a tertiary care setting and found that bacterial pathogens associated with deep SSI were skin floras [4]. The initial choice of antibiotics should cover common skin flora including methicillin-resistant *Staphylococcus aureus* (MRSA). Once the pathogen has been isolated from tissue gram stain and culture, the antibiotic regimen should be tailored to match the antibiotic sensitivities of the organism.
3. *Meningitis and encephalitis.* As with deep surgical site infections, the presence of meningitis associated with IDDS should prompt hospitalization and urgent removal of the IDDS, as IDDS salvage is unlikely. There have been case reports of the successful treatment of bacterial meningitis with intrathecal antibiotics without removal of the IDDS and other pump-salvage techniques, but there is not enough evidence at this time for their recommendation [18–20].

In a 1992 review of 22 studies, the author looked at the duration of meningitis-related symptoms prior to initiating antibiotic therapy and the development of subsequent neurologic injury and/or death [21]. He found that for patients with clinically overt bacterial meningitis, a delay in antibiotic therapy increases the likelihood of permanent neurologic injury. This, in conjunction with additional supportive evidence, suggests that bacterial meningitis is a neurologic emergency and early diagnosis with early antibiotic treatment of bacterial meningitis plays a central role in improving patient outcomes [10]. The choice of empiric antibiotic therapy

Table 34.1 Antibiotics commonly used in surgical wound infections

Antibiotics for treatment of IDDS-associated infections
Superficial SSI and deep incisional SSI
Cephalexin 500 mg every 6 h po [17] SMX-TMP 160–800 mg po every 6 h [17] Clindamycin 300–450 mg po qid [17] Vancomycin 15 mg/kg IV every 12 h (suspected MRSA) [17]
Organ/space SSI (empiric therapy for meningitis and encephalitis)
Vancomycin 30–45 mg/kg IV every 8–12 h plus cefepime 6 g every 8 h [10] Vancomycin 30–45 mg/kg IV every 8–12 h plus ceftazidime 6 g every 8 h [10] Vancomycin 30–45 mg/kg IV every 8–12 h plus meropenem 6 g every 8 h [10]

in patients with bacterial meningitis and encephalitis associated with IDDS should be broad spectrum (Table 34.1) and cover the most commonly isolated pathogens including MSSA, MRSA, coagulase-negative staphylococci (*S. epidermidis*), and aerobic gram-negative bacilli (*P. aeruginosa*) [10]. The antibiotic therapy should also be guided by community- and hospital-based bacterial resistance patterns, and an infectious disease specialist consultation is recommended. Once the bacterial pathogen is identified, antibiotic therapy should be tailored for optimal therapy while reducing resistance to broad-spectrum antibiotics.

Key Concepts

- Intrathecal drug delivery system (IDDS)-related infections are one of the most feared complications related to IDDS implantation. Infectious complications range from superficial wound infections to meningitis or encephalitis.
- Superficial surgical site infections can be treated with oral antibiotics and close observation with or without abscess drainage. If the infection is truly superficial, many times the patient can be spared having the IDDS explanted.
- Pump pocket infections require hospitalization and should be treated with removal of the IDDS and initiation of broad-spectrum antibiotic therapy.
- When meningeal signs are present, obtaining a CSF sam ple for analysis is an important first step in identifying the organism responsible for the infection. Broad-spectrum antibiotics should be started when meningitis is suspected, and one should not delay in starting antibiotic therapy.
- Deep space/organ infection such as meningitis or encephalitis should also prompt urgent removal of the IDDS in addition to appropriate antibiotic therapy.
- The diagnosis of acute bacterial meningitis is based on history, physical examination, and CSF analysis.
- Patients with significant neurologic findings should have a CT scan of the brain prior to obtaining CSF in order to rule out possible causes of elevated intracranial pressure that could result in brain herniation after dural puncture.

References

1. Koyyalagunta D, Vinh B, Chemaly R, Graviss L, LaFleur L. Infectious complications related to intrathecal drug delivery system and spinal cord stimulator implants at a tertiary care cancer center. J Pain. 2012;13(3):S65.
2. Follett KA, Ph D, Boortz-marx RL, Drake JM, Dupen S. Prevention and management of intrathecal drug delivery and spinal cord stimulation system infections. Anesthesiology. 2004;100(6):1582–94.
3. Deer TR, Provenzano DA. Recommendations for reducing infection in the practice of implanting spinal cord stimulation and intrathecal drug delivery devices: a physician's playbook. Pain Physician. 2013;16(3):E125–8.
4. Malheiro L, Gomes A, Barbosa P, Santos L, Sarmento A. Infectious complications of intrathecal drug administration systems for spasticity and chronic pain: 145 patients from a tertiary care center. Neuromodulation. 2015;18(5):421–7.
5. Neumayer L, Hosokawa P, Itani K, El-Tamer M, Henderson WG, Khuri SF. Multivariable predictors of postoperative surgical site infection after general and vascular surgery: results from the patient safety in surgery study. J Am Coll Surg. 2007;204(6):1178–87.
6. Mangram AJ, Horan TC, Pearson ML, Silver LC, Jarvis WR. Guideline for prevention of surgical site infection. ICHE. 1999;20(4):247–78.
7. de Gans J, Spanjaard L, Weisfelt M, Reitsma JB, Vermeulen M. Clinical features and prognostic factors in adults with bacterial meningitis. N Engl J Med. 2004;351(18):1849–59.
8. Durand M, Calderwood S, Weber D, et al. Acute bacterial meningitis in adults. N Engl J Med. 1993;328(1):21–8.
9. Tunkel AR, Glaser CA, Bloch KC, et al. The management of encephalitis: clinical practice guidelines by the infectious diseases society of america. CID. 2008;47:303–27.
10. Tunkel AR, Hartman BJ, Kaplan SL, et al. Practice guidelines for the management of bacterial meningitis. CID. 2004;39(1):1267–84.
11. Hasbun R, Abrahams J, Jekel J, Quagliarello V. Computed tomography of the head before lumbar puncture in adults with suspected meningitis. N Engl J Med. 2001;345(24):1727–33.
12. Minonzio G, Paolucci M, Angelo C, Davide G. Imaging of cranio-meningeal infectious and inflammatory involvement. Neurol Sci. 2008;29:279–82.
13. Friedman DP, Hills JR. Cervical epidural spinal infection: mr imaging characteristics. AJR. 1994;163:699–704.
14. Gaspari R, Blehar D, Mendoza M. Use of ultrasound elastography for skin and subcutaneous abscesses. J Ultrasound Med. 2009;28:855–60.
15. Uçkay I, Harbarth S, Peter R, et al. Preventing surgical site infections. Expert Rev Anti-Infect Ther. 2010;8(6):657–70.
16. Welsh A. Surgical Site Infection Prevention and Treatment of Surgical Site Infection. 2008.
17. Stevens DL, Bisno AL, Chambers HF, et al. Practice guidelines for the diagnosis and management of skin and soft tissue infections: 2014 update by the infectious diseases society of america. CID. 2014;59(15):147–59.
18. Kallweit U, Harzheim M, Marklein G, Welt T, Pöhlau D. Successful treatment of methicillin-resistant Staphylococcus Aureus meningitis using linezolid without removal of intrathecal infusion pump. Case report. J Neurosurg. 2007;107(3):651–3.
19. Atiyeh BS, Hayek SN, Skaf GS, Al Araj A, Roukoz B. Baclofen pump pocket infection: a case report of successful salvage with muscle flap. Int Wound J. 2006;6:23–8.
20. Zed PJ, Stiver HG, Devonshire V, Jewesson PJ, Marra F. Continuous intrathecal pump infusion of baclofen with antibiotic drugs for treatment of pump-associated meningitis. Case report. J Neurosurg. 2000;92(2):347–9.
21. Radetsky M. Duration of symptoms and outcome in bacterial meningitis: an analysis of causation and the implications of a delay in diagnosis. Pediatr Infect Dis J. 1992;11(9):694–8.

35 Intrathecal Ziconotide: Complications and Clinical Considerations

Gemayel Lee and Jeffrey Chen

35.1 Case Description

A 45-year-old female presents to the pain clinic for management of her intrathecal therapy. She has a 10-year history of post-laminectomy syndrome with low back and bilateral lower extremity pain. She had an intrathecal pump placed 2 years ago currently using morphine 4 mg/mL and bupivacaine 10 mg/mL running at 1 mg/day morphine. She uses a patient therapy manager with 0.1 mg bolus doses and a 6 h lockout. Past medical history is positive for non-insulin-dependent diabetes, depression, and hypertension. Current medications include gabapentin 800 mg po TID, venlafaxine 150 mg/day, hydrochlorothiazide, metformin, and hydrocodone/acetaminophen 5–325 every 6 h as needed. Pain is poorly controlled with a pain level on numerical rating scale (NRS) of 8/10. On exam, she is alert and oriented, neurologically unchanged with some mild pitting edema of her ankles.

The decision is made to add ziconotide to her intrathecal regimen at 10 mcg/mL running at 2.5 mcg/day. At the 2-week follow-up visit, her pain score is 6/10, but she reports some cognitive and memory impairment. Her gabapentin is reduced to 800 mg at bedtime only, and 1 week later she reports improvement in her symptoms, but pain level increased to 7/10. Her pump is refilled with morphine 4 mg/mL, bupivacaine 10 mg/mL, and ziconotide 20 mcg/mL running at 1 mg/day morphine. One week later, she returns to the clinic with a pain level of 4/10 but with significant cognitive impairment. Her husband reports that she seems confused at times and memory impairment has worsened. Vitals signs are as follows: blood pressure 124/82 with no orthostasis, pulse 70, respiratory rate 16, and temperature 98.2. She appears alert and oriented but cannot remember her home address or phone number. Neurological exam is unchanged. As the intrathecal drug delivery system was interrogated, it became apparent that while the dose of morphine and bupivacaine per day remained the same, the dose of ziconotide doubled due to inadvertent doubling of the concentration. From an initial daily dose of 1 mg/day morphine, 2.5 mg/day bupivacaine, and 2.5 mcg/day ziconotide, the patient has received in the last week same dose of morphine and bupivacaine but 5 mcg/day ziconotide. This rapid up-titration of ziconotide, while not entirely out of clinical practice, may have been contributed to patient's acute cognitive impairment; the decrease of the daily dose of ziconotide to 3.5 mcg/day achieved with slow titration of 0.2 mcg/day every 3 days from the starting dose of 2.5 mcg/day gave patient the best balance between pain relief and side effects. Cognitive dysfunction improved, and pain scores stabilized at 5/10 with a final dose of morphine 1 mg/day, bupivacaine 2.5 mg/day, and ziconotide 3.5 mcg/day.

35.2 Case Discussion

In the United States, pain has an annual cost of over $300 billion, more than heart disease, cancer, and diabetes [1]. It is estimated that about 30–50% of Americans are burdened by chronic pain, which can be substantially detrimental to their health and quality of life [2, 3]. Patients with severe chronic pain often explore multiple therapeutic options during the course of their disease and may become intolerant or refractory to systemic analgesics and adjunctive therapies [4]. Ziconotide (Prialt) was FDA approved in the United States in 2004 for use in patients with severe chronic pain in whom intrathecal therapy is warranted, and the 2012 Polyanalgesic Consensus Conference (PACC) considers it as first-line monotherapy for nociceptive and neuropathic pain [4, 5]. Randomized controlled trials investigating the efficacy and safety of ziconotide monotherapy demonstrated

G. Lee, M.D. (✉) • J. Chen, M.D., M.H.S.
Center for Pain Medicine, University of California San Diego, 9300 Campus Point Drive, Mail Code 7651, La Jolla, CA 92037, USA
e-mail: jlc021@ucsd.edu

M. Anitescu et al. (eds.), *Challenging Cases and Complication Management in Pain Medicine*, https://doi.org/10.1007/978-3-319-60072-7_35

statistically significant pain relief when compared to placebo, without the development of tolerance, addiction, or withdrawal [6–11]. However, despite these advantages, adverse effects are common, generally involve the central nervous system (CNS), and may lead patients to discontinue use of the medication [6–12]. Common side effects include confusion, dizziness, difficulty walking, and somnolence [11] and are thought to reflect the inhibition of voltage-gated calcium channels in the CNS [7, 9]. Adverse effects are related to the dose and rate of titration and resolve with discontinuation of the medication [4, 6–11]. Clinically, ziconotide is commonly used in combination with other intrathecal medications and has been shown to have additive analgesic effects with morphine, hydromorphone, clonidine, and baclofen, demonstrating a safety profile similar to its use as monotherapy [10, 13, 14]. Despite the potential favorability of ziconotide in combination therapy, experts warn that formal studies evaluating its long-term safety for this purpose are currently lacking [10].

35.2.1 Conotoxins

Ziconotide is a synthetic derivate of omega-conotoxin, which is a voltage-gated calcium channel inhibitor found in the venom of the *Conus magus* snail [11, 15, 16]. Figure 35.1 is a picture of the snail Conus magnus that produces conotoxins that are also know as conopeptides; they are a diverse group of neuroactive peptides that are found universally in the Conus genus and function to immobilize their victim during hunting and self-defense [15]. The fish-eating *Conus magus* delivers its conotoxins via percutaneous injection, and the peptides immediately act on the nervous system via the antagonism of voltage- and ligand-gated ion channels but have also been shown to act on G protein-coupled receptors and play a role in the transport of neurotransmitters [16]. Figure 35.2 is the proposed mechanism of action of conotoxin. In the 1990s, Yaksh and colleagues demonstrated significant analgesia in rats when omega-conopeptide MVIIA, a voltagc-gatcd (N-type) calcium channel inhibitor, was injected intrathecally [18]. Clinically, ziconotide exploits this same mechanism and exerts its analgesic effect by inhibiting calcium ion transport and preventing the release of proinflammatory neurotransmitters in nociceptive afferent nerve terminals [11, 16, 18].

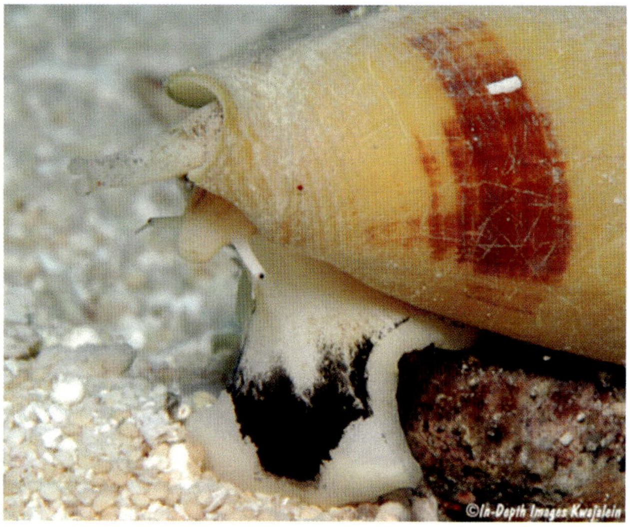

Fig. 35.1 Picture of the snail

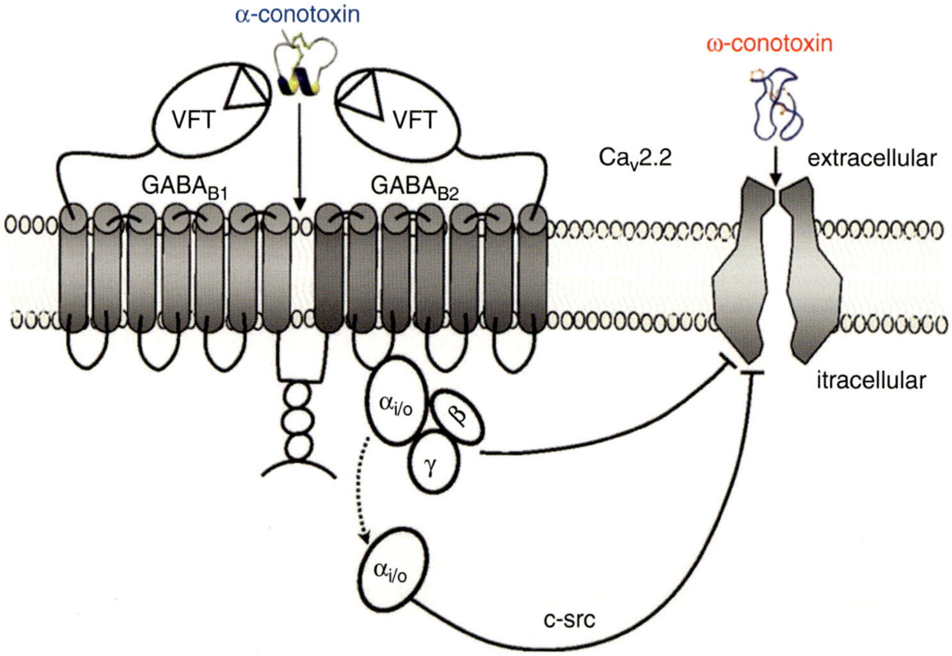

Fig. 35.2 Mechanism of action of conotoxin

35.2.2 N-Type Voltage-Gated Calcium Channel

In the nervous system, calcium is highly metabolically active and plays an important role in hormone secretion, synaptic transmission, gene expression, regulation of enzyme activity, and the modulation of synaptic plasticity [19–21]. In nociceptive pain pathways, calcium influx in response to the depolarization of nociceptors facilitates the release of proinflammatory neurotransmitters [19–21]. These neurotransmitters include substance P, glutamate, and calcitonin gene-related peptide (CGRP) [20–22], which are involved in neurogenic inflammation, nociceptor sensitization to painful stimuli, and the development of chronic pain [21]. As a result, the voltage-gated or N-type calcium channel has significant implications for the treatment and management of chronic pain and is a target for therapeutic intervention [11, 20, 21].

In rats, ziconotide has been shown to act on the N-type calcium channel, which tightly governs the transport of calcium across the cellular membrane at the afferent nerve terminal [18, 19, 21, 23]. These channels open in response to membrane depolarization from painful stimuli and are inactivated in nondepolarized states by voltage-dependent and calcium-dependent mechanisms [19–21]. In the open state, N-type calcium channels allow calcium to diffuse down its concentration gradient into the cell where it facilitates the fusion of synaptic vesicles and subsequent release of substance P, glutamate, and CGRP into the synapse of nociceptive afferent nerve terminals in the Rexed laminae I and II of the spinal dorsal horn [19–21, 23, 24]. Here, the neurotransmitters communicate with interneurons carrying afferent signals to the thalamus for interpretation [19, 21]. The N-type calcium channels are important drivers of evoked synaptic transmission and play an important role in nociceptive and neuropathic pain signaling [20, 21]. N-type calcium channels are located in the central and peripheral nervous system including the brain, spinal cord, and primary sensory neurons [19–21, 23]. The channels function at presynaptic, C fiber and A delta afferents in the spinal dorsal horn, and within the cell bodies of the dorsal root ganglia [11, 18, 19, 23]. The role of N-type calcium channel inhibition in pain pathways has been demonstrated genetically in groups of knockout mice that showed reduced pain sensitivity in models of inflammatory and neuropathic pain [11, 19], and this role has been validated clinically by multiple randomized controlled trials demonstrating the efficacy of ziconotide [6–10, 12, 25].

35.2.2.1 Pharmacodynamics and Pharmacokinetics

Ziconotide is polar, hydrophilic, and hypobaric at clinically useful concentrations [25]. It is formulated in 1 or 5 mL vials of 100mcg/mL or 20 mL of 25 mcg/mL aqueous solution diluted in preservative-free normal saline and intended for use with Medtronic SynchroMed II and CADD-Micro ambulatory infusion pumps [11, 25]. Figure 35.3 is a picture from the ziconotide packaging that holds the vials of medication that are used for the pump.

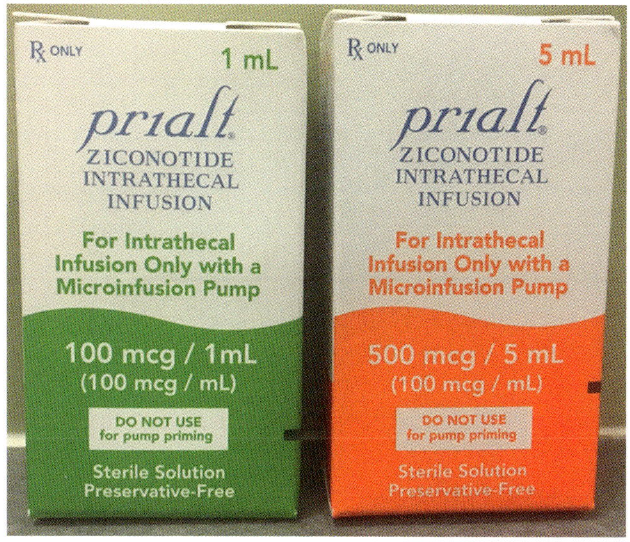

Fig. 35.3 Picture of vials by manufacturer

Ziconotide is marketed by the manufacturer for continuous intrathecal infusion [11]. The initial starting dose for ziconotide infusion is less than or equal to 2.4mcg/day or 0.1mcg/h and may be titrated by less than or equal to 2.4mcg/day or 0.1mcg/h every 2–3 days for a maximum dose of 19.2mcg/day or 0.8mcg/h on day 21 [11]. The slow titration technique described is recommended to limit the development of delayed adverse effects, and faster titrations should be restricted for situations in which urgent analgesia outweighs the risk to patient safety [11].

Ziconotide can have a delayed time of onset of ~8–24 h after initiation of infusion [6–9, 11]. The delayed onset reflects the slow distribution of ziconotide through the cerebral spinal fluid (CSF) and its slow penetration into the CNS parenchyma. Onset time may be hastened by increasing the volume and rate of infusion, which would subsequently increase the intrathecal spread of the medication [6–9, 11, 22]. The volume of distribution approximates the volume of CSF in the body at any given time (~155–260 mL), and ziconotide relies on bulk CSF flow generated by cardiac oscillations for its distribution [11, 22, 25].

The use of an intrathecal drug delivery system greatly limits the uptake of ziconotide from the CSF into the blood stream [11, 17, 22]. Its CSF half-life is 2.9–6.5 h and estimates the daily turnover of CSF [11, 12, 17, 22]. In addition, the size, polarity, and hydrophilicity of ziconotide further limit its efflux through the meninges and into the systemic circulation [22]. Potentially small amounts of medication can efflux out of the CSF through the dural puncture site, but this contribution is considered negligible [22]. Its clearance

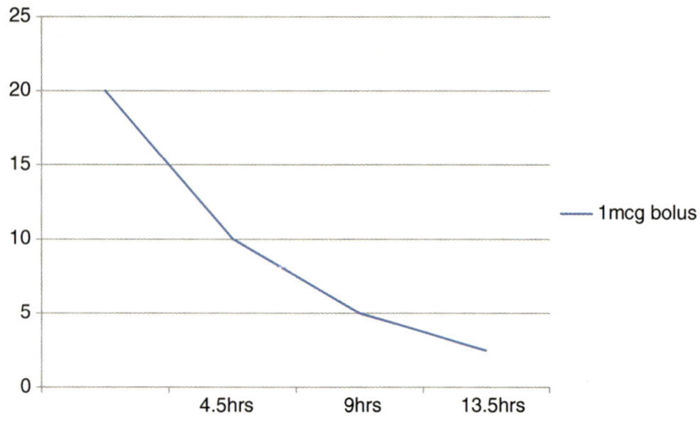

Fig. 35.4 Schematic of ziconotide clearance from the CSF following 1mcg bolus. Estimated CSF concentration of 20 ng/mL and 4.5 h half-life [17]

is described by linear kinetics whether given by bolus or infusion, and its elimination relies on bulk redistribution of CSF to the arachnoid appendages and drainage into the venous circulation [11, 22]. Once in the systemic circulation, ziconotide is cleaved into small peptides and free amino acids by endopeptidases and exopeptidases located in many tissues [11, 12, 22]. Spinal tissue uptake has a minimal contribution to the clearance of ziconotide, and protein binding is negligible in the CSF [22]. Less than 1% is excreted in the urine [12]. Figure 35.4 is a schematic of ziconotide clearance from the CSF following a 1mcg bolus. Estimated CSF concentration of 20 ng/mL and 4.5 h half-life.

35.2.2.2 Clinical Considerations

Ziconotide monotherapy is indicated for the management of moderate to severe chronic pain in patients for whom IT therapy is warranted, and who are intolerant of or refractory to systemic analgesics and adjunctive therapies, or IT morphine [8, 10–12]. Preclinical and clinical studies, including three randomized controlled trials, have established the efficacy of ziconotide intrathecal infusion for chronic malignant and nonmalignant pain of nociceptive and neuropathic origins [5–9]. Using Visual Analog Scale of Pain Intensity (VASPI) scores as efficacy measures, these RCTs demonstrated significant pain relief over placebo for ~30% of patients treated with ziconotide monotherapy, and a small portion of patients even reported complete pain relief [6–9, 12]. Of note, the early RCTs used higher doses and faster titrations than what is currently used, which led to increased pain relief but a greater incidence of adverse effects and discontinuations from treatment [6–9, 12]. Significant adverse events usually occur within 2–3 days following the initiation of therapy and are thought to reflect the slow pharmacokinetics of the medication [6–8, 11, 12]. The manufacturer recommends a slow titration over a 3-week period, and later studies utilizing the slow titration technique demonstrated a decreased, yet still significant, rate of development of adverse effects and treatment discontinuations when compared to placebo [11, 26]. Interestingly, the abrupt discontinuation of ziconotide intrathecal infusion did not result in drug withdrawal in any of the treatment subjects [6–8, 11, 12].

Despite having many advantages, such as the lack of tolerance or withdrawal, intrathecal ziconotide infusion has a narrow therapeutic window, and adverse effects are common [4, 6–14, 25–27]. Clinical studies have evaluated the use of ziconotide monotherapy in 1254 patients over 7.5 years and demonstrated that adverse effects occur in the CNS in a dose- and rate-related manner and generally resolve within 1–2 weeks after discontinuation of treatment [11, 12]. The most common adverse effects are cerebellar, cognitive, and neuropsychiatric in nature and include dizziness (46%), nausea (40%), asthenia (18%), diarrhea (18%), somnolence (17%), vomiting (16%), and confusion (15%) [11, 12]. These effects are thought to be the result of toxic inhibition of N-type calcium channels throughout the central nervous system, particularly supraspinal structures [12, 22, 23]. In addition to the spinal cord, N-type calcium channels are found in the cerebellum and basal ganglia, and inhibition at these locations is implicated for side effects like dizziness, difficulty walking, nystagmus, and confusion [12, 23]. Ziconotide also has sympatholytic activity and may inhibit central autonomic pathways, explaining the nausea, vomiting, urinary retention, and hypotension also seen in clinical use [12, 24].

35.2.3 Cognitive and Neuropsychiatric Adverse Effects

In clinical trials, confusion was the most common neuropsychiatric effect and occurred most frequently in adults >65 years (47% vs. 29%) [11]. Memory impairment was the second most frequent adverse cognitive effect reported by the manufacturer and was not related to age [11]. Other more adverse neuropsychiatric effects included hallucinations, paranoid reactions, hostility, delirium, psychosis, and mania [11]. Cognitive, psychiatric, and other CNS effects may be delayed and take 1–2 weeks to develop and usually resolve within 2 weeks of discontinuing therapy [10–12, 25]. Ziconotide can be safely discontinued without withdrawal effects [8, 10–12, 25].

The manufacturer warns of the development of severe psychiatric symptoms and neurological impairment during use and advocates patients be monitored frequently for evidence of cognitive impairment, hallucinations, and changes in mood or consciousness. Furthermore, the package insert states Prialt may cause or worsen depression, with the ultimate risk of suicide in susceptible patients [11]. Ziconotide intrathecal infusion is contraindicated in patients with a previous history of psychosis or suicidal ideations or attempts [11]. If serious psychiatric adverse effects occur during drug administration, drug dosages should be adjusted or discontinued and patients instituted on proper psychiatric therapy and/or admitted to an inpatient facility for management [11].

In addition to monitoring for neuropsychiatric adverse effects, patients, caregivers, and healthcare workers must also be diligent about monitoring for potential signs of meningitis, including headache, fever, stiff neck, altered mental status, nausea, vomiting, and seizures [11]. Meningitis was a complication in 3% (40 cases) of treatment subjects in clinical trials and predominantly occurred in patients using external delivery devices (37 cases) [11]. Strict aseptic technique should be used when preparing, placing, or refilling microinfusion delivery devices [11]. If meningitis is suspected, CSF cultures should be obtained, and the patient should be started on appropriate antimicrobial therapy [11]. Typically the drug delivery device is removed along with the intrathecal catheter and all foreign bodies in the intrathecal space [11].

35.2.4 Elevated Creatinine Kinase

In clinical trials, elevations in creatinine kinase were seen in more than 40% of patients and up to three times the upper limit of normal in some patients. There are two case reports of patients developing myopathy and even rhabdomyolysis causing acute kidney injury; however, the vast majority of cases were benign and resolved with discontinuation of therapy [11]. The elevation in CK typically occurs in the first 2 months and the etiology is unknown [11]. Serum creatinine kinase levels should be checked every other week for the first month, and then monthly thereafter, or as clinically appropriate [11].

35.2.5 Hypotension

In clinical studies using healthy volunteers, intravenous ziconotide demonstrated dose-dependent reduction in blood pressure. Ziconotide produces sympatholysis via the inhibition of N-type calcium channels and prevention of norepinephrine release in central autonomic pathways [11, 12, 26]. It is worth noting that ziconotide is delivered by intrathecal infusion and actual blood levels are minimal.

35.2.5.1 Combination Therapy

Although randomized controlled trials have focused on the use of ziconotide as monotherapy, and the manufacturer exclusively markets it for this purpose, in clinical practice ziconotide is often used as an adjunctive analgesic in combination with other intrathecal medications [10, 12–14, 28]. Other common intrathecal medications include morphine, hydromorphone, clonidine, baclofen, and bupivacaine [10, 12–14, 28]. Wallace et al. reviewed 11 preclinical and clinical studies, and the results are summarized below.

35.3 Ziconotide and Morphine

Ziconotide has distinct advantages over opiates insofar as it does not lead to the development of addiction, tolerance, dependence, or withdrawal, and it has not been shown to lead to granuloma formation [10–14, 25]. Preclinical studies demonstrated that chronic morphine does not produce cross-tolerance to ziconotide and that ziconotide has identical efficacy in opiate-tolerant and opiate-naïve individuals [10–12]. Preclinical studies in rats also demonstrated that when used together, ziconotide and intrathecal morphine have synergistic and additive antinociceptive effects [10]. Furthermore, ziconotide did not potentiate morphine-induced respiratory depression, but did potentiate morphine-induced decreased GI motility and morphine-induced hypotension [10]. Clinical studies demonstrated ~20% improvement in Visual Analog Scale of Pain Intensity (VASPI) scores with common adverse effects being dizziness and nausea [10, 13, 14]. Ziconotide may provide analgesic benefit to patients with opiate withdrawal, but otherwise will not reverse opiate withdrawal [11].

35.4 Ziconotide and Hydromorphone

Intrathecal hydromorphone is considered off-label use as it is not currently FDA approved for this purpose. It is a more lipid soluble molecule than morphine and has a small supraspinal distribution when delivered IT, potentially limiting adverse effects [10]. The data for combination therapy with IT hydromorphone and ziconotide is limited and comes from a case report involving a young woman with a spinal cord injury secondary to a fall, who reported ~90% improvement in pain scores with ziconotide and hydromorphone compared to partial relief from IT hydromorphone alone and combination of IT hydromorphone and baclofen [10, 29].

35.5 Ziconotide and Baclofen

Baclofen acts as an inhibitory neurotransmitter and blocks the GABA-B receptor in the spinal cord and CNS [30]. It is derived from gamma-aminobutyric acid and is FDA approved for intrathecal delivery in the management of severe spasticity and may be beneficial in spasticity-related pain [10]. Data from preclinical studies in rats suggests that combination ziconotide and baclofen produced additive antinociception [10, 28]. Adverse effects associated with the use of intrathecal combination therapy with baclofen and ziconotide included sedation, urinary hesitancy, and loss of bladder control. All adverse effects resolved with discontinuation of therapy [10, 28].

35.6 Ziconotide and Clonidine

Preclinical studies in rats demonstrated additive analgesia when clonidine and ziconotide were used in combination [10]. Ziconotide was not shown to exacerbate clonidine-induced hypotension or bradycardia [10]. Clonidine is FDA approved for epidural use for the management of severe cancer pain, but not currently approved for intrathecal use [10].

35.7 Ziconotide and Bupivacaine

Bupivacaine is an amide local anesthetic that binds to sodium channels and inhibits action potential propagation [31]. It is a common medication for intrathecal combination therapy despite not being FDA approved for IT use in this manner. Preclinical animal studies failed to show an increased benefit when used in combination with ziconotide [10].

Ziconotide is susceptible to proteolysis [11, 25], and its stability in combination therapy varies with different intrathecal medications. For instance, ziconotide has been shown to be more stable when mixed with morphine as opposed to hydromorphone [10, 32]. The overall clinical significance appears to be minor but may warrant more frequent dosing adjustments depending on its degradation profile when mixed with a certain intrathecal medication [10, 32–35].

35.7.1 Contraindications

Ziconotide intrathecal infusion is contraindicated in patients with a previous history of psychosis, patients with an allergy or hypersensitivity to Prialt or any of its formulation components, and in whom intrathecal therapy would be medically hazardous or unsafe, such as a bleeding diathesis or infection at the infusion site [11].

35.8 Summary

- The administration of ziconotide for the management of chronic pain requires the expertise of a physician experienced with implantable and external intrathecal drug delivery devices.
- Patients should be psychologically stable with good access to care and follow-up and suitable for intrathecal therapy.
- Ziconotide provides significant pain relief that is limited largely by the development of dose-dependent neurocognitive adverse effects that resolve with discontinuation of therapy.
- The most common adverse effects are confusion, memory impairment, elevated serum creatinine kinase, and hypotension.
- Although early data appears to favor its use as a combination therapy, formal, multicentered, randomized controlled trials are lacking to firmly establish its safety profile for this purpose.
- With these considerations in mind, ziconotide appears to be safe for use as monotherapy and combination therapy for the management of moderate to severe chronic pain in the appropriate patient.
- Ziconotide can be safely discontinued without withdrawal effects.

References

1. Gaskin DJ, Richard P. The economic costs of pain in the United States. J Pain. 2012;13(8):715–24.
2. Institute of Medicine (US) Committee on Advancing Pain Research, Care, and Education. Relieving Pain in America: A Blueprint for Transforming Prevention, Care, Education, and Research. Washington, DC: National Academies Press (US); 2011.
3. Johannes CB, et al. The prevalence of chronic pain in United States adults: results of an internet-based survey. J Pain. 2010;11(11):1230–9.
4. Rauck RL, Wallace MS, Burton AW, Kapural L, North JM. Intrathecal ziconotide for neuropathic pain: a review. Pain Pract. 2009;9:327–37.
5. Deer TR, et al. Polyanalgesic consensus conference 2012: recommendations for the management of pain by intrathecal (intraspinal) drug delivery: report of an interdisciplinary expert panel. Neuromodulation. 2012;15(5):436–66.
6. Staats PS, et al. Intrathecal ziconotide in the treatment of refractory pain in patients with cancer or AIDS: a randomized controlled trial. JAMA. 2004;291(1):63–70.
7. Rauck R, Wallace M, et al. A randomized, double-blind, placebo-controlled study of intrathecal ziconotide in adults with severe chronic pain. J Pain Symptom Manag. 2006;31(5):393–406.
8. Wallace MS, et al. The Ziconotide nonmalignant pain study 96–002 group. Intrathecal ziconotide in the treatment of chronic nonmalignant pain: a randomized, double blind, placebo-controlled clinical trial. Neuromodulation. 2006;9(2):75–86.
9. Wallace MS, et al. Intrathecal ziconotide for severe chronic pain: safety and tolerability results of an open-label, long-term trial. Anesth Analg. 2008;106(2):628–37.
10. Wallace MS, Rauck RL, Deer T. Ziconotide combination intrathecal therapy: rationale and evidence. Clin J Pain. 2010;26:635–44.
11. PRIALT® [Package Insert]. Jazz Pharmaceuticals, Inc. Palo Alto, CA.
12. Smith HS, Deer TR. Safety and efficacy of intrathecal ziconotide in the management of severe chronic pain. Ther Clin Risk Manag. 2009;5:521.
13. Wallace MS, Kosek PS, Staats P, et al. Phase II, open-label, multicenter study of combined intrathecal morphine and ziconotide: addition of ziconotide in patients receiving intrathecal morphine for severe chronic pain. Pain Med. 2008;9:271–81.
14. Webster LR, Fakata KL, Charapata S, Fisher R, MineHart M. Open-label, multicenter study of combined intrathecal morphine and ziconotide: addition of morphine in patients receiving ziconotide for severe chronic pain. Pain Med. 2008;9:282–90.
15. Olivera BM, Rivier J, Clark C, et al. Diversity of *Conus* neuropeptides. Science. 1990;249:257–63.
16. Lewis RJ, Dutertre S, Vetter I, Christie MJ. Conus venom peptide pharmacology. Pharmacol Rev. 2012;64(2):259–98.

17. Wermeling D, et al. Pharmacokinetics and pharmacodynamics of intrathecal ziconotide in chronic pain patients. J Clin Pharmacol. 2003;43(6):624–36.
18. Malmberg AB, Yaksh TL. Voltage-sensitive calcium channels in spinal nociceptive processing: blockade of N-and P-type channels inhibits formalin-induced nociception. J Neurosci. 1994;14(8):4882–90.
19. Simms BA, Zamponi GW. Neuronal voltage-gated calcium channels: structure, function, and dysfunction. Neuron. 2014;82(1):24–45.
20. Zamponi GW, et al. The physiology, pathology, and pharmacology of voltage-gated calcium channels and their future therapeutic potential. Pharmacol Rev. 2015;67(4):821–70.
21. Lee S. Pharmacological inhibition of voltage-gated Ca^{2+} channels for chronic pain relief. Curr Neuropharmacol. 2013;11(6):606.
22. Yaksh TL, et al. Pharmacokinetic analysis of ziconotide (SNX-111), an intrathecal N-type calcium channel blocking analgesic, delivered by bolus and infusion in the dog. Neuromodulation. 2012;15(6):508–19.
23. Gohil K, et al. Neuroanatomical distribution of receptors for a novel voltage-sensitive calcium-channel antagonist, SNX-230 (ω-conopeptide MVIIC). Brain Res. 1994;653(1):258–66.
24. McGuire D, et al. Sympatholysis after neuron-specific, N-type, voltage-sensitive calcium channel blockade: first demonstration of N-channel function in humans. J Cardiovasc Pharmacol. 1997;30(3):400–3.
25. Pope JE, Deer TR. Ziconotide: a clinical update and pharmacologic review. Expert Opin Pharmacother. 2013;14(7):957–66.
26. Olivier Brenet MD, et al. Ziconotide adverse events in patients with cancer pain: a multicenter observational study of a slow titration, multidrug protocol. Pain Physician. 2012;15:395–403.
27. Mohammed SI, et al. Bolus intrathecal injection of ziconotide (Prialt®) to evaluate the option of continuous administration via an implanted intrathecal drug delivery (ITDD) system: a pilot study. Neuromodulation. 2013;16(6):576–82.
28. Saulino M, et al. Intrathecal ziconotide and baclofen provide pain relief in seven patients with neuropathic pain and spasticity: case reports. Eur J Phys Rehabil Med. 2009;45(1):61–7.
29. Saulino M. Successful reduction of neuropathic pain associated with spinal cord injury via of a combination of intrathecal hydromorphone and ziconotide: a case report. Spinal Cord. 2007;45(11):749–52.
30. Coffey RJ, et al. Intrathecal baclofen for intractable spasticity of spinal origin: results of a long-term multicenter study. J Neurosurg. 1993;78(2):226–32.
31. Berde CB, Strichartz GR. Local anesthetics. In: Miller RD, Eriksson LI, Fleisher LA, et al., editors. Miller's anesthesia. 7th ed. Philadelphia: Elsevier, Churchill Livingstone; 2009.
32. Shields D, Montenegro R, Ragusa M. Chemical stability of admixtures combining ziconotide with morphine or hydromorphone during simulated intrathecal administration. Neuromodulation. 2005;8(4):257–63.
33. Shields D, Monenegro R, Aclan J. Chemical stability of admixtures combining ziconotide with baclofen during simulated intrathecal administration. Neuromodulation. 2007;10(Suppl 1):12–7.
34. Shields D, Monenegro R, Aclan J. Chemical stability of admixtures combining ziconotide and bupivacaine during simulated intrathecal administration. Neuromodulation. 2007;10(Suppl 1):1–5.
35. Shields D, Monenegro R. Chemical stability of ziconotide-clonidine hydrochloride admixtures with and without morphine sulfate during simulated intrathecal administration. Neuromodulation. 2007;10(Suppl 1):6–11.

Part V

Interventional Pain Procedures Spinal Cord Stimulator

36 Wound Dehiscence After Intrathecal Pump Implantation for Cancer Pain

Kenneth Justin Naylor and David M. Dickerson

36.1 Case Description

A 29-year-old male with stage IV appendiceal adenocarcinoma was admitted for uncontrolled pain and severe diarrhea from *C. difficile* colitis. Despite treatment for his colitis, abdominal pain worsened with chemotherapy over the following weeks. His pain was initially managed with a fentanyl patch 50 μg/h, sustained-release oxycodone 40 mg twice daily, hydrocodone-acetaminophen tablets as needed, marijuana to increase appetite, and clonidine for insomnia. The patient's history included several years of heavy alcohol consumption which he stopped when diagnosed with cancer.

After evaluation by the pain service, he was prescribed gabapentin, methadone, acetaminophen as needed, a clonidine patch, oxycodone for breakthrough pain, and naproxen. Sustained-release oxycodone and hydrocodone-acetaminophen tablets were discontinued, and he was titrated off the fentanyl patch. Marijuana was discontinued because of the potential for marijuana-induced hyperalgesia. Marinol therapy was initiated to increase appetite.

At follow-up a month after the initial evaluation, the patient's chronic abdominal pain improved. He had complaints, however, of a new unilateral, but severe, knee and lower leg pain. There were no precipitating factors, and his knee pain was described as "achy," worse with movement, and triggered by palpation of the popliteal fossa. Despite orthopedic evaluation and unremarkable imaging studies of the spine and extremity, the left lower extremity pain progressed throughout the entire left leg. At this time, the patient discontinued his gabapentin and initiated over-the-counter ibuprofen in addition to prescribed naproxen. He was self-escalating, as needed, doses of immediate-release oxycodone. He was advised to resume gabapentin, oxycodone, tizanidine, and methadone at the previous recommended dose and start diclofenac in place of naproxen and ibuprofen.

While his abdominal pain remained controlled, multiple lower extremity orthopedic complaints persisted and were thought to be associated with chemotherapy. The decision to pursue intrathecal drug delivery for his lower extremity pain was made after multidisciplinary discussion. Upon a successful 24-h intrathecal trial, the patient elected intrathecal pump implantation.

The night before implantation, the patient took a chlorhexidine bath. Two grams of cefazolin was administered intravenously before incision, and before implantation, the pump pocket was copiously irrigated with bacitracin-containing solution. The pump was secured with 2-0 nonabsorbable polyester suture (Ti-Cron) in the pocket at four points. The pocket was closed with 2-0 absorbable suture (Vicryl); the superficial layer, with 3-0 absorbable suture (Vicryl); and the skin subcuticularly, with 4-0 absorbable monofilament suture (Biosyn). Dermabond, Steri-Strips, Telfa, and Tegaderm were then applied.

Follow-up 1 week later revealed a half inch opening of the skin incision with serous drainage but an intact deep layer closure over the pump site. The area was cleaned with sterile saline, and Steri-Strips were reapplied to approximate the open end. The patient reported that he had been taking baths despite clear instructions that he was not to do so. The patient was referred to the wound care clinic that day for evaluation and treatment and again advised not to bathe, but to substitute showers instead.

The following week the patient submerged his wound underwater for the comfort of soaking in the bathtub. He was given Tegaderm films to cover the wound and again advised

K.J. Naylor, M.D.
Mercy Pain Management, Mercy Hospital,
Washington, MO 63090, USA
e-mail: naylorkj@yahoo.com

D.M. Dickerson, M.D. (✉)
Department of Anesthesia and Critical Care,
University of Chicago, Chicago, IL, USA
e-mail: DDickerson@dacc.uchicago.edu

M. Anitescu et al. (eds.), *Challenging Cases and Complication Management in Pain Medicine*,
https://doi.org/10.1007/978-3-319-60072-7_36

not to get the wound wet. A piece of Biosyn suture was removed aseptically from the wound edge. Xeroform was prescribed for the wound and bacitracin ointment for wound care, but he did not use them as directed. The wound appeared to have healthy granulation tissue without exudate or odor. When the patient returned to the wound care clinic, the wound was 1.4 × 0.8 × 0.3 cm with an opening at the center closest to midline, and yellow dried eschar was embedded in the sutures. The wound was debrided of nonviable tissue with forceps, scalpel, and scissors to pink viable granulation tissue. Round wound edges indicated a wound healing state. An endoform collagen dressing was applied to stimulate granulation tissue ingrowth. Follow-up 2 weeks later revealed a completely clean granular base and healing. When the patient kept the area dry, the wound healed without signs or symptoms of infection. The patient remained on chemotherapy throughout this time.

36.2 Case Description 2

A 48-year-old female with multiple sclerosis, stage IV non-squamous cell lung cancer after surgical resection and chemotherapy, and a pelvic mass that had been resected came to the pain clinic with severe postprandial pain. After pelvic mass resection, abdominal pain persisted and became severe with meals but was constant in the upper abdomen, radiating to the back despite continued escalation of opioid therapy. A large mass encompassing the superior mesenteric artery was found.

She underwent a continuous intrathecal drug trial with hydromorphone. After a successful trial, an intrathecal pump was placed as described in case 1. Before emergence from anesthesia, the patient exhibited blanching erythema from head to toe after intrathecal infusion of hydromorphone and clonidine. The uniform macular erythema resolved within several hours without intervention and was never associated with additional signs or symptoms. This effect was assumed to be a neuroimmune response to the intrathecal medication because of multiple sclerosis. The exact etiology was never identified.

A week later in the clinic, she reported 90% pain relief (pain of 1 on a numerical rating scale of 1–10, with 10 equal to severest pain). At this time the incision site was healing well. The patient was told that she could shower, but baths were not recommended. She continued aggressive chemotherapy throughout this time.

One month postoperatively, the patient's abdominal wound had two small areas of dehiscence. The wound was 7.2 cm in length with two sections of skin dehiscence at the medial and lateral wound edges. The wound had healed and then opened up approximately 4 weeks after surgery. The wound, at her waistline, opened up after she wore jeans. She reported that the clothing at the waistline was consistently irritating the wound, yet she had not notified the pain clinic and assumed the irritation was normal. There was no drainage or pain from the incision. The patient had been treating the wound with over-the-counter ointment and covering it with Band-Aids twice daily. The wound had erythema along the edges and required debridement to expose healthy granulation tissue. The wound was cleaned with sterile saline and gauze; Band-Aids were then applied to the medial and lateral wound borders over areas of dehiscence. The patient was referred to the wound care clinic.

Two months later, the patient went to hydrotherapy where the corner openings of the wound appeared smaller but had opening medially with straw-colored, dried exudate. She had been wearing sweatpants to decrease pressure/irritation on skin. The wound exudate was cleaned with saline on gauze and the remainder removed with forceps. New gauze was applied and secured with paper tape. The patient was instructed to put antibiotic ointment on the wound at home. At a third follow-up visit in the wound clinic, the corners of the wound were re-epithelialized. The central wound was still open. The patient was instructed not to mobilize the scar until fully healed. Total time for wound healing was just over 3 months.

36.3 Discussion

36.3.1 Etiology and Pathogenesis

Infection is a risk of any surgical procedure. Patients who undergo intrathecal drug delivery for malignant pain may be at increased risk from a poor nutritional state, which leads to poor wound healing. If they are physically debilitated, they may be unable to maintain proper wound care postoperatively. Infection at the site of pump insertion has been shown to range from 2.5 to 9% and represents the site at highest risk for infection [1]. The most common organism cultures from wounds are the *Staphylococcus* species. *Pseudomonas* is the second most common cultured organism.

Wound infection after intrathecal pump placement manifests within 2 months after surgery. Rare events have been reported well outside this window, including pump pocket infection in a non-cancer patient after unrecognized bowel injury 18 months following pump implantation [2]. In this case, *C. albicans* and *E. cloacae* were grown from cultures.

One retrospective study reported no difference in infection rate between cancer and non-cancer patients who had intrathecal drug delivery and spinal cord stimulator placement. Operative time was the main factor associated with wound infection [3].

36.4 Clinical Manifestations of Wound Dehiscence

36.4.1 Diagnosis

Pain, erythema, swelling, purulent discharge, and dehiscence or skin erosion at the pump insertion site are signs of infection. Fever may indicate deeper fascial layer involvement. After infection develops, precautions must be taken to prevent its spread to deeper tissue layers and down to the device, which may compromise function and require surgical intervention on an infected tissue bed (Fig. 36.1) [4].

Case reports describe conditions mimicking postoperative wound infection, including one case of an acute exacerbation of hereditary coproporphyria after intrathecal pump insertion [5]. In this case, symptoms developed rapidly within hours after pump placement, unusual for acute wound infection.

Four categories of complications with intrathecal pump insertion have been described: mechanical, related to medication, catheter, or procedure [6]. Procedure-related causes are the most common. They cause impaired wound infection and impair healing. The subcuticular closure technique may contribute to complications. The scar is more aesthetic, but the closure may not provide adequate prolonged approximation of skin edges under continuous tension from the underlying pump. In a population with impaired wound healing, securing the ends of the subcuticular suture may offer additional wound integrity.

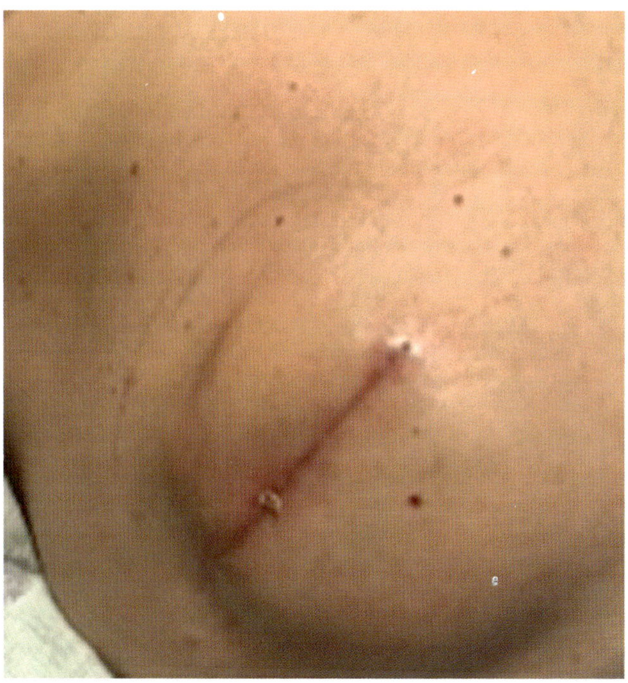

Fig. 36.1 Picture of a small area of opening 2 weeks after placement of the intrathecal drug delivery system in a patient with chronic nonmalignant pain. System was explanted as small purulent drainage was elicited; this picture is taken after initiation of intravenous antibiotic therapy upon presentation to the pain clinic and direct admission to the hospital. Image from personal library

If infection is suspected, wound cultures are obtained to guide antibiotic therapy, before incision, drainage, and washout. The wound is evaluated for possible deep fascial layer involvement, which may ultimately require pump removal. The workup should include CBC with differential, C-reactive protein, and erythrocyte sedimentation rate. Baseline values obtained before pump implantation can be compared to values when infection is suspected. Abdominal computed tomography (CT) with contrast evaluates for fluid collections, abscess, or free air.

36.5 Treatments

36.5.1 Prevention

Patients with malignancy may be malnourished and cachectic, making pump size and site selection critical in preventing wound dehiscence. The pump should not be placed over bony structures including the iliac crest or rib cage to prevent wound dehiscence and infection. A pump site over clothing friction points, such as a waistband, is not recommended because contact with the surgical wound may reduce wound healing. For surgical preparation, chlorhexidine is superior to iodine in preventing surgical site infection [7, 8]. Administering perioperative antibiotics within 1 h of skin incision minimizes infection. So does proper skin decontamination and preparation with an antiseptic agent and sterile draping [1]. For patients with penicillin allergy not listed as anaphylaxis, studies have shown less adverse reaction with cefazolin than clindamycin [9]. Specific surgical techniques may also reduce risk. Placing the surgical incision relative to the pocket so that it does not cross suture lines over the implanted device, using monofilament in place of braided suture, using antibacterial over a non-antibacterial suture, minimizing dead space within the surgical sites, and obtaining optimal hemostasis can prevent wound dehiscence and infection [10, 11]. A sufficiently large pocket must be created to minimize tension around the device. Rectus sheath implantation for patients with thin body habitus can be considered [12]. Minimizing operative time may be the single most important step taken to prevent postoperative wound infection [3].

36.5.2 Treating Pump Pocket Infection

If deep pocket infection is diagnosed, pump removal may be necessary to control and treat the infection [5]. In some cases, the pump has been salvaged with intra-reservoir antibiotic, repetitive local application of antibiotic-impregnated collagen fleece, and using rectus abdominis muscle flap and split-thickness skin graft to treat infection in a case of skin breakdown [6, 13, 14]. Timely diagnosis and treatment reduce the risk of superficial infections from penetrating deeper tissue or the pump pocket, necessitating vigilance in the postoperative period. With clear instructions for care of the incision as well as frequent follow-up visits, the healing process can be closely monitored.

Cancer patients with underlying nutritional deficiencies or infectious conditions may be at increased risk. All infections should be treated before device implantation, and nutritional status should be optimized. Obtaining albumin, prealbumin, total protein, absolute leukocyte count, and transferrin levels preoperatively may help guide nutritional status [15].

Conclusion

Targeted drug delivery via implantable devices relieves pain and improves quality of life for cancer patients. The impairments to healing from malignancy and chemotherapy should not deter practitioners from such intervention. The increased risk for impaired wound healing or infection should be assessed by the clinician and discussed with the patient. Consistent and continuous patient education, vigilant clinician monitoring, commitment to surgical best practices, and, when necessary, the expertise of wound care consultants give cancer patients access to pain relief via implantable devices.

Key Points

- Cancer diagnosis, malnutrition, diabetes, cachexia, low muscle, and fat mass in intrathecal pump patients put them at increased risk for wound dehiscence.
- Operative time is a risk factor that most increases the chance of infection in adult patients undergoing intrathecal drug delivery implantation.
- To evaluate the nutritional status of patients undergoing intrathecal pump placement, the normal ranges of values are albumin (3.4–5.4 g/dL), prealbumin (normal range, 15–35 mg/dL), total protein (6–8.3 g/dL), absolute lymphocyte count (1500–3300 cell/mm^3), and transferrin (normal range, 170–370 mg/dL).
- To prevent high-risk patients from developing wound dehiscence, the pump should be placed in an area with sufficient tissue mass and fat pad to cover it. Optimize nutritional status before insertion, use single-strand suture such as monofilament, chlorhexidine skin preparation, and perioperative antibiotics.
- The signs and symptoms of wound infection and dehiscence are pain, erythema, swelling, fever, purulent discharge, and separation of suture line or skin erosion at the pump insertion site.
- Tests to be obtained once wound dehiscence is diagnosed are CBC with differential, wound culture, C-reactive protein, erythrocyte sedimentation rate, and an abdominal CT scan with contrast.
- Intravenous antibiotics, guided by the susceptibilities of organisms from wound culture are one course of treatment for potential infection. An infectious disease specialist should be consulted if infection does not subside on antibiotic therapy. The pump may have to be removed.
- Chlorhexidine gluconate is a surgical preparation shown to be superior in preventing surgical site infections.
- Monofilament is superior to braided suture. An antibacterial suture is superior to non-antibacterial suture.
- Cefazolin is used in a patient with penicillin allergy that does not result in anaphylaxis.

References

1. Follett KA, Boortz-Marx RL, Drake JM, et al. Prevention and management of intrathecal drug delivery and spinal cord stimulation system infections. Anesthesiology. 2004;100(6):1582–94.
2. Deibert CP, Gandhoke GS, Forsythe RM, et al. Surgical site infection 18 months following intrathecal pump placement secondary to an asymptomatic bowel injury. Pain Pract. 2015;15(7):E69–71.
3. Engle MP, Vinh BP, Harun N, et al. Infectious complications related to intrathecal drug delivery system and spinal cord stimulator system implantations at a comprehensive cancer pain center. Pain Physician. 2013;16(3):251–7.
4. Malheiro L, Gomes A, Barbosa P, et al. Infectious complications of intrathecal drug administration systems for spasticity and chronic pain: 145 patients from a tertiary care center. Neuromodulation. 2015;18(5):421–7.
5. Zhou L, Villanueva J, Desai MJ, et al. Acute exacerbation of hereditary coproporphyria mimics early surgical infection following intrathecal pump implantation for chronic abdominal pain: a case report. Neuromodulation. 2010;13(4):296–8.
6. Samuel M, Finnerty GT, Rudge P. Intrathecal baclofen pump infection treated by adjunct intrareservoir antibiotic instillation. J Neurol Neurosurg Psychiatry. 1994;57(9):1146–7.
7. Levin I, Amer-Alshiek J, Avni A, et al. Chlorhexidine and alcohol versus povidone-iodine for antisepsis in gynecological surgery. J Womens Health (Larchmt). 2011;20(3):321–4.
8. Mimoz O, Lucet JC, Kerforne T, et al. Skin antisepsis with chlorhexidine-alcohol versus povidone iodine-alcohol, with and without skin scrubbing, for prevention of intravascular-catheter-related infection (CLEAN): an open-label, multicentre, randomised, controlled, two-by-two factorial trial. Lancet. 2015;386(10008):2069–77.
9. Beltran RJ, Kako H, Chovanec T, et al. Penicillin allergy and surgical prophylaxis: cephalosporin cross-reactivity risk in a pediatric tertiary care center. J Pediatr Surg. 2015;50(5):856–9.
10. Fowler JR, Perkins TA, Buttaro BA, et al. Bacteria adhere less to barbed monofilament than braided sutures in a contaminated wound model. Clin Orthop Relat Res. 2013;471(2):665–71.
11. Follett KA, Burchiel K, Deer T, et al. Prevention of intrathecal drug delivery catheter-related complications. Neuromodulation. 2003;6(1):32–41.

12. Waqar M, Ellenbogen JR, Kumar R, et al. Indwelling intrathecal catheter with subcutaneous abdominal reservoir: a viable baclofen delivery system in severely cachectic patients. J Neurosurg Pediatr. 2014;14(4):409–13.
13. Peerdeman SM, de Groot V, Feller RE. In situ treatment of an infected intrathecal baclofen pump implant with gentamicin-impregnated collagen fleece. J Neurosurg. 2010;112(6):1308–10.
14. Atiyeh BS, Hayek SN, Skaf GS, et al. Baclofen pump pocket infection: a case report of successful salvage with muscle flap. Int Wound J. 2006;3(1):23–8.
15. Lenke LG, Bridwell KH, Blanke K, Baldus C. Prospective analysis of nutritional status normalization after spinal reconstructive surgery. Spine. 1995;20(12):1359–67.

Generator and/or Lead Extrusion

37

Joseph Rabi and Magdalena Anitescu

37.1 Case Description

A 48-year-old man with a history of obesity, diabetes mellitus, and chronic low back pain presents to an outpatient pain clinic with a 2-day history of severe right gluteal pain and pruritus in the area of a previously placed spinal cord stimulator (SCS) for failed back surgery syndrome. He has a history of chronic low back pain secondary to spinal stenosis and has undergone lumbar decompression and spinal fusion which provided excellent relief for 2 years. The pain gradually recurred in the low back with radiation down both legs to his feet. Due to pain worsening, he had a SCS trial that improved his pain significantly and ability to ambulate. He subsequently had a placement of a non-rechargeable implantable pulse generator (IPG) measuring at 64 × 49 × 15 mm and weighing at 72 g with two lumbar epidural leads. The IPG was sutured in his left superior gluteal region directly below the belt line at a depth of 3 cm. He did not have any complications from the SCS, and he followed up in the pain clinic every 6 months for evaluation.

After 3 years of having the SCS in place, he went on a diet due to his obesity, and he lost over 80 lbs in a 2-month period. In addition he underwent extra shifts as a truck driver to supplement his income during the same period. Patient then gradually started to experience mild left gluteal pain and pruritus. He called the pain clinic to schedule an immediate appointment. During the visit approximately 1 week after symptoms occurred, he reported "metal sticking out of my butt" for 2 days and pain around that area. He denied having any fevers or chills. On examination, there was 0.5 cm area of the IPG exposed at the skin in the left superior buttock with the area being severely tender to palpation (Figs. 37.1 and 37.2). Given the history and presentation, it is quite clear that the IPG had extruded through the subcutaneous tissue and skin.

The area was cleaned with an antiseptic wash and topical antibiotics, and a course of oral cephalosporin was prescribed. The decision was made to remove the SCS system due to the risk of infection. Two days later, the entire SCS unit was removed without any complications. The hardware was sent to pathology and did not grow any bacteria. He completed a 10-day course of an oral cephalosporin.

Over the next 2 weeks, his pain gradually returned in the back and legs. It was decided to temporarily manage his pain with physical therapy, conservative modalities (TENS unit, back brace), and medication until a new SCS can be implanted. Three months after the removal of the first SCS, a decision was made to perform another SCS trial with the plan to implant in the right gluteal region. Patient was instructed about the risks associated with excessive weight loss which he acknowledged. In addition a smaller, rechargeable IPG was also used. The trial and implantation both took place without any complications and relieved his pain back to his original pain level when he had the initial SCS.

J. Rabi, M.D.
Pain Treatment Centers of Illinois,
Orland Park, IL, USA
e-mail: jrabi1@gmail.com

M. Anitescu, M.D., Ph.D. (✉)
Department of Anesthesia and Critical Care,
University of Chicago Medical Center, Chicago, IL, USA
e-mail: MAnitescu@dacc.uchicago.edu

M. Anitescu et al. (eds.), *Challenging Cases and Complication Management in Pain Medicine*,
https://doi.org/10.1007/978-3-319-60072-7_37

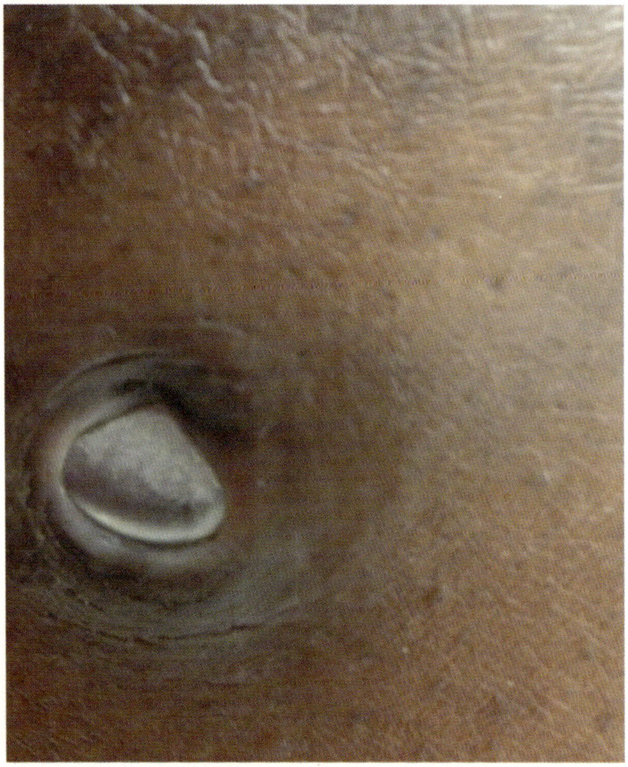

Fig. 37.1 Initial presentation of the implantable pulse generator (IPG) extrusion. Image from personal library

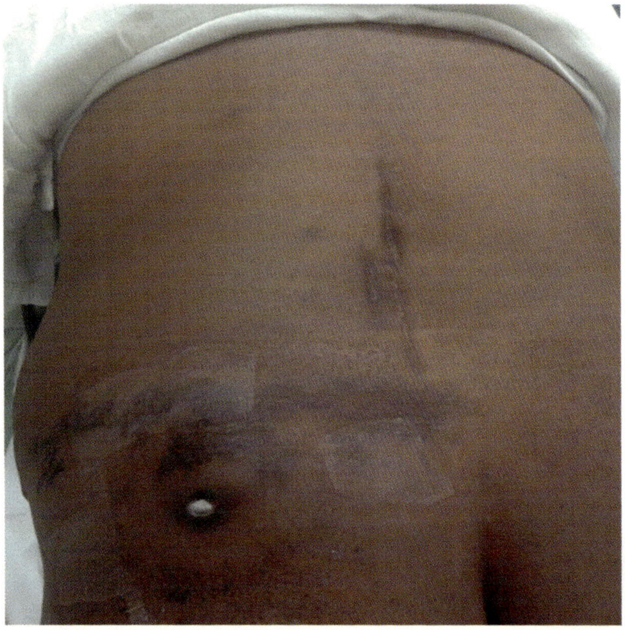

Fig. 37.2 Extrusion of the IPG immediately before explantation. As seen in this image, the original implant was toward the superior border of the gluteal area, possible pressurized during long drives as a truck driver and as a consequence of weight loss. Image from personal library

37.2 Battery and Lead Extrusion

The rate of implantations and utilization of spinal cord stimulators for pain is ever increasing. Battery and lead extrusion are rare complications that can be seen after spinal cord stimulation implantation. Extrusion refers to a component of the spinal cord stimulator protruding outside of the skin. It is usually preceded by skin erosion in which there is skin breakdown allowing the component to extrude. Typically, an extrusion occurs after superficial lead placement. The actual incidence of this occurring in the neuromodulation literature is unknown, but there is up to 1% incidence in cardiac pacemakers which uses similar components (leads/battery) to the SCS [1]. The sources used for this chapter are gathered from both the cardiac electrophysiology and neuromodulation literature as the complication of extrusion can occur in both in a similar manner.

37.3 Etiology and Pathogenesis

An extrusion of the implantable pulse generator (IPG) can be due to a number of factors (Table 37.1) [2]. First, an infection at the site can lead to skin erosion leading to an extrusion. Wound infections that involve the IPG, incision site, or tunneled area occur in up to 4% of patients [3]. Infections generally occur in the acute phase after implantation from unsterile techniques. The administration of prophylactic antibiotics during the implantation can diminish the risk of infection. The clinical manifestation of infection can be with mild systemic signs or symptoms (leukocytosis, fever, elevated sedimentation rate, or C-reactive protein) or more severe with fulminant life-threatening sepsis. Second, in the absence of infection, pressure necrosis of the soft tissue and skin can lead to an extrusion. Pressure necrosis is influenced by the size and design of the IPG. There are certain IPGs that have bigger dimensions and different architecture design that may lead to local tension on the dermis. Older versions and non-rechargeable

Table 37.1 Etiology of IPG extrusion

Etiology
Infection
Pressure necrosis size/design of IPG, occupational hazard
Technical skill in which the pocket is created
Excessive weight loss
Tissue vulnerability—elderly, diabetes, poor hygiene, depressed immunity

IPGs tend to be larger and may have sharp edges which may theoretically cause more local tension. Third, technical skill with which the pocket is created is important. The pocket in which an IPG is placed is vital in the prevention of an extrusion occurring as inadequate size or a paucity of subcutaneous tissue can contribute to local tension. A small pocket may lead to poor wound closure, pressure on the tissue, and eventual erosion. A large pocket size can potentially lead to flipping of the device, tissue irritation causing pain, or a seroma in the remaining pocket space. The pocket should be created on the surface of the gluteal muscle with enough overlying soft tissue and placed at a depth of 3 cm as superficial pockets can lead to an erosion. To ensure appropriate depth placement, telemetry and impedance testing can be done in the pocket prior to closure. Fourth, abrasive action exerted on the skin from external agents such as an occupational hazard (i.e., truck driver from prolonged sitting) can lead to extrusion [4]. The pocket location is important as it should not be placed where a long duration of pressure can be applied such as sitting for prolonged periods; therefore, the best placement of the pocket is generally in the superior gluteal area and in some instances in the abdomen. Next, excessive weight loss can cause the subcutaneous tissue to diminish leading to tension on the skin [5]. Lastly, elderly patients are at an increased risk of an erosion due to subcutaneous tissue fat loss and tissue fragility that occurs with aging. As patients age, the skin becomes more fragile causing loss of the protective fat layer.

Lead extrusion is a very rare complication as opposed to lead migration. There are only a few case reports describing extrusion occurring involving the leads [6]. The causes can include weight loss, multiple revisions, loosening of the sutures or anchors allowing the lead to float freely within a fascia tear, and patient's movement causing excessive tension on the anchor lead.

37.4 Treatment for Battery or Lead Extrusion

In the event that an extrusion occurs, the system is considered contaminated, and most practitioners favor the removal of the generator and leads [7]. The extrusion should be sterilely cleaned, covered with topical antibiotics and a sterile dressing in order to prevent exposure to the environment until explantation occurs. A course of oral antibiotics should be given in order to avoid a secondary infection. An extensive debridement of the pocket might be necessary during the removal. In addition, there should be prolonged antibiotic irrigation during the removal. An antibiotic should be given for a 1–2-week course post-explantation depending on the severity and growth of an organism. Aerobic and anaerobic cultures of the skin, blood, leads, and IPG should be taken to determine organism growth, if any, and sensitivities to antibiotics. The antibiotic choices should cover *Staphylococcus* organisms which include a cephalosporin, fluoroquinolone, or TMP-SMX. If methicillin-resistant *Staphylococcus aureus* is grown, the antibiotic given should be doxycycline, clindamycin, TMP-SMX, or linezolid. In special circumstances (colostomy, sacral hiatus, bacteremia), the antibiotic choice should also cover a gram-negative organism. It is best to seek a consultation from an infectious disease expert regarding duration and optimal antibiotic regimen. After the spinal cord stimulator system is removed, the cause should be determined in order to prevent a future extrusion. The clinician should allow the erosion site to heal prior to reimplantation. The IPG can be reimplanted either in the abdomen although this requires longer leads or connected extensions and is technically difficult to position the patient during the procedure or the opposite gluteal site.

It is imperative for the clinician and patient to be able to recognize the period of erosion preceding IPG extrusion with warning signs such as pruritus, discomfort, discoloration, thinning, and a tensely stretched appearance of the skin. If the skin is intact, surgical revision of the pocket is often sufficient to protect the hardware from contamination and infection and eventual extrusion.

Patients that undergo multiple revisions have higher risk of wound dehiscence due to local trauma to the area. A clinician may have to make revisions for lead migration, epidural fibrosis, current CSF leak, or infection. The risk factors of wound dehiscence include obesity, diabetes, poor-quality sutures, and trauma to the wound after surgery. Wound dehiscence can lead to erosion of the SCS system resulting in the necessity of removal.

The clinical vignette describes a middle-aged man that had excellent relief of his failed back syndrome after having the spinal cord stimulator implanted. As SCS alleviates pain, it allows patients to be more active and participate in more exercise. As a result, patients may lose weight as the patient in the vignette lost 80 lbs over 2 months. Weight loss can potentially cause the positioning of the IPG to shift. Also, weight loss causes a decrease in subcutaneous tissue between the IPG and the surface of the skin. Therefore, patients need to be educated on excessive weight loss prior to implantation of a spinal cord stimulator as dramatic weight loss can lead to a decrease in subcutaneous fat and potentially increase the risk of extrusion of the IPG through the skin. In thin patients or in patients with excessive weight loss, it may be necessary to perform a revision to a different location or to a tissue plane below the fascia.

Key Concepts

- The extrusion of an implantable pulse generator and leads of a spinal cord stimulator system are uncommon.
- Extrusion occurs due to an infection, pressure necrosis, superficial implantation, or excessive weight loss.
- The clinical symptoms a patient presents with include discoloration of the skin, pruritus, and discomfort prior to the extrusion of the IPG or leads.
- An urgent diagnosis is necessary and is based on history and physical exam.
- Treatment consists of removal of the IPG and a course of antibiotics. Reimplantation should be performed once the site heals into a different site.

References

1. Harcombe AA, Newel SA, Ludman PF, et al. Late complications following permanent pacemaker implantation or elective unit replacement. Heart. 1998;80:240–4.
2. Santarpia G, Sarubbi B, D'Alto M, et al. Extrusion of the device: a rare complication of the pacemaker implantation. J Cardiovasc Med. 2009;10:330–2.
3. Deer TR, Stewart CD. Complications of spinal cord stimulation: identification, treatment, and prevention. Pain Med. 2008;9:S93–101.
4. Rabi J, Anitescu M. Late extrusion of an implantable pulse generator of a spinal cord stimulator. Pain Physician. 2016;19(4):E671–4.
5. Nold CJ, McLennan MT. Spontaneous extrusion of sacral nerve implant secondary to massive weight loss. Int Urogynecol J Pelvic Floor Dysfunct. 2007;18(1):105–7.
6. Soliman S, Wang J, Kim D, Cipta A, Pang G. Percutaneous extrusion of an implanted spinal cord stimulator. Pain Med. 2015;16(2):407–8.
7. Shapiro M, Hanon S, Schweitzer P. A rare, late complication after automated implantable cardioverter-defibrillator placement. Indian Pacing Electrophysiol J. 2004;4(4):213–6.

Spinal Cord Stimulator Complications: Lead Migration and Malfunction

38

Mikiko Murakami, Imanuel Lerman, and R. Carter W. Jones III

38.1 Case Description

A 55-year-old male, with a past medical history significant for multilevel cervical and lumbar degenerative disease, presents to the pain clinic with chronic axial neck and radicular low back pain after cervical and lumbar spine surgery consistent with cervical and lumbar post-laminectomy syndrome. After successful trial, he had a spinal cord stimulation (SCS) system placed to treat his low back pain without complications. He reported alleviation of this pain using conventional paresthesia stimulation via two percutaneous eight contact leads positioned with the tips at the middle of the T6 vertebral body level. The patient had adequate analgesia for over a year and was able to return to employment, which he hadn't been able to do for 6 months prior to the implant. One year later, he experienced a reduction in analgesia with inadequate coverage of his previously painful areas. In addition, he noticed increased paresthesias migrating to above the nipple line that were now bothersome. He also complained of insomnia refractory to conservative regimen. Reprogramming the stimulator did not resolve these issues. Imaging studies obtained at that time confirmed a cephalad and lateral migration of one of the stimulation leads. During the surgical revision to reposition the migrated lead, both leads were found to be frayed at the distal tips. The leads were replaced and repositioned to obtain adequate coverage of his painful areas. The patient reported adequate pain relief after the revision, without any adverse events.

M. Murakami, D.O. • I. Lerman, M.D.
R.C.W. Jones III, M.D., Ph.D. (✉)
Department of Anesthesiology, Center for Pain Medicine, University of California San Diego, San Diego, CA, USA
e-mail: c0jones@ucsd.edu

38.2 Case Discussion

38.2.1 Overview of Spinal Cord Stimulation

SCS is a well-established neuromodulatory technique used to address refractory chronic pain. The implantable device is part of an overall pain treatment strategy and is implemented only after more conservative treatments have failed. It has been shown to decrease pain and improve functionality, enabling some patients to go back to work, and, ultimately, SCS implantation has proven to be cost-effective despite relatively high initial costs of implantation [1]. This invasive treatment typically involves two steps, first a trial of stimulation for one or more days (typically 4–7) to verify adequate pain relief and lack of adverse side effects, including unwanted paresthesias. During this step, one or more stimulation leads are placed percutaneously in the posterior epidural space and are driven by an external IPG. If successful (more than 50% reduction of the pain with the system on), the trial leads are removed and replaced by surgical implantation of a permanent, subcutaneous stimulation system. The system consists of stimulation leads, either paddle or percutaneous, that are placed into the posterior epidural space with or without laminectomy, respectively, and tunneled subcutaneously to an IPG secured in a subcutaneous pocket, typically on the posterior flank or buttock. SCS is FDA approved for the management of chronic, intractable pain of the trunk or limbs, including post-laminectomy syndrome, and the device has been shown to successfully treat various neuropathic pain syndromes [2, 3]. Although off-label, SCS has also been shown to successfully treat cancer-related pain in adults [4], ischemic pain from peripheral vascular diseases [5], chronic visceral abdominal pain [6], and even refractory angina, although recent randomized controlled studies have shown small improvement effects [7].

Despite clinically positive results, mechanisms supporting its efficacy have not been well elucidated. Parameters such as lead design, stimulation mode, and stimulation

M. Anitescu et al. (eds.), *Challenging Cases and Complication Management in Pain Medicine*,
https://doi.org/10.1007/978-3-319-60072-7_38

intensity can all effect outcomes with likely differing mechanisms, and the exact nerve fibers and neural pathways that are activated through the highly conductive cerebrospinal fluid remain unclear [8, 9]. SCS has been shown to inhibit both nociceptive and non-nociceptive myelinated sensory afferents at segmental spinal or supraspinal levels [10]. Several studies of SCS used resting-state functional MRI to investigate changes in cortical networks and cortical processing involved in stimulation-induced analgesia; they revealed that SCS can reduce the affective component of pain [11]. The sympatholytic effect of SCS is considered to be responsible for the effectiveness of SCS in peripheral ischemia [12] and complex regional pain syndrome [13]. This effect has also been considered part of the management of other chronic pain states such as failed back surgery syndrome, phantom pain, diabetic neuropathy, and post-herpetic neuralgia [13–15].

38.2.2 Factors Influencing Success of Spinal Cord Stimulator Implantation

38.2.2.1 Patient Selection

As with any pain treatment, proper patient selection includes a comprehensive history and physical examination. In addition, a detailed psychological assessment is necessary to identify psychosocial factors that could limit efficacy. Ultimately, the goal is for the patient to achieve therapeutic success while minimizing adverse events. Patients who meet the following criteria are most likely to benefit [16]:

- Chronic, intractable pain for more than 6 months.
- Objective evidence of pathology concordant with pain complaint.
- Lack of adequate relief from more conventional treatments.
- Initial or further surgical intervention not indicated.
- No contraindications to therapy or surgery.
- Patient can properly understand how to operate the system and is able to operate it.
- Patient understands therapy risks.
- Therapy and function goals have been established.
- Satisfactory results from the screening test.
- Patient is not pregnant.
- No untreated drug abuse.
- Clearance and completion of psychological evaluation.
- 18 years of age or older.

38.2.2.2 Perioperative Preparation and Procedure

Anatomical, medical, and psychological considerations are taken into account prior to considering SCS trial in all patients. Spinal abnormalities such as spondylosis, scoliosis, prior surgery, and spinal stenosis can pose technical difficulties for successful placement of the stimulator leads within the epidural space. Medical assessment includes evaluation of functional and neurologic status, excluding sources of active infection, and identifying coagulopathy, impaired immune response, and other factors that would affect tissue healing, such as diabetes and tobacco abuse [17]. Psychological evaluation is essential, as negative psychosocial factors have been found to predict poor outcome with SCS [18]. Patients benefit from being educated about the procedural and postoperative expectations of SCS prior to the trial [17]. Presurgical psychological preparation, detailed informed consent, and post-procedural information should also be given. Intraoperative medical considerations include holding anticoagulant medications for the appropriate length of time [19] and the administration of antibiotics.

38.2.2.3 SCS Device Comparisons

Various vendors have different hardware components that may affect treatment outcomes. Things to consider include:

- System type (e.g., voltage, power sources)
- Coverage (e.g., number of contacts, percutaneous versus paddle lead, maximum pulse width, maximum voltage, maximum frequency)
- Software (e.g., programming algorithm, upgradeable, positional shock)
- Battery (e.g., cordless recharge, battery life)
- Warranty and accessibility to SCS device representative

38.2.3 Overview of Complications

As with any sophisticated medical device, complications can and do occur with SCS (Table 38.1). In a 2014 review of complications, electrode (lead) migration was found to be the most

Table 38.1 Approximate rate of complications of SCS: compilation of published data from Zan et al. [22] and Bendersky et al. [20]

Complication	Frequency (%)
Electrode migration	1.5–13.2
Hardware malfunction	
• Electrode	3–9
• IPG	3–25
Infection	2.5–14
Cerebrospinal fluid leakage	0.3–8
Pain at the incisions, IPG site	0.9–12
Subcutaneous hematoma or seroma	9
Epidural hematoma	4
Electrode fracture	
Intraoperative neurologic injury	Case reports
Unexplained temporary paralysis	1.8
Others (e.g., skin erosion, aseptic meningitis, allergic dermatitis, activation of pyramidal tract)	Case reports

frequent complication of SCS, with a greater incidence involving percutaneous compared to paddle leads [20]. Other complications include infection, electrode fracture, extension wire or implantable pulse generator failures, cerebrospinal fluid leakage, pain over the stimulator components, and spinal epidural hematoma [20]. A recent retrospective study of 345 SCS patients concluded that it is a safe, minimally invasive procedure with good long-term outcomes but with high rates of hardware malfunction particularly, comprising 74.1% of all complications and leading to surgical revision and explant rates of 23.9% each [21]. In a different 5-year retrospective review, review of radiologic imaging studies obtained in patients with SCS systems found that hardware complications comprised 50% of all complications while infectious complications comprised 29.1% (Table 38.1) [22]. In a systematic review that analyzed the effectiveness and complications of this device for failed back surgery syndrome and complex regional pain syndrome, 34% of the patients experienced some type of an adverse event, and pain relief decreased over time [23].

38.2.4 Surgical Complications

Complications may be avoided or at least diminished by good surgical technique and strict sterile precautions, as well as optimizing patient selection before the implantation according to published recommendations [20].

38.2.4.1 Seroma and CSF Hygromas

Seromas and hematomas can occur in up to 9% of patients with SCS implants [20]. Seromas, a collection of serous fluid beneath the wound, are one of the most benign surgical complications. Early detection is key in order to prevent infection complicating a seroma. Seromas present early after surgery similarly to hematomas with acute, afebrile, swelling and pain at the surgical site. If the seroma is very tender or large, it can be aspirated under sterile conditions. Empiric antibiotics are not recommended for seromas to avoid complicating the diagnosis: seromas can be managed conservatively with abdominal binder and serial aspirations if necessary, whereas infected hardware warrants explantation [17].

CSF leakage can occur in 0.3–7% of patients [20]. If the fluid collection is due to CSF accumulation (hygroma), the initial care is to observe and treat similarly as a seroma, but if the wound is tense and painful, it should be aspirated under sterile conditions. If laboratory analysis of the aspirate is consistent with CSF and the hygroma does not respond to conservative management, an epidural blood patch can be performed near the site of catheter entry into the intrathecal space to theoretically seal the leak. Rarely, referral for surgical exploration is necessary for large or persistent hygromas. If the patient has systemic symptoms and signs of infection and hygroma is present, urgent evaluation and treatment for meningitis should be initiated [17].

38.2.4.2 Hematoma

A hematoma is a blood collection in the subcutaneous tissues. They are associated with an increased risk of infection compared to seromas [17], which can best be mitigated by careful surgical technique and meticulous attention to hemostasis, as well as appropriate perioperative management of coagulation issues; any anticoagulant should be held an appropriate amount of time prior to surgery to aid in their prevention. There is a greater risk in exploring a small, stable hematoma compared to watchful waiting, as usually a hematoma will usually resolve on its own. Larger volume or expanding hematomas should be evacuated under sterile conditions to prevent wound dehiscence [17]. Basic laboratory studies of aspirated fluid and ultrasound imaging can be helpful to differentiate between seroma, hematoma, and infection.

38.2.4.3 Wound Dehiscence

Wound dehiscence (Fig. 38.1) occurs when one or more layers of the surgical wound separate. This most often occurs between 5 and 8 days after surgery [17]. It is more common in patients prone to poor wound healing, such as patients with diabetes, immunosuppression, and cancer. Wound closure with excessive tension on the wound itself can lead to ischemia and subsequent separation of tissue layers due to necrosis. Failure to sufficiently close tissue layers will also lead to dehiscence. In the absence of infection, the patient with a partially dehisced wound can be managed conservatively with regular decontamination of the wound and dressing changes to allow the wound to heal by secondary intention.

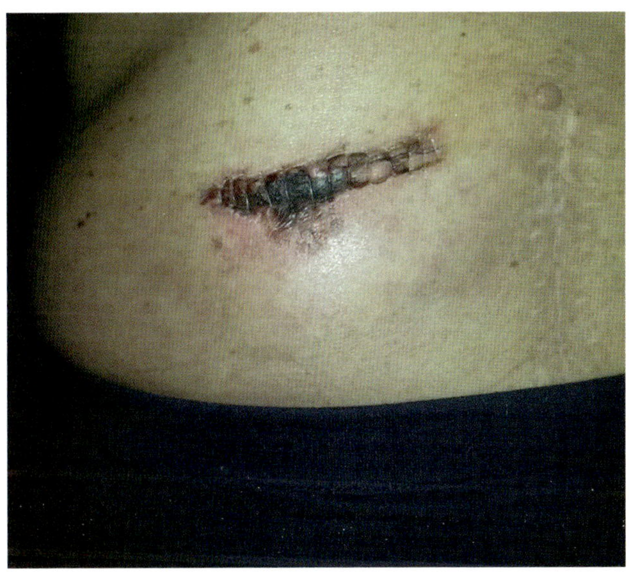

Fig. 38.1 Postoperative wound dehiscence. Photo courtesy of the University of California San Diego Anesthesia Department

38.2.4.4 Infection or Epidural Abscess

Infection or epidural abscess after an SCS trial or implantation calls for explantation of the device as well as decompression and drainage of the abscess. Infection rates after SCS implantation range from 2.5 to 14% [21]. The symptoms of an epidural abscess can be similar to an epidural hematoma, including fever, new neurologic deficits, leukocytosis, and severe pain and are all strong indications for emergent surgical decompression. Suspicion of an epidural abscess warrants an emergent CT scan and an infectious laboratory workup, including ESR, CRP, CBC, and blood cultures.

A recent international survey examined current reported infection control practices for SCS trials and implants and compared them to evidence-based recommendations obtained from standard surgical guidelines and recommendations of the Centers of Disease Control and Prevention (CDC), the National Institute for Health and Care Excellence (NICE), and the Surgical Care Improvement Project (SCIP) [24]. The authors identified multiple areas with high levels of noncompliance, including weight-based antibiotic dosing, hair removal strategies, double gloving, surgical dressing, skin antiseptic agent selection, and postoperative continuation of antibiotics [24]. Improved compliance with established infection control practices can significantly reduce reported rates of infection after SCS procedures.

38.2.4.5 Dural Puncture and Spinal Cord Injury

Although dural puncture is a very rare complication of SCS, it can occur, as noted in a case study of electrode placement into the spinal cord itself causing tetraparesis in a patient [25]. One of the most common causes of a "wet tap" is an unrecognized blood clot obstructing the lumen of the Tuohy needle during lead placement. With a clot in the needle, it is difficult to appreciate the loss of resistance when entering the epidural space. If blood drips back out of the hub, the physician should stop, flush the needle with saline, and withdraw the needle to make sure it is patent prior to proceeding [17]. Judicious use of multiple fluoroscopic angles (AP, lateral, and oblique), cautious needle advancement, and entering the epidural space below the termination of the spinal cord can help to prevent inadvertent dural puncture and potential spinal cord injury.

38.2.5 Hardware Complications

Although the available SCS systems are very reliable and most hardware malfunctions can be readily corrected, device malfunctions and complications should not be trivialized, as surgery is still required to repair them. Complications also interfere with the patient's pain therapy, are costly, and are associated with all the attendant risks of surgery and anesthesia.

38.2.5.1 Lead Migration

After epidural placement, percutaneous leads are typically secured into the prevertebral fascia. Nonetheless, lead migration commonly occurs after implant, resulting not just in loss of analgesia but also potential for onset of new pain due to electrical stimulation of other structures, including the ligamentum flavum and/or the dorsal root entry zone (DREZ) [26]. Percutaneous spinal cord stimulation (SCS) electrodes are prone to migration even after scar tissue encapsulation [27] and are the most common mechanical reason for SCS failure [28]. In a retrospective review that examined records of SCS implantation between 2008 and 2011, 2.1% of the patients required a surgical revision due to clinically significant lead migration. Some investigators have estimated a 13–22% revision rate due to lead migration [29], with others reporting up to 30–40% [30]. Proper anchoring of the lead will lessen the chance of lead migration. Different manufacturers provide several different types of lead anchors; a simple "figure-of-eight" anchoring suture tie is also effective for securing stimulation leads [17]. A recent retrospective review of a novel fixation device demonstrated no lead migration at extended follow-up (10–68 weeks), suggesting that these types of devices may reduce the incidence of lead migration [30]. Another group showed the utility of bone cement to prevent lead migration with minimally invasive placement of spinal cord stimulator leads via laminectomy [31] (Fig. 38.2).

38.2.5.2 Lead Fraying, Pulse Generator Failure, and Losing Coverage

As illustrated in the case presentation, lead fraying (Fig. 38.3) is a known complication of SCS systems. A patient may experience increased pain, dysesthesias, and/or paresthesias. Commonly, the patient may report a prior traumatic event causing strain on the lead itself. Spontaneous lead breakage and insulation failures have also been reported [32] (Fig. 38.4). On rare occasions the IPG can also fail. All of these scenarios require surgical replacement and revision of the system.

If the patient reports loss of analgesia, reprogramming of the device is a viable first option. This can be done in the outpatient clinic setting. There are several published cases where a patient treated with SCS develops a new pain complaint, and device reprogramming provides an additional pain control of the new region. For example, a patient with complex regional pain syndrome type I with lower extremity radiculopathy reported 1 month of pain relief with the use of an SCS. However, she developed slipping rib syndrome after thoracotomy, and reprogramming her SCS covered her newly developed pain condition [33].

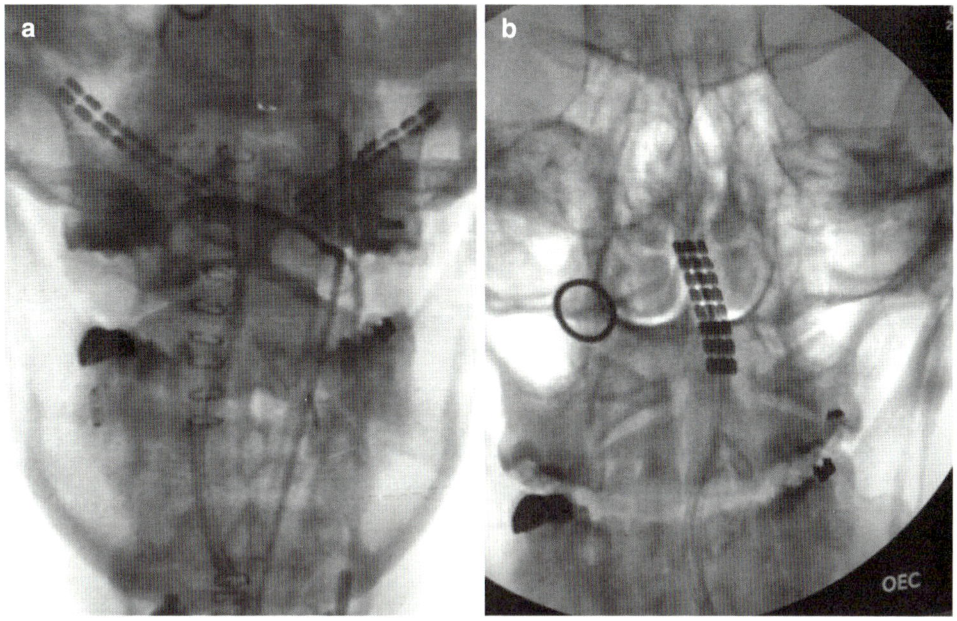

Fig. 38.2 Migration of occipital nerve stimulator leads. Panel **a**: proper intraoperative positioning of leads. Panel **b**: postoperative lead migration. Photo courtesy of the University of California San Diego Anesthesia Department

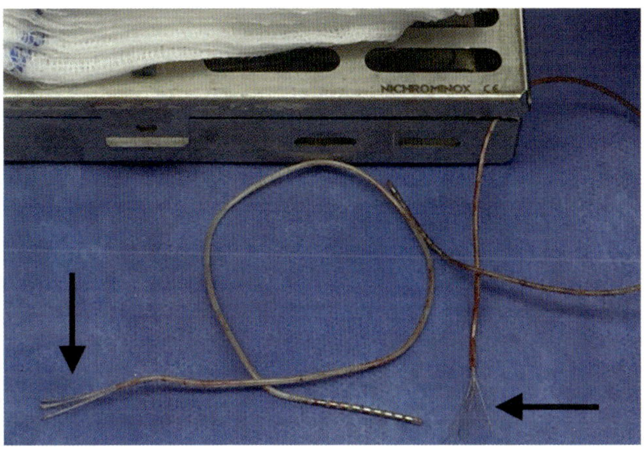

Fig. 38.3 Frayed spinal cord stimulator leads. Arrows point to frayed ends. Photo courtesy of the University of California San Diego Anesthesia Department

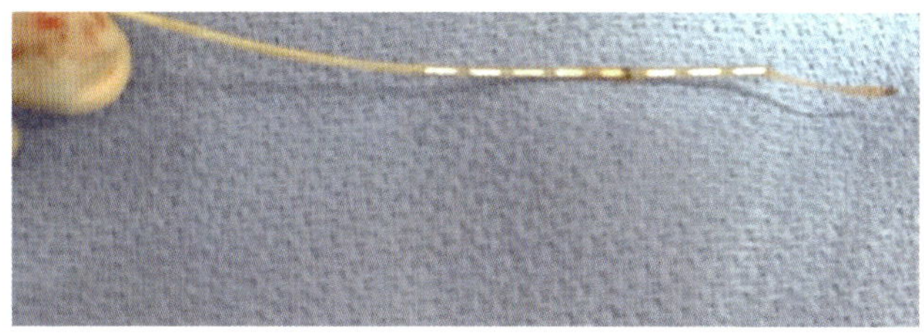

Fig. 38.4 Defected spinal cord stimulator lead. Contact number 4 with charring and different color; when on, patient felt electric shock in the mid-thoracic area. Photo courtesy of the University of Chicago Medicine, Department of Anesthesia and Critical Care

38.2.5.3 Hardware Complications due to Perioperative Procedures: MRI and Electrocautery

Perioperative hardware complications can also occur in patients with SCS systems. Prior to July 2013, SCS systems were not MRI compatible [34], requiring explantation prior to imaging. Now, based on the hardware specifications, certain SCS systems are compatible with MRI imaging of the brain and full body (conditional) MRI. Before performing an MRI, it is important to know which device a patient has implanted and if it is compatible with an MRI and to assess that the device is functioning properly and fully intact prior to the procedure, as these issues may result in heating of the device and potential injury to the patient. Electrocautery is another process that may damage SCS systems, and it is generally not recommended. If cautery is deemed necessary by the surgeon, bipolar electrocautery is recommended, and the electrocautery units should be used with caution to avoid damage to the system and thermal injury to the patient. Similar to MRI, electrocautery use in patients with impaired SCS systems, such as systems with suspected breaks or abnormal impedances, is unsafe and may cause injury [35].

Key Concepts

- Spinal cord stimulators are cost-effective in the long term and aid people with chronic, intractable pain.
- Surgical complications include seroma, hematoma, hygroma, wound dehiscence, infection, dural puncture, and cord injury.
- Hardware complications include lead migration (most common), lead fraying, and IPG failure.
- Prompt workup of any suspected complication is based on history, physical exam, appropriate laboratory studies, and imaging.

References

1. Kumar K, Malik S, Demeria D. Treatment of chronic pain with spinal cord stimulation versus alternative therapies: cost-effectiveness analysis. Neurosurgery. 2002;51(1):106–15; discussion 115–6.
2. Health Quality O. Spinal cord stimulation for neuropathic pain: an evidence-based analysis. Ont Health Technol Assess Ser. 2005;5(4):1–78.
3. Yampolsky C, Hem S, Bendersky D. Dorsal column stimulator applications. Surg Neurol Int. 2012;3(Suppl 4):S275–89.
4. Peng L, et al. Spinal cord stimulation for cancer-related pain in adults. Cochrane Database Syst Rev. 2015;6:CD009389.
5. Wu M, Linderoth B, Foreman RD. Putative mechanisms behind effects of spinal cord stimulation on vascular diseases: a review of experimental studies. Auton Neurosci. 2008;138(1–2):9–23.
6. Kapural L, et al. Spinal cord stimulation for chronic visceral abdominal pain. Pain Med. 2010;11(3):347–55.
7. Tsigaridas N, et al. Spinal cord stimulation in refractory angina. A systematic review of randomized controlled trials. Acta Cardiol. 2015;70(2):233–43.
8. Guan Y, et al. Spinal cord stimulation-induced analgesia: electrical stimulation of dorsal column and dorsal roots attenuates dorsal horn neuronal excitability in neuropathic rats. Anesthesiology. 2010;113(6):1392–405.
9. Guan Y. Spinal cord stimulation: neurophysiological and neurochemical mechanisms of action. Curr Pain Headache Rep. 2012;16(3):217–25.
10. de Andrade DC, et al. Neurophysiological assessment of spinal cord stimulation in failed back surgery syndrome. Pain. 2010;150(3):485–91.
11. Deogaonkar M, et al. Spinal Cord Stimulation (SCS) and Functional Magnetic Resonance Imaging (fMRI): modulation of cortical connectivity with therapeutic SCS. Neuromodulation. 2016;19(2):142–53.
12. Pedrini L, Magnoni F. Spinal cord stimulation for lower limb ischemic pain treatment. Interact Cardiovasc Thorac Surg. 2007;6(4):495–500.
13. Vannemreddy P, Slavin KV. Spinal cord stimulation: current applications for treatment of chronic pain. Anesth Essays Res. 2011;5(1):20–7.
14. Katayama Y, et al. Motor cortex stimulation for phantom limb pain: comprehensive therapy with spinal cord and thalamic stimulation. Stereotact Funct Neurosurg. 2001;77(1–4):159–62.
15. Viswanathan A, Phan PC, Burton AW. Use of spinal cord stimulation in the treatment of phantom limb pain: case series and review of the literature. Pain Pract. 2010;10(5):479–84.
16. Medtronics Spinal Cord Stimulation: Patient Selection. http://professional.medtronic.com/pt/neuro/scs/edu/patient-selection/index.htm. kQZEmSrQ1h.
17. Kreis PG, Fishman S. Spinal cord stimulation: percutaneous implantation techniques. Oxford: Oxford University Press; 2009.
18. Block AR, Ben-Porath YS, Marek RJ. Psychological risk factors for poor outcome of spine surgery and spinal cord stimulator implant: a review of the literature and their assessment with the MMPI-2-RF. Clin Neuropsychol. 2013;27(1):81–107.
19. Narouze S, et al. Interventional spine and pain procedures in patients on antiplatelet and anticoagulant medications: guidelines from the American Society of Regional Anesthesia and Pain Medicine, the European Society of Regional Anaesthesia and Pain Therapy, the American Academy of Pain Medicine, the International Neuromodulation Society, the North American Neuromodulation Society, and the World Institute of Pain. Reg Anesth Pain Med. 2015;40(3):182–212.
20. Bendersky D, Yampolsky C. Is spinal cord stimulation safe? A review of its complications. World Neurosurg. 2014;82(6):1359–68.
21. Hayek SM, Veizi E, Hanes M. Treatment-limiting complications of percutaneous spinal cord stimulator implants: a review of eight years of experience from an academic center database. Neuromodulation. 2015;18(7):603–9.
22. Zan E, et al. Spinal cord stimulators: typical positioning and postsurgical complications. AJR Am J Roentgenol. 2011;196(2):437–45.
23. Turner JA, et al. Spinal cord stimulation for patients with failed back surgery syndrome or complex regional pain syndrome: a systematic review of effectiveness and complications. Pain. 2004;108(1–2):137–47.
24. Provenzano DA, et al. An international survey to understand infection control practices for spinal cord stimulation. Neuromodulation. 2015.
25. Meyer SC, Swartz K, Johnson JP. Quadriparesis and spinal cord stimulation: case report. Spine (Phila Pa 1976). 2007;32(19):E565–8.
26. Jang SS, et al. Case series on variable presentation of ligamentum flavum stimulation following percutaneous cylindrical spinal cord stimulator lead implants. Pain Physician. 2014;17(3):E397–403.
27. Renard VM, North RB. Prevention of percutaneous electrode migration in spinal cord stimulation by a modification of the standard implantation technique. J Neurosurg Spine. 2006;4(4):300–3.
28. Stojanovic MP, Abdi S. Spinal cord stimulation. Pain Physician. 2002;5(2):156–66.
29. Gazelka HM, et al. Incidence of clinically significant percutaneous spinal cord stimulator lead migration. Neuromodulation. 2015;18(2):123–5; discussion 125.
30. Justiz R 3rd, Bentley I. A case series review of spinal cord stimulation migration rates with a novel fixation device. Neuromodulation. 2014;17(1):37–40; discussion 40–1.
31. Connor DE Jr, et al. The utility of bone cement to prevent lead migration with minimally invasive placement of spinal cord stimulator laminectomy leads. Neurosurgery. 2012;71(1):157–63.
32. Kim TH, et al. Spontaneous lead breakage in implanted spinal cord stimulation systems. Korean J Pain. 2010;23(1):78–81.
33. Knezevic NN, et al. Reprogramming of in situ spinal cord stimulator for covering newly developed postthoracotomy pain. J Clin Anesth. 2015;27(5):411–5.
34. Moeschler SM, et al. Spinal cord stimulator explantation for magnetic resonance imaging: a case series. Neuromodulation. 2015;18(4):285–8; discussion 288.
35. Walsh KM, Machado AG, Krishnaney AA. Spinal cord stimulation: a review of the safety literature and proposal for perioperative evaluation and management. Spine J. 2015;15(8):1864–9.

Epidural Infection

39

David R. Walega

39.1 Case Description

A 41-year-old female with type 2 diabetes mellitus, GERD, and asthma presents to the outpatient pain management practice 3 weeks following the surgical implantation of a single electrode spinal cord stimulator and internal pulse generator. She is reporting worsening low back pain, malaise, fevers, poorly controlled glucose levels, and 24 h of urinary retention. She missed her scheduled, postoperative follow-up appointment and wound check at 1 week due to transportation problems. The indication for SCS implantation was intractable, and refractory left buttock and radicular left leg pain was present for the past 2 years. Prior to her treatment with you, she had been diagnosed with S1 radiculopathy from a large L5–S1 herniated disc and had undergone an uncomplicated L5–S1 microdiscectomy. Initially after her decompressive surgery, she had a nearly complete resolution of pain symptoms, but 4 months later, she developed worsening radicular pain of the same pattern and distribution. A subsequent MRI showed profound epidural fibrosis on the left L5–S1 region, the prior surgical site. Under your care, she failed to improve with trials of membrane stabilizers, physical therapy, and selective spinal nerve injections of steroid. She had undergone a 9-day percutaneous trial of dorsal columns stimulation with 90% reduction in buttock and leg pain prior to the surgical implantation of the permanent system. The permanent SCS implantation was performed on the same day the trial electrode was removed.

She works as a nursing assistant in a rehabilitation facility and has been unable to return to work since her SCS was implanted, 3 weeks prior to the current postoperative visit. She does not use alcohol, and she smokes one-half pack of cigarettes per day but stopped during her SCS trial.

D.R. Walega, M.D.
Feinberg School of Medicine Northwestern University,
Chicago, IL, USA
e-mail: d-walega@northwestern.edu

Her vital signs show a blood pressure of 108/57, a heart rate of 108, respirations of 22, and a temperature of 101.9 °F. She reports 8/10 central back and bilateral buttock pain using the numerical rating scale (NRS). The back pain is well localized to the surgical incision at the midline upper lumbar region. She is in moderate to severe distress with any movement. She has a slow, guarded, antalgic gait. Her motor and sensory examination of the lower extremities demonstrates no focal deficits, but there is decreased sensation in the S2, S3, and S4 dermatomes bilaterally. Rectal tone is normal. Straight leg raise causes profound back and buttock pain. The internal pulse generator (IPG) site on the right gluteal region shows an intact incision, resolving ecchymosis and a mild seroma. The midline incision where the electrode was implanted is partially dehisced with a purulent exudate and erythema in the surrounding tissues (Fig. 39.1). On closer inspection of this wound, the infection is deep to the skin layer, and a portion of the electrode is visible within a purulent fluid collection.

Clearly, a wound infection has occurred, but you suspect an epidural infection given her worsening back pain and new neurologic findings. While in the office, you have her blood drawn for analysis and culture:

- WBC 12.5 K/UL
- Differential: segmented neutrophils 81%, lymphocytes 14%, basophils 2%, and eosinophils 3%
- Hemoglobin 13.4 g/dL and platelets 318 K/UL
- Hemoglobin A1C (glycohemoglobin) 7.7%
- Erythrocyte sedimentation rate (ESR) 44 mm/h
- C-reactive protein (CRP) 108 mg/L

The MRI shows an enhancing fluid collection in the posterior epidural space at the T11–T12 level. See Figs. 39.2, 39.3, 39.4, and 39.5 for examples of epidural abscesses on MRI. Neurosurgery is consulted, and they agree that the abscess necessitates surgical drainage. Culture samples of

M. Anitescu et al. (eds.), *Challenging Cases and Complication Management in Pain Medicine*,
https://doi.org/10.1007/978-3-319-60072-7_39

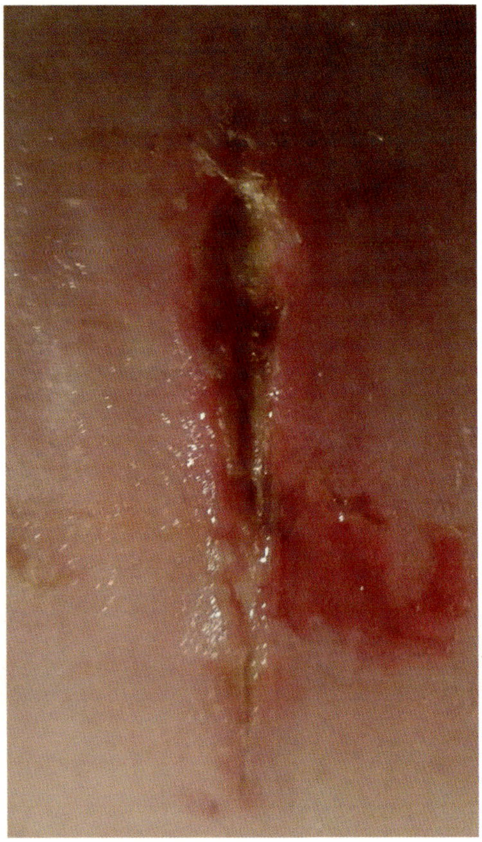

Fig. 39.1 Epidural electrode implantation scar at midline thoracolumbar junction. The superior edge of the wound is dehisced with thick purulent drainage. A deep pocket of pus was identified on closer inspection, and the contaminated electrode could be visualized

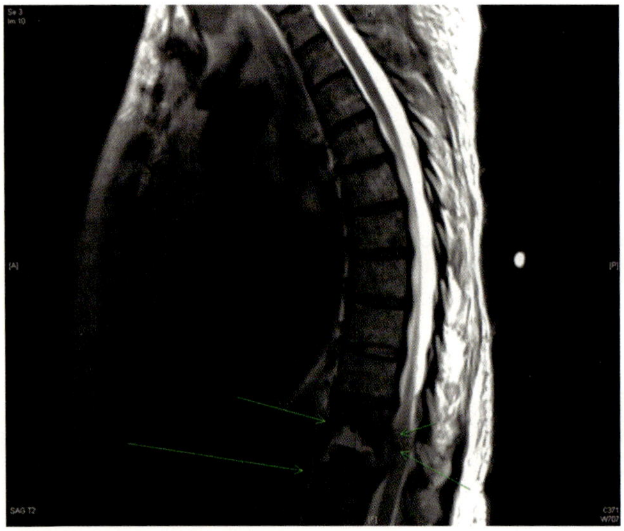

Fig. 39.2 T2 sagittal MRI image of a 78-year-old female with a large ventral epidural abscess at the T11–T12 level, surrounded by green arrows. This extensive infection extends into the vertebral body and intervertebral disc. The patient, in contrast to the patient presented in this case study, presented with profound neurologic deficits

the abscess material return with abundant gram-positive cocci. Given the patient's risk factors for methicillin-resistant *Staphylococcus aureus* (MRSA), (recent surgery,

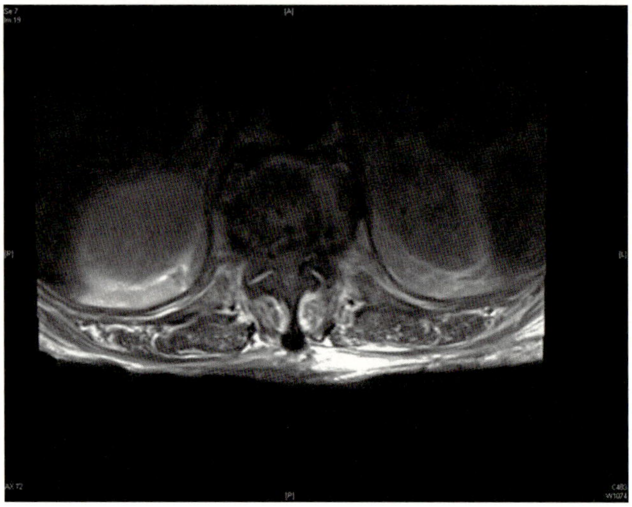

Fig. 39.3 T2 axial image of this same patient. The spinal canal is essentially obliterated with abscess at this level

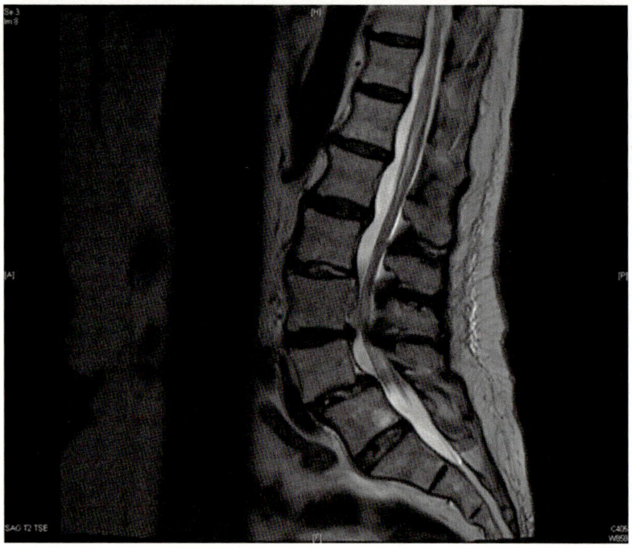

Fig. 39.4 A 69-year-old female with known L45 anterolisthesis presented with worsening back and right thigh pain following an LESI at L34. This T2 sagittal image confirms a ventral epidural fluid collection consistent with an epidural abscess

works in an inpatient healthcare facility), vancomycin is initiated to treat the infection until antibiotic sensitivity testing is completed. The following day, she is afebrile, and she remains neurologically intact, and urinary retention symptoms improve. Blood cultures are found to be positive for MRSA with sensitivity to vancomycin. She is hospitalized for an additional 4 days during which her glucose level is stabilized and serial ESR and CRP continue to decrease. A PICC line is placed, and she is sent home for an additional 5-week course of vancomycin. Despite this nearly catastrophic complication, the patient requests that you reimplant the SCS again, as she had profound pain relief and improved function during her trial and immediately after the initial implant.

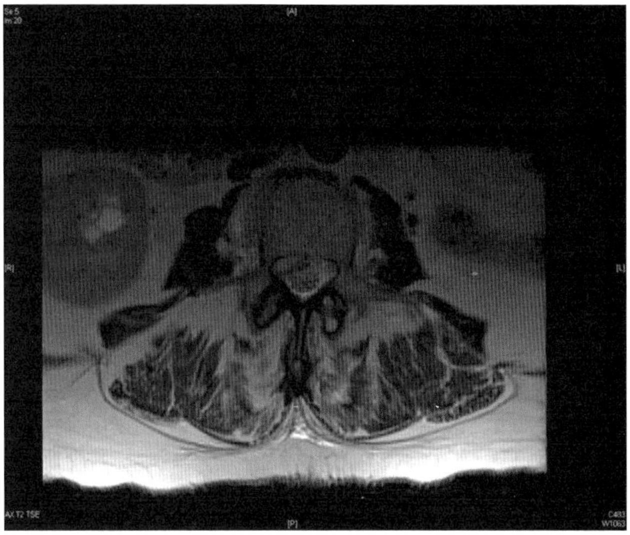

Fig. 39.5 T2 axial image at the L3 level in this same patient. A fluid collection in the ventral epidural space on the right is seen

39.2 Case Discussion

Spinal epidural abscess (SEA) following SCS implantation is a rare but life-threatening complication that will require surgical explantation of the device, evacuation of the abscess, and parenteral antibiotic therapy. Early diagnosis is essential to limit the neurologic compromise that can occur in these cases. In 1948, Heusner et al. classically described four distinct stages of SEA: Stage 1, which includes back pain and tenderness to spine palpation; Stage 2, in which spinal nerve root findings, radicular pain, nuchal rigidity, and hyperreflexia are seen; Stage 3, in which sensory findings, motor weakness, and bladder or bowel dysfunction are found; and finally Stage 4, paralysis [1]. In reality, the progression of symptoms may not be so linear and concrete. Recent studies have shown that the classic triad of "back pain, fever, and neurological deficit" is actually present in only 10% cases of SEA, but when present, it predicts poor outcomes [2].

In the case presented here, the diagnosis is straightforward, but in cases of spontaneous SEA in the absence of a recent spinal procedure or recent surgery, severe back pain with leukocytosis is the most common presenting scenario. A chief complaint of back pain is present in 70–95% of patients with SEA [2–4]. Fever was seen in about 20% of cases in one 10-year retrospective study [2] of patients with SEA and in 54% of cases in another [3]. Motor deficits may be present in 30% of cases of SEA, and bladder dysfunction or frank paresis is seen in about 25% of cases [5]. The mortality rate from SEA is less than 10% and is usually related to overwhelming sepsis or meningitis as a result of the abscess [3, 5, 6]. Approximately 50% of those who are treated for SEA are left with permanent neurologic deficits, including 15% with paresis or complete paralysis [7]. Motor deficits at the time of diagnosis highly correlate with permanent residual motor deficits after treatment [3].

The most common pathogens found in blood and wound cultures are *Staphylococcus aureus* and *Streptococcus* species [4]. MRSA was found in 20% of cases in a recent meta-analysis of SEA [4]. Cost of treatment is high. In one recent analysis, the mean total charges incurred for SEA inpatient treatment was $160,000 [5]. Risk factors for rapid clinical deterioration and poor outcomes include a history of diabetes mellitus, C-reactive protein >115, WBC > 12, age > 65, positive blood cultures, and the presence of MRSA [4].

The causes of SEA include hematogenous spread, direct inoculation, or contiguous spread of bacteria from a primary source. Skin and soft tissue infections are common sources of hematogenous spread of bacteria, in addition to urinary tract and respiratory tract infections. The vertebral column is highly vascularized, so hematogenous spread to this region is not unlikely. In this case, dehiscence of the surgical incision from a wound infection may have allowed spread of bacteria into the deeper tissue layers or contiguous spread of bacteria from a wound infection into the epidural space. Optimally, a wound check within 1 week after surgery and better patient vigilance could have mitigated this case, as a superficial wound infection after SCS can usually be treated successfully with antibiotics and not require explantation of the entire SCS system. Alternatively, poor aseptic technique or contamination of the introducer needle or electrode at the time of trial or permanent implantation may have been causes, but direct inoculation would likely cause abscess formation and clinical symptoms more immediately after implantation. In patients with diabetes and a history of smoking, it may be best to stage the percutaneous trial and allow complete healing of the skin prior to proceeding with the permanent implantation of an SCS system in the same region. In one case report, a patient developed back pain and an epidural abscess 3 days following a percutaneous SCS trial [8] and required surgical drainage. In most spontaneous cases of SEA, the bacterial infection is unimicrobial.

The incidence of SEA with SCS implantation is not well studied and is limited to case reports [8, 9]. In a recent retrospective analysis of 131 patients with 142 SCS or programmable pumps at a single institution by Engle et al., the overall infection rate was 2.8% in the first 12 months following implantation. In two of the 59 SCS systems implanted (3.4%), a postoperative infection occurred. In all cases in this series, the infections were at the IPG or pump site, and there were no cases of epidural abscess [10]. Longer operative time was an independent risk factor for these infections. Kumar et al. reported an 8% incidence of infection or wound breakdown following SCS implantation [11]. Follett et al. reviewed medical device reports from 2000 to 2002 from a single SCS manufacturer and analyzed 114 cases of infections related to SCS implantation. In all cases, the indication for SCS implant was non-cancer pain, and 38% of the patients had a medical condition that was a risk factor for increased infection risk. The majority of the infections occurred at the IPG pocket site. Wound cultures were positive for a *Staphylococcus* species in 48% of cases; a *Pseudomonas* species was identified in 3%; wound cultures were negative for bacterial growth in 18% of cases [12]. Infections were most likely to occur within the first month following surgical implantation, and in 91% of cases, the infection resolved without complications after treatment [12]. In another large, 20-year literature review of SCS publications by Cameron et al., an infection rate of 3.4% in 2972 SCS procedures was seen [13]. One case of psoas abscess related to implantation of an epidural electrode has also been described [14].

39.2.1 Risk Factors for Spinal Epidural Abscess

Patients with DM and poorly controlled glucose levels are more prone to wound infections, especially with spine surgery [15]. DM is the most common medical morbidity seen in patients with SEA [4]. In a recent meta-analysis of 12 SEA studies, 27% of patients with SEA were diabetic [4]. Other risk factors for SEA include renal failure, liver failure, recent spinal procedure or spinal instrumentation, an immunocompromised or debilitated state, poor nutritional status, intravenous drug use, alcoholism, smoking, and chronic steroid use [4, 16]. Many of these risk factors can be addressed, mitigated, or otherwise controlled preoperatively prior to the implantation of an SCS system with proper screening and patient education. Advanced age and pulmonary disease were independent risk factors of poor outcomes after SEA was diagnosed in an analysis by Schoenfeld et al. [5].

Chronic pain patients may be more prone to MRSA infections, related to exposure to this bacteria during multiple hospitalizations or surgeries. In this case, the patient may have been a MRSA carrier since she worked in an inpatient rehabilitation facility and was in contact with chronically ill patients. In situ MRSA inoculation at the time of surgery and a contiguous MRSA wound infection are other possibilities.

Surgical technique and compliance with infection control procedures to prevent surgical site wound infections have strong effects on infection risk. Surgical site infections are known to occur in 2–5% of all surgical cases, regardless of location [17]. The Centers for Disease Control and Prevention recommends that intravenous antibiotics be administered before surgical incision, so a bactericidal concentration of the drug is present when the skin is incised. The North American Spine Society has developed evidence-based guidelines on the administration of antibiotics for spine surgery and recommends a single-dose broad-spectrum coverage of gram-positive organisms be given prior to skin incision [18]. Diabetes, smoking, bed confinement, blood glucose levels above 120 mg/dL, longer lengths of incisions, and longer hospital stays are all risk factors for surgical wound infections following spine surgery [15]. A recent survey of over 500 SCS-implanting physicians assessed the self-reported compliance rates for surgical infection control practice recommendations (i.e., CDC, SCIP, etc.). Overall, compliance rates with these standard recommended practices in this cohort were low. Weight-based antibiotic dosing, hair removal strategies, double gloving, surgical dressing, skin antiseptic agent selection, and postoperative continuation of antibiotics were specific areas of common noncompliance [19]. Updated recommendations for the control of surgical site infections should be reviewed by all SCS implanters [20].

In addition to following evidence-based guidelines for infection prevention and control, the use of vancomycin powder in surgical wounds prior to closure can, in theory, decrease the rate of surgical site infections and has gained recent popularity. In one meta-analysis, surgical wound infection rate following spine surgery was 7.5% in a control group that did not receive intra-wound vancomycin, whereas the treated group wound infection rate was only 1.4% in comparison. Adverse events were rare, occurring 0.3% of the time, but included nephrotoxicity and ototoxicity [21]. One prospective case-control study showed a decrease in the incidence of postoperative wound infections following laminectomy for paddle electrode placement performed with intra-wound vancomycin as wound closure [22], but, in general, there are few high-quality prospective trials assessing the efficacy and safety of intra-wound vancomycin powder in the context of routine SCS implantation.

In less severe or superficial wound infections, complete explantation of the costly SCS system may not be necessary. Superficial infections can be managed solely with antibiotic therapy, but deeper infections generally require incision, drainage, or surgical revision of the SCS components. If any of the SCS components are exposed in an infected or necrotic area, they must be removed [23]. Once the infection has cleared, a new device can be reimplanted but at a site distant from the prior infection.

39.2.2 Diagnostic Studies

In patients presenting with increasing back pain following a spine intervention procedure like SCS implantation or spinal steroid injections, vigilance for SEA should be high. Screening tools to assess the likelihood of an infection include erythrocyte sedimentation rate (ESR), C-reactive protein levels (CRP), and white blood cell count (WBC) with differential. In one large retrospective series, 98% of patients with SEA had an ESR > 20 mm/h at presentation to an emergency department [2]. Although fever is not uncommon, SEA can present without this finding. In this same large retrospective series, only 17–38% of patients were febrile at presentation [2]. An elevated ESR and an elevated CRP are both more sensitive screens for SEA as compared to WBC [24].

As MRI-compatible SCS systems are increasingly common, MRI is the imaging study of choice in assessing SEA whenever possible. CT scans can be performed when MRI is contraindicated [25]. Myelography and diagnostic lumbar puncture are not recommended for diagnosis, as these can cause a spread of an infection to the intrathecal space. MRI is 91–100% sensitive and highly specific in identifying the extent of nerve root or spinal cord compression from an SEA; a T1 hypointense and T2 hyperintense soft tissue mass in the epidural space with displacement of the dura will be seen. The use of contrast enhancement allows one to differentiate CSF from purulent extradural fluid collections. A ring-enhancing fluid collection in the epidural space on a contrast-enhanced MRI is pathognomonic for SEA; vertebral spondylodiscitis adjacent to the abscess is seen in 86% of cases [16]. Air is rarely seen within the mass [24]. A subdural abscess can also occur but is extremely rare.

Imaging of the entire spine is recommended when SEA is suspected, in order to rule out skip lesions or noncontiguous infections in the epidural space, especially when hematogenous spread is suspected. The posterior thoracic or lumbar epidural space is the most common site for spontaneous SEA [4, 24].

39.2.3 Treatment

Once the diagnosis of SEA has been confirmed, surgical evacuation is key when the SEA is related to infected or contaminated spinal hardware or instrumentation, as in an epidural electrode in this case. Depending on the size and extent of the abscess, simple drainage, laminectomy, or multilevel decompression with segmental stabilization may be required [26]. In addition to consultation with a spine surgeon, consultation with infectious disease specialists is recommended to direct the duration of antibiotic treatment, as well as dosing, route, and antibiotic selection [25]. Cefazolin provides coverage against most *Staphylococcus* species, although penicillin allergy is a relative contraindication to its use, as there is a 10% incidence of cross reactivity between these two antibiotic classes [27]. Clindamycin can be substituted in these cases. Intravenous vancomycin is required when MRSA is identified as the pathogen.

Risk factors for failed antibiotic treatment of these spinal infections include persistently high ESR and CRP after 4 weeks of antibiotic treatment [28]. Hyperbaric oxygen treatment has been used in refractory spine infections with good success rates [29].

Key Concepts

- Epidural abscess is a rare but life-threatening sequela of spine procedures like SCS implantation. Diabetes is an important risk factor. Delays in diagnosis result in poor clinical outcomes. Patient and provider vigilance in the postoperative period are critical. Preoperatively, patient health status assessment and patient education are equally important.
- Patients with SEA present most commonly with localized back pain accompanied by fever or elevated ESR or CRP. WBC may not be significantly elevated. Sensory deficits, weakness, reflex changes, and loss of sphincter tone occur less commonly but predict a poor neurologic outcome. Imaging of the entire spine to identify the size and extent of the abscess and to rule out skip lesions. Contrast-enhanced MRI (or CT scan if MRI is contraindicated) is essential to confirm the diagnosis of SEA.
- Although some spontaneous SEA can be treated medically when no neurologic deficits are seen, in cases of infected or contaminated hardware like electrodes, explantation of the infected device is required. Emergent consultation with a spine surgeon and an infectious disease specialist at the time of diagnosis are strongly recommended.
- Adherence to evidence-based infection control measures is key to prevention of surgical site infections and SEA. Pain management physicians should be familiar with the CDC and SCIP guidelines for reducing surgical site infections (SSI) and practice proper sterile technique and surgical technique when implanting SCS systems. The CDC has a SSI "toolbox" available at http://www.cdc.gov/HAI/ssi/ssi.html.
- Prolonged operative time is an independent risk factor for infections following SCS implant. See Table 39.1 for summary of recommendations.

Table 39.1 Summary of recommendations to prevent surgical site infections and epidural abscess

1.	Follow CDC guidelines to reduce infection risks, including weight-based prophylactic antibiotic administration within 1 h prior to incision
2.	Proper surgical technique is essential
3.	Limit OR traffic during implant procedures
4.	Proper hand hygiene prior to gloving. Use double gloves and change gloves during surgery when appropriate
5.	Patients should shower with chlorhexidine prior to surgery. Nasal antibiotic ointment for several days prior to surgery in those at risk of being a MRSA carrier
6.	If hair removal at surgical site is necessary, use clippers in lieu of razors
7.	Chlorhexidine with alcohol should be used for skin prep at time of surgery. Use adhesive iodophor incise drapes
8.	Use a "no touch" or "minimal touch" technique when handling implants
9.	Select suture that does not promote bioadhesive properties of bacteria; avoid silk suture; use monofilament when possible
10.	Avoid excessive electrocautery and minimize tissue handling
11.	Irrigate wounds with copious antibiotic irrigation prior to closure. Use antibiotic different form the parenteral antibiotics given at the beginning of the case
12.	Close wounds in multiple fascial layers and avoid dead space. Continuous closure has less infection risk than interrupted sutures
13.	Use occlusive dressings for the first 48 h
14.	Keep patients warm during and after surgery
15.	Optimize patient health status prior to surgery, specifically with 4 weeks of smoking cessation and maintenance of glucose levels below 150 mg/dL in diabetics
16.	Maintain proper surveillance of surgical wounds, specifically in the first few weeks after implant

References

1. Heusner AP. Nontuberculous spinal epidural infections. N Engl J Med. 1948;239(23):845–54.
2. Davis DP, Wold RM, Patel RJ, et al. The clinical presentation and impact of diagnostic delays on emergency department patients with spinal epidural abscess. J Emerg Med. 2004;26(3):285–91.
3. Joshi SM, Hatfield RH, Martin J, Taylor W. Spinal epidural abscess: a diagnostic challenge. Br J Neurosurg. 2003;17(2):160–3.
4. Arko L, Quach E, Nguyen V, Chang D, Sukul V, Kim BS. Medical and surgical management of spinal epidural abscess: a systematic review. Neurosurg Focus. 2014;37(2):E4.
5. Schoenfeld AJ, Wahlquist TC. Mortality, complication risk, and total charges after the treatment of epidural abscess. Spine J. 2015;15(2):249–55.
6. Rigamonti D, Liem L, Sampath P, et al. Spinal epidural abscess: contemporary trends in etiology, evaluation, and management. Surg Neurol. 1999;52(2):189–96. discussion 197
7. Reihsaus E, Waldbaur H, Seeling W. Spinal epidural abscess: a meta-analysis of 915 patients. Neurosurg Rev. 2000;23(4):175–204; discussion 205.
8. Rauchwerger JJ, Zoarski GH, Waghmarae R, et al. Epidural abscess due to spinal cord stimulator trial. Pain Pract. 2008;8(4):324–8.
9. Arxer A, Busquets C, Vilaplana J, Villalonga A. Subacute epidural abscess after spinal cord stimulator implantation. Eur J Anaesthesiol. 2003;20(9):755–7.
10. Engle MP, Vinh BP, Harun N, Koyyalagunta D. Infectious complications related to intrathecal drug delivery system and spinal cord stimulator system implantations at a comprehensive cancer pain center. Pain Physician. 2013;16(3):251–7.
11. Kumar K, Taylor RS, Jacques L, et al. Spinal cord stimulation versus conventional medical management for neuropathic pain: a multicentre randomised controlled trial in patients with failed back surgery syndrome. Pain. 2007;132(1–2):179–88.
12. Follett KA, Boortz-Marx RL, Drake JM, et al. Prevention and management of intrathecal drug delivery and spinal cord stimulation system infections. Anesthesiology. 2004;100(6):1582–94.
13. Cameron T. Safety and efficacy of spinal cord stimulation for the treatment of chronic pain: a 20-year literature review. J Neurosurg. 2004;100(3 Suppl Spine):254–67.
14. Gutierrez Vall de Cabres V, Solans Laque R, Pigrau Sarrallach C, Pahissa Berga A. Psoas abscess due to an epidural spinal cord stimulation catheter. Scand J Infect Dis. 1992;24(1):119.
15. Saeedinia S, Nouri M, Azarhomayoun A, et al. The incidence and risk factors for surgical site infection after clean spinal operations: a prospective cohort study and review of the literature. Surg Neurol Int. 2015;6:154.
16. Boody BS, Jenkins TJ, Maslak J, Hsu WK, Patel AA. Vertebral osteomyelitis and spinal epidural abscess: an evidence-based review. J Spinal Disord Tech. 2015;28(6):E316–27.
17. Barie PS, Eachempati SR. Surgical site infections. Surg Clin North Am. 2005;85(6):1115–35, viii–ix
18. Watters WC 3rd, Baisden J, Bono CM, et al. Antibiotic prophylaxis in spine surgery: an evidence-based clinical guideline for the use of prophylactic antibiotics in spine surgery. Spine J. 2009;9(2):142–6.
19. Provenzano DA, Deer T, Luginbuhl Phelps A, et al. An international survey to understand infection control practices for spinal cord stimulation. Neuromodulation. 2016;19(1):71–84.
20. Alexander JW, Solomkin JS, Edwards MJ. Updated recommendations for control of surgical site infections. Ann Surg. 2011;253(6):1082–93.
21. Ghobrial GM, Cadotte DW, Williams K Jr, Fehlings MG, Harrop JS. Complications from the use of intrawound vancomycin in lumbar spinal surgery: a systematic review. Neurosurg Focus. 2015;39(4):E11.
22. Amrani J. Intraoperative powdered vancomycin use with paddle lead placement. Neuromodulation. 2015;18(3):177–80; discussion 181.
23. Bendersky D, Yampolsky C. Is spinal cord stimulation safe? A review of its complications. World Neurosurg. 2014;82(6):1359–68.
24. Tali ET, Oner AY, Koc AM. Pyogenic spinal infections. Neuroimaging Clin N Am. 2015;25(2):193–208.
25. Sans N, Faruch M, Lapegue F, Ponsot A, Chiavassa H, Railhac JJ. Infections of the spinal column–spondylodiscitis. Diagn Interv Imaging. 2012;93(6):520–9.
26. Martin RJ, Yuan HA. Neurosurgical care of spinal epidural, subdural, and intramedullary abscesses and arachnoiditis. Orthop Clin North Am. 1996;27(1):125–36.
27. Hall WA. Vancomycin powder in spine surgery: still a work in progress. World Neurosurg. 2015;83(6):1051–2.
28. Yoon SH, Chung SK, Kim KJ, Kim HJ, Jin YJ, Kim HB. Pyogenic vertebral osteomyelitis: identification of microorganism and laboratory markers used to predict clinical outcome. Eur Spine J. 2010;19(4):575–82.
29. Onen MR, Yuvruk E, Karagoz G, Naderi S. Efficiency of hyperbaric oxygen therapy in iatrogenic spinal infections. Spine (Phila Pa 1976). 2015;40(22):1743–8.

Part VI

Interventional Pain Procedures: Kyphoplasty

Kyphoplasty in Fibrous Dysplasia

40

Christina C. Moore, Matthew V. Satterly, and Magdalena Anitescu

40.1 Case Description

A 48-year-old physically fit male complains of back pain that interferes with his daily activities. He has a history of FD, affecting the axial skeleton presumably a condition diagnosed 10 years ago. He underwent a cervical fusion for neck instability with excellent results. For the last 5 years, he has had a documented space-occupying lesion in the L2 vertebral body considered stable. He is very motivated to maintaining mobility and pursues a vigorous exercise routine with aerobic and weight-bearing exercises.

After a minor car accident 9 months ago, he suffered acute-onset back pain, not alleviated by rest or anti-inflammatory medication, and was rendered almost immobile. His endocrinologist recommended a second infusion of zoledronic acid (Reclast) to which he responded favorably in the past. The infusion was not successful. Imaging studies again identified the space-occupying lesion which was considered stable when compared to the previous images. He was no longer able to perform his regular exercises and experienced a steep decline in his perceived quality of life.

Medications like tramadol (25 mg in the morning and 50 mg at night) were discontinued because of sedating effects. Ibuprofen 800 mg every 8 h was ineffective for his pain. Physical therapy was instituted with minimal success (Fig. 40.1).

The patient described the pain as a 10/10 at its worst, typically after 10–15 min of exercise. He experienced tenderness to palpation over the upper lumbar spinous processes. He also described radicular pain over the anterior thigh bilaterally, correlating with coexisting multilevel degenerative disk disease, worse at L3–L4, and mild disk protrusion at L5–S1, consistent with MRI findings. Physical therapy provided no relief of pain. A lumbar epidural steroid injection was performed 1 month after his first visit. It had no effect on his back pain but decreased his radicular pain to a 3–4/10 for approximately 2 weeks. A TENS unit and back brace brought minor back pain relief. The patient's exercise regimen was limited because of continuous back pain, and he perceived his overall physical function as rapidly deteriorating.

With weight gain, the axial pain increased. Long-acting therapies including OxyContin and a fentanyl patch were discontinued because of nausea and constipation.

Given the characteristics of his pain and physical examination, we thought that the patient had an unhealed fracture, not radiographically visible at the L2 level, in the fibrous material. Multidisciplinary and contradictory discussions with the patient's endocrinologist were conducted with disagreement between the pain physician and endocrinologist on the medical necessity of the performing kyphoplasty. Given the patient's rapid deterioration in functional status and after carefully weighing the risks and benefits, kyphoplasty was eventually seen as a valid option. The patient underwent balloon kyphoplasty of the L2 vertebral body. Under monitored anesthesia care and after thorough vertebral body periosteal infiltration with an 18-gauge spinal needle, the kyphoplasty trocar was advanced under fluoroscopic guidance within the L2 vertebral body. The placement of the trocars and the balloons was limited to the lateral aspect of the vertebral body, given the near-complete apposition of the superior and inferior end plates in the mid third of the vertebral body. The balloon was inserted and inflated within the L2 vertebral body under low pressure. It was then deflated and methylmethacrylate was injected within the vertebral body. The distribution of cement within the L2 vertebral body followed the concavity seen in the MR image.

This technique was used to avoid disruption of the cortex after inflating the balloon and depositing methylmethacrylate.

C.C. Moore, M.D.
Department of Anesthesia, Medical Colege of Wisconsin, Milwaukee, WI, USA
e-mail: christina.gavrilos@gmail.com

M.V. Satterly, M.D.
Western Anesthesia Associates, St Louis, MO, USA

M. Anitescu, M.D. Ph.D. (✉)
Department of Anesthesia and Critical Care, University of Chicago, Chicago, IL, USA
e-mail: cgavrilos1@dacc.uchicago.edu; manitescu@dacc.uchicago.edu

M. Anitescu et al. (eds.), *Challenging Cases and Complication Management in Pain Medicine*, https://doi.org/10.1007/978-3-319-60072-7_40

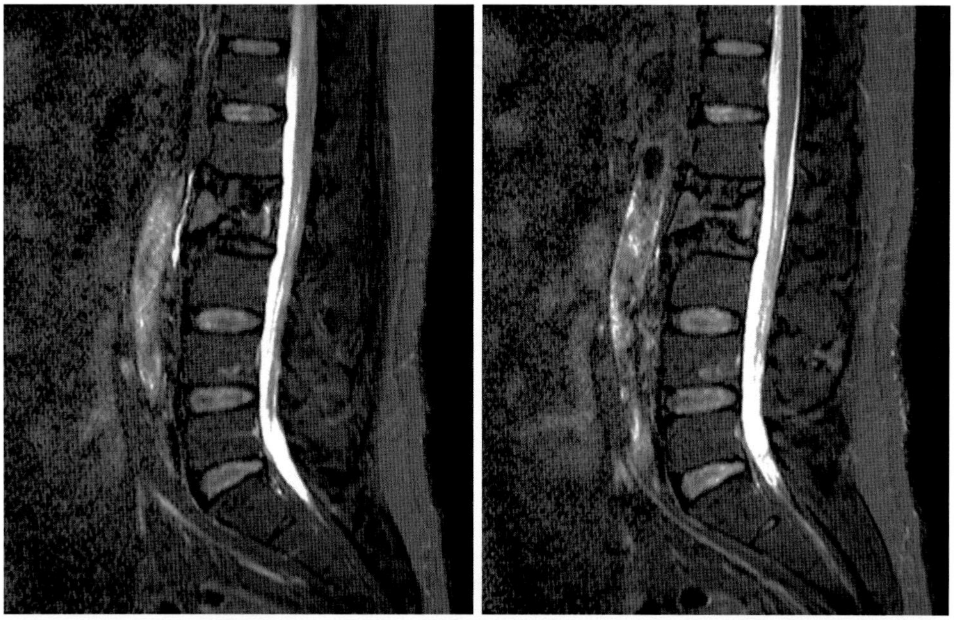

Fig. 40.1 Sagittal MRI STIR lumbar spine demonstrating decreased height and biconcave deformity of the L2 vertebral body (personal library)

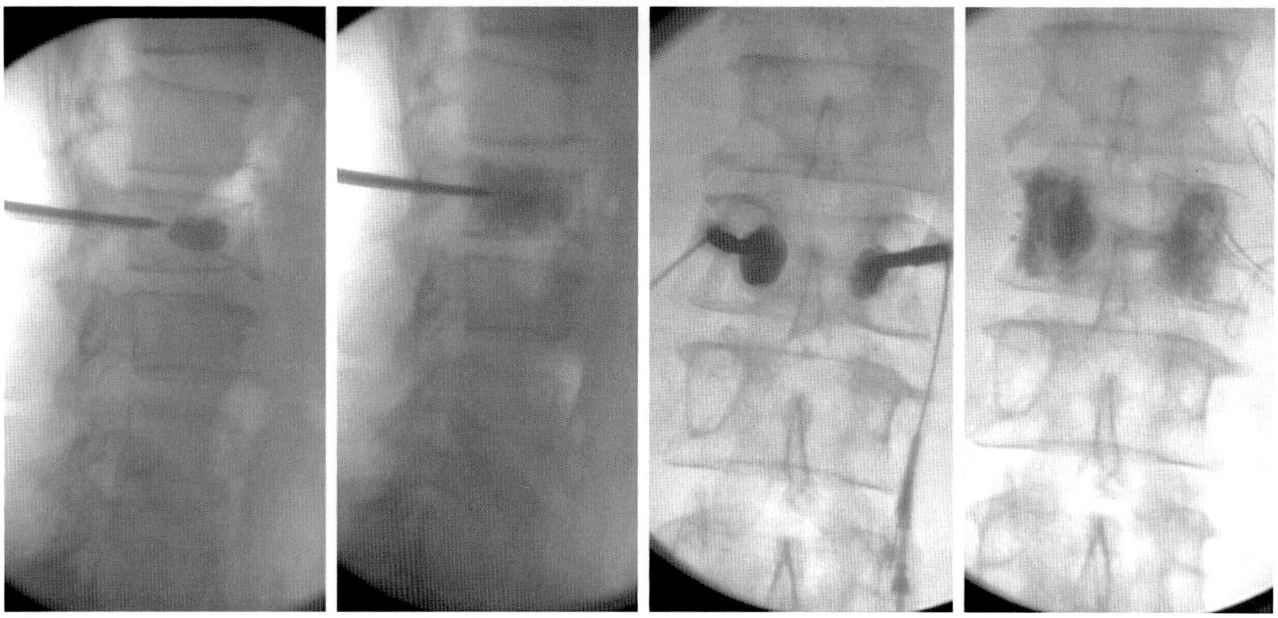

Fig. 40.2 Kyphoplasty at L2 demonstrating distribution of cement within the dysplastic lesion (personal library)

Posterior wall entry was strong, but there was no need for mallotting while passing the 2 mm posterior wall, suggesting replacement of osseous material with fibrous material consistent with known fibrous dysplasia (Fig. 40.2).

The patient experienced immediate and near-complete resolution of his acute and chronic pain. He was able to walk without pain in the recovery room, and 1 week after the procedure, he resumed an aggressive exercise regimen including 300 sit-ups, jogging several miles, and kickboxing three to four times per week. He lost weight, his functional status improved rapidly, and his medical comorbidities were alleviated. With weight loss, obstructive sleep apnea improved dramatically that he no longer required nocturnal CPAP. He continued to complain of a radicular pain in the left lower extremity from a disk protrusion at L5/S1, but this was mild overall and responded well to repeat steroid injections.

40.2 Discussion: The Syndrome of Axial Fibrous Dysplasia

40.2.1 Etiology and Pathogenesis

First described as a benign intramedullary fibro-osseous lesion by Lichtenstein and Jaffe [1, 2], fibrous dysplasia (FD) is currently defined as a genetic, non-inherited disease that affects men and women equally [3]. In this benign process, the normal bone is replaced with fibrous connective tissue. The result is ineffective remodeling of poorly mineralized, immature trabecular bone, widening of the affected bones, and subsequent cortical bone thinning. These changes cause a loss in mechanical strength and increased pain and fracture [4].

The process takes place in the medullary marrow cavity and is thought to result from a mutation of the guanine nucleotide stimulatory protein (*GNAS1*) gene, which encodes the alpha subunit of the stimulatory G protein (G1) located on chromosome 20q13.2–13.3.

This protein is responsible for stimulating guanine nucleotide-binding protein Gsα, leading to high levels of cyclic adenosine monophosphate and, in turn, overexpression of the c-fos proto-oncogene, which regulates expression and differentiation of osteoblasts and osteoclasts [5, 6].

The cell mutation seems to take place after fertilization in somatic cells; as a consequence all affected cells carry the same dysplastic feature from that moment on. Depending on where the affected cells are located during embryogenesis and numbers of cells affected, the clinical presentation of the disease is variable. The disease can manifest at any age, but the majority of lesions are detected around the third or fourth decade of life. Following the original genetic mutation, the primitive bone fails to remodel into mature trabecular lamellae. The resultant immature trabeculae enmeshed in dysplastic fibrous tissue, although turning over constantly, never achieve the complete remodeling process of mature bone that offers stability to the skeleton. The immature matrix also lacks effective and normal mineralization. As a consequence, the combination of insufficient mineralization coupled with lack of stress alignment from immature trabeculae results in significant loss of mechanical strength, subsequent pain, and pathological fractures [4]. The Office of Rare Diseases of the National Institutes of Health lists FD as a rare disease, meaning that fewer than 200,000 people in the USA are affected. The true prevalence is difficult to determine given the rarity of the disease and the likelihood of people being affected without experiencing symptoms. It is estimated that 1:15,000–1:30,000 Americans are affected with a lifetime incidence of 1:9000–1:18,000 [7].

FD comprises roughly 7% of all nonmalignant bone tumors and 2.5% of all bone lesions [8]. There are two forms: monostotic and polyostotic. The appendicular and axial skeletons have been implicated in each form [4] (Tables 40.1 and 40.2).

Of patients with FD, 3% have McCune-Albright syndrome [9] (a triad of precocious puberty, café au lait skin pigmentation, and fibrous dysplasia of the bone). FD also exists with Mazabraud syndrome (fibrous dysplasia with soft tissue myxomas), 80 cases of which have been described to date [10]. Mazabraud syndrome is seen in 70% of females, and the onset of fibrous dysplasia typically precedes myxomas.

The two main forms of FD differ by the location of bone involvement. The monostotic form (70% of cases) involves a single bone; the polyostotic form (30% of cases) involves two or more bones [9]. The appendicular skeleton is much more commonly affected, with only a few case reports involving the axial skeleton. In one survey of monostotic FD, the skull was affected in 20% of cases, the lower limbs in 34%, upper limbs in 10%, and the axial skeleton in just 2% [11]. Malignant transformation is rare, occurring less than 5% of the time [4].

The exact incidence and prevalence of spinal pathology in FD are unknown. In two studies of more than 100 FD patients, evidence suggests that spinal pathology is almost exclusively seen in the polyostotic form [12–14]. In 62 patients with polyostotic FD, 39 (63%) had 76 lesions in the spine, the overwhelming majority lumbar or thoracic [12, 13]. Of 56 patients with FD, the spine was affected in 6 of

Table 40.1 Types of fibrous dysplasia

	Characteristics
Monostotic	• The replacement of normal bone with fibrous connective tissue, causing a loss in mechanical strength and increased pain and fracture • Most prevalent form • Involves a single bone, may include multiple lesions on one bone • Rarely, can involve the spine—only 2% of monostotic FD cases • Lesions evolve in parallel with skeletal growth. Rarely progress past adolescence • Most often found incidentally
Polyostotic	• Identical pathophysiology • Less prevalent form • Involves two or more bones • Higher incidence of spinal involvement than the monostotic form • Lesions continue to grow after bone maturity, leading to deformity and fracture

Table 40.2 Categories of known fibrous dysplasia personal table based on Hoffman et al. [8]

	Bone involvement	% of FD cases	Spinal involvement	Associated pathology
Monostotic	Single	70	Yes	
Polyostotic	Multiple	30	Yes	
McCune-Albright syndrome	Single (monostotic) or multiple (polyostotic)	3	Yes	Precocious puberty, café au lait skin pigmentation ± hyperthyroidism, acromegaly [10]
Mazabraud syndrome	Single (monostotic) or multiple (polyostotic)	Unknown (80 total cases of Mazabraud syndrome described to date)	Yes	Soft tissue myxomas

Table 40.3 Skeletal involvement of fibrous dysplasia personal table based on Refs. [9–12]

	Appendicular	Axial
Monostotic fibrous dysplasia	Skull (20%), lower limbs (34%), upper limbs (10%)	3%
Polyostotic fibrous dysplasia	Femur (91%), tibia (81%), pelvis (78%)	21–63%

24 patients with McCune-Albright syndrome. In polyostotic patients, spinal involvement was noted in 7 of 33 (21.2%) patients [13]. FD in the spine was also significantly more frequent in patients with FD in the skull or pelvis (Table 40.3).

40.2.2 Clinical Manifestations

In the monostotic type, the dysplastic lesions are incidental findings, with diagnosis made usually when radiographs are performed as part of an examination of the region affected [4]. When symptomatic, the monostotic lesions seem to enlarge parallel to skeletal growth [15].

The rarer polyostotic form has a different clinical presentation and natural history. Severe deformities by late adolescence accompany this form. Those lesions tend to enlarge even after skeletal maturity is achieved and commonly progress to fractures [4].

When symptomatic, by age 30 fibrous dysplasia causes localized bone pain and deformity frequently related to fatigue or stress fractures. Diagnosis is made by radiographic findings in typical FD image. Otherwise, biopsy is indicated [4]. FD is found in long bones of the legs, arms, pelvis, and craniofacial bones, with spinal involvement estimated in 1.4%–5.5% of lesions [16]. Sole spinal involvement is rare. Differential diagnosis includes simple bone cyst, fibroma, metastasis, osteoblastoma, multiple myeloma, chronic infectious spondylitis, hemangioma, giant cell tumor, and Paget's disease [17]. Upon diagnosis, osteomalacia from vitamin D deficiency, hypophosphatemia, hypothyroidism, Cushing's, and hyperparathyroidism must also be ruled out, given bone turnover with FD.

Localized pain is often the first symptom of FD, especially if the disease affects the femoral neck. In addition to pain, patients may also experience limping. Women affected may have increased pain during pregnancy. Pain during the menstrual cycle is also possible because of more estrogen receptors in the fibrous dysplastic bone [4].

Bone deformity is also common. Deformity depends on the site of the lesion, age of the patient, severity of disease, and the type of FD. In the appendicular skeleton, the classical deformity is at the level of the proximal femur. The pathognomonic, so-called shepherd crook that appears in the polyostotic form, occurs as a result of an abnormal remodeling process in the proximal femur that continues even after the skeleton reaches maturity. Large weight-bearing bones such as the femur appear as bowing deformities and are accompanied by a shortened ipsilateral leg and widened hip region as a result of fatigued fractures of the dysplastic bone. Sudden pathological fractures and pain result from underlying swelling and deformity. In addition to limb length discrepancies and pain, approximately 50% of patients with monostotic disease have pathological fractures (most commonly of the femur).

Monostotic lesions are often indolent and stop progressing at the time of the completion of bone development in late adolescence, but in polyostotic lesions, the dysplasia may continue into adulthood.

Though less common, the first sign may be axial. In one study of 22 patients with axial disease, 16 complained of pain (6 of which were precipitated by trauma), 2 had symptoms of spinal cord compression, and 1 patient had a tumor mass [18]. In this study, three of the adult patients had progressive bony destruction after diagnosis and before treatment.

Axial fibrous dysplastic lesions may also cause deformities. Pain in polyostotic FD of the spine is a less common symptom. However, close to 40% of patients with FD have scoliosis from multiple fractures of diseased vertebrae [12]. The dysplastic process may also affect the transverse process and pedicles with added instability to the spine (Fig. 40.3).

Patients with McCune-Albright syndrome typically present with unilateral café au lait spots and endocrine disorders such as precocious puberty along with polyostotic fibrous dysplasia. The early onset of secondary sexual characteristics is the most common endocrinopathy in McCune-Albright syndrome. The hyperpigmentation lesions, primarily on the trunk or proximal parts of the extremities, have irregular borders and thus differ from lesions with smooth borders seen in neurofibromatosis. The osseous lesions are generally larger, persistent, and associated with more complications when compared with poly- or monostotic fibrous dysplasia [15, 17].

An even rarer form of FD, Mazabraud syndrome, combines osseous lesions commonly seen in FD with intramuscular myxomas.

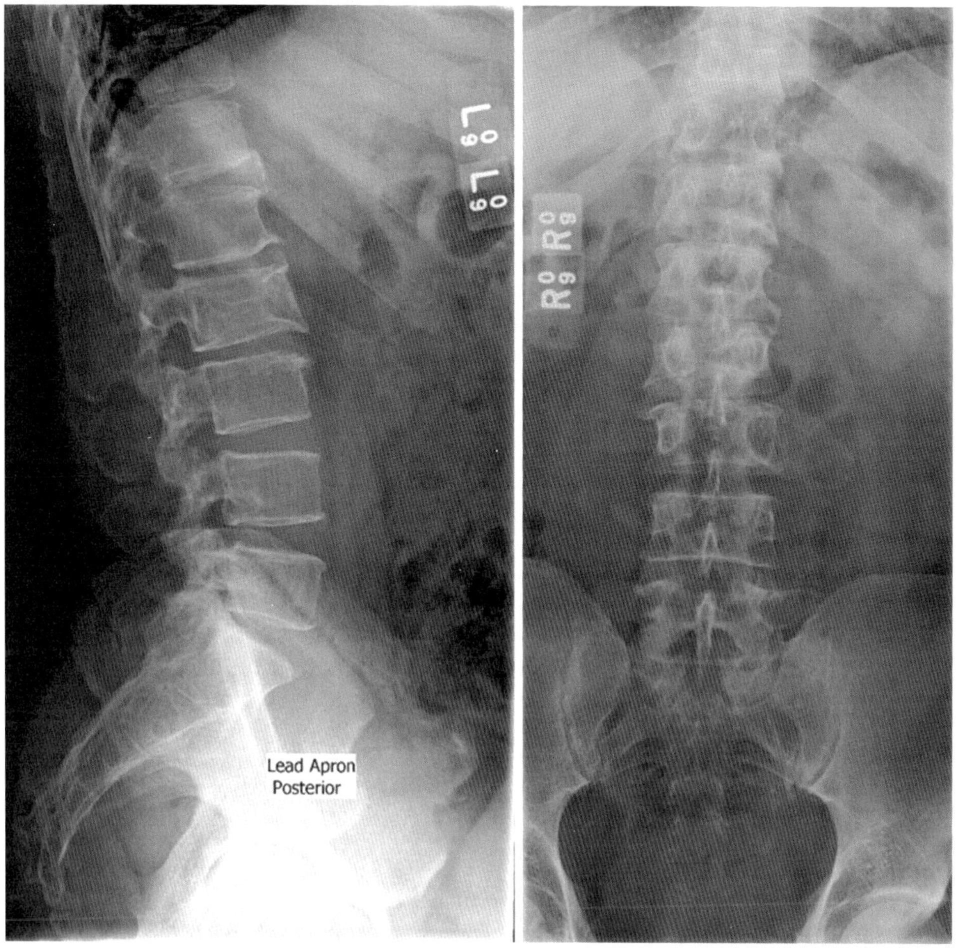

Fig. 40.3 Radiographic image with evidence of FD in pedicles and in the right transverse process of L3. Multiple mild lumbar vertebral compression deformities and L3 posterior element expansile remodeling (personal library)

40.2.3 Diagnostic Modalities

Imaging studies are valuable in the diagnosis of FD. Simple radiographs may show a well-defined lesion with smooth sclerotic margins and a hazy matrix, primarily in the big, weight-bearing bones such as the femur. Bone deformities can also be appreciated during simple radiographic exam, especially in larger polyostotic lesions in the appendicular skeleton.

In fibrous dysplasia, normal bone is replaced by a radiolucent material that appears as a gray "ground-glass" like picture with no visible trabecular pattern. The lesion arises in the intramedullary canal and eventually replaces both the cancellous and the cortical bone. The dysplastic lesion, however, is bounded by a shell of reactive bone that gives the appearance of the sclerotic margin. In axial FD, vertebral body height decreases as part of vertebral collapse [17]. An expansile process is seen with pedicle involvement.

MRI findings include varying signal intensities on T1- and T2-weighted images according to the components within the cellular matrix of fibrous tissue within the lesion [18]. MRI is best used as complementary to CT imaging. The lesions with high fibrous and low water content display a low-intensity signal on the T1-weighted images. Most often, MRI will show an intermediate to high signal on T2-weighted images and heterogenous enhancement after gadolinium administration [20]. The T2 higher-intensity signal is less bright than the signal from tumors, fat, or fluid. Areas of heterogeneity are also seen when hemorrhage, cysts, or cartilaginous degeneration occurs concomitant with the dysplastic lesion (Fig. 40.4).

CT findings include lytic lesions that can be expansile in nature and have a sclerotic rim and contour deformities. The

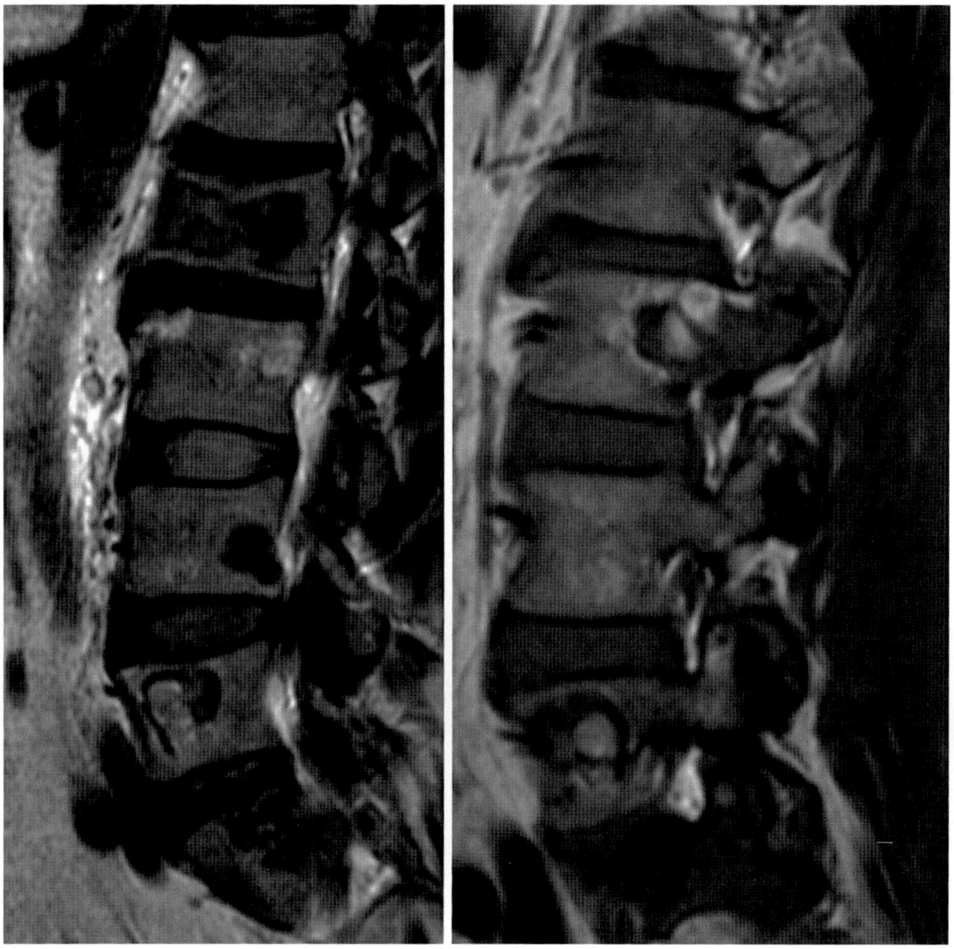

Fig. 40.4 MRI view of lumbar spine demonstrates dysplastic lesions with enhancement in T2 view (*image 1*); T1 view of pedicle lesion at the L3 vertebrae (*image 2*) (personal library)

lesional tissue enhances with contrast because of vascularity [4]. A diagnostic CT study displays a clearly visible, poorly mineralized lesional tissue with well-defined cortical boundary and increased thickness of the native cortex with new periosteal bone formation. The CT image is the best technique to reveal lesions in FD (Fig. 40.5).

Positron emission tomography scan and scintigraphy show activity at lesion sites [20]. A bar-shaped pattern, whole bone involvement, and close correlation between the area of uptake and the lesion are seen on radiography [4]. The increased uptake of the tracer diminishes gradually as the lesions mature. This diagnostic test is sensitive for detecting lesions but non-specific (Fig. 40.6).

If only some radiologic features are seen or there is a history of cancer or aggressive growth, bone biopsy may be warranted [19]. Grossly, trabeculae can be seen throughout the lesion, which is yellow-white with a gritty texture. Histologically, dysplastic cells are spindle-shaped without osteoblastic rimming and with capillaries throughout. The microscopic examination of a dysplastic lesion shows many immature mesenchymal cells with virtually no collagen bathing immature, non-stress-oriented, disconnected dysplastic trabeculae [4].

40.2.4 Treatment

Given the rarity of this condition, there is no consensus on treatment based upon randomized controlled trials, and regimens vary widely. Treatment focus is on relief of symptoms and correction of disease manifestations. The patient is monitored for disease progression, bisphosphonate therapy, and surgical correction.

Monitoring of the disease is via serial radiography after incidental diagnosis. Upon diagnosis, a bone scan is performed to identify the extent of the disease. If polyostotic disease is confirmed, patients are referred to endocrinology

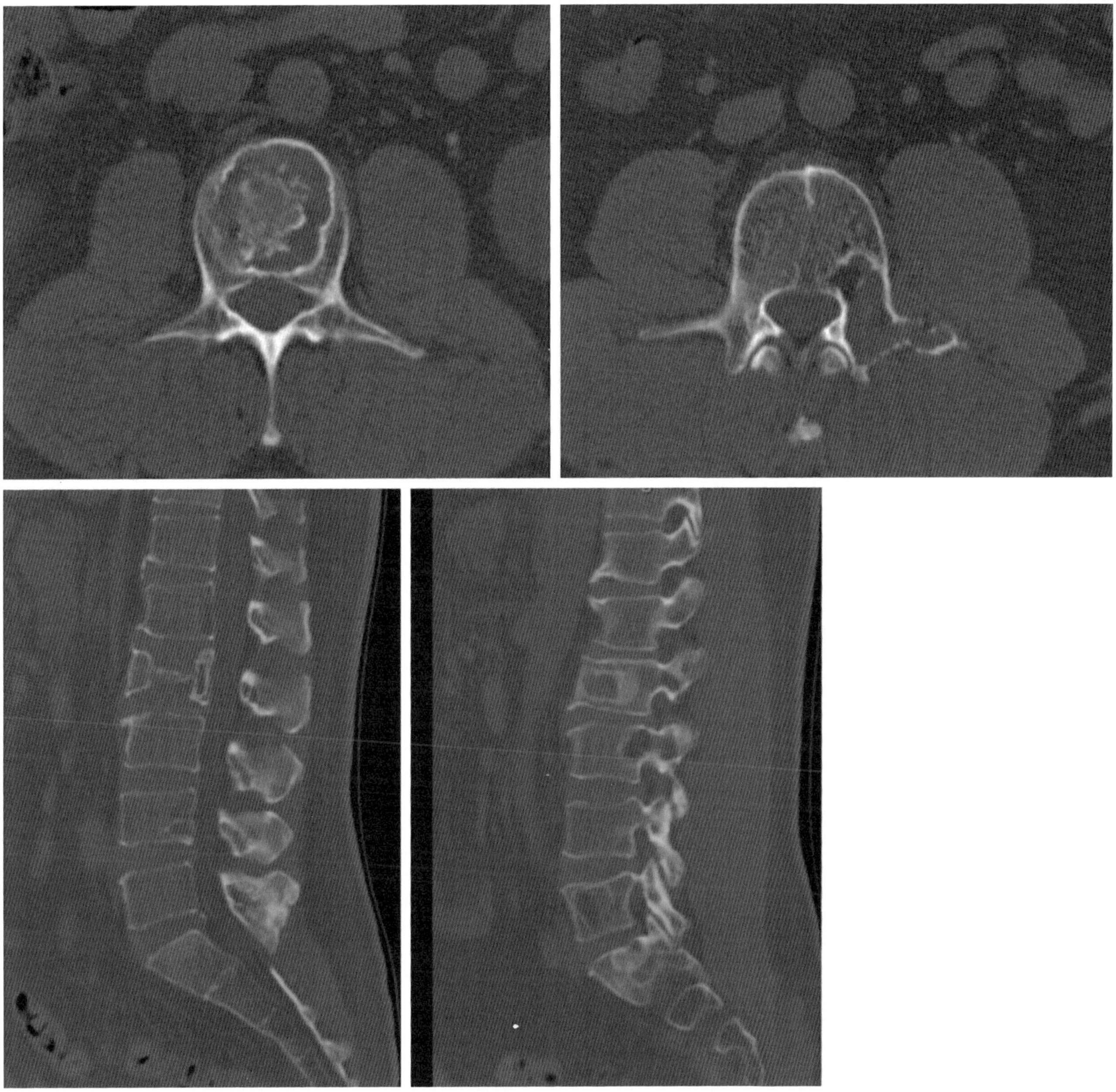

Fig. 40.5 CT showing a lytic process and thinning of the cortex. *Images 1 and* 2, axial views of lesions of vertebral body and right pedicle. *Images 3 and 4*, sagittal view of the same lesions (personal library)

to rule out associated endocrine disorders [4]. Radiographic surveys every 6 months measure progression.

Relief of symptoms is paramount to successful treatment. While many cases can be discovered incidentally after an indolent course of the disease, a number of patients, both adults and children, suffer with significant pain [21]. Contrary to the initial belief that pain in FD dissipates with age, it has recently been shown that it actually persists and transitions to severe pain with age [22].

The exact mechanism of pain in FD is unknown, but research in the last decade suggests that pain comes from changes in select sensory fibers that innervate the skeleton. The bone is innervated by A delta fibers (thinly myelinated sensory nerve fibers) and CGRP+ nerve fibers that express

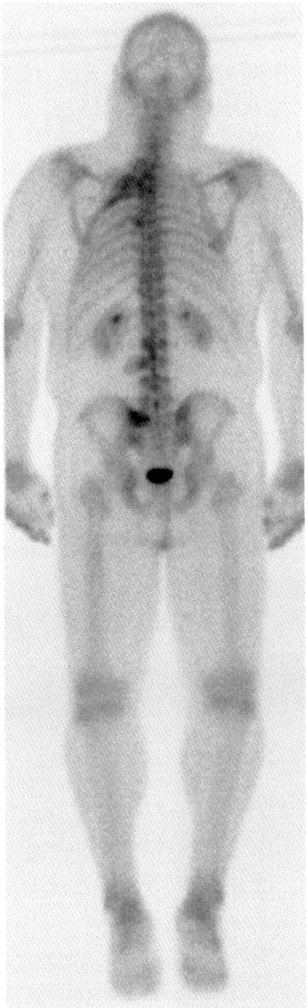

Fig. 40.6 Bone scintigraphy demonstrating increased uptake at multiple levels, L2 and L3 vertebrae consistent with lesions of fibrous dysplasia (personal library)

high affinity for the nerve growth factor (NGF) receptor, TrkA, that affect neuronal differentiation and survival. In malignant states, the pain generator is not only bone remodeling but also alteration of the nerve endings within the osseous structure that contributes to the refractory and severe pain of osseous metastases [22]. In this osteosarcoma model, the nerve sprouting and neuroma-like structure formation in the sensory and sympathetic nerve fibers of the bone are blocked by sustained administration of anti-NGF factors. In nonmalignant skeletal pain states, similar findings were observed. Human discogenic pain is the result of excessive growth of TrkA nerve fibers into the normally aneural and avascular intervertebral disks, while significant sprouting of CGRP+ of nerve fibers has been observed in rat fractures and in arthritic joints in humans and animals [23–25]. It is possible that similar alterations in the innervation of the affected bone structures may contribute to pain.

Medications to treat pain in FD are bisphosphonates, NSAIDS, and opiates [21].

Bisphosphonates reduce bone pain and decrease markers of bone turnover. They do not change appearance on radiographies, reduce fracture incidence, or prevent the progression of bony lesions [21]. They are potent inhibitors of bone resorption. Pamidronate, a second-generation bisphosphonate, is administered as an intravenous infusion over 3 days at 60 mg/day and then repeated every 6 months. Treatment with bisphosphonates is supplemented with vitamin D and calcium [4]. In a study of 91 patients, up to 81% of adults with FD had bone pain, with a mean pain score of 4.1 out of 10. Many of the patients who relapsed after bisphosphonate therapy had a history of multiple fractures [21]. Side effects of the bisphosphonate treatments are usually mild and transient and include fever, diffuse bone pain, and mild hypocalcemia [26]. Some patients, given intravenous zoledronic acid, suffered osteonecrosis of the jaw, so preventative dentistry is recommended [27, 28]. Markers of bone turnover, such as alkaline phosphatase and N-telopeptide, are measured at 6 months, and bone mineral density is measured yearly to assess the efficacy of bisphosphonate therapy.

Surgical intervention is reserved for correction of serious deformity or fracture, pain refractory to medical treatment, or restoration of spinal stability. Histological evaluation of segments excised confirms the diagnosis. Stabilization of the spine is needed in progressive neurological deficits in scoliotic and kyphotic deformities of the spine from fatigue and pathological fractures.

Some pathology may progress beyond what medication alone may treat. Surgery can confirm diagnosis, correct deformity, and eradicate symptomatic lesions. In some patients, however, surgical options are limited given the anatomical distribution of the dysplastic and adjacent stable bone. Possible surgical interventions include curettage and grafting, intramedullary fixation, fusion, or tumor resection with arthrodesis. Many of these options are not options in the spine where the only treatment may be multilevel fusion, assuming stable bone is available for fixation.

Fractures from FD tend to heal on their own, but with dysplastic and fibrotic bone, increasing the risk of subsequent fracture at the same site [20]. This may be especially detrimental in axial presentation, where compression fractures may appear chronic or unchanging, yet are in fact unstable and therefore continue to result in pain. Untreated vertebral compression fracture in FD leads to vertebral collapse with consequences such as severe cord compression and neurologic deficit [8].

There are reports of progression and recurrence after curettage and surgical correction. With incompletely treated or untreated vertebral fractures in particular, lesions have an affinity for progressive enlargement and possibly graft destruction [18]. With remodeling, the graft is once again replaced by dysplastic bone and returned to preoperative sta-

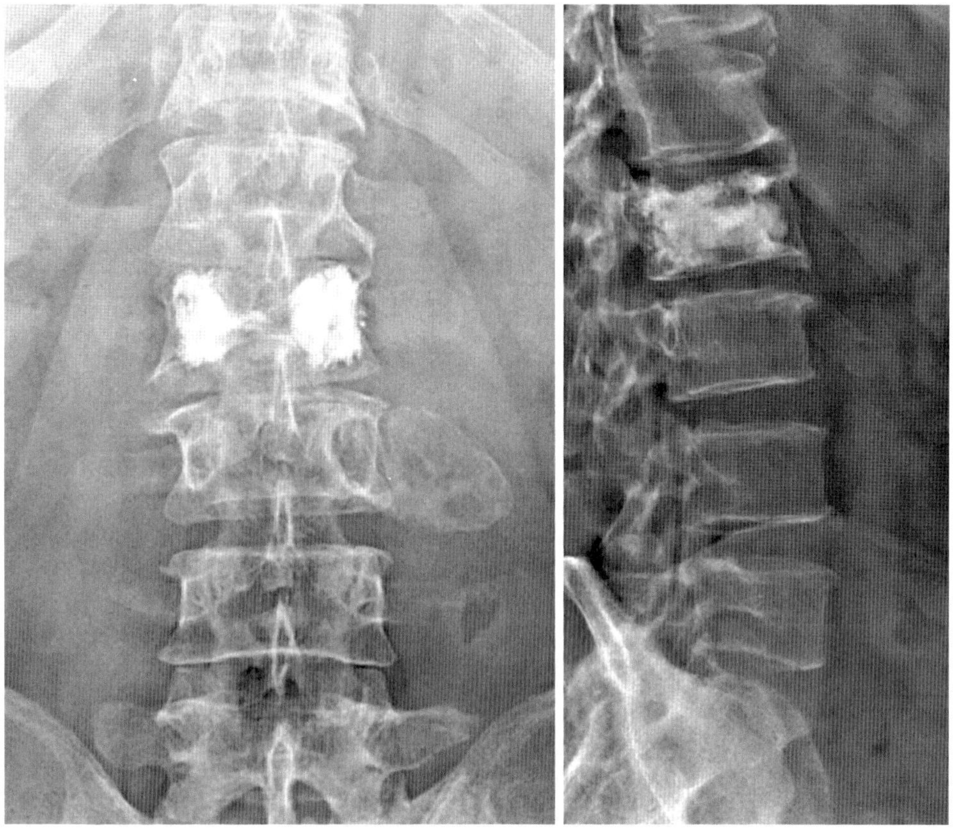

Fig. 40.7 Plain radiographs after kyphoplasty at L2 in a patient with fibrous dysplasia of the spine; cement filled the bone void with good stabilization and significant decrease in pain (personal library)

tus [4]. Obtaining clear margins during resection is required to prevent recurrence of this type.

Kyphoplasty is considered in patients with axial pathology in the form of compression fractures and pain. Chronic pathology may obscure an acute fracture after a traumatic event or cause pain without an identifiable cause. Based upon this case report and others, we recommend careful consideration of the use of kyphoplasty in the management of pain and compression fractures in fibrous dysplasia (Fig. 40.7).

Whether the success of kyphoplasty is a result of stabilization of the non-healing chronic compression fracture or of destruction of nociceptive fibers from a cascade of factors after compression fracture is unknown. It is becoming increasingly clear, however, that kyphoplasty helps to reduce or even eliminate pain resulting from compression fracture.

Conclusion

In our FD patient, acute destabilization of a dysplastic spine in conjunction with a chronic non-healed compression fracture, obscured by degenerative changes, resulted in chronic pain. A traumatic event led to an acute exacerbation of pain, likely from fatigue fracture. Both the acute and chronic pain were successfully treated by our procedure. In this case, we proceeded with kyphoplasty, suspecting that the chronic vertebral compression fracture was at least in part responsible for the chronic pain and an occult change for the exacerbation.

Despite no apparent changes in vertebral architecture, patients may benefit from kyphoplasty with immediate and lasting relief of acute, chronic, or acute-on-chronic pain. The pain relief may come from stabilization of the spine or the destruction of nociceptors within the dysplastic bone; remodeling is no longer present when cement replaces the dysplastic bone. More research is needed to determine the overall efficacy of this application, but the clinician should consider kyphoplasty as a valuable treatment option for patients with compression fractures and pain related to axial fibrous dysplasia, whether acute, chronic, or both.

Key Concepts

- Axial lesions are found in both monostotic and polyostotic fibrous dysplasia, as well as in McCune-Albright syndrome and Mazabraud syndrome.
- Axial fibrous dysplasia can lead to acute and chronic pain, particularly with vertebral fracture.
- The dysplastic changes of fibrous dysplasia can obscure imaging.
- Although medical management may be sufficient in most cases, some pathology may progress beyond what medication alone may treat.

- Untreated vertebral compression fractures may lead to further collapse and severe cord compression.
- Surgical correction of fibrous dysplasia may not always be an option.
- Vertebrogenic pain from fibrous dysplasia can be successfully treated using balloon kyphoplasty.

References

1. Lichtenstein L. Polyostotic fibrous dysplasia. Arch Surg. 1938;36:874–98.
2. Lichtenstein L, Jaffe HL. Fibrous dysplasia of bone: a condition affecting one, several or many bones, the graver cases of which may present abnormal pigmentation of skin, premature sexual development, hyperthyroidism or still other extraskeletal abnormalities. Arch Pathol. 1942;33:777–816.
3. Chapurlat RD, Orcel PO. Fibrous dysplasia of bone and McCune-Albright syndrome. Best Pract Res Clin Rheumatol. 2008;21(1):55–69.
4. Dicaprio MR, Enneking WF. Fibrous dysplasia pathophysiology, evaluation, and treatment. J Bone Joint Surg Am. 2005;87(8):1848–64.
5. Candeliere GA, Glorieux FH, Prud'homme J, St-Arnaud R. Increased expression of the c-fos proto-oncogene in bone from patients with fibrous dysplasia. N Engl J Med. 1995;332(23):1546–51.
6. Kashima TG, Nishiyama T, Shimazu K, et al. Periostin, a novel marker of intramembranous ossification, is expressed in fibrous dysplasia and in c-Fos-overexpressing bone lesions. Hum Pathol. 2009;40(2):226–37.
7. Fibrous Dysplasia Foundation. https://www.fibrousdysplasia.org/index.php?page=16#12. Accessed 20 Dec 2015.
8. Hoffman KL, Bergman AG. Kohler S Polyostotic fibrous dysplasia with severe pathologic compression fracture of L2. Skelet Radiol. 1995;24:160–2.
9. Ozdemir Kutbay N, Sarer Yurekli B, Kartal Baykan E, et al. Characteristics and treatment. Results of 5 patients with fibrous dysplasia and review of the literature. Case Rep Endocrinol. 2015;2015:670809.
10. Samper Wamba JD, Fernandez Bermudez MJ, Damiaguez TL, Pascua LR, et al. Polyostotic fibrous dysplasia associated with intramuscular myxomas: Mazabraud syndrome. Indian J Radiol Imaging. 2015;25:280–3.
11. Parekh SG, Donthineni-Rao R, Richetti E, Lackman RD. Fibrous dysplasia. J Am Acad Orthop Surg. 2004;12(5):305–13.
12. Kransdorf MJ, Maser RP Jr, Gilkey FW. Fibrous dysplasia. Radiographics. 1990;10:519–37.
13. Leet AI, Magur E, Lee JS, et al. Fibrous dysplasia in the spine: prevalence of lesions and association with scoliosis. J Bone Joint Surg Am. 2004;86-A(3):531–7.
14. Mancini F, Corsi A, De Maio F, Riminucci M, Ippolito E. Scoliosis and spine involvement in fibrous dysplasia of bone. Eur Spine J. 2009;18(2):196–202.
15. Henry A. Monostotic fibrous dysplasia. J Bone Joint Surg Br. 1969;51:300–6.
16. Wu FL, Liu ZJ, Liu XG, et al. Polyostotic fibrous dysplasia involving the thoracic spine with myelopathy: case report and review of the literature. Spine J. 2014;14(1):E11–5.
17. Park S, Lee I. CT and MRI of fibrous dysplasia of the spine. Br J Radiol. 2012;85:996–1001.
18. Chow LT, Griffith J, Chow WH, Kumta SM. Monostotic fibrous dysplasia of the spine: report of a case involving the lumbar transverse process and review of the literature. Arch Orthop Trauma Surg. 2000;120:460–4.
19. Bousson V, Rey-Jouvin C, Laredo JD, et al. Fibrous dysplasia and McCune Albright syndrome: imaging for positive and differential diagnosis, prognosis, and follow up guidelines. Eur J Radiol. 2014;83:1828–42.
20. Fitzpatrick KA, Taljanovic MS, Speer DP, et al. Imaging findings of fibrous dysplasia with histopathologic and intraoperative correlation. Am J Roentgenol. 2004;182:1389–98.
21. Chapurlat RD, Gensburger D, Jimenez-Andrade JM, et al. Pathophysiology and medical treatment of pain in fibrous dysplasia of bone. Orphanet J Rare Dis. 2012;7(suppl 1):S3.
22. Kelly MH, Brilante B, Collins MT. Pain in fibrous dysplasia of bone: age-related changes and anatomical distributions of skeletal lesions. Osteoporos Int. 2008;19:57–63.
23. Freemont AJ, Watkins A, Le Maitre C, et al. Nerve growth factor expression and innervation of the painful intervertebral disc. J Pathol. 2002;197(3):286–92.
24. Ashraf S, Wibberley H, Mapp PI, et al. Increased vascular penetration and nerve growth in the meniscus: a potential source of pain in osteoarthritis. Ann Rheum Dis. 2011;70:523–9.
25. Suri S, Gill SE, Massena de Camin S, et al. Neurovascular invasion at the osteochondral junction and in osteophytes in osteoarthritis. Ann Rheum Dis. 2007;66:1423–8.
26. Kiens D, Delmas PD, Meunier PJ. Long term effects of intravenous pamidronate in fibrous dysplasia of bone. Lancet. 1994;343:953–4.
27. US Food and Drug Administration. MedWatch. The FDA Safety Information and Adverse Event Reporting Program. Zometa (zoledronic acid) injection. www.fda.gov/medwatch/SAFETY/2004/safety2004.htm#zometa. Accessed 20 Dec 2015.
28. Collins M, et al. McCune Albright syndrome and the extraskeletal manifestations of fibrous dysplasia. Orphanet J Rare Dis. 2012;7(Suppl 1):S4.

41 Epidural Cement Leak in Kyphoplasty

Neil Malhotra, Nitin Malhotra, and Magdalena Anitescu

41.1 Case Report

A 75-year-old male with known history of renal cell carcinoma suffers from new-onset back pain without a history of trauma. He describes his pain as achy, constant, worse with every move, and localized primarily over the mid-lumbar spine. Recently he experienced sharp pain over the left leg from the knee down. However he has no sensory or motor deficits and walks well without assistance. An MRI of the lumbar spine reveals 50% compression of the L4 vertebrae with a suspicious space-occupying lesion consistent with metastatic disease. Minimal retropulsion with facet arthropathy and ligamentum flavum hypertrophy cause moderate left L4 foraminal stenosis without cord signal change. The patient's severe pain responds minimally to conservative therapy. Because radiation therapy of the space-occupying lesion is not possible due to previous treatments in the area, kyphoplasty is planned. The MRI shows extension of the metastatic process toward the left pedicle, an intact right pedicle, and an extensive metastatic process close to the posterior vertebral wall (Fig. 41.1).

Patient is scheduled for kyphoplasty. During procedure, after placement of the cannulas, the balloons are inflated in the targeted position.

Upon cement injection, it is clear that the posterior and superior walls are compromised, likely by the infiltrative metastatic process. Cement of a more paste-like consistency is deposited carefully to limit leak of the injectate toward the L3–L4 intervertebral disc or the epidural space. Posterior leak of cement in the epidural, although minimal, is noted. After the procedure, the patient's back pain is resolved, but radicular pain increases with slight, new right quadriceps weakness 4+/5. A second radiographic image performed in the recovery room confirms tracking of the cement toward the posterior vertebral wall and shows only minimal epidural leak (Figs. 41.2 and 41.3).

The patient is admitted for observation. His pain and weakness improve with an IV steroid taper, and a repeat MRI shows the right-sided cement leak that, together with underlying degenerative changes, contributes to the severity of right L4 foraminal stenosis. After a neurosurgery consultation, the patient is not considered a surgical candidate. The patient is discharged home, pain-free with a minor burning sensation in the right L4 distribution, and full motor strength. He is instructed to enroll in outpatient physical therapy. Following an aggressive physical therapy session, the patient complains of severe positional headache and severe back pain. When he returns to the hospital 2 days later, a CT of the lumbar spine with contrast is performed. It confirms a cerebrospinal fluid (CSF) leak and fluid accumulation around the L4 vertebra, likely from dural proximity to the hardened cement during aggressive physical therapy. CT also confirms end plate depression of the vertebrae adjacent to the kyphoplasty-treated L4, likely from cement leak in the intervertebral disc. The patient's headache responds well to a subsequent epidural blood patch, and his back pain improves with a conservative regimen and a back brace. He is able to enroll in a chemotherapy trial given his improved functional status after the interventions.

N. Malhotra, M.D. • N. Malhotra, M.D.
Expert Pain Physicians, Pain and Wellness Center, Orland Park, IL, USA
e-mail: neil.malhotra07@gmail.com

M. Anitescu, M.D., Ph.D. (✉)
Department of Anesthesia and Critical Care
University of Chicago, Chicago, IL, USA
e-mail: MAnitescu@dacc.uchicago.edu

M. Anitescu et al. (eds.), *Challenging Cases and Complication Management in Pain Medicine*, https://doi.org/10.1007/978-3-319-60072-7_41

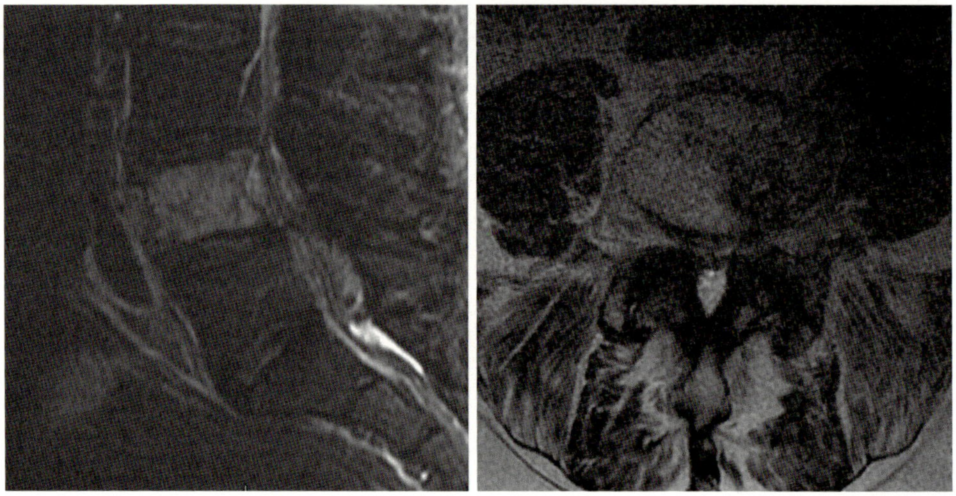

Fig. 41.1 MRI sagittal view of active infiltrative metastatic process as evidenced by STIR (short tau inversion recovery) images. STIR is an MRI image that causes loss of fat signal (bone marrow) from the relaxation properties of fat protons. STIR imaging is the most sensitive modality for visualization of edema and thus of acute fractures. MRI axial view in T2-weighted images shows invasive of the infiltrative metastatic process in the left pedicle. Images from personal library

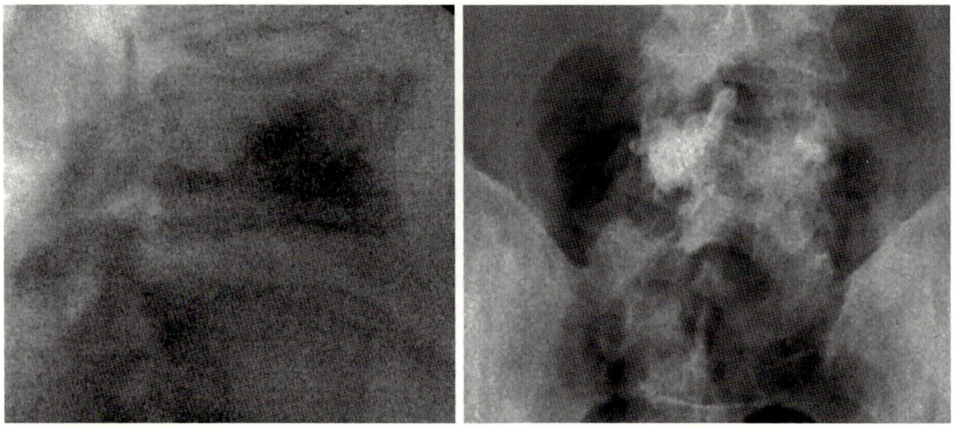

Fig. 41.2 Intraoperative fluoroscopy, lateral view, showing back track of cement toward the posterior elements; portable anteroposterior image does not clearly show cement leak. Images from personal library

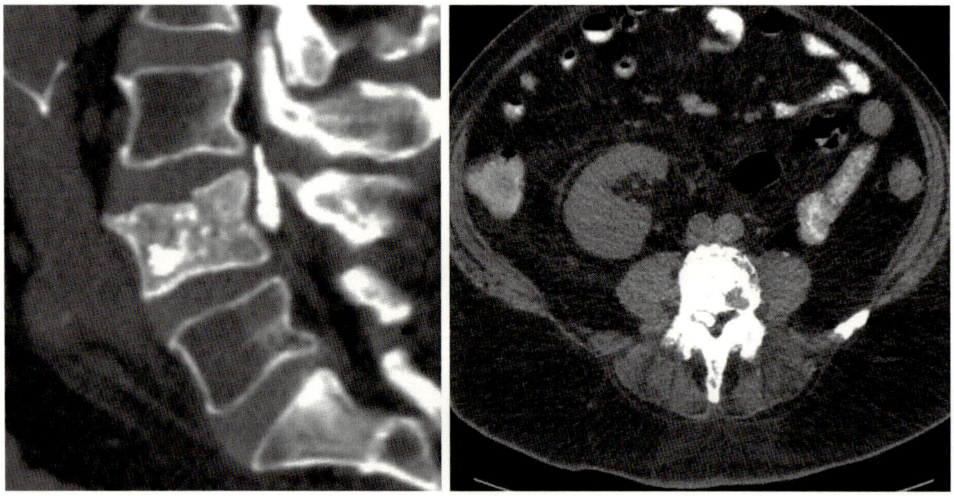

Fig. 41.3 Sagittal CT scan showing cement extravasation in the epidural space; after initial radiculitis, patient became asymptomatic after conservative treatment. In the axial view, the cement is seen toward the right L4 nerve root. Images from personal library

41.2 Case Discussion

41.2.1 Background

Vertebral compression fractures (VCFs) are associated with severe pain even with only minimal movement. In severe cases, pain from a VCF can be debilitating, leaving patients bedridden. The annual incidence of vertebral compression fractures has been reported to be 1.21% in women and 0.68% in men in those 50–79 years old, worsening with age and in women of all age groups [1]. When a VCF is identified, conservative management of pain is first attempted with medication, support braces, and in some cases gentle physical therapy. A normal course for a noncomplicated, stable vertebral compression fracture is gradual decrease of pain with healing of the fracture within 3 months. When pain is debilitating, functional capacity decreases, or when initial conservative measures are ineffective, interventional treatments such as vertebral augmentation procedures are involved earlier after the diagnosis.

The first percutaneous vertebroplasty was performed in France in 1984. The procedure has been improved since then. Although an excellent technique to treat VCF, vertebroplasty has been associated with several complications: adjacent-level fracture, pulmonary embolism, cement leak, systemic toxicity, infection, CSF leak, and epidural hematoma [2]. Recently, the advent of kyphoplasty has decreased the incidence of some of these complications such as cement extravasation [3].

With regard to technique, vertebroplasty and kyphoplasty are similar with a few notable exceptions. During vertebroplasty, fluoroscopic guidance is used to advance a needle into the cancellous bone of a vertebra to inject cement at the site of a fracture. In kyphoplasty, the needle is guided with the same technique, but a balloon is inflated in the vertebral body before injecting cement. Inflation is thought to compress the bone and create a cavity for injecting the cement under low pressure to minimize extravasation [4]. If the working kyphoplasty cannula and balloon are close to a compromised wall of a vertebra, an "egg shell technique" recreates the defected wall. Details of this technique are described later in this chapter.

Currently, polymethylmethacrylate (PMMA) is widely accepted as the standard cement type for both kyphoplasty and vertebroplasty. In some studies that have compared PMMA with calcium phosphate cement (CPC), loss of correction at 6 weeks was found on radiographic images in CPC compared to PMMA. CPC may have lower resistance to flexing, tractive, and sheer forces than PMMA. In burst fractures, CPC had a higher risk of cement failure, and patients' pain scores approached preoperative levels after 1 year. With PMMA pain levels were lessened 1 year post-procedure [5]. Other studies argue that CPC is equally safe and effective, but because there is no literature to date proving its superiority to PMMA, PMMA remains the standard cement used [6].

Kyphoplasty also may have the added benefit of correcting prevalent kyphosis. A VCF follows an increase of anterior column load in response to hyperflexion forces that ultimately contribute to the progressing kyphosis often present in VCFs. With the added benefit of "fracture reduction" and kyphosis correction, kyphoplasty may offer an advantage over vertebroplasty in select cases [7]. Thus far, kyphoplasty has been successfully utilized by practitioners in thousands of patients who have improvement in short-term pain, quality of life, and function [8]. Improvements in pulmonary function also have been noted with respect to forced vital capacity and maximum voluntary ventilation [9]. Based on a comparison of transcortical and vascular extravasation of contrast, the risk of cement extravasation is lower with kyphoplasty than with vertebroplasty [3].

The two most common causes of vertebral compression fractures are osteoporosis and malignancy. Symptoms are almost indistinguishable between the two forms, but they differ depending on a patient's medical history. A diagnosis of either osteoporosis or cancer is helpful in determining the type of fracture. Risk factors for osteoporotic fractures include alcohol or tobacco use, early menopause, dementia, frailty, and vitamin D deficiency [10]. Osteoporotic fracture is by far the more common of the two, often presenting after trivial events such as lifting objects, a vigorous sneeze, or turning in bed especially in cases of severe disease [11]. In moderate osteoporosis, trauma after falling off a chair or tripping can precipitate fracture. For patients younger than age 55, undiagnosed malignancy also should be considered [11]. During a vertebral augmentation procedure, the diagnosis is confirmed with an intraoperative bone biopsy. MRI distinguishes an osteoporotic from a malignant compression fracture. Studies of imaging have reported 100% sensitivity and 93% specificity for diagnosing metastatic compression fractures [12]. Lesions on the convex posterior border of vertebral bodies, abnormal signal intensity of the pedicle of the posterior element, epidural extension, encasing epidural mass, focal paraspinal mass, and other spinal metastases suggest a metastatic compression fracture.

Low signal intensity band on T1- and T2-weighted images, spared normal bone marrow signal intensity of vertebral body, retropulsion of posterior bone fragment, and multiple compression fractures suggest an osteoporotic compression fracture [12]. Adding axial diffusion-weighted imaging to standard spine MRI improves diagnostic accuracy in osteoporotic and malignant compression fractures [13]. For patients with osteoporotic VCF, the risk factors for developing more fractures are smoking, female gender, and history of treated or untreated VCF [14]. Indications for treatment of both types of fractures are pain refractory to conservative measures, but some patients with malignant fractures may have a better prognosis with radiation therapy.

41.3 Cement Extravasation

Despite advancements in vertebral augmentation techniques, the procedures are not risk-free. Rates of cement extravasation in kyphoplasty may be higher than originally postulated. Many case reports of significant spinal cord injury and nerve damage have been linked to vertebroplasty; recently, several reports document injury with kyphoplasty as well. In a study that reviewed 100 radiographs of consecutive balloon kyphoplasties, the overall cement leakage rate was 31%, with most leakages being anterior and superior [15]. Only 2% were posterior, and most leakages were below 3 mm. Of the

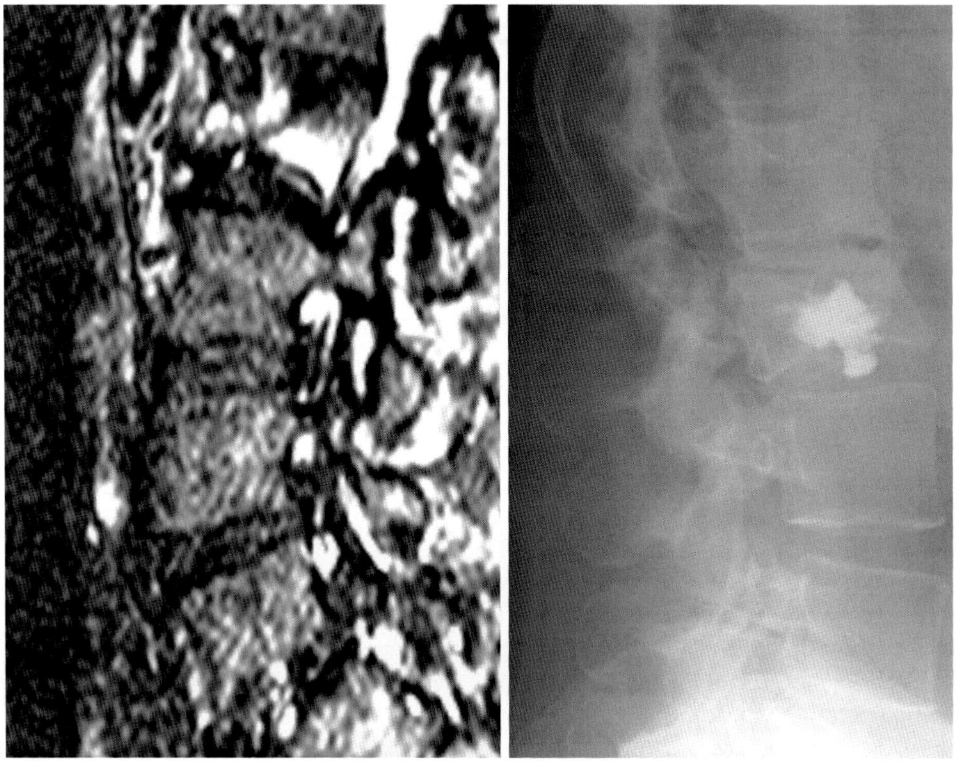

Fig. 41.4 MRI STIR images showing a fracture line over the L2 vertebral body; post-kyphoplasty portable fluoroscopic image showing escape of the cement through the fractured vertebral end plate into the inferior vertebral disc. Images from personal library

distribution of leakages reported from kyphoplasty, 48% were paraspinal, 38% intradiscal, 11% epidural, 1.5% pulmonary, and 1.5% foraminal [16]. Epidural cement leakage has had the worst neurological outcomes [17]. Paraspinal and intradiscal leakages have been less harmful, although some describe intradiscal leakage as one of the most significant predictors of adjacent vertebral fracture [18] (Fig. 41.4).

After performing kyphoplasty, the proceduralist must ask the patient about any new symptoms postoperatively. With an epidural cement leak, the patient may experience improvement in back pain but complain of new-onset radicular pain in the lower extremities, in addition to weakness and numbness. Patients may not be able to ambulate and have a positive straight leg raise. There have been reports of epidural cement leakage after pedicle breakage that causes neurological damage after kyphoplasty [2].

Monitoring cement leakages can be difficult, especially since fluoroscopy under a C-arm is the only practical method of imaging during the procedure. Patients are often under deep sedation for the procedure, making intraoperative neurological assessment difficult. Some believe that it is difficult to confirm a cement leak on simple radiogram, and oftentimes a leak can be observed only in a lateral and not anteroposterior view [2]. Furthermore, leakage through the pedicle wall can be difficult to assess, and some report that oblique images would be helpful for prompt detection of leakages after pedicle wall perforation [15]. For these reasons, urgent CT scan post-procedure is recommended if neurological symptoms occur [2]. In a study of 76 vertebrae in 49 patients who underwent vertebroplasty for osteoporotic VCF, more leaks were identified on CT scans than on radiographs by a factor of 1.5 [19].

Cement extravasation into the paravertebral veins may lead to pulmonary embolism or cardiovascular distress [16]. Despite the lower incidence of cement leak in kyphoplasty than in vertebroplasty, there was no correlation between cement embolism to the lungs and the type of procedure performed when post-procedure radiographs in 64 patients were obtained to assess for the presence of pulmonary cement emboli [20]. All patients with pulmonary cement emboli remained asymptomatic. Occasionally, patients have mild dyspnea and rarely experience cardiopulmonary instability making surgical embolectomy necessary.

41.4 Prevention and Treatment

Preventing epidural cement leaks begins with patient selection. Vertebral augmentation should be reserved for patients with intractable, debilitating pain that requires high-dose IV or oral opiates. Similarly, the procedure should be considered in patients for whom conservative management such as physical therapy, oral analgesics, bracing, and epidural steroid injections has failed.

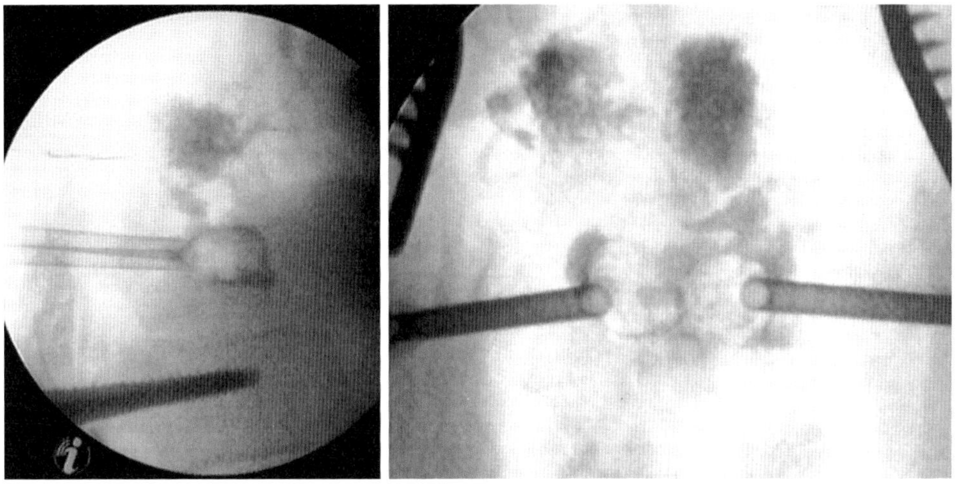

Fig. 41.5 "Eggshell" technique. Small amount of higher-viscosity PMMA is placed after the initial balloon deflation. Balloon is then reinserted and inflated several minutes, allowing the thin layer of cement to harden. Subsequently, the balloon is deflated, and the cavity is filled with the rest of the cement that is now protected inside the "eggshell" barrier of hardened cement, thus preventing leakage in adjacent structures [22]. Permission granted by Springer http://link.springer.com/chapter/10.1007/978-3-211-74221-1_9

In addition to proper patient selection, when a vertebral wall is not intact, several experts recommend a technique known as the "egg shell" method. It is also useful when the cannula and balloon inflation are positioned very close to the lateral or posterior vertebral wall. The technique was first described in 2007; anteroposterior and lateral images are obtained if cortical bone is violated during initial balloon inflation [21]. Next, the balloon is deflated and removed, and a small amount of doughy cement is injected to cover the defect. The balloon is then reinserted, slowly inflated, and expands against the cement. Once hardened, a barrier of cement prevents subsequent cement injection from extravasating [21]. For this technique to work, it is essential that cement consistency is paste-like and not runny (Fig. 41.5).

Other preventative methods focus on the type of cement injected. Even in vertebroplasty, high-viscosity bone cement (PMMA) was associated with a lower incidence of cement extravasation [23]. If injection of the cement via the working cannula does not reach all areas of fracture, results are mixed.

With regard to preventing cement leak via pedicle breakage, one study recommended placing a trocar in the center on the lateral margin of the pedicle in the anteroposterior (AP) view and in the middle of the pedicle in the lateral view. When the trocar reaches the posterior border of the vertebral body in the lateral view, the AP view should be obtained, and the trocar should not cross the middle of the oval pedicle shape. This technique will help prevent advancing the trocar across the medial wall of the pedicle [2].

Understanding the advantages and disadvantages of common vertebral augmentation procedures may help in the selection of appropriate patients and techniques [24] (Table 41.1).

Table 41.1 Comparison of percutaneous vertebroplasty and balloon kyphoplasty for the treatment of a single-level vertebral compression fracture—personal table based on and modified from Wang et al. [24]

	Vertebroplasty	Kyphoplasty
Long-term pain relief	Comparable	Comparable
Short-term pain relief	Inferior	Superior
Functional outcome	Comparable	Comparable
New adjacent vertebral compression fracture	Comparable	Comparable
Injected cement volume	Higher	Lower
Improvement kyphotic angle	Inferior	Superior
Cement extravasation rate	Higher	Lower
Procedure time	Shorter	Longer
Material cost	Lower	Higher

If severely symptomatic cement leak has occurred, immediate surgical decompression is indicated, with possible removal of the cement causing compression [15].

In multiple case reports, patients are unable to bear weight or ambulate immediately postoperatively after surgical decompression. Muscle strength recovery is 5/5 at 1-month follow-up, emphasizing the importance of prompt and early surgical intervention in symptomatic cases of cement leak [2]. Should the symptoms be more consistent with a lumbar radiculitis than true lumbar radiculopathy with weakness and unremitting radicular pain, conservative management with epidural steroid injection could be considered.

The significance of intervertebral disc cement leak is still debatable. Several practitioners reported an increase in the risk of fracture of the adjacent vertebrae with cement extravasation in the intervertebral disc during vertebroplasty [25]. The cement leak during the vertebral augmentation procedures occurs either through perforation of the end plate by the needle tip or a vacuum cleft; lack of vertebral end plate integrity by either malignancy or shattered fracture also may contribute [26]. In laboratory animals, the presence of cement in the intervertebral disc also has been associated with disc degeneration. When either polymethylmethacrylate (PMMA) or calcium phosphate cement (CPC) was injected in the intervertebral discs of dogs, disc degeneration observed was greater with PMMA than with CPC and seemed to correlate with volume of cement injected and time period after injection [27]. Although the animal model studied may not entirely match a true accidental cement leak, it does raise questions regarding potential serious, long-lasting complications of inadvertent cement extravasation in the intervertebral disc.

Of note that posterior cement leak also can occur with lack of integrity of the posterior vertebral wall; this may happen more often when radio-frequency ablative procedures are used to sterilize single lesion spine metastases. Two systems have been described, the DFINE system by Stryker and the OsteoCool RF by Medtronic; both allow kyphoplasty at the end of radio-frequency treatment.

In the DFINE system, the introducer cannula is placed close to the metastatic lesion, allowing the ablation instrument that has a curved tip to allow steering within the lesion to be placed directly into the lesion. The system uses conventional radio-frequency ablation and as such may need repositioning of the probe during the procedure to create multiple ablation zones and thus completely cover the area of tumor; at the conclusion of the radio-frequency procedure, cement is administered via vertebroplasty, using more liquid cement; therefore, direct fluoroscopic images in real time are needed to identify any possible cement leak toward the spine, especially if the metastatic lesion is close to the posterior vertebral wall that can be engulfed in the metastatic process.

OsteoCool RF system uses two internally water-cooled probes heated to 70 degrees Celsius (Fig. 41.6). During the radio-frequency ablation process, heat extends between the two probes in a synergistical manner, thus creating a sizable, bigger lesion inside the spine metastases. Because of the internally cooled technology, the probes never char as is the case in the conventional systems. Built-in safety measures allow the probes to shut off during heat application when impedance related to tissue structure changes (i.e., when heating extends further than the bone margins). As in any lesion that is close to posterior vertebral border, careful monitoring for impedance change or sudden drop to 0 will alert the clinician of the integrity break of the vertebral wall, allowing appropriate measures for the subsequent cement augmentation (Fig. 41.7). OsteoCool RF is coupled with balloon kyphoplasty to stabilize the vertebrae after lesioning. In kyphoplasty, following balloon inflation and removal, physicians use more cured, pasty cement to fill in the vertebral defect from the radio-frequency ablation (Figs. 41.8, 41.9, and 41.10). Therefore, cement leak, if it happens, tends to be more localized. Early identification of vertebral wall break is another important feature to present cement leak.

In conclusion, cement extravasation, although rare, is associated with a devastating neurologic deficit when the leak reaches the spinal canal. A leak contributes to delayed complications such as disc degeneration and adjacent vertebral compression fractures when the cement escapes in the intervertebral disc from a fractured vertebral body end plate. Special preventative and containment techniques are considered when cement extravasation is suspected to limit the development of severe side effects and complications.

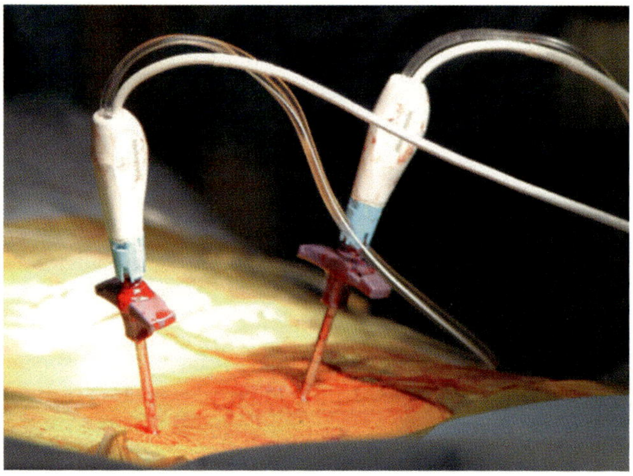

Fig. 41.6 The OsteoCool RF system with the water-cooled probes placed through the kyphoplasty working cannula. Image from personal library

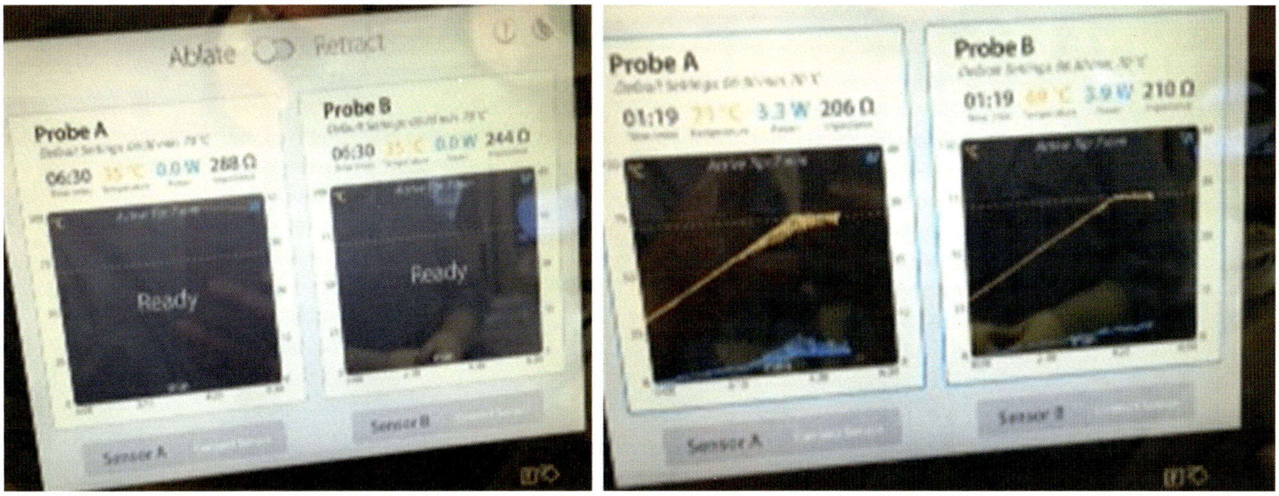

Fig. 41.7 The ablation system with built-in fail-safe mechanisms. System is ready when impedance reads 200–400 Ohms (*image 1*). The impedance is constant with small downward variation during ablation. Image from personal library

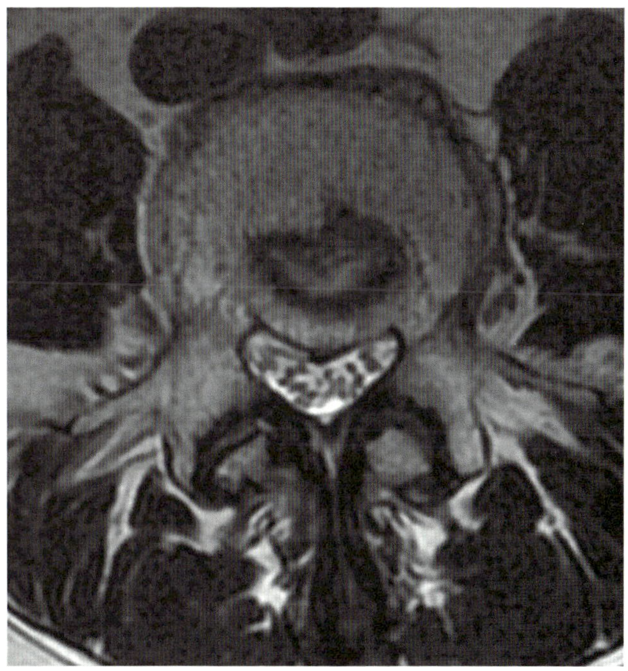

Fig. 41.8 Multiple myeloma spine lesion. Lesion is close to the posterior vertebral wall; OsteoCool RF followed by kyphoplasty was used in this case with good results and resolution of back pain. Image from personal library

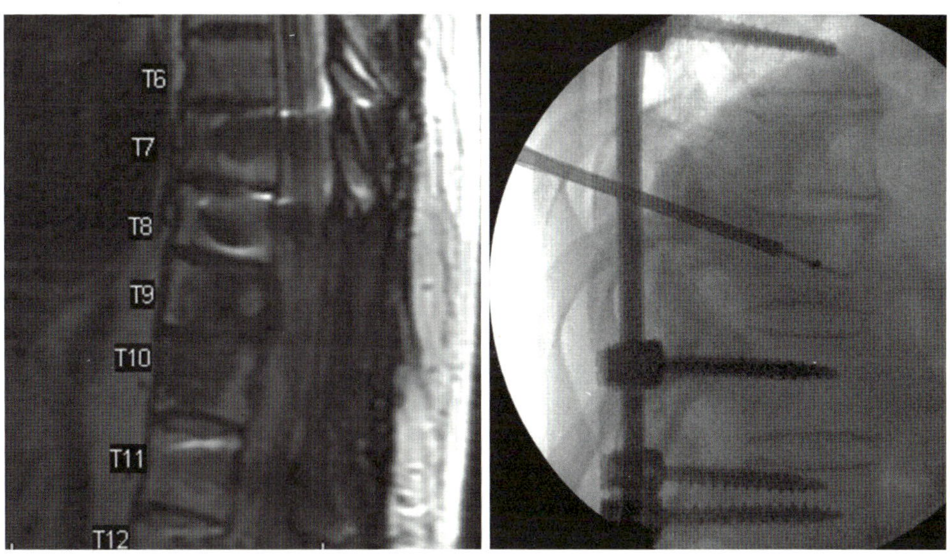

Fig. 41.9 Metastatic renal cell carcinoma with significant back pain due to vertebral metastases. MRI of the thoracic spine (*first image*) shows integrity of the vertebral wall at T10 but tumor invasion with no posterior wall at T9. OsteoCool RF was performed at the T10 level. *Image 2* shows positioning of the water-cooled probes in the middle of T10 (*black* dot is the site of maximum heat to 90–95 °C). Image from personal library

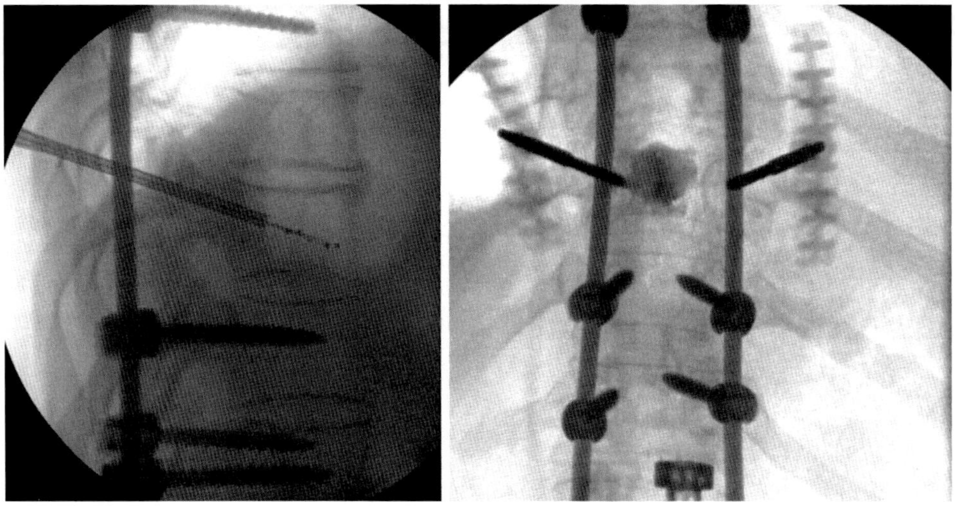

Fig. 41.10 Following OsteoCool RF, kyphoplasty is performed as usual using balloons and cement. Image from personal library

References

1. Felsenberg D, Silman AJ, et al. Incidence of vertebral fracture in europe; results from the European prospective osteoporosis study. J Bone Miner Res. 2002;17(4):716–24.
2. Park SY, Modi HN, Suh SW, Hong JY, Noh W, Yang JH. Epidural cement leakage through pedicle violation after balloon kyphoplasty causing paraparesis in osteoporotic vertebral compression fractures—a report of two cases. J Orthop Surg. 2010;5:54.
3. Phillips FM, Todd Wetzel F, Lieberman I, Campbell-Hupp M. An in vivo comparison of the potential for extravertebral cement leak after vertebroplasty and kyphoplasty. Spine. 2002;27(19):2173–9.
4. McCall T, Cole C, Dailey A. Vertebroplasty and kyphoplasty: a comparative review of efficacy and adverse events. Curr Rev Musculoskelet Med. 2008;1(1):17–23.
5. Blattert TR, Jestaedt L, Weckbach A. Suitability of a calcium phosphate cement in osteoporotic vertebral body fracture augmentation: a controlled, randomized, clinical trial of balloon kyphoplasty comparing calcium phosphate versus polymethylmethacrylate. Spine. 2009;34(2):108–14.
6. Grafe IA, Baier M, Noldge G, et al. Calcium-phosphate and polymethylmethacrylate cement in long-term outcome after kyphoplasty of painful osteoporotic vertebral fractures. Spine. 2008;33(11):1284–90.
7. Robinson Y, Tschoke SK, Stahel PF, Kayser R, Heyde CE. Complications and safety aspects of kyphoplasty for osteoporotic vertebral fractures: a prospective follow-up study in 102 consecutive patients. Patient Saf Surg (electronic resource). 2008;2:2.
8. Van Meirhaeghe J, Wardlaw O, Bastian L, et al. An international multicentre randomised comparison of balloon kyphoplasty and nonsurgical care in patients in patients with acute vertebral body compression fractures. Orthopaedic Proccedings. 2012;94-B(Suppl 4)
9. Yang HL, Zhao L, Liu J, Sanford CG Jr, Chen L, Tang T, et al. Changes of pulmonary function for patients with osteoporotic vertebral compression fractures after kyphoplasty. J Spinal Disord. 2007;20:221–5.
10. Old JL, Calvert M. Vertebral compression fractures in the elderly. Am Fam Physician. 2004;69(1):111–6.
11. Alexandru D, So W. Evaluation and management of vertebral compression fractures. Perm J. 2012;16(4):46–51.
12. Jung HS, Jee WH, McCauley TR, Ha KY, Choi KH. Discrimination of metastatic from acute osteoporotic compression spinal fractures with MR imaging. Radiographics. 2003;23(1):179–87.
13. Sung JK, Jee WH, Jung JY, et al. Differentiation of acute osteoporotic and malignant compression fractures of the spine: use of additive qualitative and quantitative axial diffusion-weighted MR imaging to conventional MR imaging at 3.0 T. Radiology. 2014;271(2):488–98.
14. Ning L, Wan S, Liu C, Huang Z, Cai H, Fan S. New levels of vertebral compression fractures after percutaneous kyphoplasty: retrospective analysis of styles and risk factors. Pain Physician. 2015;18(6):565–72.
15. Becker S, Meissner J, Tuschel A, Chavanne A, Ogon M. Cement leakage into the posterior spinal canal during balloon kyphoplasty: a case report. J Orthop Surg. 2007;15(2):222–5.
16. Hulme PA, Krebs J, Ferguson SJ, Berlemann U. Vertebroplasty and kyphoplasty: a systematic review of 69 clinical studies. Spine. 2006;31(17):1983–2001.
17. Patel AA, Vaccaro AR, Martyak GG, et al. Neurological deficit following percutaneous vertebral stabilization. Spine. 2007;32(16):1728–34.
18. Komemushi A, Tanigawa N, Kariya S, et al. Percutaneous vertebroplasty for osteoporotic compression fracture: multivariate study of predictors of new vertebral body fracture. Cardiovasc Intervent Radiol. 2006;29(4):580–5.
19. Yeom JS, Kim WJ, Choy WS, Lee CK, Chang BS, Kang JW. Leakage of cement in percutaneous transpedicular vertebroplasty for painful osteoporotic compression fractures. J Bone Joint Surg Br. 2003;85(1):83–9.
20. Choe DH, Marom EM, Ahrar K, Truong MT, Madewell JE. Pulmonary embolism of polymethyl methacrylate during percutaneous vertebroplasty and kyphoplasty. AJR Am J Roentgenol. 2004;183(4):1097–102.
21. Greene DL, Isaac R, Neuwirth M, Bitan FD. The eggshell technique for prevention of cement leakage during kyphoplasty. J Spinal Disord Tech. 2007;20(3):229–32.

22. Becker S, Ogon M. Special indications and techniques of balloon kyphoplasty. In: Becker S, Ogon M, editors. Balloon Kyphplasty. New York: Springer Wien; 2008. p. 85–98.
23. Anselmetti GC, Zoarski G, Manca A, Masala S, Eminefendic H, Russo F, et al. Percutaneous vertebroplasty and bone cement leakage: clinical experience with a new high-viscosity bone cement and delivery system for vertebral augmentation in benign and malignant compression fractures. Cardiovasc Intervent Radiol. 2008;31(5):937–47.
24. Wang H, Sribastav SS, Ye F, et al. Comparison of percutaneous vertebroplasty and balloon kyphoplasty for the treatment of single level vertebral compression fractures: a meta-analysis of the literature. Pain Physician. 2015;18(3):209–22.
25. Chen WJ, Kao YH, Yang SC, Yu SW, Tu YK, Chung KC. Impact of cement leakage into discs on the development of adjacent vertebral compression fractures. J Spinal Disord Tech. 2010;23(1):35–9.
26. Mirovsky Y, Anekstein Y, Shalmon E, Blankstein A, Peer A. Intradiscal cement leak following percutaneous vertebroplasty. Spine. 2006;31(10):1120–4.
27. Zhao H, Ni CF, Huang J, et al. Effect of bone cement on intervertebral disc degeneration. Exp Ther Med. 2014;7(4):963–9.

Vascular Uptake of PMMA After Spinal Procedures

42

Khalid Malik

42.1 Case Description

A 67-year-old male presented with severe mid-back pain of 3 months duration after a minor fall. His past medical history included well-controlled diabetes mellitus and hypertension, and his only medications were oral antihypertensive and antihyperglycemic drugs. He was treated conservatively with acetaminophen, ibuprofen, and hydrocodone for 3 months but with continued pain. On examination, he was acutely tender over the upper lumbar and lower thoracic vertebral spinous processes, and his neurological examination was grossly intact. A plain roentgenograph of his thoracic and lumbar spine showed L1 vertebral body compression fracture. Magnetic resonance imaging (MRI) of his thoracic and lumbar spine showed edema of the L1 vertebral body on short T1 inversion recovery (STIR) images, confirming the acute nature of the fracture, and there was absence of any retropulsed bone fragments. Due to the intense and persistent pain unrelieved with conservative measure and MR images confirming acute vertebral body fracture conducive to augmentation, decision was made to proceed with L1 vertebroplasty (VP).

The procedure was performed under monitored anesthesia care (MAC) in the pain medicine department procedure room. Transpedicular approach for VP using biplanar fluoroscopy was employed. After placing bipedicular trocars and confirming their adequate positioning on anteroposterior and lateral fluoroscopic images, a total of 4 cc of PMMA was injected with ease under live fluoroscopy. No venous, discal, or epidural extravasation of the cement was observed during the injection, and the patient remained hemodynamically stable throughout the procedure. After completion of the procedure, the MAC anesthesia was concluded, and the patient was transferred to the recovery area. Upon arrival in the recovery room, the patient complained of shortness of breath and chest tightness. He was tachycardic and tachypneic and his neurological examination was grossly intact. The patient was given supplemental oxygen and an urgent EKG was obtained. The latter showed ST segment depression and T wave inversion in precordial leads V1 to V3 and in leads II, III, and AVF. Due to the continued shortness of breath, unrelenting chest pain, tachycardia, tachypnea, and EKG pattern suggestive of right heart strain, a preliminary diagnosis of pulmonary cement embolism (PCE) was rendered, and the patient was transferred to the cardiovascular intensive care unit (CV-ICU). In CV-ICU, the laboratory studies showed elevated serum troponin and creatine kinase (CK), and a chest computed tomographic (CT) scan with contrast enhancement and three-dimensional image reconstruction showed PMMA in both major pulmonary arterial trunks. After a failed attempt at minimally invasive embolectomy by interventional radiology, pulmonary embolectomy using cardiopulmonary bypass was performed, and a PMMA embolus straddling bifurcation of the main pulmonary artery was extracted. Patient's postoperative recovery was uneventful, and he was discharged home a week after the surgery.

42.2 Case Discussion

VP and KP are routinely performed minimally invasive techniques for a variety of pathological or osteoporotic vertebral body compression fractures. The use of these procedures is widespread due likely to their minimally invasive nature, ease of performance, and a well-reputed efficacy. Even though the stated risk of VP and KP is minimal, a number of serious complications have been reported. These include pedicular fractures, segmental nerve and spinal cord injury, spinal canal and intra-discal extravasation of the bone cement, infection, and vascular PMMA uptake. Of the various complications cited, vascular PMMA uptake

K. Malik
Department of Anesthesiology, Feinberg School of Medicine
Northwestern University, Chicago, IL 60611, USA
e-mail: kmalikmd@yahoo.com

M. Anitescu et al. (eds.), *Challenging Cases and Complication Management in Pain Medicine*,
https://doi.org/10.1007/978-3-319-60072-7_42

appears to be the most common. PMMA extravasation occurs into the perivertebral and azygos veins and can extend to the inferior vena cava (IVC) and ultimately into the pulmonary veins [1, 2]. A number of procedure-related factors may contribute to vascular PMMA uptake and include (1) injection of large cement volume, (2) PMMA injection under significant pressure, and (3) relatively liquescent cement injection. Host factors also may contribute to greater PMMA vascular uptake and include greater vertebral body vascularity such as from invasive vascular tumors and the presence of osteoporosis. The ensuing cement embolic phenomenon includes IVC thrombosis [3], cardiac tamponade from cement penetration of the right ventricle, renal artery cerebral and other peripheral arterial embolism, and PCE. Among the various cement embolic phenomena, PCE appears to be the most common. The majority of reported cases of PCE are asymptomatic. Two studies of routine imaging—plain X-rays and CT—after vertebroplasty showed PMMA in pulmonary vasculature in 3.5–23% of the patients, respectively [4, 5]. Symptoms of PCE range from mild to life-threatening and may occur days to weeks after the procedure [6].

No clear treatment guidelines for suspected PCE exist. To ascertain the presence of asymptomatic PCE, routine chest X-rays after the procedure have been recommended [4]. No treatment is generally recommended in asymptomatic patients with PCE. In symptomatic patients treatment depends on their severity. Antithrombotic and/or thrombolytic therapy with intravenous heparin followed by oral anticoagulation therapy for 6 months may be considered in symptomatic but otherwise stable patients [7]. After 6 months the intravascular PMMA is likely endothelialized, and the risk of thrombosis is reduced obviating the need for further anticoagulation. Invasive embolectomy by interventional radiologist or surgical embolectomy by median sternotomy carries high mortality and should be reserved for cases of PCE with significant hemodynamic instability. Many patients are prone to delayed complications of vascular PMMA uptake and should be clinically reevaluated for several weeks after the procedure. The risks of various possible complications of VP and KP, especially PCE, should be clearly explained to the patient before the procedure, and an appropriate informed consent should be obtained. Recommendations to reduce the risk of vascular PMMA uptake during VP and KP include:

1. Prone positioning with adequate abdominal support to maintain sufficiently elevated intrathoracic and intra-abdominal pressure during the procedure
2. The use of blush venography before cement injection [8]
3. Injection of appropriate cement volume
4. Cement injection without undue pressure
5. Avoidance of excessive cement liquescency during the injection
6. Vigilance of cement extravasation during the injection and abort the procedure if this occurs

The patient should be cautiously monitored after the procedure for various respiratory symptoms such as chest pains and shortness of breath for extended period of time. The patients should be instructed to notify immediately if such symptoms occur even days and weeks after the procedure.

Key Concepts

- Vascular uptake of PMMA after spinal procedures involving bone cement injection such as VB and KP is common.
- PCE is the most frequent embolic complication.
- Majority of PCE patients are asymptomatic.
- Symptoms of PCE may be delayed for days to weeks.
- The symptom can vary extensively in severity.
- The treatment of PCE is mainly supportive.
- Symptomatic patients may require anticoagulation for extended period of time.
- Invasive treatment for PCE is indicated only in rare cases with systemic hemodynamic instability.
- Vigilance and meticulous technique of cement injection into the vertebral body may reduce this incidence of vascular PMMA uptake.

References

1. Choe D, Marom E, Ahrar K, Truong M, Madewell J. Pulmonary embolism of polymethyl methacrylate during percutaneous vertebroplasty and kyphoplasty. AJR Am J Roentgenol. 2004;183:1097–102.
2. Krueger A, Bliemel C, Zettl R, Ruchholtz S. Management of pulmonary cement embolism after percutaneous vertebroplasty and kyphoplasty: a systematic review of the literature. Eur Spine J. 2009;18:1257–65.
3. Kao F, Tu Y, Lai P, Yu S, Yen C, Chou M. Inferior vena cava syndrome following percutaneous vertebroplasty with polymethylmethacrylate. Spine. 2008;33:E329–33.
4. Anselmetti G, Corgnier A, Debernardi F, Regge D. Treatment of painful compression vertebral fractures with vertebroplasty: results and complications. Radiol Med. 2005;110:262–72.
5. Kim Y, Lee J, Park K, et al. Pulmonary cement embolism after percutaneous vertebroplasty in osteoporotic vertebral compression fractures: incidence, characteristics, and risk factors. Radiology. 2009;251:250–9.
6. Nooh A, Abduljabbar FH, Abduljabbar AH, Jarzem P. Pulmonary artery cement embolism after a vertebroplasty. Case Rep Orthop. 2015;2015:582769. doi:10.1155/2015/582769.
7. Righini M, Sekoranja L, Le Gal G, Favre I, Bounameaux H, Janssens JP. Pulmonary cement embolism after vertebroplasty. Thromb Haemost. 2006;95:388–9.
8. Peh WC, Gilula LA. Additional value of a modified method of intraosseous venography during percutaneous vertebroplasty. AJNR Am J Neuroradiol. 2003;180:87–91.

43 Increased Pain After Kyphoplasty

Tariq Malik

43.1 Case Report

A 70-year-old female is admitted to the hospital for pain control after 3 weeks of worsening back pain. She has a long-standing history of pain, managed with Tylenol. She was walking independently at home until she fell in her bathroom. Now the pain is worse and limits her mobility. She had fallen before, but the fall never worsened her pain. Pain is localized to her back, non-radiating, with no obvious neurological deficit. Her medical history is significant for hypertension, coronary artery disease, and osteoarthritis of the knees. Before this admission, her primary care physician ordered an x-ray of the spine after noticing a localized tender spot in her back. The spine x-ray was negative for a fracture, so the patient was treated for muscle pain and lumbago with a muscle relaxant and an opioid prescription. The pain medications made her light-headed and constipated with no improvement in her pain. This condition forced her to go to the ER as she lives alone and could not function alone at home. In the hospital, she was given an intravenous opioid for better pain relief. The physical therapy service was consulted to improve her mobility. There was no improvement, prompting a pain service consult. After evaluating the patient, the pain service ordered an MRI of the spine, which revealed a subacute L2 compression fracture. Kyphoplasty was recommended for immediate pain relief and improved ambulation. The patient agreed. Kyphoplasty was performed using a bi-pedicular approach, and the intraoperative course was uneventful. In the recovery area, the patient complained of right leg pain. She was able to wiggle her toes and move her leg. CT scan of the lumbar spine revealed that cement had leaked into the spinal canal, pressing on L2 nerve root. The neurosurgery service was consulted and advised against surgery. The leg pain made the patient miserable, and her ambulation did not improve. The patient was taken to the pain clinic for a lumbar epidural injection at the L2/L3 level. Her leg pain improved, and she started participating in physical therapy. Back pain still prevented her from independent ambulation. She was discharged to an inpatient rehabilitation facility for muscle conditioning and strengthening. She was readmitted to the hospital a week later with worsening back pain. Repeat MRI showed an acute L1 compression fracture. The patient was hesitant to undergo another kyphoplasty. Pain did not diminish with opioid analgesia, and the patient opted for kyphoplasty for the new compression fracture. The procedure was uneventful. Afterward, the patient felt pain relief in the postanesthesia care unit. She was able to ambulate with an assist and was sent back to a rehabilitation facility. She did well for a week. Then she noticed an increase in her back pain again; the pain began slowly, without an inciting event, but rapidly became intense. The pain was present at rest and even when lying flat. An x-ray of the spine revealed no fracture. Elevated C-reactive protein led to another MRI of the spine, which revealed presence of cement in L1 from the recent treatment of the fracture with kyphoplasty as well as persistent edema in the body of L1. Accompanying changes in the endplate raised the suspicion of infection in the L1 body. The patient was started on an IV antibiotic. Both the infectious disease service and neurosurgery were consulted. The intravenous antibiotic treatment was unsuccessful, and the patient was taken to the operating room for surgical treatment of the infected body. The rest of the hospital course was unremarkable, and she was finally discharged to an inpatient rehabilitation facility.

T. Malik, M.D.
University of Chicago Hospitals,
5841 S. Maryland Avenue, Chicago, IL 60637, USA
e-mail: tmalik@dacc.uchicago.edu

M. Anitescu et al. (eds.), *Challenging Cases and Complication Management in Pain Medicine*,
https://doi.org/10.1007/978-3-319-60072-7_43

43.2 Discussion

It is estimated that up to ten million individuals in the USA have osteoporosis, and almost 34 million more have low bone mass, placing them at a significant risk for a fracture later in life [1]. With improved life expectancy for the elderly, the number of persons with osteoporosis, as defined by bone mass density measurement, will become even greater. Vertebral compression fracture (VCF) is a major hazard of osteoporosis. The prevalence in the eighth decade is 20–25% in women and 15–20% in men. The lifetime risk of a clinical vertebral fracture at the age of 50 years is 3.1% for women and 1.2% for men [2]. In the USA, osteoporosis is responsible for more than 1.5 million fractures annually, half of which happen in the spine. In 1998 in the UK, it was estimated that osteoporotic fractures cost £942 million annually, of which only £12 million was owing to the acute cost of vertebral fractures. Once a patient suffers a vertebral fracture, the risk of another vertebral or hip fracture goes up many folds [3]. Quality of life is most affected by a lumbar compression fracture [4]. Back pain may arise either directly from vertebral fracture or indirectly from the consequences of spinal deformity, secondary degenerative change, and disc disease [5]. Nerve root compression may cause additional pain in the buttocks and legs. Vertebral fractures associated with osteoporosis rarely cause spinal cord compression. Cord compression was seen in only 2% of a series of 497 older patients admitted with acute vertebral fractures [6]. The two aims of treating acute VCF are pain relief and ambulation. During bed rest, virtually every organ system is adversely affected. These effects tend to be more pronounced in older patients, who have less reserve than younger patients. Bone mass decreases approximately 2% per week, a serious concern in patients with osteoporosis. These patients are unlikely to ever regain the lost bone mass. A bone loss tends to occur in stages, with the most dramatic changes occurring in the first 12 weeks of immobilization. Muscle strength decreases 1–3% per day or 10–15% per week. The benefit of vertebral augmentation in providing immediate analgesia is apparent [7, 8, 9]. The mechanism of analgesic relief, however, is unclear. It is believed that kyphoplasty can reduce the pain resulting from hardening of the fractured vertebra, and it eliminates microscopic motion at the fracture site [10, 11]. Other postulated mechanisms include chemical and thermal neurolytic effects of polymethyl methacrylate and partial denervation of the bone matrix caused by heat generated during the course of cement hardening. One of the outcomes of this therapy is insufficient or poor pain relief, partly because of the multifactorial nature of pain in elderly patients with compression fracture who tend to have other spine morbidities.

The post-procedure pain after kyphoplasty/vertebroplasty needs systematic evaluation. Pain may be patient or procedure related. Patient-related factors are poor patient selection, degenerative disc disease, spinal stenosis, facet arthropathy, or myofascial pain from severe kyphosis.

Persistent pain may be due to a recurrence of a new compression fracture as the underlying disease of osteoporosis still exists. History and physical examination along with an MRI of the spine will help to eliminate the possibility of a new fracture as the cause of pain. In the presence of an unremarkable MRI, localized back pain points to facet arthropathy or myofascial pain, both of which can be confirmed using a local anesthetic injection followed by a course of physical therapy. Procedure-related complications include soft tissue damage from frequent needling or redirections, cement leak into the disc or neural canal, pedicle fracture from the trocar insertion, rib fractures, and adjacent level fracture. There is always a risk of infection at the injection site [11, 12].

The optimal time for kyphoplasty is unknown. In general, vertebral augmentation therapy gives the best analgesic response within 1–2 months of fracture. The natural healing pattern of a compression fracture is unknown, but it generally takes a few months to heal. Kyphoplasty is best reserved for an acute fracture [7]. An acute fracture is best assessed with an MRI with a short-TI inversion recovery (STIR) sequence. In this sequence, fat is suppressed to bring out edema in the vertebral body, which is a sensitive marker for a non-healed fracture. The role of augmentation therapy in a fracture that is more than 6 months old is less clear despite quite a few case reports of good outcome in fractures more than a year old [13]. A fracture with no edema on MRI is not a good candidate for kyphoplasty. The fracture has already healed, and back pain will persist after the procedure. Pain in such a situation most likely may come from facet arthropathy or other spine pathologies. Facet joints contribute significantly to back pain in compression fracture because of mechanical strain (Fig. 43.1). Part of the pain relief from vertebral augmentation therapy comes from neurotomy of the medial branch of dorsal ramus during cannula placement [14]. Performing a diagnostic medial nerve branch block before kyphoplasty may prove effective in relieving back pain. The block may relieve pain if kyphoplasty does not. The nerves should be blocked two levels: one at the level of the fracture and another one level above. If effective, radiofrequency neurotomy of the medial branch should be performed. In patients with a compression fracture, poor ambulation because of pain quickly leads to back muscle deconditioning and is perhaps one of the most important factors contributing to back pain. Early ambulation and physical therapy are the cornerstones of any compression fracture management plan. A patient who does not respond to kyphoplasty should be carefully evaluated for rehabilitation therapy to improve core muscle strengthening and balance.

Persistent post-procedure pain prompts an x-ray or CT evaluation of the injected site, especially if the pain has changed or gets worse with movement or in a certain

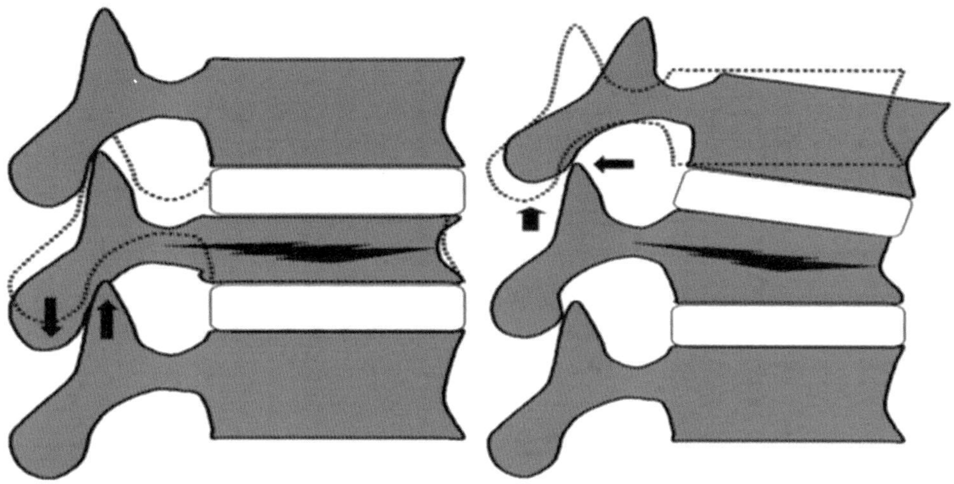

Fig. 43.1 Facet strain causing back pain after compression fracture

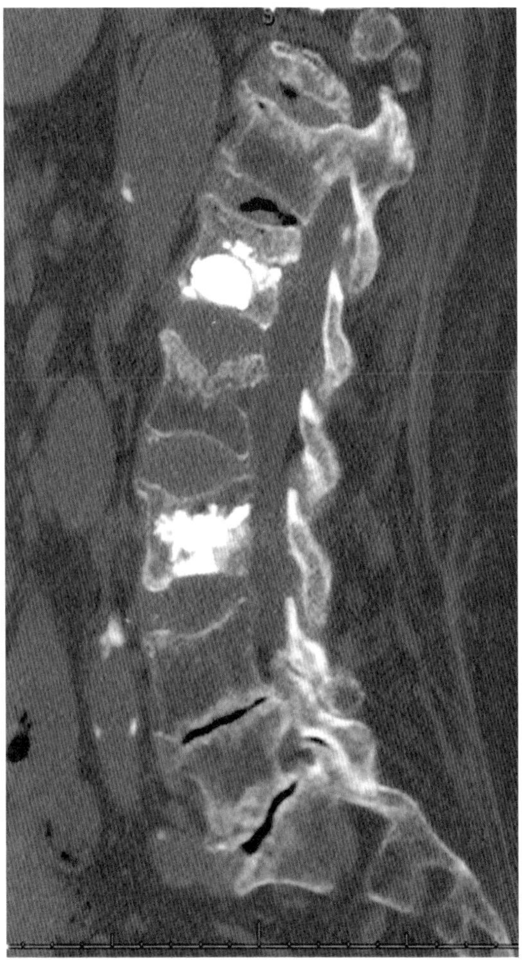

Fig. 43.2 Adjacent level fracture causing new or return of pain

position. Fracture of the pedicle and ribs has been reported with kyphoplasty.

A new compression fracture is a common occurrence after kyphoplasty (Fig. 43.2). The bone cement (polymethyl methacrylate) does not have the same resilience as natural cancellous bone, probably contributing to an adjacent level vertebral compression fracture [15]. The evidence for this phenomenon is suggestive but not conclusive. Patients with preexisting vertebral compression fracture are at much higher risk for another fracture. A new fracture produces back pain or worsening of preexisting back pain. There may not be an inciting event for a new fracture. A physical examination may or may not reveal a focal tender point over the fractured vertebra. An MRI is still the best imaging modality to evaluate the spinal anatomy as well as to time the fracture. Leaking of bone cement outside the body of the vertebra also is common.

The incidence is as high as 70%, depending upon the definition of leak and imaging modality used. Clinically not all leaks are equally significant. A leakage into the spinal canal resulting in cord compression can be devastating, requiring emergent decompressive surgery. Cement leak into a neural foramen can cause nerve root irritation or compression. The symptom is radicular pain after the procedure. If there is no sign of nerve root compression, i.e., motor weakness or loss of deep tendon reflexes, a leak is treated conservatively with an oral steroid or epidural steroid injection. Cement leak into the disc may accelerate degeneration of the disc or elicits an inflammatory response within the disc, leading to persistent back pain. A cement leak is prevented by injecting bone cement slowly and limiting the volume of injection.

Back pain also can arise from soft tissue damage or hematoma. Minimizing cannula manipulation will prevent these problems. In the absence of coagulopathy, hematoma formation is unlikely. Holding pressure at the injection site minimizes hematoma formation. Infection is rare but a reported complication. Infection may result in discitis, osteomyelitis, or epidural abscess. Common risk factors are a preexisting infection, diabetes mellitus, and immunosuppression. *Staphylococcus aureus* is often the isolated organism. Symptoms are worsening back pain and fever usually within a week to a month after the procedure. Inflammatory markers

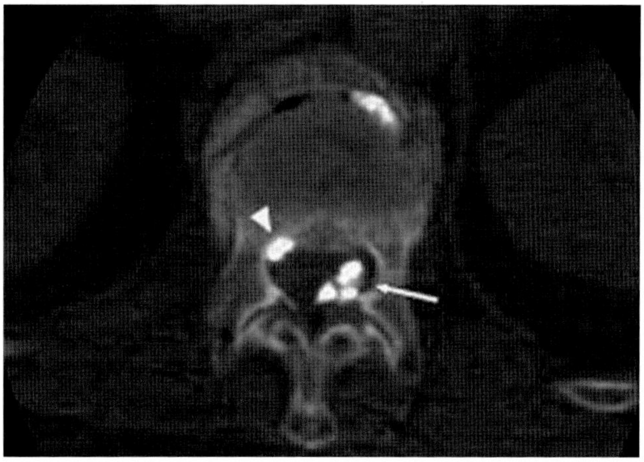

Fig. 43.3 Cement leakage into the foraminal space/epidural space

like C-reactive protein, erythrocyte sedimentation rate, and white cell count are elevated. MRI in the context of proper clinical picture confirms the diagnosis, but in some cases, a biopsy may be needed. Treatment is often surgery along with prolonged antibiotic therapy as many patients failed to improve with antibiotic alone. Cement laced with antibiotic as well as the periprocedure use of antibiotic has been suggested in immunocompromised patients. Patients with preexisting infections should be cleared of infection before getting kyphoplasty.

Vertebral augmentation therapy is a benign but not risk-free procedure. It relieves pain in selected patients [16]. Persistent pain after kyphoplasty requires systematic evaluation. If the pain is in the back and focal, then a physical examination rules out hematoma or bruising. A neurological deficit should be ruled out. If the pain is radicular or a neurological deficit cannot be ruled out, a prompt CT of the spine is obtained to rule out cement leak into the spinal canal or neural foramen or a rib or pedicle fracture (Fig. 43.3). Pain beginning days to weeks after a procedure may represent a new fracture or infection.

43.2.1 Algorithm for Persistent Back Pain

1. Immediate onset with no radiation
   (a) Localized/non-radiating
   (b) No neuro-deficit
   (c) Localized tenderness
      Differential: muscle pain, pedicular fracture, hematoma, rib fracture
      Treatment: trigger point injection, intercostal block, heat therapy
2. Immediate onset with radiation down the leg
   (a) No tender points
   (b) No localized swelling
   (c) No weakness
      Differential: cement leak, mechanical irritation of the nerve root during procedure
      Treatment: epidural steroid injection
3. Immediate onset with radiation
   (a) No tender point
   (b) Motor weakness
   (c) Loss of sensation or reflexes
      Differential: cement leak causing cord or nerve root compression, damage to nerve root during cannula placement
      Treatment: immediate CT of the spine, consult with neurosurgery
4. Delayed onset pain
   (a) Localized pain
   (b) Fever
   Differential: new fracture, recurrent fracture, discitis, epidural abscess
   Treatment: MRI of spine, kyphoplasty, consult with neurosurgery or infectious disease service

References

1. National Osteoporosis Foundation: http:/www.nof.org/osteoporosis.
2. Genant HK, Cooper C, Poor G, et al. Interim report and recommendations of the World Health Organization task force for osteoporosis. Osteoporos Int. 1999;10:259–64.
3. Cooper C, Atkinson EJ, Jacobsen SJ, et al. Population-based study of survival after osteoporotic fractures. Am J Epidemiol. 1993;137:1001–5.
4. Silverman SL, Minshall ME, Shen W, et al. The relationship of health-related quality of life to prevalent and incident vertebral fractures in postmenopausal women. Arthritis Rheum. 2001;44:2611–9.
5. Lyritis GP, Mayasis B, Tsakalakos N, et al. The natural history of the osteoporotic vertebral fracture. Clin Rheumatol. 1989;2:66–9.
6. Silverman SL. The clinical consequences of vertebral compression fracture. Bone. 1992;13:S27–31.
7. Jensen ME, McGraw JK, Cardella JF, Hirsch JA. Position statement on percutaneous vertebral augmentation: a consensus statement developed by the American society of interventional and therapeutic neuroradiology, society of interventional radiology, American association of neurological surgeons/congress of neurological surgeons, and American society of spine radiology. AJNR Am J Neuroradiol. 2007;28:1439–43.
8. Robinson Y, Olerud C. Vertebroplasty and kyphoplasty—a systematic review of cement augmentation techniques for osteoporotic vertebral compression fractures compared to standard medical therapy. Maturitas. 2012;72:42–29.
9. Humes PA, Krebs J, Ferguson S, Berlemann U. Vertebroplasty and kyphoplasty: a systematic review of 69 clinical studies. Spine. 2006;31:1983–2001.
10. Han S, Shuanglin W, Ning L, Tong Y, Zhang J, Fan S. Percutaneous vertebroplasty versus balloon kyphoplasty for treatment of osteoporotic vertebral compression fracture: a meta-analysis of randomised and non-randomised controlled trials. Int Orthop. 2011;35:1349–58.
11. Taylor RS, Taylor RJ, Fritzell P. Balloon kyphoplasty and vertebroplasty for vertebral compression fractures: a comparative systematic review of efficacy and safety. Spine. 2006;31:2747–55.
12. Nussbaum DA, Gailloud P, Murphy K. A review of complications associated with vertebroplasty and kyphoplasty as reported to the

Food and Drug Administration medical device related web site. J Vasc Interv Radiol. 2004;15:1185–92.
13. Eck JC, Nachtigall D, Humphreys SC, et al. Comparison of vertebroplasty and balloon kyphoplastsy for treatment of vertebral compression fractures: a metaanalysis of the literature. Spine J. 2008;8:488–97.
14. Bliemel C, Ludwig O, Beucking B, Timmesfeld T, Ruchholtz S, Kreuger A. Higher incidence of new vertebral fractures following percutaneous vertebroplasty and kyphoplasty—fact or fiction? Acta Orthop Belg. 2012;78:220–9.
15. Kallmes DF, Comstock BA. Commentary: no comparison: conservative management of painful spontaneous osteoporotic compression fractures is the way to go. Spine J. 2012;12:1006–7.
16. Nikolai B, John M, James B. The Pain of Vertebral Compression Fractures Can Arise in the Posterior Elements. Pain Med. 2010;11(11):1666–73.

Part VII
Miscellaneous

Pneumothorax After Serratus Anterior Trigger Point Injection

44

Paul M. Scholten

44.1 Case Description

A 22-year-old female sprinter presents to an outpatient pain clinic with intermittent, 4/10 deep, aching pain at the medial border of the inferior portion of the right scapula that radiates down the medial portion of the right arm into the fourth and fifth digits. Her symptoms began 2 weeks prior without any obvious trauma. Her symptoms are exacerbated during her running workouts. She finds it is particularly bothersome with heavy breathing during interval sprints, and she has developed a "stitch" in her side during these workouts that is affecting her performance. She is unable to identify any other clear triggers, but her symptoms are associated with shortness of breath. She does not report any numbness, tingling, or other neurological symptoms in her hands or feet.

On examination she appears well nourished and is in no obvious distress. Inspection of the spine does not reveal any abnormal curvature, and there are no rashes, erythema, or signs of trauma. Shoulder range of motion is full and pain-free, but reveals scapulothoracic dyskinesis. Palpation of tissue overlying the right fifth and sixth ribs in the midaxillary line reveals taut, exquisitely tender bands that cause radiation of pain to the inferomedial portion of the scapula and the anterior chest wall. She is neurologically intact. Movement of the shoulders and chest wall do not exacerbate her symptoms.

A chest radiograph is ordered to rule out a rib fracture as well as any pulmonary causes for her symptoms such as a spontaneous pneumothorax given her respiratory symptoms. Treatment is initiated with oral nonsteroidal anti-inflammatory drugs, and the patient is taught stretching/self-massage techniques for a suspected diagnosis of serratus anterior trigger point.

P.M. Scholten, M.D.
Pain Management Center, Shirley Ryan AbilityLab, Chicago, IL, USA
e-mail: paul.scholten@northwestern.edu

The patient returns for follow-up 2 weeks later at which time she reports no improvement in her symptoms, and she is having ongoing difficulty fully participating in her track workouts. The results of the radiograph were normal and are reviewed with the patient. On examination, there remains a palpable trigger point that has the same referral pattern as at the time of her initial evaluation. Further treatment options are discussed with the patient, and the decision to proceed with serratus anterior trigger point injections is made.

The patient is placed in a left side-lying position with the right arm extended and the right scapula adducted. Flat palpation technique is used to locate the trigger point, and a 25-gauge, 1.5″ needle is inserted into the trigger point eliciting a twitch response. At this location, 0.4 cc of local anesthetic is injected after which the needle is withdrawn to the subcutaneous tissue and then redirected into additional regions of the trigger point where this process is repeated. Upon entering the third such trigger point, the patient develops severe pain that radiates down her arm as it typically does, but this increased discomfort improves upon injection of anesthetic. She is discharged home in stable condition.

Six hours later the patient calls complaining of increasingly worsening shortness of breath and a dry cough. Deep inspiration worsens the symptoms, and she has difficulty answering questions over the phone due to the severity of her dyspnea. She is referred to the emergency department (ED) for a possible pneumothorax.

Upon arrival in the ED, she appears in moderate distress and is tachypneic, but vital signs are otherwise normal, including oxygen saturation which is 96%. There are mildly decreased breath sounds on the right compared to the left. A chest radiograph demonstrates a moderate pneumothorax. A chest tube is placed and she is admitted to the hospital for treatment. Three days later her symptoms and radiographs are improving and the chest tube is removed. A repeat chest radiograph is obtained and confirms resolution of the pneumothorax after tube removal. She is discharged home in stable condition.

M. Anitescu et al. (eds.), *Challenging Cases and Complication Management in Pain Medicine*,
https://doi.org/10.1007/978-3-319-60072-7_44

She returns to clinic 2 weeks later for follow-up. She has some residual pain and a small area of paresthesias at the site at which the chest tube was inserted. The pain she was initially evaluated for is no longer bothersome. She has not been running, but plans to begin a conditioning program and hopes to return to competition by the end of the season.

44.2 Case Discussion

A trigger point (TP) is a hyperirritable nodule of spot tenderness in a taut contracted band of skeletal muscle that reproduces the patient's characteristic symptoms and causes referred pain [1]. The finding of referred pain is important, because this differentiates TPs from tender points, which only cause tenderness at the site of palpation. TPs are typically classified as either latent or active. Latent TPs are tender to palpation and may be associated with restricted range of motion and stiffness but are not associated with spontaneous complaints of pain. Active TPs, by definition, are associated with clinical complaints of pain and produce symptoms including local tenderness and pain that radiates to distant sites [1]. The specific patterns of referred pain from TPs have been described in detail by Janet Travell, David Simons, and Lois Simons in their two-volume textbook *Myofascial Pain and Dysfunction: The Trigger Point Manual* [1].

44.2.1 Etiology and Pathogenesis

Myofascial pain is a common presenting complaint with prevalence rates as high as 75–95% being reported in specialty pain management centers [2, 3]. It is believed that TPs and the pain associated with them are the result of a positive feedback loop. The primary dysfunction in the "integrated hypothesis" proposed by Simons et al. [1] is the pathologic increase in release of acetylcholine (ACh) by nerve terminals at abnormal motor endplates under resting conditions. Increased sustained release of ACh produces sustained depolarization of the muscle fiber which produces sustained sarcomere shortening and muscle contraction. Clinically, this is identified as the taut band associated with TPs. The sustained contraction consumes energy in the form of ATP and also produces local ischemia and hypoxia by compressing arterioles traveling through the contracted muscle. This localized ischemia triggers release of prostaglandin, bradykinin, capsaicin, serotonin, and histamine, producing an inflammatory milieu that works to sensitize peripheral afferent nerve fibers. This is proposed to produce local TP tenderness. The referred pain associated with trigger points can be explained by central convergence and facilitation and is driven by peripheral sensitization. Sensitized peripheral afferent nerve fibers chronically depolarize second-order neurons in the dorsal horn of the spinal cord that lead to neuroplastic changes and eventually results in central sensitization. In addition, the so-called inflammatory soup consisting of substances such as bradykinin, substance P, serotonin, and histamine also stimulates activity of the local autonomic nervous system to release more ACh perpetuating the positive feedback loop.

44.2.2 Clinical Features

Myofascial pain may either be acute or insidious in onset and is often experienced as localized or regional deep aching sensations that vary in intensity from mild to severe. Serratus anterior trigger point activation may occur with deep breathing (i.e., a "stitch in the side") while running, severe coughing due to pulmonary disease, push-ups, lifting heavy weights overhead, as well as psychogenic factors [4]. This muscle originates from the outer surface of the upper eight or nine ribs and inserts on the costal aspect of the medial margin of the scapula. Under normal circumstances, it protracts the scapula and upwardly rotates it while abducting the arm in addition to stabilizing it by holding it to the chest wall to prevent winging [4]. The tonic contraction characteristic of TPs may restrict these motions. A sense of air hunger with short panting respirations due to pain may be seen in patients with serratus anterior TPs. In addition to the localized pain present at the site of the TP, serratus anterior TPs typically cause radiation of pain anterolaterally at the midchest level, posteriorly to the medial border of the inferior angle of the scapula, as well as laterally down the arm extending into the palm and fourth and fifth digits [4]. Given this referral pattern, the differential diagnosis includes cardiac causes of anterior chest pain, which should be ruled out with an EKG and further workup as appropriate. In addition, referral of pain down the arm extending into the fourth and fifth digits is similar to that seen in a C7 or C8 radiculopathy or radiculitis. Serratus anterior trigger point palpation, however, would reproduce patients' characteristic pain including radiating symptoms, which is not expected to occur with nerve root pathology (Fig. 44.1).

General and musculoskeletal physical exam findings in a patient with a serratus anterior trigger point may include reduced chest wall expansion, rounded shoulder posture, and limited scapular adduction with disruption of scapulohumeral rhythm. The palpatory portion of the examination for TPs is performed using either the flat technique in which the taut band of the trigger point is compressed between the examiner's finger and underlying bone or the pincer technique in which the affected tissue is held

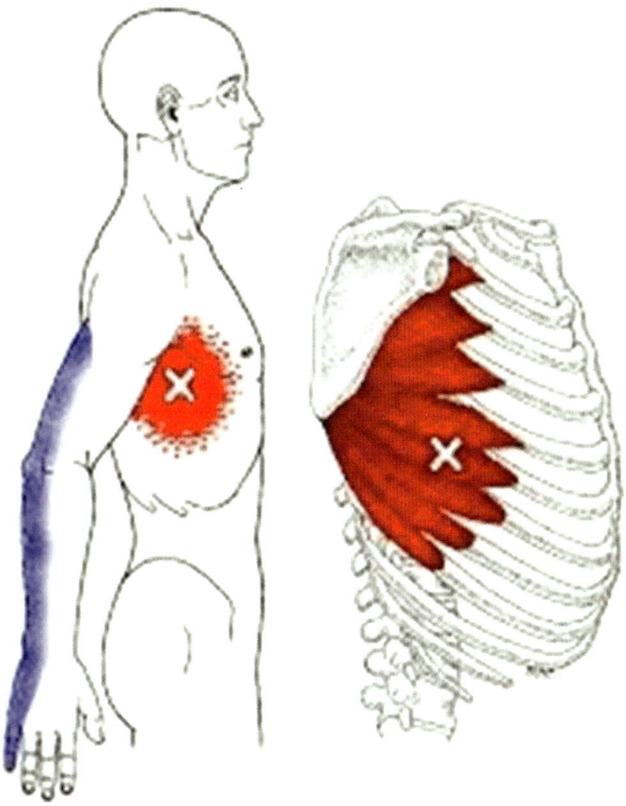

Fig. 44.1 Serratus anterior muscle with common trigger point. Image based on web open-source material: https://www.quora.com/What-causes-side-stitch-while-running-and-what-are-good-ways-to-deal-with-this-pain

between the clinician's finger and thumb. The minimum criteria for identification of an active trigger point are the presence of a taut band with exquisite spot tenderness and patient-recognized pain [5]. Such findings are expected along the upper two-thirds of the midaxillary line around the fifth or sixth rib with referred pain expected in the distribution previously described when the TP is in the serratus anterior muscle.

44.2.3 Diagnostic Studies

There is no specific laboratory test, imaging study, or intervention for diagnosing trigger points, although the use of ultrasonography, electromyography, thermography, and muscle biopsy have been studied as potential diagnostic tools. The diagnosis relies on careful palpation, but there remain no research-validated diagnostic criteria [5]. Depending on the study, the most reliable physical exam indicators are presence of a taut band associated with tenderness or presence of a jump sign and pain referral patterns [6, 7].

44.2.4 Treatment

Initial treatments for trigger points include prescription of oral nonsteroidal anti-inflammatory medications for improved analgesia, and activity modification to eliminate chronic overuse or stress in the affected muscle. Spray and stretch techniques are commonly employed to inactivate trigger points, relieve muscle spasm, and reduce referred pain [8]. This technique involves spraying either dichlorodifluoromethane-trichloromonofluoromethane or ethyl chloride spray topically to produce temporary anesthesia, which then allows the muscle to be passively stretched to interrupt the chronic contraction and break the vicious cycle perpetuating the TP. For spray and stretch of the serratus anterior, the patient lies on the uninvolved side with the back to the clinician and the upper arm extended. This initiates a stretch of the muscle which can be further increased by the clinician placing the scapula in greater adduction and by the patient taking a deep breath to enlarge the lower rib cage [4]. One effective self-stretch of the serratus anterior requires the patient to sit sideways on a chair with the affected side toward the backrest with the arm on the affected side positioned over the backrest. The patient then rotates the upper trunk in the opposite direction toward the front of the chair [4]. The ultimate goal of such manual methods is to train the patient to effectively self-manage their pain [9].

Alternatively, or if failure with manual techniques occurs, a more invasive approach utilizing trigger point injection (TPI) can provide prompt symptomatic relief. Contraindications to TPI include anticoagulation or bleeding disorders, local or systemic infection, allergy to anesthetic agents, acute muscle trauma, or extreme fear of needles [1, 10]. The patient should be positioned in a comfortable position, preferably recumbent to minimize muscle tension at the site of injection and protect against injury from fall should the patient have a vasovagal reaction. For serratus anterior injection, this is the same position as for spray and stretch with the patient side lying with the unaffected side on the examination table and the arm extended posteriorly. Typically a 22-gauge, 1.5-in. needle is sufficient to reach the trigger point. Most often, a solution of 1% lidocaine is injected, but other substances such as diclofenac, botulinum toxin type A, and corticosteroids have been used, but are associated with myotoxicity [1, 11]. First, the trigger point is identified and prepped to establish a sterile field. The practitioner then inserts the needle 1–2 cm away from the TP and advances it at an angle of 30° to the skin. Proper technique when injecting muscles of the chest wall requires fixing the TP against the rib between two fingers and directing the needle tip directly toward the rib to avoid deeper than intended penetration through the intercostal space resulting in a pneumothorax. To confirm that the needle has not entered a blood vessel or lung, negative pressure should be applied to the syringe while observing for withdrawal of blood or air. Once satisfied, a small amount of injectate is delivered. Then, the needle is withdrawn to the level of the subcutaneous tissue and redirected to a different region of the TP. This process is repeated superiorly, inferiorly, laterally, and medially until the local twitch response is no longer elicited or resisting muscle tautness is no longer perceived [1]. Stretching the affected muscle group immediately after injection can help increase the efficacy of TPIs.

44.2.5 Complications of Treatment

Potential complications of TPI include vasovagal syncope, skin infection, needle breakage, hematoma formation, and pneumothorax. Although rare, the consequences of a pneumothorax can be devastating if not identified and treated in a timely fashion.

A pneumothorax may occur spontaneously, often in cases of underlying lung pathology such as chronic obstructive pulmonary disease, tuberculosis, cystic fibrosis or severe asthma, or due to trauma. Traumatic causes may either be iatrogenic (as in this case) or non-iatrogenic such as with penetrating chest trauma, rib fractures, and barotrauma during flight or while diving. Other common iatrogenic causes of pneumothorax include thoracentesis, transthoracic needle biopsy, central venous subclavian vein catheterization, transbronchial lung biopsy, intercostal nerve block, suprascapular nerve block, nasogastric tube placement, cardiopulmonary resuscitation, and positive pressure ventilation [12–15]. Less common causes include injection of prolotherapy, botulinum toxin, and anesthetic or steroid solutions into tissues of the thoracic wall [16–18].

Early identification of a pneumothorax is essential to providing prompt treatment. Signs and symptoms include dyspnea on exertion, tachypnea, chest pain, dry cough, cyanosis, diaphoresis, and decreased breath sounds over the affected region. If a tension pneumothorax develops, mediastinal structures may become displaced and result in cardiopulmonary compromise. The onset of symptoms may be delayed up to several hours and may remain relatively mild after an iatrogenic pneumothorax, especially if a small diameter needle was used. If suspected, a plain chest x-ray should be obtained to confirm or rule out the diagnosis. A pneumothorax can be identified on upright, supine (least sensitive), or lateral decubitus (most sensitive) films. Characteristic findings include a white visceral pleural line, which is separated from the parietal pleura by a collection of gas. Typically there are no pulmonary vessels visible beyond the visceral pleural line. Computed tomography offers an alternative and is able to detect even small amounts of intrapleural gas but is typically reserved for more complicated cases or situations in which cross-sectional chest imaging is desired. Several techniques have been described to estimate the size of the pneumothorax described as a percentage [19, 20] but are difficult to apply, and most often clinicians simply use the terms small or large. A pneumothorax has been defined as small by the British Thoracic Society if the distance from the chest wall to the visceral pleural line is less than 2 cm and large if this distance is 2 cm or greater [21]. In otherwise healthy patients with a small pneumothorax, treatment includes monitoring to ensure appropriate lung reinflation, which can be done on either an inpatient or outpatient basis depending on the clinical situation. If a large pneumothorax develops, placement of a chest drain (pigtail catheter or tube thoracostomy) should be performed to facilitate re-expansion of the lung.

Prevention of this complication relies on careful technique when performing trigger point injections. Needle depths of 10–20 mm parasternally and in the midclavicular line or 15–20 mm posteriorly could result in pneumothorax. When performing the injection, inserting the needle over intercostal spaces should be avoided. Instead, it should be inserted into tissue directly overlaying a rib. A useful technique is to straddle the rip over which injection is planned with the index and middle finger keeping the tissue taut and providing the clinician with proprioceptive feedback as to the borders of the bony landmark. Alternatively, if possible, the tissue to be injected may be lifted away from the chest wall and the needle inserted in an oblique trajectory away from the underlying lung tissue [22].

Key Concepts

- Serratus anterior trigger points typically refer pain to the inferomedial border of the scapula and the anterior chest wall and may mimic cardiopulmonary causes of chest pain. These more serious diagnoses should be ruled out.
- Initial treatment of trigger points should include an active stretching program to put the patient in control of managing their symptoms.
- Pneumothorax is a rare but serious complication of TPI over the chest wall.
- Patients experiencing signs and symptoms consistent with pneumothorax such as shortness of breath, tachypnea, dry cough, or decreased breath sounds following TPI over any portion of the lung should have a chest radiograph to evaluate for a pneumothorax.
- Mild pneumothoraces associated with mild symptoms may be managed with close observation, but moderate or severe pneumothoraces require admission to the hospital and chest tube placement for lung re-expansion.

References

1. Travel J, Simons D, Simons L. Myofascial pain and dysfunction: the trigger point manual-upper half of body. 1999.
2. Gerwin R. A study of 96 subjects examined both for fibromyalgia and myofascial pain. J Musculoskel Pain. 1995;3(Suppl 1):121.
3. Fishbain DA, Goldberg M, Meagher BR, Steele R, Rosomoff H. Male and female chronic pain patients categorized by DSM-III psychiatric diagnostic criteria. Pain. 1986;26(2):181–97.
4. Simons DG, Travell JG, Simons LS. Chapter 46: Serratus anterior muscle. In: Travell & Simons' myofascial pain and dysfunction: upper half of body. 2nd ed. Baltimore: Lippincott Williams & Wilkins; 1999. p. 887–99.
5. Dommerholt J, Shah JP. Chapter 35: Myofascial pain syndrome. In: Bonica JJ, Fishman S, Ballantyne J, Rathmell JP, editors. Bonica's management of pain. 4th ed. Philadelphia, PA: Lippincott Williams & Wilkins; 2010.
6. Bron C, Franssen J, Wensing M, Oostendorp RA. Interrater reliability of palpation of myofascial trigger points in three shoulder muscles. J Man Manip Ther. 2007;15(4):203–15.
7. Gerwin RD, Shannon S, Hong C-Z, Hubbard D, Gevirtz R. Interrater reliability in myofascial trigger point examination. Pain. 1997;69(1):65–73.
8. Han SC, Harrison P. Myofascial pain syndrome and trigger-point management. Reg Anesth Pain Med. 1997;22(1):89–101.
9. Alvarez DJ, Rockwell PG. Trigger points: diagnosis and management. Am Fam Physician. 2002;65(4):653–60.
10. Ruoff G. Technique of trigger point injection. In: Pfenninger J, Fowler G, editors. Procedures for primary care physicians. St Louis: Mosby; 1994.
11. Fischer AA. New approaches in treatment of myofascial pain. Phys Med Rehabil Clin N Am. 1997;8:153–70.
12. Despars JA, Sassoon CS, Light RW. Significance of iatrogenic pneumothoraces. Chest J. 1994;105(4):1147–50.
13. Noppen M, De Keukeleire T. Pneumothorax. Respiration. 2008;76(2):121–7.
14. Sanchez HB, Mariano ER, Abrams R, Meunier M. Pneumothorax following infraclavicular brachial plexus block for hand surgery. Orthopedics. 2008;31(7):709.
15. Zhan C, Smith M, Stryer D. Accidental iatrogenic pneumothorax in hospitalized patients. Med Care. 2006;44(2):182–6.
16. Chiou-Tan FY, Miller JS, Goktepe AS, Zhang H, Taber KH. Sectional neuroanatomy of the upper thoracic spine and chest. J Comput Assist Tomogr. 2005;29(2):281–5.
17. Dorman T. Prolotherapy: a survey. J Orthop Med. 1993;15(2):49–50.
18. Miller JS, Chiou-Tan F, Zhang H, Taber KH. Sectional neuroanatomy of the lower thoracic spine and chest. J Comput Assist Tomogr. 2007;31(1):160–4.
19. Rhea JT. Determining the size of pneumothorax in the upright patient. Radiology. 1982;144(4):733–6.
20. Noppen M, Alexander P, Driesen P, Slabbynck H, Verstraete A. Quantification of the size of primary spontaneous pneumothorax: accuracy of the light index. Respiration. 2001;68(4):396–9.
21. MacDuff A, Arnold A, Harvey J. Management of spontaneous pneumothorax: British Thoracic Society pleural disease guideline 2010. Thorax. 2010;65(Suppl 2):ii18–31.
22. McCutcheon L, Yelland M. Iatrogenic pneumothorax: safety concerns when using acupuncture or dry needling in the thoracic region. Phys Ther Rev. 2011;16(2):126–32.

45 Complications of Occipital Nerve Block

Dalia Elmofty

45.1 Case Description

A 26-year-old female complains of chronic migraine headaches and new onset left-sided occipital pain. The patient reports a long-standing history of migraine headaches occurring two to three times per week associated with blurry vision and a preceding aura. She describes paroxysmal attacks of severe shooting and sharp pain on the left side of her neck as well as in the occipital region, worsening over the last few weeks. The symptoms are triggered and exacerbated by touch on the ipsilateral scalp and posterior neck region. Physical examination demonstrates decreased range of motion and tenderness throughout the cervical spine, most prominently at the left occiput with ipsilateral brush allodynia and reproduction of headache upon palpation. She had an unremarkable magnetic resonance imaging (MRI) of the brain. Based on her history and physical examination, the diagnosis is occipital neuralgia. The patient has been offered a multimodal approach to symptom management: massage therapy, myofascial release, anti-inflammatory medications, and muscle relaxants. Pain relief was minimal and she was referred to an interventional pain clinic. Given the debilitating nature of her pain, the decision is made to perform an ultrasound-guided left-sided occipital nerve block. Sonoanatomy was identified, including the occipital artery, and a 22 gauge 1 and 1/2 inch needle was utilized to inject a 4 mL solution containing 0.25% bupivacaine (Marcaine) and 40 mg of triamcinolone (Kenalog). She reported 6 months of relief from her headaches and occipital pain. The patient returned to clinic 10 months later with a recurrence of pain but noted a deformity that she described as a "divot" over the base of her skull, at the location of the block. She was referred to the dermatology clinic where a diagnosis of steroid-induced myonecrosis was confirmed by MRI, demonstrating atrophy of the left splenius capitis muscle. She received treatment with Botulinum toxin (Botox) injections and was advised to discontinue steroids.

D. Elmofty, M.D.
Department of Anesthesia and Critical Care,
University of Chicago, 5841 S. Maryland Ave., M.C. 4028,
Chicago, IL 60637, USA
e-mail: DElmofty@dacc.uchicago.edu

45.2 Case Discussion

45.2.1 Occipital Neuralgia

Occipital neuralgia is defined by the International Headache Society as a "paroxysmal jabbing pain in the distribution of the greater (GON) or lesser (LON) occipital nerves or of the third (TON) occipital nerve, sometimes accompanied by diminished sensation or dysaesthesia in the affected area" [1]. The GON is most commonly involved, as of the LON, less commonly, and the TON, rarely [2]. Occipital neuralgia is associated with tenderness over the affected nerve. The attacks last from seconds to minutes, but the pain can be persistent between attacks. The occipital nerve also may have a role in the pathogenesis of migraine headaches. Migraine headaches are a disabling medical condition affecting 12% of the US population [3]. It is estimated that approximately 3–14% of migraine patients will experience chronic migraines [4]. The underlying pathophysiology of migraine headaches remains unclear, but the trigeminocervical complex has been implicated: fibers from trigeminal afferents along with fibers from cervical spinal nerve 2 [5].

Thorough history taking and physical and neurological examination are necessary for the diagnosis of occipital neuralgia. Diagnostic testing may be required to rule out primary or secondary causes of occipital neuralgia. Computed tomography scan, magnetic resonance imaging, or X-ray imaging of the head and cervical spine may be indicated to rule out underlying pathologies. Tumors, infection, and congenital anomalies, such as Arnold-Chiari malformation, should be excluded.

M. Anitescu et al. (eds.), *Challenging Cases and Complication Management in Pain Medicine*,
https://doi.org/10.1007/978-3-319-60072-7_45

Despite advances in understanding the pathogenesis, patients remain intractable to conservative therapy: massage, physical therapy, anti-inflammatory medications, muscle relaxants, gabapentinoids, and antidepressants. Interventional procedures such as occipital nerve blocks may be appropriate in the management occipital neuralgia. Occipital nerve blocks also are efficacious in treating migraine, cluster and cervicogenic headache, hemicrania continua, and short-lasting unilateral neuralgiform headache attacks with conjunctival injection and tearing. The distribution of the pain (GON vs. LON vs. TON) determines the treatment.

45.2.2 Anatomy

The GON originates from the medial branch of the dorsal ramus of the cervical spinal nerve 2. It ascends after emerging from below the inferior oblique capitis and semispinalis capitis muscles. It then passes deep to the trapezius muscle and pierces the aponeurosis where it becomes subcutaneous, lying medial to the occipital artery. It provides sensory innervations from the external occipital protuberance to the vertex of the posterior scalp [6]. The LON is a cutaneous spinal nerve that arises from the lateral branches of the ventral rami of the cervical spinal nerve 2 and cervical spinal nerve 3. It travels superiorly along the posterior border of the sternocleidomastoid muscle and innervates the lateral scalp along with the area just posterior to the auricle [6]. The TON (also known as the least occipital nerve) is the medial branch of the posterior division of the cervical spinal nerve 3. It innervates the upper neck and lower occipital scalp [6].

45.2.3 Technique

The occipital nerve block can be performed using landmark anatomy (blind approach) or ultrasonography. The blind approach identifies the mastoid process, the greater occipital protuberance and the superior nuchal line. After the occipital arterial pulse is identified, an injection of 5 mL solution containing local anesthetic with or without steroid is administered medial to the arterial pulsation, at the medial third of the distance between the occipital protuberance and the mastoid process, at the level of the superior nuchal line. An ultrasound-guided method has been described using a proximal or distal technique [7]. In the proximal technique, the GON is identified at the level of the C2 spinal process, while the probe is moved laterally to the inferior obliquus capitis muscles. In the distal technique, the ultrasound probe is placed at the medial third of the distance between the occipital protuberance and the mastoid process, at the level of the superior nuchal line, in a short axis plane.

45.2.4 Complications

Occipital nerve blocks are generally without side effects although infection and bleeding are possible complications of any percutaneous procedure. Among the rare side effects are cutaneous adverse reactions, myonecrosis, intra-arterial injections (leading to local anesthetic systemic toxicity), and subarachnoid injections resulting in brain stem anesthesia (Table 45.1).

45.2.5 Cutaneous Adverse Reactions

Depot steroid preparations are commonly used for occipital nerve blocks. Rare but well recognized, cutaneous side effects of local corticosteroid injections have been reported. Side effects include full-thickness soft tissue atrophy, alopecia, hyperpigmentation, and folliculitis (Fig. 45.1) [8–11]. The incidence of soft tissue atrophy after corticosteroid injection has been reported as <1% [12]. The risk of cutaneous adverse reactions appears to correlate with the quantity and solubility of the corticosteroid injected. Insoluble, particulate corticosteroids such as triamcinolone are more likely

Table 45.1 Occipital nerve block complications

Complication	Presentation
Cutaneous adverse reactions	Atrophy, alopecia, hyperpigmentation, folliculitis
Myonecrosis/ myotoxicity	Attributed to local anesthetic or corticosteroid
Intra-arterial injection	Central nervous system manifestations Cardiovascular manifestations
Subarachnoid injection	Brain stem anesthesia

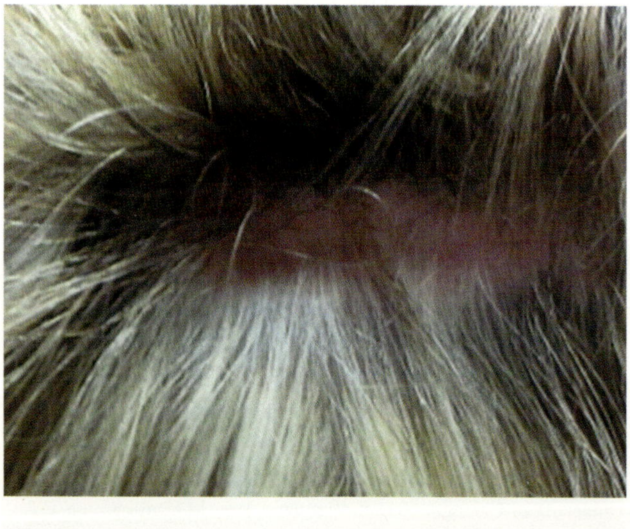

Fig. 45.1 Alopecia and cutaneous atrophy following an occipital nerve block

to cause adverse outcomes compared to soluble agents such as methylprednisolone or betamethasone. The underlying mechanism is associated with vasoconstriction of the surrounding vessels and deposit of insoluble crystals at the site, which results in atrophy of the skin and interruption of hair growth [12].

45.2.6 Myonecrosis

The exact mechanism of analgesia induced by corticosteroids is unknown but is attributed to their anti-inflammatory effects, which reduce chemical mediators that stimulate nociception. Intramuscular injection of local anesthetics and corticosteroid can lead to myonecrosis (Fig. 45.2). Lidocaine, bupivacaine, and mepivacaine have been found to be myotoxic. The pathogenesis of myotoxicity is complex. The muscle fibers hypercontract, degenerate, and swell with inflammatory cell infiltration and necrosis after injection. The underlying mechanism is thought to be the interaction of the local anesthetic with the sarcoplasmic reticulum. Intracellular calcium increases and further reuptake of calcium is inhibited, subsequently causing cell death [13]. Histological changes in the muscle are reversed between 2 to 5 weeks after initial insult to the muscle. Although muscle regeneration is expected, late-stage scarring has been reported. Concentration of local anesthetic correlates with degree of damage. The evidence that triamcinolone alone is myotoxic is limited, but a combination of triamcinolone and bupivacaine was more myotoxic than bupivacaine alone. A synergistic effect has been suggested with the two-drug combination. Corticosteroids seem to delay the regenerative process after bupivacaine-induced myonecrosis [14].

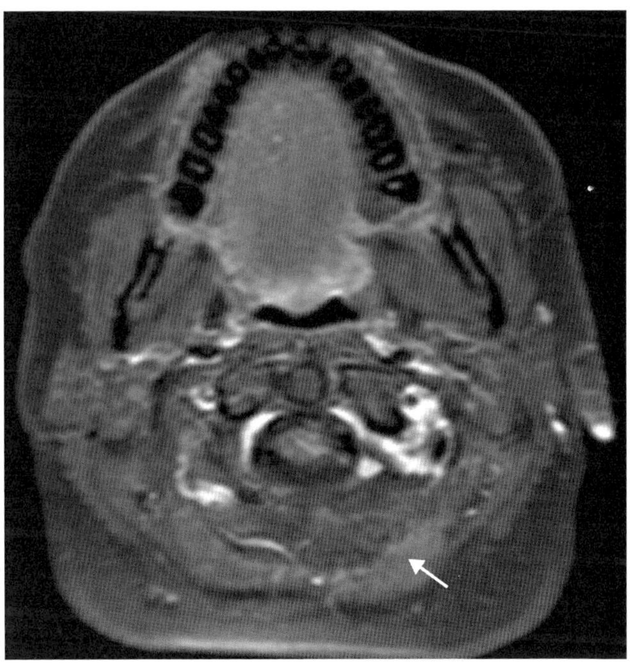

Fig. 45.2 Magnetic resonance imaging revealing atrophy of the left splenius capitius muscle (*white arrow*) after an occipital nerve block

45.2.7 Intra-arterial Injection

Intra-arterial injection of local anesthetic into the occipital artery can result in local anesthetic systemic toxicity. Substantial plasma concentrations of local anesthetics are required to produce central nervous system manifestations. Retrograde vascular spread along the occipital artery and then anterograde spread in the internal carotid artery makes the brain concentrations of local anesthetic high [15]. The classic symptoms of local anesthetic systemic toxicity are tinnitus, perioral numbness, agitation, confusion, seizures, and loss of consciousness (Table 45.2). Bradycardia and hypotension may progress to asystole and prolongation of the QTc interval and ventricular arrhythmia. In a review of published cases from 1979 to 2009, one study identified a total of 93 events of local anesthetic systemic toxicity, central nervous system toxicity in 89% of the cases, and cardiovascular toxicity in 51%. Simultaneous toxicity of both was 44%. The time of onset of symptoms ranged from less than 1 min to greater than 10 min after a single injection of local anesthetic [16].

Lipid infusion has been described to treat local anesthetic systemic toxicity. Intralipid 20% is administered as an initial bolus of 1.5 mL/kg before an infusion of 0.25 mL/kg/min with a maximum of 10 mL/kg over 30 min. Intralipid acts as a "lipid sink" by extracting the lipophilic local anesthetic and by providing fatty acids for aerobic metabolism in cardiac mitochondria. Data regarding the side effect profile of intralipid are lacking. In 2010, the American Society of Regional Anesthesia and Pain Medicine published a practice advisory for the treatment of systemic toxicity from local anesthetics.

Table 45.2 Local anesthetic systemic toxicity

Symptoms	Perioral numbness, metallic taste, tinnitus, agitation, coma
Signs	Central nervous system: Seizure Cardiovascular system: Hyper- or hypotension, tachy- or bradycardia, ventricular arrhythmia, cardiac arrest
Treatment	1. Intralipid 2. Advanced cardiac life support: Low dose epinephrine 10–100 mcg. Do not use lidocaine, procainamide, calcium channel blockers, beta-blockers, or vasopressin. Coronary pulmonary bypass if measures fail 3. Benzodiazepine or small doses of propofol for seizures

Calling for help, airway management, seizure suppression, basic life support, advanced cardiac life support, and infusion of lipid emulsion are recommended. Ultrasound-guided nerve blocks may decrease the incidence of unintended vascular puncture [17].

45.2.8 Subarachnoid Injection

Patients with cranial abnormalities or a history of cranial surgery are at greater risk of inadvertent injection of local anesthetics into the cranial vault. Subarachnoid injection of local anesthetic has been reported in the presence of an occipital bony defect [18]. Puncturing the dura can result in a potentially life-threatening complication. In brain stem anesthesia, the patient is unarousable and apneic and needs support. A detailed medical history should elicit any previous craniotomies. Imaging may be warranted to identify and detail cranial defects. Posterior fossa craniotomies are contraindication for the blind approach to the occipital nerve block. Ultrasound in combination with fluoroscopic guidance is recommended to help identify an area of body defect.

45.3 Summary

Occipital nerve blocks are a simple procedure when performed by a properly trained physician. They are safe and possibly more favorable for treatment than other options. Complications are rare but can be devastating. Additional research is needed to clarify the potential risk of repeated nerve blocks.

Key Concepts

- Occipital nerve blocks are commonly performed for headache management in the outpatient setting.
- Rare complications have been reported which include cutaneous side effects and myonecrosis.
- Intra-arterial injections of local anesthetic can cause systemic toxicity, and subarachnoid injections in patients with cranial defects have also been reported.
- Physicians should anticipate these complications and incorporate safety measures in their practice to prevent them.

References

1. Headache Classification Committee of the International Headache Society (IHS). The international classification of headache disorders, 3rd edition (beta version). Cephalalgia. 2013;33:629Y808.
2. Hammond SR, Danta G. Occipital neuralgia. Clin Exp Neurol. 1978;15:258.
3. Lipton RB, Stewart WF, Diamond S, Diamond ML, Reed M. Prevalence and burden of migraine in the United States: data from the American migraine study II. Headache. 2001;41:646–57.
4. Goadsby PJ, Hargreaves R. Refractory migraine and chronic migraine: pathophysiological mechanisms. Headache. 2008;48:799–804.
5. Katsarava Z, Schneeweiss S, Kurth T, et al. Incidence and predictors for chronicity of headache in patients with episodic migraine. Neurology. 2004;62:788–90.
6. Dougherty C. Occipital neuralgia. Curr Pain Headache Rep. 2014;18:411.
7. Greher M, Moriggl B, Curatolo M, Kirchmair L, Eichenberger U. Sonographic visualization and ultrasound-guided blockade of the greater occipital nerve: a comparison of two selective techniques confirmed by anatomical dissection. Br J Anaesth. 2010;104:637–42.
8. Mutagi H, Boger A, Kapur S. Full thickness local soft tissue atrophy following steroid injection to greater occipital nerve. Pain Pract. 2011;11(6):582–4.
9. Lambru G, Lagrata S, Matharu S. Cutaneous atrophy and alopecia after greater occipital nerve injection using triamcinolone. Headache. 2012;52:1596–9.
10. Shields KG, Levy MJ, Goadsby PJ. Alopecia and cutaneous atrophy after greater occipital nerve infiltration with corticosteroid. Neurology. 2004;63:2193–4.
11. Degerli S, Gulec H, Koc F. Folliculitis following greater occipital nerve block. Agri Derg. 2015;27(2):121–2.
12. Papadopoulous PJ, Edison JD. The clinical picture: soft tissue atrophy after corticosteroid injection. Cleve Clin J Med. 2009;76:373–4.
13. Zink W, Graf BM, Sinner B, Martin E, Fink RH, Kunst G. Differential effects of bupivacaine on intracellular Ca^{2+} regulation: potential mechanisms of its myotoxicity. Anesthesiology. 2002;97(3):710–6.
14. Reurink G, Goudswaard GJ, Moen MH, Weir A, Verhaar J, Tol JL. Myotoxicity of injections for acute muscle injury: a systematic review. Sports Med. 2014;44:943–56.
15. Okuda Y, Matsumoto T, Shinohara M, Kitajima T, Kim P. Sudden unconsciousness during a lesser occipital nerve block in a patient with an occipital bone defect. Eur J Anaesthesiol. 2001;18:829–32.
16. Di Gregorio G, Neal J, Rosenquist RW, Weinberg GL. Clinical presentation of local anesthetic systemic toxicity: a review of published cases, 1979 to 2009. Reg Anesth Pain Med. 2010;35:181–7.
17. Neal J. Ultrasound-guided regional anesthesia and patient safety: an evidence-based analysis. Reg Anesth Pain Med. 2010;35(suppl 1):S59–67.
18. Sprenger T, Seifert CL. Coma after greater occipital nerve blockade in a patient with previous posterior fossa surgery. Headache. 2013;53:548–50.

Septic Knee

46

Paul M. Scholten

46.1 Case Description

An 82-year-old male with a history of diabetes mellitus presents with recent worsening of his chronic right knee pain. His typical pain is 4/10 on average, is achy in nature, and worsens with activity and improves, but does not resolve with rest. Functionally, he is able to walk four to five blocks before the pain limits him. He had x-rays nearly 1 year ago that showed lateral joint space narrowing. He was referred for a course of physical therapy, but he was unable to fully participate due to the level of his pain. He subsequently had two intra-articular injections with corticosteroid and local anesthetic over the last 12 months. Each of these allowed him to better participate in his rehabilitation program, and he reports approximately 5 months of near-complete pain relief after each injection. Over the last 6–8 weeks, he has had gradual return of symptoms, and he is requesting a repeat injection. His examination remains unchanged from when he was last seen with tenderness over the lateral joint line, mild crepitus with passive range of motion, and an intact neurological examination. After discussing the risks and benefits of the procedure with the patient, he is prepped and draped in the usual sterile fashion before an ultrasound-guided intra-articular right knee injection is performed with 1 cc of triamcinolone 40 mg/mL and 4 cc of 0.25% bupivacaine. There are no complications and he is discharged in stable condition.

The patient returns to the clinic 3 days later complaining of worsening pain in the right knee that he rates as a constant 9/10 and is severe enough to keep him from sleeping at night. He has difficulty bending the knee because of the pain and maintains it in a fully extended position. He also believes he may have had a fever but did not measure his temperature.

P.M. Scholten, M.D.
Pain Management Center, Shirley Ryan AbilityLab, Chicago, IL, USA
e-mail: paul.scholten@northwestern.edu

On examination his temperature is 38.5 °C, but all other vital signs are within normal limits, and he appears to be in a moderate amount of pain. The right knee is erythematous and swollen and there is a moderate effusion. There are no rashes or signs of trauma, but it is diffusely tender to palpation and warm to touch. He maintains the right knee in an extended position, and active and passive range of motion are significantly restricted due to the severity of his pain. Strength testing at the knee is limited by pain, but in all other tested muscle groups, strength is intact. There are no sensory deficits, and he has 2+ pulses at the dorsalis pedis and posterior tibialis bilaterally.

Laboratory work including complete blood count, C-reactive protein, erythrocyte sedimentation rate, and two sets of blood cultures are drawn for analysis. In addition, radiographs of the right knee are obtained. Right knee arthrocentesis is performed, and 6 cc of synovial fluid is drained and sent for Gram stain and culture, leukocyte count with differential, and assessment for crystals. When aspirated, the fluid appears purulent.

The radiograph demonstrates mild worsening of his known unicompartmental osteoarthritis and soft tissue swelling. The white blood cell count, C-reactive protein, and erythrocyte sedimentation rate are all elevated. Initial joint fluid analysis reports opaque, yellow-green very low-viscosity fluid without crystals, >100,000 WBCs/mm^3, and 83% polymorphonuclear leukocytes. Both blood and synovial fluid stainings reveal Gram-positive cocci.

The patient is admitted to the hospital immediately after obtaining initial laboratory tests, and empiric treatment with vancomycin is initiated. Three days later synovial fluid and blood cultures reveal *Staphylococcus aureus* as the causative organism. Based on antibiotic susceptibility profiles, the patient is transitioned to IV clindamycin and discharged with home infusion services. After 2 weeks of parenteral treatment, he is transitioned to oral therapy for a total duration of treatment of 4 weeks.

He returns to the office 4 weeks after completing his course of antibiotics. His pain is back to baseline and his

M. Anitescu et al. (eds.), *Challenging Cases and Complication Management in Pain Medicine*,
https://doi.org/10.1007/978-3-319-60072-7_46

range of motion has returned, but he continues to have ongoing difficulty ambulating long distances and plans to see an orthopedic surgeon to discuss what surgical options he has to hopefully return to his previous level of pain-free walking.

46.2 Case Discussion

Septic arthritis is the direct invasion of the joint space by an infectious microorganism. Most commonly it is caused by bacteria, but viruses, mycobacteria, and fungi may also result in this orthopedic emergency. Bacteria can cause rapid destruction of the joint space, and significant morbidity including subchondral bone loss and permanent joint dysfunction can occur if it is not diagnosed and treated with the appropriate antibiotic therapy within 24–48 h [1, 2]. The incidence of bacterial septic arthritis has been reported to be between 4 and 29 cases per 100,000 person-years [2].

46.2.1 Etiology and Pathogenesis

Septic arthritis is most commonly the result of hematogenous spread of an infection to the joint, but may also be due to a bite or other trauma, direct inoculation of bacteria during joint surgery, or rarely following preexisting osteomyelitis through the cortex into the joint. Infective endocarditis should be considered in patients who use injection drugs or when the causative organism is *S. aureus*, enterococci, or streptococci. Although most cases are the result of hematogenous spread of bacteria to the joint, many of these patients may have only had a transient self-limited bacteremia, and as a result blood cultures may not be positive.

Bacteria have the potential to rapidly destroy intra-articular cartilage. Synovial tissue has no basement plate, and as a result bacterial organisms quickly gain access to the synovial fluid where an inflammatory process takes place releasing cytokines and proteases that cause cartilage degradation and inhibit cartilage synthesis. If a large synovial effusion is present, pressure necrosis can cause further cartilage and bone loss.

Nearly any microorganism may cause septic arthritis, but typically it is a monomicrobial infection, except in cases of penetrating trauma or hematogenous spread in patients with polymicrobial bacteremia. *S. aureus* (including methicillin-resistant *S. aureus*) is the most common organism to affect adult joints, although other Gram-positive organisms such as streptococci are also common. Gram-negative bacilli can be seen following trauma, in intravenous drug users, neonates, older adults, and immunosuppressed patients or those with urinary or skin infections. Mycobacteria, Gram-negative cocci, Gram-positive bacilli, anaerobes, fungi, and viruses represent important but less common causes.

46.2.2 Clinical Manifestations

Septic arthritis typically presents as acute-onset monoarticular arthritis with a single painful, warm, swollen joint with restricted range of motion. The majority of patients with bacterial arthritis are febrile. Typically the patient maintains the joint in such a position to maximize intra-articular space and thus minimize pain from the increased volume of purulent fluid within it. At times there may be evidence of an associated skin, urinary tract, or respiratory infection, which may help identify the source of bacteria.

The knee is involved in 50% of cases with other commonly affected joints including the wrists, ankles, and hips [3]. Less commonly, axial joints such as the sternoclavicular or sacroiliac joint may be involved, but often these patients will have a history of intravenous drug abuse [4, 5]. Although monoarthritis is most commonly seen, oligoarticular or polyarticular infection occurs in ~20% of septic joint infections, often in those with rheumatoid arthritis, those with systemic connective tissue disease, or those with severe sepsis [6].

Eighty-four percent of adults with septic arthritis have an underlying medical condition, and 59% have a previous joint disorder [7]. Risk factors for septic arthritis include age greater than 80, diabetes mellitus, rheumatoid arthritis, presence of a prosthetic joint, recent joint surgery, skin infection, intravenous drug abuse, alcoholism, and prior intra-articular corticosteroid injection. Existing joint damage is also an important risk factor. One study showed 40% of patients with bacterial arthritis have preexisting joint disease, usually rheumatoid arthritis or osteoarthritis [8]. Patients with rheumatoid arthritis are 4–15× more likely to develop bacterial arthritis [7, 9, 10] and are even more likely to do so if they have had a prior intra-articular steroid injection, or are on immunosuppressive medications or antitumor necrosis factor therapy [11–14]. Other processes affecting the joint including gout, pseudogout, and Charcot arthropathy also increase risk [15, 16]. Bacterial arthritis was found to be iatrogenic in 41.8% of cases in one study in Europe [17]. Furthermore, intra-articular steroids [18] and hyaluronate injections [19] may increase the risk of joint infection and can be the source of inoculation if the steroids are contaminated as has been reported in at least one case [20].

Gonococcal arthritis caused by the Gram-negative diplococci *Neisseria gonorrhoeae* characteristically occurs in young, healthy sexually active patients and presents clinically as a migratory pattern of arthralgias, tenosynovitis, or nonerosive arthritis rather than the monoarticular presentation typical of nongonococcal septic arthritis.

Fungal and mycobacterial joint injections typically have a more insidious onset and slowly progressive course than cases caused by more common organisms.

46.2.3 Diagnostic Methods

Initial diagnostic workup typically includes serum markers of infection and inflammation including white blood cell (WBC) count, erythrocyte sedimentation rate, and C-reactive protein levels. These may be normal in cases of septic arthritis but, when abnormal, are useful to follow for response to treatment. In addition, blood cultures should be obtained given the high coincidence of bacteremia and hematogenous spread to the joint.

Septic arthritis cannot be diagnosed with imaging studies, but they can provide additional helpful clinical information. Plain radiographs obtained at the time of presentation establish a baseline to which posttreatment films can be compared and may identify osteomyelitis or other concurrent joint pathology that is amenable to treatment. Ultrasonography can help establish the presence of an effusion, particularly in joints such as the hip, which are difficult to examine, and can be used to guide a needle during joint aspiration for synovial fluid analysis. Alternatively, fluoroscopy and CT can also be used to guide needle placement for joint aspiration but provide less useful information about the surrounding soft tissue and presence of effusion. Magnetic resonance imaging is rarely obtained specifically for suspected cases of septic arthritis, but if findings such as bone erosions with marrow edema are seen concurrently, the diagnosis should be considered.

The definitive diagnostic study for septic arthritis is synovial fluid analysis and is required to identify the causative infectious agent and rule out other causes of acute arthritis including gout and pseudogout. When performing arthrocentesis, bedside analysis of the fluid should be performed to note the volume of fluid as well as its color, viscosity, and clarity. Laboratory testing of the fluid should include WBC count with differential, crystal analysis, Gram stain, and culture.

Classification of effusions as physiologic, noninflammatory, inflammatory, hemorrhagic, or septic based on fluid analysis is helpful (Table 46.1). A small volume (<3.5 mL in the knee) of fluid may be present in normal joints and is considered physiologic. Typically this fluid is clear, acellular, and highly viscous and has a protein concentration that is one-third of that for plasma and a glucose concentration near that of plasma. Noninflammatory effusions are usually transparent, yellow in color with high viscosity, WBC counts ranging from 0 to 2000 cells/mm^3 with less than 25% polymorphonuclear leukocytes (PMLs) and often caused by degenerative joint disease or trauma. Inflammatory effusions may be present in conditions such as rheumatoid arthritis, acute crystal-induced synovitis, reactive arthritis, psoriatic arthritis, arthritis associated with inflammatory bowel disease, rheumatic fever, systemic lupus erythematosus, and sarcoidosis and are characterized by opaque, yellow to green colored low-viscosity fluid with 2000–100,000 WBCs/mm^3 and greater than 50% PMLs. Hemorrhagic effusions may be found in patients with hemophilia, those on anticoagulation or with hemorrhagic diathesis as well as following trauma, or in the presence of a tumor and are characterized by bloody-appearing fluid with 200–2000 WBCs/mm^3 with 50–75% PMLs. A white blood cell count of more than 50,000 mm^{-3} and a polymorphonuclear cell count greater than 90% are correlated with infectious arthritis, although values in these ranges may also be found in crystalline disease. Furthermore, the higher the synovial fluid WBC count, the more likely the patient is to have septic arthritis. Among patients presenting with acute mono- or oligoarthritis having WBC counts less than 25,000 mm^{-3}, the likelihood ratio of septic arthritis was 0.32 which increased to 2.9 with leukocyte counts above 25,000 mm^{-3}, to 7.7 when over 50,000 mm^{-3}, and to 28 when over 100,000 mm^{-3} [3]. Synovial white blood cell counts may be less elevated in patients with disseminated gonococcal disease, peripheral leukopenia, or joint replacement.

Septic effusions are also unique compared to other effusions by the fact that Gram stain and culture are often positive. When positive, Gram stain provides information about the presence of Gram-positive versus Gram-negative organisms that should help guide initial antibiotic treatment. Culture and sensitivity results establish the pathogenic organism and help guide subsequent treatment. Routine aerobic and anaerobic bacterial culture is typically sufficient

Table 46.1 General guidelines for the classification of synovial fluid (data should always be interpreted in light of all available clinical information)

	Volume, mL (knee)	Clarity	Color	Viscosity	WBC/mm^2	PML (%)	Culture
Normal	<3.5	Transparent	Clear	High	<200	<25	Negative
Noninflammatory	Often >3.5	Translucent-opaque	Yellow	High	0–2000	<25	Negative
Inflammatory	Often >3.5	Translucent -opaque	Yellow	Low	2000–100,000	≥50	Negative
Hemorrhagic	Usually >3.5	Bloody	Red	Variable	200–2000	50–75	Negative
Septic	Often >3.5	Opaque	Yellow to green	Variable	>50,000[a]–>100,000	≥75	Often positive

WBC white blood cells, *PML* polymorphonuclear leukocytes
[a]May be as low as 15,000 if organisms are low virulence

unless there is a clinical suspicion of gonococcal, mycobacterial, or fungal infection in which case unique cultures may be required.

Other common causes of acute mono- or oligoarthritis include crystal arthropathies such as gout and pseudogout. Clinically these can be difficult to differentiate from septic arthritis with patients presenting with chills, high fever, and leukocytosis with a painful joint. Synovial fluid crystal analysis is very helpful in differentiating between these. Monosodium urate crystals, characteristically seen in gout, are needle-shaped and negatively birefringent. Calcium pyrophosphate crystals observed in pseudogout are positively birefringent and typically rhomboid or rectangular in shape. Septic arthritis may also occur concurrently with crystal arthropathy so the presence of crystals does not necessarily exclude the diagnosis.

46.2.4 Treatment

Treatment of septic arthritis should be initiated with empiric antibiotics as soon as initial blood and synovial fluid cultures have been drawn and should be based on the findings of the Gram stain (Table 46.2). Initial treatment generally begins with vancomycin for Gram-positive cocci. If Gram-negative cocci are found, treatment is typically begun with ceftriaxone. When Gram-negative rods are present, ceftazidime, cefepime, piperacillin/tazobactam, or carbapenems are considered as first-line treatment unless the patient has a penicillin or cephalosporin allergy in which case aztreonam or fluoroquinolones can be considered as alternatives. If the Gram stain is negative but suspicion of septic arthritis remains high, a regimen of both vancomycin and either ceftazidime or an aminoglycoside should be given [21]. If clinical suspicion for another organism not covered by this regimen is high such as *Pseudomonas aeruginosa* among injection drug users or *N. gonorrhoeae* in those at risk for sexually transmitted causes, additional therapy should be added accordingly. Once culture and susceptibility results become available, the antibiotic coverage should be narrowed appropriately.

Table 46.2 Initial antibiotic therapies based on Gram stain results

Stain result	Initial antimicrobial agent
Gram-positive cocci	Vancomycin
Gram-negative cocci	Ceftriaxone
Gram-negative rods	Ceftazidime, cefepime, piperacillin/tazobactam, or carbapenems. If penicillin or cephalosporin allergic: aztreonam or fluoroquinolones
Negative Gram stain	Vancomycin + ceftazidime or an aminoglycoside

The duration of therapy is variable and depends on the organism, severity of infection, and physician preference as there is limited data to inform this decision. Generally, gonococcal arthritis is treated for 7–14 days, and nongonococcal bacterial arthritis requires 2–4 weeks of parenteral antibiotics. Many physicians give an initial course of parenteral antibiotics followed by additional oral therapy. One study from the United Kingdom defined an adequate duration of intravenous treatment as at least 7 days in adults and an adequate oral duration as 14 days [22]. Retrospective review demonstrated a mean duration of therapy of 10.2 days with IV therapy and 55.3 days with oral therapy [22]. Others have recommended a minimum duration of treatment of 3 weeks for injections due to staphylococci and Gram-negative bacilli and at least 10–14 days for streptococci, meningococci, and *Haemophilus* but emphasize that these are minimums, and actual duration must be adjusted based on clinical response to therapy [23].

In addition to antibiotic treatment, drainage of the septic joint is typically performed. This may be done using arthrocentesis or surgery. If arthrocentesis is used, daily joint aspiration, particularly for the first 5 days of treatment, may be required. Synovial fluid should be analyzed to confirm an appropriate response to the selected treatment. Arthroscopic or open surgical techniques may also be utilized to rapidly drain the joint and debride any necrotic tissue that is present.

Prosthetic joint injections may lead to failure of the replacement and require special attention to diagnosis, selection of antibiotics, duration of therapy, and method of drainage that are beyond the scope of this discussion.

46.2.5 Complications

Death and prolonged disability are both possible outcomes from septic arthritis if it is not treated appropriately. Mortality among patients with bacterial arthritis can be as high as 10–20%, particularly in older patients with coexisting renal or cardiac disease or those who are immunosuppressed [4, 8, 22]. Patients older than 65 with an infection in the shoulder, elbow, or at multiple sites are the most likely to die [8]. The morbidity associated with septic arthritis even after appropriate antibiotic therapy can still be severe and depends to a certain extent on the responsible organism. Patients with *S. aureus* septic arthritis have been reported to regain 46–50% of their baseline joint function [22], whereas adults who survive the 20% mortality associated with pneumococcal septic arthritis return to 95% of their baseline joint function [24]. In addition, amputation, arthrodesis, prosthetic surgery, or severe functional deterioration occurs in one-third of patients with bacterial arthritis with older patients with preexisting joint disease and those with synthetic intra-articular material being affected most often [8].

Key Concepts

- Septic arthritis is an orthopedic emergency that requires rapid identification, diagnosis, and treatment to avoid cartilage destruction and long-term morbidity.
- Hematogenous spread is the most common mechanism by which the joint becomes infected and *S. aureus* is the most common organism.
- The knee is the most commonly affected joint.
- Synovial fluid analysis, Gram stain, and culture is the definitive diagnostic test and shows opaque, yellow-green, low-viscosity fluid (bacterial) with >50,000 WBC/mm^3, >75% polymorphonuclear leukocytes, and positive cultures.
- Prompt empiric antibiotic treatment based on Gram stain results immediately following collection of blood and synovial fluid for culture is the first step in treatment followed by joint drainage and eventual narrowing of antibiotic coverage according to culture and sensitivity results.

References

1. Goldenberg DL. Septic arthritis. Lancet. 1998;351(9097):197–202.
2. Mathews CJ, Weston VC, Jones A, Field M, Coakley G. Bacterial septic arthritis in adults. Lancet. 2010;375(9717):846–55.
3. Margaretten ME, Kohlwes J, Moore D, Bent S. Does this adult patient have septic arthritis? JAMA. 2007;297(13):1478–88.
4. Ross JJ, Shamsuddin H. Sternoclavicular septic arthritis: review of 180 cases. Medicine. 2004;83(3):139–48.
5. Goldenberg D. Bacterial arthritis. In: Ruddy S, Harris ED, Sledge CB, Kelley WN, editors. Kelly's textbook of rheumatology. 6th ed. Philadelphia, PA: Saunders; 2001. p. 1469–83.
6. Dubost JJ, Fis I, Denis P, Lopitaux R, Soubrier M, Ristori JM, et al. Polyarticular septic arthritis. Medicine (Baltimore). 1993;72(5):296–310.
7. Kaandorp CJ, Dinant HJ, van de Laar MA, Moens HJB, Prins APA, Dijkmans BA. Incidence and sources of native and prosthetic joint infection: a community based prospective survey. Ann Rheum Dis. 1997;56(8):470–5.
8. Kaandorp CJ, Krijnen P, Moens HJB, Habbema JDF, van Schaardenburg D. The outcome of bacterial arthritis. A prospective community-based study. Arthritis Rheum. 1997;40(5):884–92.
9. Doran MF, Crowson CS, Pond GR, O'Fallon WM, Gabriel SE. Frequency of infection in patients with rheumatoid arthritis compared with controls: a population-based study. Arthritis Rheum. 2002;46(9):2287–93.
10. Edwards CJ, Cooper C, Fisher D, Field M, van Staa TP, Arden NK. The importance of the disease process and disease-modifying antirheumatic drug treatment in the development of septic arthritis in patients with rheumatoid arthritis. Arthritis Rheum. 2007;57(7):1151–7.
11. Katsarolis I, Tsiodras S, Panagopoulos P, Giannitsioti E, Skarantavos G, Ioannidis T, et al. Septic arthritis due to *Salmonella enteritidis* associated with infliximab use. Scand J Infect Dis. 2005;37(4):304–5.
12. Mor A, Mitnick HJ, Greene JB, Azar N, Budnah R, Fetto J. Relapsing oligoarticular septic arthritis during etanercept treatment of rheumatoid arthritis. J Clin Rheumatol. 2006;12(2):87–9.
13. Nadarajah K, Pritchard C. *Listeria monocytogenes* septic arthritis in a patient treated with etanercept for rheumatoid arthritis. J Clin Rheumatol. 2005;11(2):120–2.
14. Schett G, Herak P, Graninger W, Smolen JS, Aringer M. Listeria-associated arthritis in a patient undergoing etanercept therapy: case report and review of the literature. J Clin Microbiol. 2005;43(5):2537–41.
15. Goldenberg DL, Reed JI. Bacterial arthritis. N Engl J Med. 1985;312(12):764–71.
16. Goldenberg DL. Septic arthritis and other infections of rheumatologic significance. Rheum Dis Clin N Am. 1991;17(1):149–56.
17. Geirsson ÁJ, Statkevicius S, Víkingsson A. Septic arthritis in Iceland 1990–2002: increasing incidence due to iatrogenic infections. Ann Rheum Dis. 2008;67(5):638–43.
18. Ostensson A, Geborek P. Septic arthritis as a non-surgical complication in rheumatoid arthritis: relation to disease severity and therapy. Br J Rheumatol. 1991;30(1):35–8.
19. Albert C, Brocq O, Gerard D, Roux C, Euller-Ziegler L. Septic knee arthritis after intra-articular hyaluronate injection: two case reports. Joint Bone Spine. 2006;73(2):205–7.
20. Kainer MA, Reagan DR, Nguyen DB, Wiese AD, Wise ME, Ward J, et al. Fungal infections associated with contaminated methylprednisolone in Tennessee. N Engl J Med. 2012;367(23):2194–203.
21. Ohl C. Infectious arthritis of native joints. In: Mandell GL, Bennett JE, Dolin R, editors. Principles and practice of infectious diseases. 6th ed. Philadelphia, PA: Elsevier; 2010. p. 1443–56.
22. Weston V, Jones A, Bradbury N, Fawthrop F, Doherty M. Clinical features and outcome of septic arthritis in a single UK Health District 1982–1991. Ann Rheum Dis. 1999;58(4):214–9.
23. Syrogiannopoulos GA, Nelson JD. Duration of antimicrobial therapy for acute suppurative osteoarticular infections. Lancet (London, England). 1988;1(8575-6):37–40.
24. Ross JJ, Saltzman CL, Carling P, Shapiro DS. Pneumococcal septic arthritis: review of 190 cases. Clin Infect Dis. 2003;36(3):319–27.

47 Bupivacaine-Induced Myonecrosis

David Gordon and Magdalena Anitescu

47.1 Case Description

A 27-year-old female is admitted to the hospital with a severe headache. She describes the pain as a generalized throbbing, with localized right supraorbital pain that has lasted for 1 week. Her medical history is significant for migraine headaches and Chiari malformation, treated with decompression surgery. She has been evaluated in the pain clinic for ongoing occipital neuralgia from a long-standing ventriculoperitoneal (VP) shunt. Neuralgia has been controlled with oral pain medications and has never required hospitalization. When asked about this current episode, she describes it as a sharp, burning, cramping, pain over the right supraorbital notch, superimposed over the occipital neuralgia. Topiramate and sumatriptan were ineffective in controlling the pain, which she rates as severe. Because of concerns of shunt malfunction, butalbital-acetaminophen-caffeine is prescribed which provides partial relief of the generalized headache but has no effect on the frontal region. The relief lasts for 12 h. The patient's throbbing, generalized headache intensifies with standing. CT and MRI studies confirm severe intracranial hypotension from excessive shunt drainage; the positional headache improves with adjustments of the shunt setting. Right frontal burning continues and a stabbing pain is consistent with supraorbital neuralgia.

With ultrasound guidance and anatomical landmarks, a right supraorbital nerve block is performed using 3 mL of 0.25% bupivacaine combined with 10 mg of triamcinolone over the right supraorbital notch. Pain is relieved completely 20 min after the procedure. At subsequent appointments, the patient reports excellent pain relief lasting approximately 10 weeks after which the pain returns with similar intensity and distribution. Since the patient's occipital pain is manageable with a muscle relaxant, a repeat supraorbital nerve block is performed using the same technique and medications. The second block lasts only 8 weeks and pain is again severe. The patient is persistent in requesting a third supraorbital nerve block. Upon a detailed discussion of the risks and benefits of repeating this procedure including the general effects of glucocorticosteroids in systemic uptake, possible nerve damage, and infection, a third procedure is performed using 3 mL of 0.25% bupivacaine alone. Full pain relief lasts for approximately 6 weeks, after which the patient again insists on another block. She refuses other medications because of concern about sedation, nausea, and dizziness from opiates and membrane stabilizers in the past. She says that after the third nerve block without the steroid, the pain relief did not last long and she requests a repeat block with steroid. After a second thorough discussion of the side effects of steroids, with emphasis on adrenal suppression, demineralization, water retention, and hypertension, the patient agrees to have the fourth block with local anesthetic only. Upon return in 4 weeks for a fifth supraorbital nerve block, the patient reports that her pain is still relatively well controlled. Examination of the forehead shows a small indentation over the supraorbital notch. It developed 1 week after the most recent injection and seems to be slowly enlarging over time. It is not painful to touch but it becomes tender with deeper palpation over the site of the previous injection. There is no associated paresthesia. The area measures roughly 3 cm × 3 cm with uneven borders; the depression is 4–5 mm. The patient is referred to a dermatologist who confirms an area of decreased muscle mass likely associated with repeat use of bupivacaine. Since the condition is usually self-limiting and likely reversible, observation with close follow-up is recommended.

Approximately 6 weeks later, the patient returns, devastated, complaining of severe supraorbital pain, and afraid of

D. Gordon, M.D.
Section of pain management, Department of Anesthesia, University of California at San Francisco, San Francisco, CA, USA
e-mail: Dmgordon.dg@gmail.com

M. Anitescu, M.D., Ph.D. (✉)
Department of Anesthesia and Critical Care, University of Chicago Medical Center, Chicago, IL, USA
e-mail: MAnitescu@dacc.uchicago.edu

M. Anitescu et al. (eds.), *Challenging Cases and Complication Management in Pain Medicine*,
https://doi.org/10.1007/978-3-319-60072-7_47

the new deformity. Her friends notice it and she feels self-conscious. A plastic surgeon confirms that the area represents myonecrosis. The plan is to watch the area for regeneration which may be a lengthy process. The patient does not agree to watchful waiting. The surgeon fills in the defect with a fat transfer and the patient is pleased with the results. Her pain, however, persists. Since no additional blocks are to be performed and the patient is not interested in neuromodulation, a ketamine infusion provides 50% pain relief for supraorbital neuralgia. Her pain is reasonably well controlled with a multimodal analgesic regimen and ketamine infusions.

47.2 Case Discussion

47.2.1 Common and Uncommon Side Effects of Local Anesthesia

There are several commonly known, well documented, and thoroughly studied adverse events of local anesthetics. The signs of central nervous system toxicity are perioral numbness and tingling, tinnitus, and progression through the "sense of impending doom" culminating in seizure. By now, every medical provider administering local anesthetics should reflexively answer "intralipid" to the question of how to treat the cardiac collapse brought on by inadvertent intravascular injection of bupivacaine. Other less common effects, however, may remain underdiagnosed and underappreciated in clinical practice.

47.2.2 Myotoxicity

Local anesthetic myotoxicity has been recognized as a clinical entity since 1959 [1]. The effects have been reproduced in rats, rabbits, pigs, and humans in multiple clinical and experimental studies [1–5]. In fact, bupivacaine has been used in laboratory studies as a reliable method to produce myotoxicity to study this phenomenon. In humans, the problem is thoroughly described in ophthalmological surgery where atrophic effects were noted in the extraocular muscles after retrobulbar or peribulbar block [6].

All local anesthetics produce some degree of myotoxicity, bupivacaine causing the worst effects, and procaine the least [7]. Recent case reports have revisited the effects of local anesthetics on striated muscle fibers. Emerging evidence suggests that local anesthetic myotoxicity, once thought to be limited to the realm of laboratory rats whose muscle fibers were bathed in high concentrations of local anesthetic drugs, is likely not a rare event. In regional anesthesia and analgesia, even with the decreasing volumes afforded by the transition from "volume blocks" guided by paresthesia to "targeted blocks" using ultrasound, muscle weakness continues to be reported after surgical procedures. Even after a single-shot block, weakness may not be attributed entirely to the surgical intervention.

A recent review article of complications of peripheral nerve blocks did not report myotoxicity, although the researchers acknowledged its existence [8]. Despite reproducible and profound myotoxic effects in laboratory studies, only a few case reports detailing complications in humans exist in the literature [9]. Most are related to diplopia and other complications from ophthalmologic administration during cataract removal or other eye surgeries. Others discuss the effects after trigger point injections, wound infiltration, or with peripheral nerve catheters for prolonged local administration [10].

47.2.2.1 Diagnosis

The initial sensation of myotoxicity may be pain and tenderness around the site of the injection [11]. Pain in the muscle may be elicited by palpation and active and passive range of motion indicating muscle irritation. The time course after injection offers clues to the cause of the pain. Inflammation begins in the first day and peaks 3–4 days after the injection when the inflammatory response is maximal [11]. Swelling and edema may be seen on MRI during this time. After 4 weeks, myopathy may be revealed by EMG abnormalities including small, brief polyphasic motor action potential [11]. Although rarely indicated, a muscle biopsy would provide a definitive diagnosis with the histological changes discussed below [11]. After retrobulbar blocks, symptoms of extraocular muscle dysfunction including diplopia after retrobulbar or peribulbar injections may suggest various degrees of local anesthetic myotoxicity.

47.2.2.2 Differential Diagnosis

The differential diagnosis for the acute inflammation with local anesthetic myotoxicity includes infection and hematoma. The possible cause of myotoxicity depends upon the agents that were administered. Local anesthetics, especially bupivacaine cause myotoxicity. However, triamcinolone could also contribute toxicity. In a systematic review that examined myotoxicity of steroid injections for acute muscle injury, a single study met the eligibility criteria [12]. In a study in rats, no histological changes were found after intramuscular corticosteroid injection. Injection of triamcinolone and bupivacaine combinations resulted in greater damage to muscle tissue compared to bupivacaine alone [13]. In our patient, the injection of a low dose of triamcinolone more than 3 months before myotoxicity suggests that her myotoxicity was associated with the local anesthetic and not the steroid.

47.2.2.3 Pathogenesis

There is a predictable pattern to the histological effects and time course of myonecrosis from administration of local anesthetics. Initially, the myofibrils hypercontract, before myocyte edema and calcified necrosis. Eventually the tissues undergo signs of regeneration. The basal lamina and connective tissue elements typically remain intact, which facilitates regeneration via myoblasts after about 4 weeks [7].

Myotoxicity results from the disruption of mitochondria in muscle cells. Multiple mechanisms have been suggested for myonecrosis: uncoupling of oxidative phosphorylation, inhibition of ATP synthase, reduction of respiratory chain protein content, and mediation through reactive oxygen species [14, 15]. The sarcoplasmic reticulum (SR) is also thought to play a role, given its association with regulation of calcium homeostasis [14]. Local anesthetics act not only on sodium channels but also on the sarcoplasmic reticulum where action at the calcium release channel ryanodine receptors (RyR) results in an excess of calcium by inhibitory reuptake. This effect on the RyR receptor and resulting hypercontractility stirred a theoretical debate about a linkage to malignant hyperthermia (MH), but it has long been established that local anesthetics are safe for patients susceptible to MH. It is also thought that production of reactive oxygen species may lead to depletion of calcium in the SR. Other studies have shown that high concentration of local anesthetics increases cytosolic calcium attributed to cell death [15].

In laboratory animals, myotoxicity results from doses in excess of those used in clinical practice in humans. In rabbit extraocular muscles, the effect of concentration correlated with the degree of myotoxicity [16] (Fig. 47.1).

When the histological changes 5 days after injection of either saline or bupivacaine were compared, normal appearing muscle fibers were seen with saline and 0.19% bupivacaine. Injection of 0.38% bupivacaine showed degenerative changes at 5 days. The most pronounced effects were at

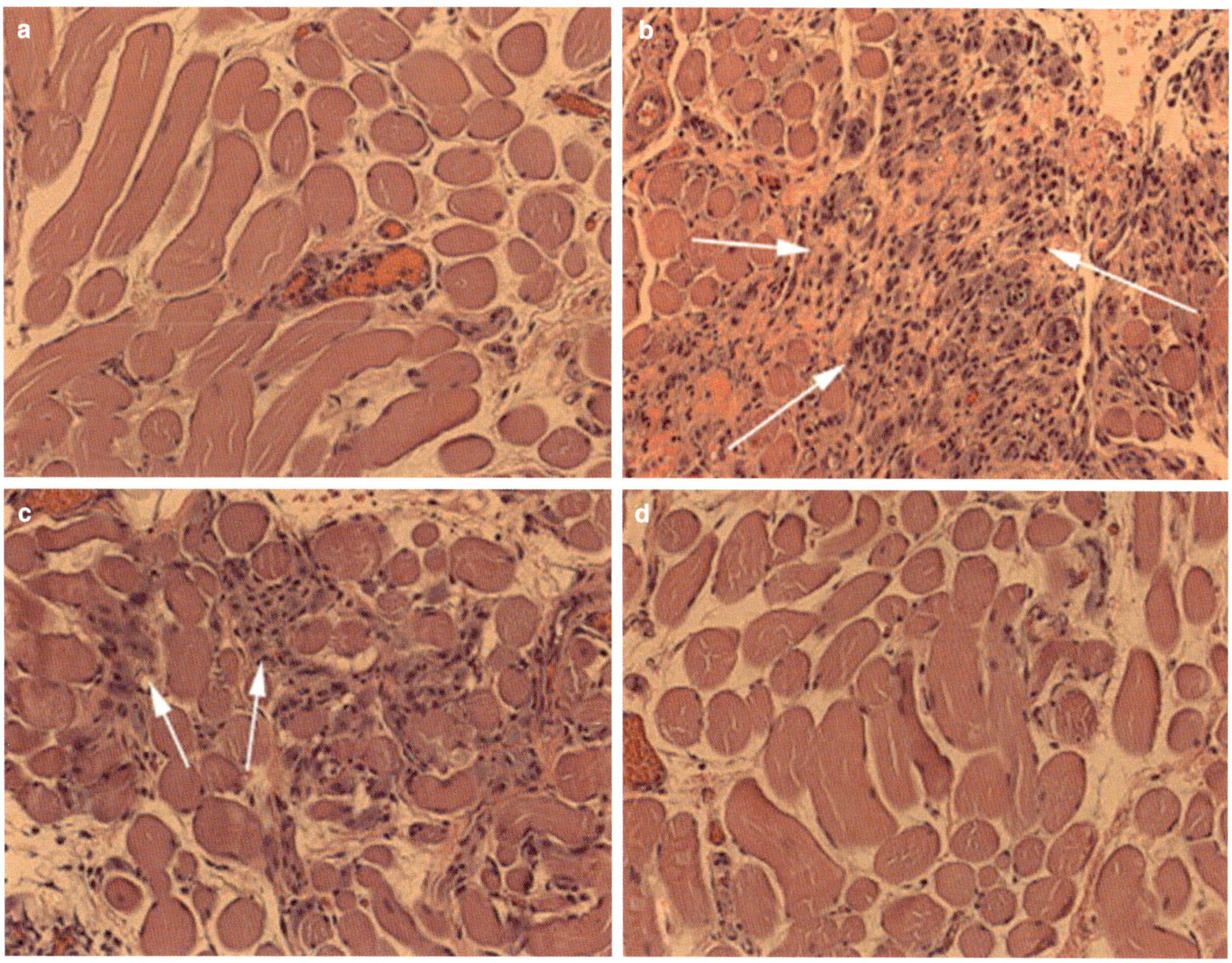

Fig. 47.1 Concentration-dependent bupivacaine myotoxicity. Rabbit extraocular muscles at 5 days after injection of bupivacaine or saline. (**a**) Saline injection: normal-appearing muscle fiber cells displayed regular arrangement with the nuclei in the periphery of the fiber cells. (**b**) Bupivacaine 0.75% injection: large areas of degenerated muscle tissue with regenerating muscle fibers and inflammatory cell infiltrate and fibrous tissue formation between these cells (*between arrows*). (**c**) Bupivacaine 0.38% injection: scattered degenerated areas showed regenerating muscle fibers (*arrows*). (**d**) Bupivacaine 0.19% injection: normal-appearing muscle fibers were seen. Reproduced with permission from Elsvier [16]

bupivacaine concentrations of 0.75% with large areas of degenerated muscle tissue, inflammation, and fibrous tissue.

The severity of myotoxicity from bupivacaine and ropivacaine was demonstrated in a study in pigs. In the study, 0.5% bupivacaine or 0.75% ropivacaine was injected through a catheter inserted next to the femoral nerve. Then an infusion of 0.25% bupivacaine or 0.375% ropivacaine was administered at 8 mL/h for 6 h. At 7 and 28 days, the biopsied muscle samples showed varying stages of necrosis and regeneration with calcium deposits and necrotic clusters of myocytes and signs of fiber regeneration with proliferation of myoblasts with myotubes. The greatest damage was along the surface of the muscle fascicles, presumably along the path of local anesthetic spread. Scars were formed and in each case, the degree of damage was greater with bupivacaine [10]. In another study in humans findings were similar. Muscle damage was confirmed in lesions obtained after radical neck dissection where 1.8 mL of 2% lidocaine with 1:100,000 epinephrine was injected before surgery [3].

The mechanism of myotoxicity, thought to be related to the concentration of local anesthetic, is time dependent, enhanced by preexisting altered metabolism, and is often associated with young age [14]. Thus, it is expected that effects are more pronounced with peripheral nerve catheters with prolonged duration at high concentrations. It has been proposed that continued release or "depo" preparations increase myonecrosis. More evidence is needed before the effects of time and concentration in humans are known. Consistent with its use in trigger point injections, the effects of local anesthetics combined with glucocorticoids are known to increase muscle breakdown. The co-administration of epinephrine is believed to increase the incidence of myotoxicity.

For several decades, the theoretical risk of needle and catheter-induced mechanical trauma in patients with preexisting neural compromise made regional techniques a rarity in various surgical procedures. There may be a component of a double-insult phenomenon with local anesthetic myotoxicity as well. Certainly, patients with rare mitochondrial disorders may suffer more from local anesthetics than other patients. Patients who have a defect in the basal lamina, connective tissue, muscle-related neuronal structure, myotubules, and similar structures of regeneration may experience a greater degree and possibly permanent effects from administration of local anesthetics.

47.2.2.4 Prevention

To decrease the risk and magnitude of myotoxicity, the "As Low As Reasonably Achievable" or ALARA principle should be adopted from our experience with radiation exposure. Given the strong correlation between concentration and time of exposure, the lowest effective concentration should be used, and the duration of administration should be limited to the shortest time possible. The widespread problems of chronic opioid use should not be unfamiliar to anyone in the practice of medicine today. Respiratory depression and the risk of dependence will likely outweigh the risk of local anesthetic-induced myotoxicity. For certain patients, the scales may tip in the other direction. Knowing even the rarest of side effects helps to set one apart as a true consultant and practitioner of the art of medicine.

Table 47.1 Factors that decrease risk of myotoxicity

Tetracaine, procaine < lidocaine, ropivacaine, prilocaine < bupivacaine [13]
Lowest effective concentration
Inject outside the muscle
Avoid serial injections
Avoid injection of epinephrine and steroid
Coadminister dexmedetomidine

There are several possible strategies that may reduce or even prevent local anesthetic-induced myotoxicity. When co-administered, dexmedetomidine has been shown to decrease the degree of bupivacaine-induced neurotoxicity and extend the duration of the block. Given the degree of involvement of Ca^{2+} discussed above, it should be no surprise that Ca^{2+} channel antagonists are preventative in in vitro studies. Antioxidants decrease the presence of reactive oxygen species, and recombinant human erythropoietin is thought to mitigate mitochondrial damage. In preclinical studies, both those agents had a protective effect when co-administered with bupivacaine [14].

Ropivacaine and levobupivacaine have fewer cardiotoxic effects and are less myotoxic than bupivacaine. Both agents have an onset and duration of action similar to that of bupivacaine. Bupivacaine is off-patent unlike the others, which decreases cost. It is difficult to demonstrate an overall cost savings using expensive medications when the incidence of myotoxicity is low or under-acknowledged and underreported.

Care should be taken to evaluate the potential effects of long-term or repeated administration of local anesthetics, especially at higher concentrations. Further studies are needed, but ultrasound may allow a decrease in the volume of local anesthetic to achieve effective neural blockade. Patients with certain mitochondrial disorders, although rare indeed, may suffer a large "first hit" and there may be many other phenotypes which predispose patients to local anesthetic-induced myonecrosis. The preventative measures that can be taken to reduce the risk of myonecrosis are summarized in Table 47.1.

47.2.2.5 Treatment

Treatment of myotoxicity is rarely necessary and muscles usually regenerate with time. During myonecrosis additional muscle injury may be prevented by discontinuing repeat injections, and using nonsteroidal anti-inflammatory drugs, or a course of systemic steroids [11]. Depending on the muscles affected, rehabilitation therapy may be necessary.

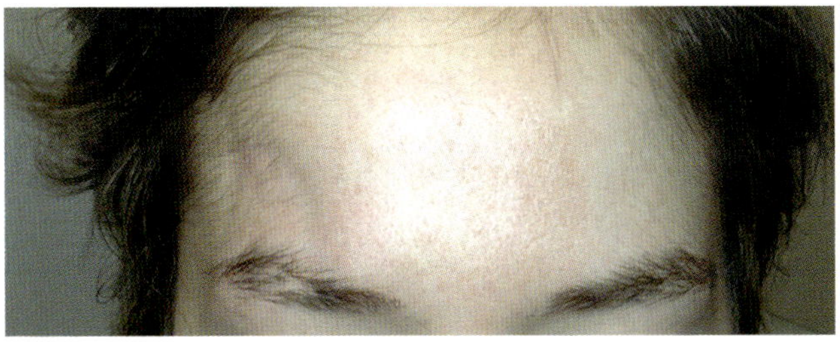

Fig. 47.2 Patient with signs of myonecrosis in response to bupivacaine injection. Image from personal library

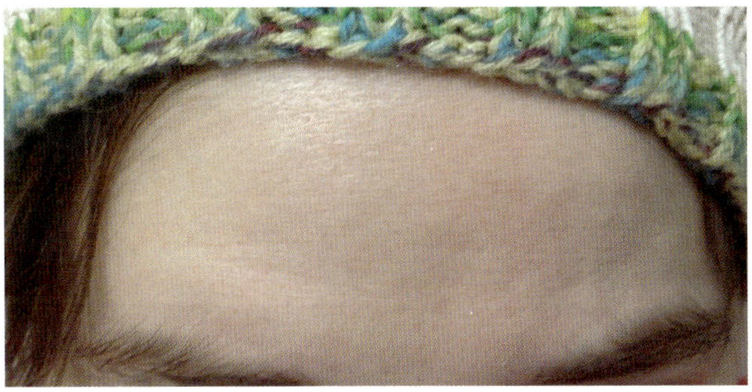

Fig. 47.3 Same patient status post fat transfer, 2 years after the myonecrosis episode. Image from personal library

Conclusion

Although muscles generally regenerate, repeated injections of myotoxic medications may put patients at risk for irreversible myonecrosis, especially when muscles are thin, small, or part of a limited structural network (Figs. 47.2 and 47.3).

Some defect in the neuronal architecture or structural framework may prevent muscle regeneration. Chronic, neuropathic pain predisposes patients to untoward effects after repeated nerve blocks. Each clinical situation must be evaluated to provide an informed consent. The possible consequences of myotoxic medications must be appreciated to prevent them and to produce favorable outcomes.

Key Concepts

- All local anesthetics have some degree of myotoxicity, with bupivacaine causing the worst effects.
- Myotoxicity results from the disruption of mitochondria in muscle cells.
- The mechanism of myotoxicity, thought to be related to the concentration of local anesthetic, is time dependent, enhanced by preexisting altered metabolism, and is often associated with young age.
- The effects of local anesthetics combined with glucocorticoids are known to increase muscle breakdown.
- Although muscles generally regenerate, repeated injections of myotoxic medications may put patients at risk for an irreversible myonecrosis.

References

1. Brun A. Effect of procaine, carbocaine and xylocaine on cutaneous muscle in rabbits and mice. Acta Anaesthesiol Scand. 1959;3:59–73.
2. Zink W, Seif C, Bohl JR, et al. The acute myotoxic effects of bupivacaine and ropivacaine after continuous peripheral nerve blockades. Anesth Analg. 2003;97:1173–9.
3. Yagiela JA, Benoit PW, Buoncristiani R, et al. Comparison of myotoxic effects of lidocaine with epinephrine in rats and humans. Anesth Analg. 1981;60:471–80.
4. Carlson BM, Shepard B, Komorowski TE. A histological study of local anesthetic-induced muscle degeneration and regeneration in the monkey. J Orthop Res. 1990;8:485–94.
5. Karpie JE, Chu CR. Lidocaine exhibits dose and time dependent cytotoxic effects on bovine articular chondrocytes in vitro. Am J Sports Med. 2007;25:1621–7.
6. Guyton DL. Strabismus complications from local anesthetics. Semin Opthalmol. 2008;23(5):298–301.
7. Zink W, Graf BM. Local anesthetic myotoxicity. Reg Anesth Pain Med. 2004;29(4):333–40.
8. Berg AP, Rosenquist RW. Complications of peripheral nerve blocks. Tech Reg Anesth Pain Manag. 2007;11(3):133–40.
9. Hogan Q, Dotson R, Erickson S, et al. Local anesthetic myotoxicity: a case and review. Anesthesiology. 1994;80:942–7.
10. Zink W, Bohl J, Hacke N, et al. The long term myotoxic effects of bupivacaine and ropivacaine after continuous peripheral nerve blocks. Anesth Analg. 2005;101(2):548–54.
11. Neal JM, Rathmell JP. Complications in regional anesthesia and pain medicine. Philadelphia: Lippincott Williams & Wilkins; 2013. p. 170–3.
12. Reurink G, Goudswaard GJ, Maen MH, et al. Myotoxicity of injections for acute muscle injuries: a systematic review. Sports Med. 2014;44(7):943–56.
13. Guttu RL, Page DG, Laskin DM. Delayed healing of muscle after injection of bupivacaine and steroid. Ann Dent. 1990;49:5–8.
14. Nouette-Gauhlain K, Jose C, Capdevila X, et al. From analgesia to myopathy: when local anesthetics impair the mitochondrion. Int J Biochem Cell Biol. 2011;43(1):14–9.
15. Nouette-Gauhlain K, Capdevila X, Rossignol R. Local anesthetic 'in-situ' toxicity during peripheral nerve blocks: update on mechanisms and prevention. Curr Opin Anesthesiol. 2012;25(5):589–95.
16. Zhang C, Phamanvaechavan P, Rajan R, et al. Concentration-dependent bupivacaine myotoxicity in rabbit extraocular muscle. J AAPOS. 2010;14(4):323–7.

Migration of a Supraclavicular Catheter for Complex Regional Pain Syndrome

48

Tariq Malik

48.1 Case Description

A 40-year-old male was injured at work when a heavy object fell on his left hand. He required immediate surgery. After surgery, his forearm was placed in a cast for a few weeks. When the cast was removed, he had symptoms that suggested complex regional pain syndrome. He participated in physical therapy, but when he failed to make progress, he was referred to the pain clinic for pain management. His main complaints were intense pain, swelling of the hand, intense sensitivity, and decreased range of motion. He was treated with sympathetic chain blocks. After series of three stellate ganglion blocks, there was no improvement. As there was no progress in pain relief, a supraclavicular tunneled catheter was placed under ultrasound guidance. The plan was to leave the catheter in for 2 weeks to facilitate physical therapy. In the first week, he made progress in physical therapy sessions. Ten days after the placement of the tunneled supraclavicular catheter, the patient presented to the ER with a new onset of shortness of breath and chest discomfort with sharp shooting pain every time he tried to take a deep breath. After ruling out cardiac dysfunction, the ER team concerned of pleuritic pain ordered a plain chest radiograph. When the film revealed no evidence of pneumothorax but the wire-reinforced catheter close to the apex of the left lung, a CT of the chest was ordered to evaluate the position of the catheter more accurately. The newly performed scan showed the tip of the catheter was still close to the parietal pleura. The on-call pain team was unable to remove the catheter. Since the catheter was stuck and in what appears to be in close contact to the pleura, a thoracic surgery consult was called, and the patient was scheduled for thoracotomy the next day as an add-on for removal of the catheter under direct vision (Fig. 48.1).

However, during the morning hours, another attempt was made to remove the catheter under fluoroscopic guidance. In the pain clinic, the catheter was clearly visible under fluoroscopic guidance. The area around the catheter was cleaned with an alcohol-based chlorhexidine solution and draped. Lidocaine 1% was injected to numb the area around the catheter. The injection was done under fluoroscopy guidance to ensure that the needle did not contact the catheter to avoid catheter shearing or breakage. A 16 g angiocath cannula was threaded over the catheter, under fluoroscopy guidance, up to the hub, in order to mobilize the tissue around it, ensuring again that catheter did not break under the skin. Under fluoroscopic guidance, we verified that that catheter did not kink or that a piece of it did not break off during tugging or mobilization maneuvers (Figs. 48.2 and 48.3).

After repeated gentle tugging, the catheter was withdrawn with the tip intact. The thoracotomy was canceled, and the patient was discharged home from the pain clinic (Figs. 48.4 and 48.5).

T. Malik, M.D.
University of Chicago Hospitals,
5841 S. Maryland Avenue, Chicago, IL 60637, USA
e-mail: tmalik@dacc.uchicago.edu

M. Anitescu et al. (eds.), *Challenging Cases and Complication Management in Pain Medicine*,
https://doi.org/10.1007/978-3-319-60072-7_48

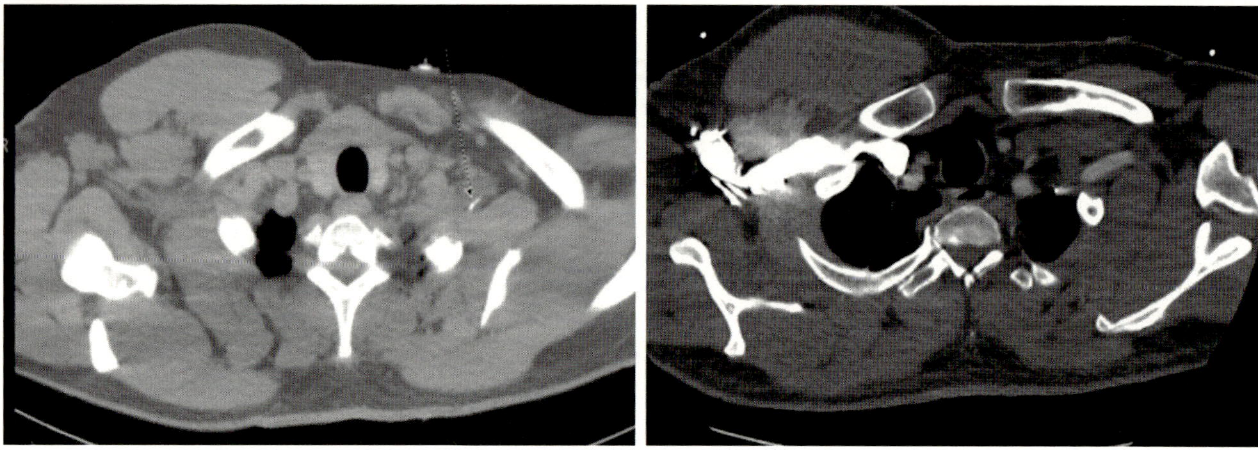

Fig. 48.1 CT scan of the chest; *arrow* points out the catheter in first image; second image shows bright-smeared impression of the catheter abutting the parietal pleura; patient with pleuritic pain from irritation of pleura by the migrated catheter. The *arrows* point toward the catheter and its proximity to the pleura. Image from personal library

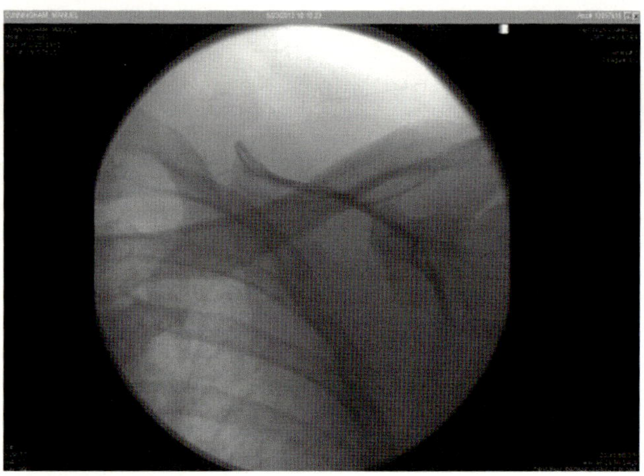

Fig. 48.2 Catheter as seen under fluoroscopy when removing efforts started. Image from personal library

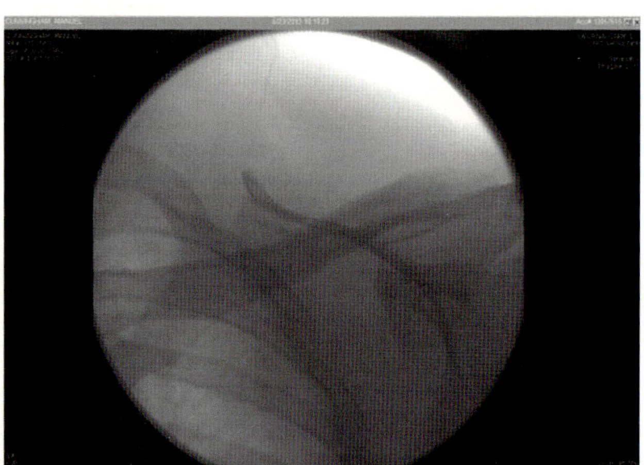

Fig. 48.3 Fluoroscopic image after catheter has been removed. There is no piece left behind in the patient's body; all pieces were removed. Image from personal library

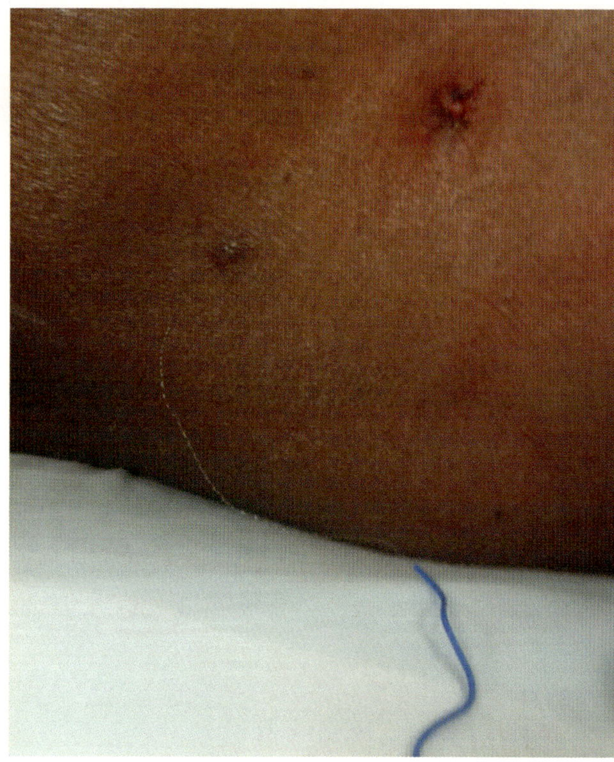

Fig. 48.4 Sheered catheter from attempt to remove it in the ER. Image from personal library

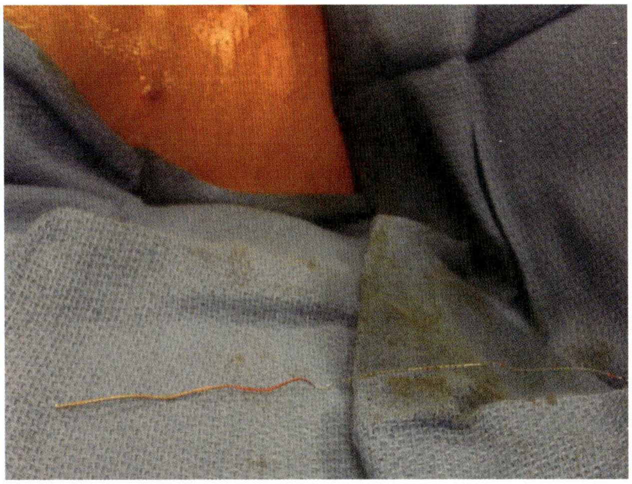

Fig. 48.5 Catheter removed from patient body with tip intact after procedure performed under direct fluoroscopy. Image from personal library

48.2 Case Discussion

Complex regional pain syndrome (CRPS) is a chronic painful condition. Its prevalence is reportedly around <2% in most retrospective series [1]. A study from the Netherlands reported an incidence of 26.2 cases per 100,000 person-years; a study from the United States estimated the incidence at 5.5 cases per 100,000 person-years [2, 3].

CRPS is a complicated condition to manage. No abnormal diagnostic test proves or disproves the diagnosis. Currently the diagnosis is made from the Budapest criteria, which rely on the presence of symptoms and signs in four different categories [4] (Table 48.1).

In the absence of any other explanation and the presence of any symptoms in three out of four categories and any sign in two of the four other categories, the diagnosis is made [4] (Table 48.2).

These criteria have a sensitivity of 85% and a specificity of 69%. Once a diagnosis is established, the mainstay is physical and desensitization therapy to slowly and steadily restore function. In the acute phase, the condition is treated with steroids for anti-inflammatory effect, tricyclic antidepressants for sleep restoration and central anti-analgesic effect, and cation channel blockers for analgesic effect. These medications, however, are not effective in many patients. CRPS is considered a sympathetically mediated condition, but not all patients respond to sympathetic blocks. Since some patients do, a series of blocks is warranted as long as a patient responds sufficiently to make progress in physical therapy. If there is no response to medication or to sympathetic block, a continuous plexus block helps with pain control and physical therapy. The catheter can be placed using ultrasound guidance or nerve stimulation. It is left in place for 1–2 weeks. To secure the catheter and to guard against infection, the catheter is tunneled under the skin and secured with a chlorhexidine patch and transparent sterile dressing. The patient is sent home with a solution strong enough for pain relief while preserving motor function, usually a bupivacaine solution 0.0625–0.125% at 5–8 mL/h. The physical therapist must be mindful of the effect of the solution on sensory perception to prevent injury. The focus is preservation of range of motion and desensitization. Even though successful in providing analgesia, the long-term benefits of a continuous plexus are unknown. Once the catheter is removed, many patients cannot make progress with therapy (Fig. 48.6).

The common drawbacks with this method for pain control are insufficient analgesia, slipping out of the catheter, and

Table 48.1 Clinical diagnostic criteria for complex regional pain syndrome—Budapest criteria

1. Continuing pain disproportionate to the inciting event
2. At least one symptom in one of three of the four following categories Sensory Motor/trophic Sudomotor/edema Vasomotor
3. At least one sign at the time of evaluation in two or more of the following categories Sensory Motor/trophic Sudomotor/edema Vasomotor
4. No other diagnosis explains the signs and symptoms
CRPS I = no major nerve damage; CRPS II = major nerve damage

Table 48.2 Common clinical characteristics of complex regional pain syndrome

Diagnostic categories	Symptoms	Signs
Sensory	Hyperesthesia and/or allodynia	Hyperalgesia (to pinprick) and/or allodynia (to light touch and/or temperature sensation and/or deep somatic pressure and/or joint movement)
Motor/trophic	Decreased range of motion and/or motor dysfunction (weakness, tremors, dystonia) and/or trophic changes (hair, nail, skin)	Decreased range of motion and/or motor dysfunction (weakness, tremor, dystonia) and/or trophic changes (hair, nail, skin)
Vasomotor	Temperature asymmetry and/or color changes and/or color asymmetry	Temperature asymmetry (>1 °C) and/or skin color changes and/or asymmetry
Sudomotor/edema	Reports of edema and/or sweating changes and/or sweating asymmetry	Edema and/or sweating changes and/or sweating asymmetry

Fig. 48.6 Treatment algorithm

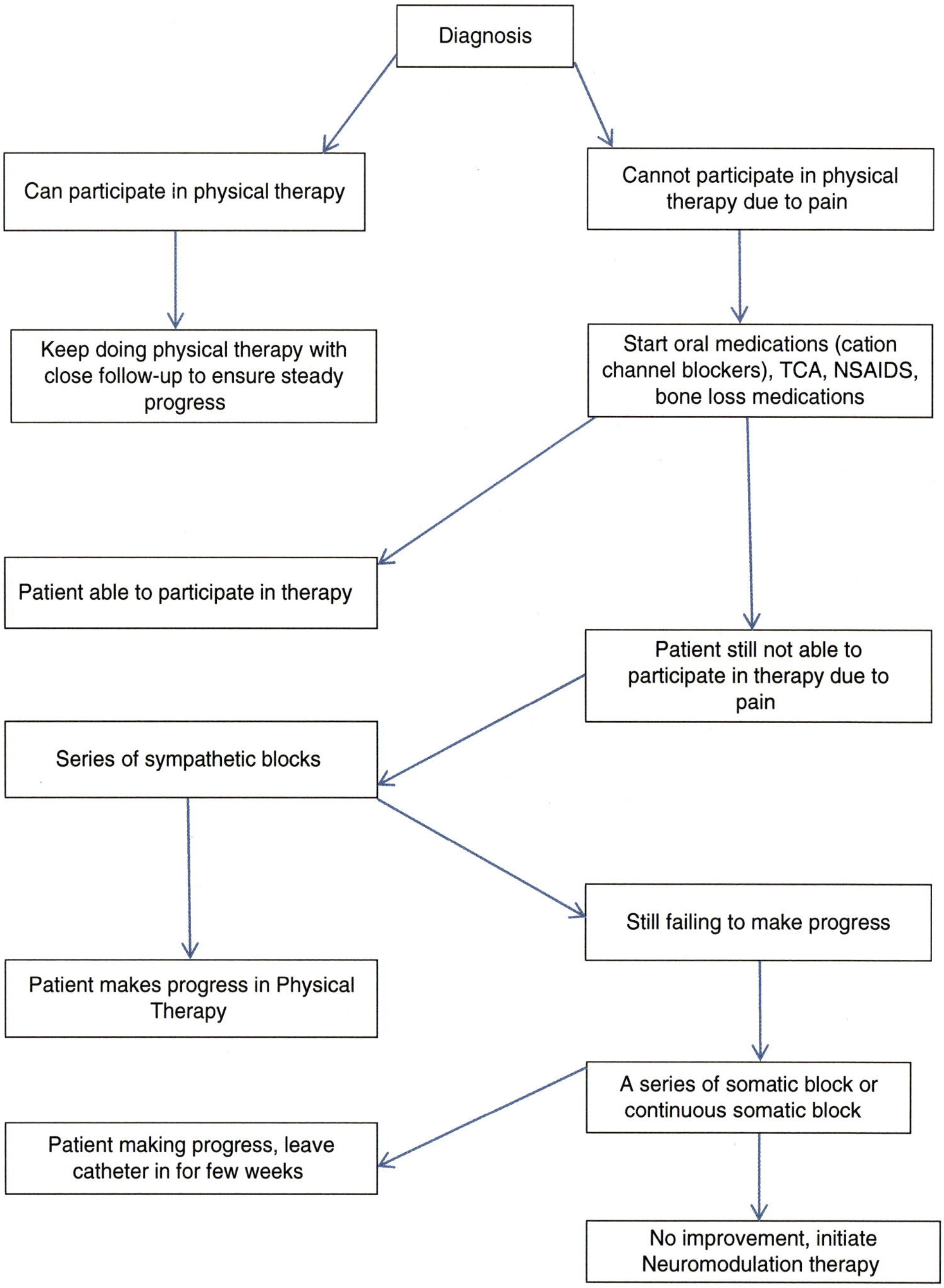

leakage of the infused solution. Less common complications are infection and nerve damage [5]. Insufficient analgesia or leakage often requires catheter replacement. Infection is minimized by placing the catheter with sterile methods and using a chlorhexidine-soaked patch. Patient selection is of utmost importance as the dressing must be kept clean and dry. The tunneling of the catheter does not prevent infection but helps to diagnose it before it becomes widespread. Most infections start at the skin. By tunneling the catheter, infection can be diagnosed as cellulitis around the catheter skin entry site before it spreads to deeper structures, which can result in mediastinitis [6]. Catheter infection is proportional to the time course of use. Longer periods are often not recommended [7]. Catheter migration is possible with long-term placements and may result in erosion of the catheter into another anatomical plane. The published reports of catheters for postsurgical pain control discuss a malposition or stuck catheter, but the discussions are not comprehensive, and complications may be underreported [8]. Catheter management requires vigilance. Before a patient is discharged, physical examination is carefully documented. Change in pain level or motor function means the catheter tip has moved. If analgesia is lost and no other symptoms (i.e., chest pain, shortness of breath, or hypotension) are present, the

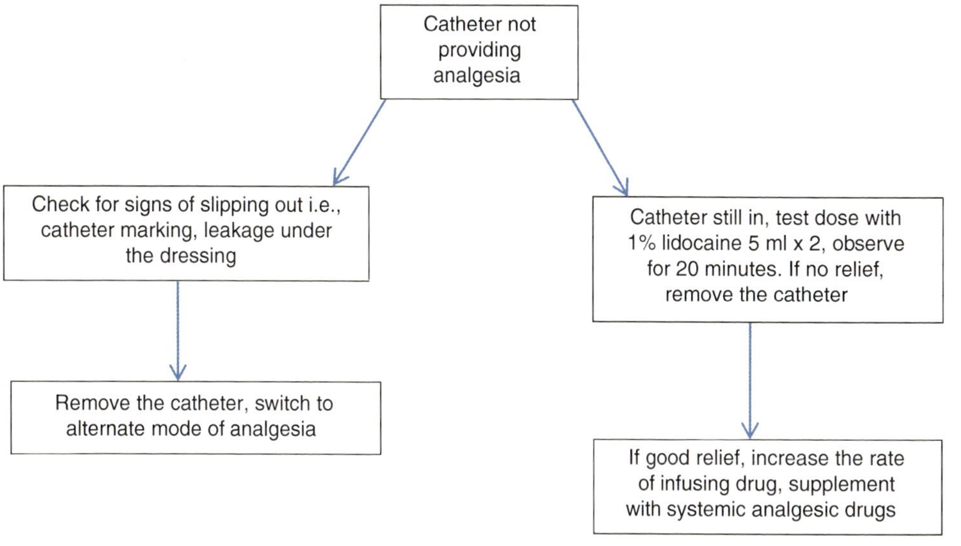

Fig. 48.7 Trouble shooting a catheter

next step depends upon the patient's location. If at home, the most likely possibility is that the catheter has slipped out or the patient is transitioning from surgical block to analgesic block. The analgesic block is best managed by increasing the rate of infusing medication, supplemented with oral analgesics. If the catheter has slipped out, fluid around the catheter may leak confirming that catheter has slipped out. In this case, patient is advised to remove the catheter and rely on oral analgesics. With new onset of shortness of breath or increasing weakness, the concern is spread of local anesthetic to the cervical epidural space. The result is an extensive somatic or cardiac sympathetic block, causing cardiac autonomic imbalance. The anesthetic infusion is discontinued and the patient is evaluated (Fig. 48.7).

If the catheter has a reinforced wire, the position of the catheter tip can be viewed, and its proximity to the cervical epidural space or a pneumothorax can be ruled out. Lobe atelectasis is common or the ipsilateral diaphragm is higher than usual from a phrenic nerve block. This condition should not be confused with a lung infection. For catheters without a wire and that are radiolucent, radiopaque solution such as omnipaque is injected under fluoroscopy so that the tip of the catheter can be identified. The spread of the dye reveals epidural spread that can explain a change in symptoms. When the decision is made to remove the catheter, force should not be needed for removal. Gentle pulling allows catheter to be removed with ease in majority of cases. A catheter should be removed only when all the anesthetic effect has worn off. Should catheter removal tug on a nerve or knot around a nerve, the patient will feel pain. The person tugging on the catheter then needs to stop immediately as nerve injury can occur with further force. If a catheter is MRI compatible, an MRI of the catheter area rules out abnormal kinking or knotting of the catheter around the nerves. A radiopaque catheter can be removed in a procedure suite under fluoroscopic guidance. This procedure requires a sterile technique, numbing of the area around the catheter, and blunt dissection around the catheter using a regular intravenous, angiocath cannula which can be threaded over the catheter. The catheter is mobilized from the surrounding soft tissue for easy removal. If an MRI or CT scan shows that the catheter is knotted around a nerve or plexus, a surgical consult may be warranted. A catheter may get stuck if its tip is bent into a hook shape. This happens generally when catheter is threaded against resistance. The metal tip of a nerve-stimulating catheter, for example, can bend during threading to become a hook. If a stylet can be successfully inserted, the tip may be straightened for removal without open exploration. If stylet insertion fails to straighten the tip, plastic angiocath or a dilator from a central line kit, threaded over the stuck catheter up to the bent tip, can help remove the stuck catheter. The most difficult removal is for a catheter that has been placed intraneurally. Tugging on the catheter causes severe paresthesia. An MRI of the brachial plexus along with strong paresthesia will confirm intraneural catheter placement. Shearing of a nerve on tugging is a real possibility. Avulsion of the nerve has been reported [9]. If only a minimal part of the catheter is intraneural, its removal can be attempted with careful monitoring. In the procedure suite, the catheter insertion site is prepped and draped. The area around the catheter is numbed using 1% lidocaine. Then using blunt dissection, an 18 or 16 g intravenous angiocath cannula is threaded over the catheter up to the plexus using ultrasound guidance. The cannula frees the catheter from adhesions and stabilizes the plexus, minimizing any stretch of the nerves during tugging, while the angiocath cannula is held in a fixed position. Gentle persistent traction may help the catheter slip out. Key in this maneuvering is an awake patient who can complain of pain or paresthesia. No force should be applied. If the maneuvers are unsuccessful, a surgical consult is needed (Fig. 48.8).

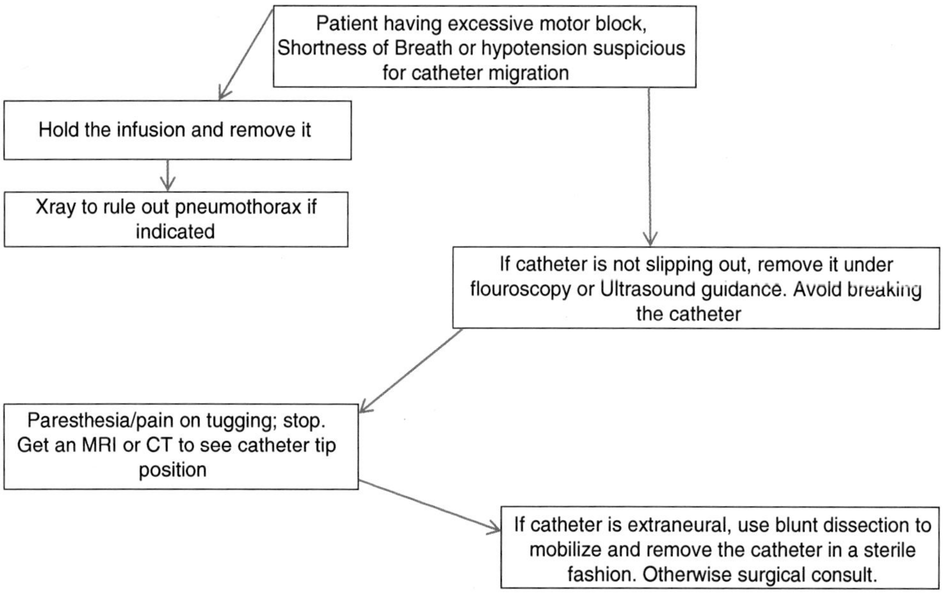

Fig. 48.8 Catheter with suspected malposition

Conclusion

A stuck peripheral nerve catheter is uncommon but not a rare complication. A systematic approach is needed. The catheter can be removed without surgical exploration most of the time if done methodically, but surgical approach should never be discounted.

References

1. Albazaz R, Wong YT, Homer-Vanniasinkam S. Complex regional pain syndrome: a review. Ann Vasc Surg. 2008;22(2):297–306.
2. de Mos M, de Bruijn AG, Huygen FJ, Dieleman JP, Stricker BH, Sturkenboom MC. The incidence of complex regional pain syndrome: a population-based study. Pain. 2007;129(1–2):12–20.
3. Sandroni P, Benrud-Larson LM, McClelland RL, Low PA. Complex regional pain syndrome type I: incidence and prevalence in Olmsted county, a population-based study. Pain. 2003;103(1–2):199–207.
4. Harden RN, Bruehl S, Stanton-Hicks M, Wilson PR. Proposed new diagnostic criteria for complex regional pain syndrome. Pain Med. 2007;8:326–31.
5. Capdevila X, Pirat P, Bringuier S, et al. Continuous peripheral nerve blocks in hospital wards after orthopedic surgery. A multicenter prospective analysis of the quality of postoperative analgesia and complications in 1,416 patients. Anesthesiology. 2005;103:1035–45.
6. Capdevila X, Jaber S, Pesonen P, Borgeat A, Eledjam JJ. Acute neck cellulitis and mediastinitis complicating a continuous interscalene block. Anesth Analg. 2008;107(4):1419–21.
7. Capdevila X, Bringuier S, Borgeat A. Infectious risk of continuous peripheral nerve blocks. Anesthesiology. 2009;110(1):182–8.
8. Burgher AH, Hebl JR. Minimally invasive retrieval of knotted nonstimulating peripheral nerve catheters. Reg Anesth Pain Med. 2007;32(2):162–6.
9. Adhikary SD, Armstrong K, Chin KJ. Perineural entrapment of an interscalene stimulating catheter. Anaesth Intensive Care. 2012;40(3):527–30.

Buprenorphine Challenges in the Perioperative Period

49

Katherine Kozarek and David M. Dickerson

49.1 Case Description

A 67-year-old female with a medical history of hypertension, fibromyalgia, and right hip osteoarthritis was scheduled for right total hip arthroplasty under neuraxial anesthesia. Her fibromyalgia and chronic hip pain were managed by a pain physician at another institution. Her pain regimen included gabapentin 100 mg nightly and a 10 μg/h transdermal buprenorphine (Butrans®) patch. On the day of surgery, a lumbar epidural was placed in the preoperative area. Upon initial dosing of the epidural catheter, the anesthesia provider found the buprenorphine patch on the patient's shoulder. The medication was not included on her preoperative preparation instructions. Because the epidural was to be discontinued on postoperative day 1 for thromboembolic prophylaxis and because of a concern for potentially severe, difficult to control pain, surgery was canceled. Therefore, the already placed epidural catheter was discontinued, and patient was discharged from the preoperative area; patient and the family perfectly understood the rationale behind this action plan. However, since no other cases were available to be added on, the operating room was not utilized and remained closed for the duration of the day.

The patient was sent that same day to the pain clinic for conversion to a full opioid agonist pain regimen: sustained-release oxycodone 10 mg every 8 h and hydrocodone-acetaminophen every 6 h as needed for breakthrough pain. Upon discussion between the attending surgeon, attending pain physician, and attending anesthesiologist in the perioperative medicine clinic, it was felt that 1-week duration of replacement therapy would have been sufficient for the effects of buprenorphine patch to dissipate.

K. Kozarek, M.D. • D.M. Dickerson, M.D. (✉)
Department of Anesthesia and Critical Care,
University of Chicago, Chicago, IL, USA
e-mail: kkozarek8@gmail.com; DDickerson@dacc.uchicago.edu

The patient returned 7 days later and underwent an uneventful right total hip arthroplasty under epidural anesthesia. On the evening after surgery, her self-reported pain scores were generally less than or equal to 4, and she was discharged home on postoperative day 2. On follow-up 1 month after surgery, the patient was no longer taking opioids and was recuperating well.

49.2 Case Discussion

49.2.1 Pharmacodynamics

Several pharmacologic properties determine the function and mechanism of action of buprenorphine. A partial mu opioid receptor agonist and kappa receptor antagonist, buprenorphine exhibits high affinity for opioid receptors, dissociates slowly from the receptor, and has high potency. As a partial mu agonist, it binds and activates the receptor but has low intrinsic activity in comparison to full agonists such as methadone, fentanyl, and hydromorphone. Receptor stimulation results in weak mu opioid effects including analgesia, euphoria, sedation, respiratory depression, cough suppression, miosis, constipation, nausea, and urinary retention [1–3]. The kappa receptor mediates sedation, dysphoria, and psychotomimetic effects, so antagonism by buprenorphine may have beneficial effects on mood and maintenance of sobriety [3]. In doses less than 8 mg daily, it is an opioid receptor agonist with low intrinsic activity. Opioid receptor antagonism predominates at doses greater than 32 mg daily. Partial mu agonism results in a ceiling effect, meaning large dose escalations provide minimal additional analgesia or respiratory depression. Therefore, buprenorphine has a broader therapeutic index compared to full mu agonists because incremental doses are less likely to result in deleterious side effects. Weak receptor activation and the ceiling effect diminish the euphoria associated with opioid abuse when compared to full agonists [3]. Partial agonism and high

M. Anitescu et al. (eds.), *Challenging Cases and Complication Management in Pain Medicine*,
https://doi.org/10.1007/978-3-319-60072-7_49

affinity for the mu opioid receptor result in opioid tolerance. Thus, considerable doses of full mu agonists may be needed to achieve analgesia during acute pain episodes. Such doses may not be feasible in higher-dose buprenorphine regimens.

Buprenorphine's affinity for the mu and kappa opioid receptors is 1000 times that of morphine [2, 4]. Avid binding inhibits other opioids from interacting with and activating these receptors so that subsequently administered opioids, including illicit drugs, are less efficacious [3]. Similarly, buprenorphine may displace full mu agonists from the receptor, potentially precipitating withdrawal because of weaker intrinsic activity. Slow dissociation of buprenorphine from the mu opioid receptor results in a long duration of action so that dosing can be infrequent. Buprenorphine's potency is approximately 25–50 times that of morphine [4].

These pharmacologic properties make buprenorphine a valuable option for opioid replacement therapy. The same characteristics, however, complicate acute pain management. Partial mu agonism results in opioid tolerance, and buprenorphine's high receptor affinity further decreases the efficacy of full mu agonists. All buprenorphine doses, however, do not preclude surgery for all patients.

49.2.2 Pharmacokinetics

Buprenorphine is highly lipophilic, which enhances sublingual and parenteral administration. Oral bioavailability is poor because of first pass hepatic metabolism [5].

The time to onset of the intravenous formulation is 5–15 min; onset of the sublingual formulation is 30–60 min with peak effect at 90–100 min and bioavailability of 60–70% [6]. Several factors contribute to buprenorphine's long half-life. With a large volume of distribution, 96% protein binding, high lipophilicity, and slow receptor dissociation, the half-life of the sublingual form ranges from 24 to 60 h [3].

The long duration of action may complicate perioperative pain management. Even 5–7 days after discontinuation, buprenorphine may still impede full opioid agonist activity [7]. Smaller doses may have a shorter half-life of 3–27 h, but then more frequent dosing is needed to maintain therapy. Sublingual doses of buprenorphine have an elimination half-life ten times longer than intravenous doses because release of drug from the buccal mucosa is slow.

49.2.2.1 Metabolism and Clearance

Buprenorphine is metabolized by the liver via the cytochrome P450 enzyme system. It is primarily metabolized by the CYP3A4 isozyme with minor contributions from CYP2C8, CYP3A5, and CYP3A7. Patients concurrently taking CYP3A4 inducers or inhibitors may require dose adjustments to prevent opioid withdrawal or toxicity. Buprenorphine is metabolized via N-dealkylation to norbuprenorphine and via glucuronidation to buprenorphine glucuronide. Norbuprenorphine, the only active metabolite, is one fourth as potent as buprenorphine. Of buprenorphine metabolites, 85% undergo glucuronidation to form conjugated byproducts, which are excreted via the biliary route. The remaining 15% are inactive metabolites excreted unchanged in the urine. Buprenorphine is safe to administer in patients with compromised renal function and does not require dose adjustment since only inactive metabolites are excreted renally. Patients with hepatic injury may require dose reductions and close laboratory monitoring of hepatic function [4, 8].

49.2.2.2 Dosing

The maximum recommended buprenorphine dose is 32 mg for opioid replacement therapy, administered once every 2–3 days. Therapeutic efficacy is limited at doses larger than 32 mg because of partial mu receptor agonist activity and ceiling effect [7, 9]. The effective analgesic dose depends on the indication and the patient's pathophysiology. Some patients require low doses of 5 μg/h (120 μg daily) transdermal buprenorphine; others require 6–8 mg daily with other formulations for effective therapy.

Patients with acute pain may be at increased risk of respiratory depression since buprenorphine may be present at receptors for up to 72 h, and large opioid doses are needed for adequate analgesia. While the likelihood of sedation with buprenorphine alone is low, when it is administered with other central nervous system depressants, respiratory depression may occur. Because of the high receptor affinity and slow receptor dissociation, effective opioid reversal may require higher than expected naloxone doses [5]. Therefore, patients should be closely monitored with continuous pulse oximetry and apnea and cardiac monitoring for at least 72 h after the last dose of buprenorphine [10].

49.2.3 Buprenorphine Formulations

Buprenorphine is available in several formulations; each has distinct clinical applications (Table 49.1). At low doses it is an analgesic. Parenteral buprenorphine (Buprenex®) treats acute and chronic pain. Butrans®, the transdermal patch, is indicated for the treatment of severe chronic pain. The dosing range for Butrans® is 5–20 μg/h (120–480 μg daily). Buprenorphine has anti-hyperalgesic effects possibly due to kappa receptor antagonism. Kappa antagonism blocks spinal dynorphin activity, an opioid ligand that has been implicated in opioid-induced hyperalgesia. Buprenorphine may also attenuate central pain sensitization in chronic pain treatment [3].

In 2002, the US Federal Drug Administration approved two sublingual buprenorphine preparations for the treatment of opioid abuse. Subutex, a tablet, is approved for opioid maintenance therapy or initial induction during detoxification

Table 49.1 Buprenorphine formulations

Formulation	Administration	Dose	Half-life	Indication
Buprenex	IM, IV	0.3 mg/mL	1.2–7.2 h	Moderate to severe pain
Butrans	Transdermal patch	5, 7.5, 10, 15, 20 µg/h	24–46 h	Chronic pain
Subutex	Sublingual tablet	2, 8 mg	31–44 h	Opioid dependence, induction
Suboxone (buprenorphine/naloxone)	Sublingual film	2 mg/0.5 mg, 4 mg/1 mg, 8 mg/2 mg, 12 mg/3 mg	24–60 h	Opioid dependence, maintenance

Table 49.2 Physician requirements to prescribe buprenorphine

• Complete 8 h of continuing medical education courses on the treatment of patients with opioid dependence
• Hold a license under state law
• Register with the Drug Enforcement Administration to dispense opioids
• Treat 30 patients or fewer during the first year of qualification
• Have the resources to refer patients to counseling services

from illicit opioids. Suboxone is a film of buprenorphine/naloxone in a 4:1 ratio [11]. The drug has also been used off-label as a combination maintenance therapy and analgesic for patients with chronic pain and a history of opioid dependence. Naloxone, a full mu receptor antagonist, has poor sublingual bioavailability. The parenteral bioavailability of naloxone, however, is high. If the tablet is crushed and injected, naloxone induces withdrawal symptoms in opioid-dependent users. The naloxone addition deters misuse of the medication [2, 3]. Buprenorphine/naloxone should not be used for the detoxification phase of opioid replacement therapy because naloxone may precipitate withdrawal.

Buprenorphine and buprenorphine/naloxone formulations used in opioid replacement therapy may be managed in the outpatient setting because of low abuse potential, favorable safety profile, and the long duration of action. The Drug Addiction Treatment Act categorized buprenorphine as a Schedule III drug that can be used on an outpatient basis. Patients are provided a 1-month supply to self-administer the medication (unlike methadone, which typically requires daily witnessed distribution in methadone clinics). Outpatient management of opioid dependence has increased patient access to treatment and mitigates the social stigma frequently associated with methadone maintenance programs. Physicians are licensed to prescribe buprenorphine by completing 8 h of continuing medical education courses on buprenorphine before submitting an application to the Substance Abuse and Mental Health Services Administration. Physicians must also be able to refer patients to counseling and other consulting services and be qualified by the Drug Enforcement Agency to prescribe controlled substances. Once approved, physicians may prescribe buprenorphine/naloxone to 30 patients during the first year, then up to 100 patients after the first year [3, 4, 12]. Table 49.2 summarizes the requirements to prescribe buprenorphine therapy.

49.3 Perioperative Buprenorphine Management

Evidence-based guidelines for the perioperative management of buprenorphine are not available, but four succinct recommendations exist within the literature. These are based on case reports, expert opinion, and pharmacologic principles.

49.3.1 Continuing Buprenorphine Therapy

In lower-dose regimens, the patient's daily maintenance dose of buprenorphine may be continued perioperatively, and short-acting full opioid receptor agonists are supplemented to treat acute pain. Because of opioid tolerance and partial mu receptor blockade by buprenorphine, large doses of opioids should be anticipated to compete with buprenorphine at the receptor. Intravenous patient-controlled analgesia (IV-PCA) requirements should be titrated to effect but may be three times higher in these patients than in opioid naïve patients [13]. The effective opioid dose results in adequate analgesia without worrisome opioid-related adverse effects including respiratory depression. The preferred supplemental full opioid agonist should be titratable and have high affinity for the mu receptor to effectively compete with buprenorphine. Fentanyl, hydromorphone, and morphine are candidates; codeine and hydrocodone are not [14]. Fentanyl, highly lipophilic with a rapid onset and short duration of action, is ideal for rapid titration of analgesia without narcosis. Continuing buprenorphine perioperatively prevents buprenorphine withdrawal, and the drug does not need to be resumed after surgery, which can be a complicated process. Case reports document successful perioperative analgesia in patients continued on buprenorphine. In five patients with uninterrupted buprenorphine therapy during general surgical procedures, adequate analgesia was achieved on self-reported or subjective pain scores. All received full mu agonists; two patients also received epidural opioids/bupivacaine, and one received ketamine [15]. In two other cases of obstetric patients on buprenorphine therapy, post-cesarean section pain was adequately managed with an opioid IV-PCA, opioid/local anesthetic epidural solution, and NSAIDs [16]. The disadvantage of continuing buprenorphine perioperatively is the exceptionally high doses of opioids required for adequate pain control. In other case studies, achieving sufficient analgesia was difficult in patients who continued buprenorphine perioperatively, possibly because of partial mu receptor blockade and inability of full agonists to displace buprenorphine from the receptor [7, 17].

The addition of full agonists to provide analgesia for a patient on buprenorphine requires vigilant monitoring of effect. The supplemental dosing of non-titratable agents such as methadone or sustained-release opioids may result in delayed toxicity from gradual displacement of buprenorphine with effector-site concentrations still rising hours after the analgesic threshold is reached. Reducing pain and nociception with non-opioid therapies, such as regional anesthesia and ketamine infusions, may be optimal for continuing buprenorphine perioperatively.

49.3.2 Continuing Buprenorphine with Supplemental Buprenorphine

Buprenorphine can be the sole agent for perioperative pain control because low-dose buprenorphine is predominantly analgesic [4]. The analgesic elimination half-life is 2–6 h. The total daily dose of buprenorphine is divided and administered in equal doses every 6–8 h. In one case of a patient maintained on buprenorphine/naloxone for opioid dependence who also underwent removal of breast implants, pain was adequately controlled postoperatively with her regular maintenance dose and supplemental buprenorphine every 6 h [18]. This method may be useful only for patients with moderate pain who take less than 32 mg buprenorphine daily. There is a ceiling effect on analgesia once doses exceed 32 mg in a 24-h period. Higher doses of buprenorphine are not more analgesic but will block full mu opioid receptor agonists from binding the receptor. This approach prevents exposure to full agonist opioids in patients with a history of opioid abuse. Clinical expertise is needed in buprenorphine supplementation. Patients may take their home buprenorphine if the medication is not on formulary, but any dose increase should be discussed preoperatively and throughout the titration phase with a buprenorphine expert if the primary clinicians do not possess this expertise.

49.3.3 Rotate to Full Opioid Agonist Therapy Preoperatively, Methadone-Based Regimen

A third option is to replace buprenorphine with a full receptor agonist preoperatively, typically methadone, to maintain opioid replacement therapy while adding short-acting opioids for analgesia [4]. When converting from buprenorphine to methadone, the first dose of full opioid agonist is administered 24 h after the last dose of buprenorphine. Methadone, 20 mg daily, may be substituted for 4 mg daily or less of buprenorphine. For buprenorphine doses of more than 4 mg daily, 40 mg methadone is substituted to prevent acute withdrawal. If withdrawal symptoms are experienced, methadone is increased by 5–10 mg daily until symptoms resolve. If patients have breakthrough pain on methadone, short-acting full agonist opioids may be titrated to effect [5, 19]. Opioid rotation from buprenorphine to methadone is considered for patients who are at high risk of relapse and should continue opioid replacement therapy perioperatively or who are expected to have moderate to severe postoperative pain. Conversion to methadone prevents the buprenorphine ceiling effect so that short-acting full agonists can be titrated without buprenorphine-induced opioid blockade. Because buprenorphine and methadone have long and fairly unpredictable half-lives, careful patient monitoring is necessary during the transition to methadone and postoperatively. Converting back to buprenorphine after surgery will result in withdrawal if a patient is simultaneously taking full opioid agonists [4]. Full opioid agonists must be discontinued, and the patient should be in mild withdrawal before resuming buprenorphine [14, 17].

49.3.4 Rotate to Full Opioid Agonist Therapy, Non-methadone-Based Regimen

Buprenorphine may be discontinued completely and full agonist opioids titrated. This option is for patients undergoing surgical procedures expected to have moderate to severe postoperative pain. The anticipated duration of treatment with full agonists should be brief so that the lack of opioid replacement therapy does not increase the patient's risk of relapse. To limit the risk of withdrawal, buprenorphine is tapered slowly over 2 weeks. If a slow taper is not possible, buprenorphine may be discontinued over 3 days, but the patient will likely experience withdrawal symptoms or relapse. For low-dose buprenorphine, the last dose of buprenorphine is ideally at least 72 h before surgery or as many as 7 days before for higher doses to ensure minimal residual partial mu receptor blockade. In one case report, a patient with Chiari I malformation rotated off buprenorphine to hydromorphone before gynecologic surgery. Adequate pain control was ultimately achieved with large amounts of full agonist opioids, which reflects potential residual activity of buprenorphine at the receptor [20]. In a case of a trauma patient (maintained on buprenorphine/naloxone for opioid dependence) who developed significant postoperative pain when his maintenance dose was resumed 4 days after surgery, discontinuation in favor of treatment with full mu agonists was successful [17]. Discontinuing buprenorphine prevented the ceiling effect and partial agonist effect that interfered with full mu receptor agonists. Patients taking buprenorphine, however, may still require large amounts of opioids because of opioid tolerance. Discontinuing buprenorphine may risk relapse in patients on opioid replacement therapy. Buprenorphine is resumed once full agonists have been discontinued and the patient is experiencing mild withdrawal symptoms.

49.3.5 Multimodal Analgesia

The unanticipated nature of trauma and emergent surgery may preclude rotation or cessation of buprenorphine. In all surgical patients taking buprenorphine, consideration of broad multimodal analgesia techniques including regional anesthesia is necessary. Infiltration of local anesthetic at the incision site and the use of non-opioid analgesics such as ketamine, ketorolac, NSAIDs, tricyclic antidepressants, and dexmedetomidine and systemic local anesthetics such as lidocaine infusions and corticosteroids may be beneficial in decreasing postoperative pain [13]. Regional and neuraxial anesthesia may decrease opioid requirements and have been successfully incorporated into the analgesic regimens of buprenorphine-maintained patients [1, 14]. Non-pharmacologic interventions such as transcutaneous electric nerve stimulation, aromatherapy, acupuncture, and massage also may be beneficial in treating myofascial and neuropathic pain [5].

Conclusion

Patients taking buprenorphine often have complicated pain syndromes or a history of substance abuse. They may benefit from an interdisciplinary approach to their pain treatment and medical care. Communication with the patient's buprenorphine prescriber should be continued, especially with regard to the buprenorphine dose and postoperative analgesic regimens. Other consultants who may facilitate the patient's postoperative recovery include a psychiatrist, addiction medicine specialist, social worker, pain specialist, and physiotherapist [5]. Open communication should be maintained with the patient regarding the medical care plan, and clinicians should work to set realistic expectations for postoperative analgesia. Preoperative coordination and planning for these patients are necessary to ensure positive outcomes and a high quality of recovery.

References

1. Bryson EO. The perioperative management of patients maintained on medications used to manage opioid addiction. Curr Opin Anaesthesiol. 2014;27:359–64.
2. Bryson E, Lipson S, Gevirtz C. Anesthesia for patients on buprenorphine. Anesthesiol Clin. 2010;28:611–7.
3. Chen KY, Chen L, Mao J. Buprenorphine-naloxone therapy in pain management. Anesthesiology. 2014;120:1262–74.
4. Gevirtz C, Frost EAM, Bryson EO. Perioperative implications of buprenorphine maintenance treatment for opioid addiction. Int Anesthesiol Clin. 2011;49:147–55.
5. Roberts MD, Meyer-Witting M. High-dose buprenorphine: perioperative precautions and management strategies. Anaesth Intensive Care. 2005;33:17–25.
6. Vadivelu N, Mitra S, Kaye AD, Urman RD. Perioperative analgesia and challenges in the drug-addicted and drug-dependent patient. Best Pract Res Clin Anaesthesiol. 2014;28:91–101.
7. Huang A, Katznelson R, de Perrot M, Clarke H. Perioperative management of a patient undergoing Clagett window closure stabilized on Suboxone for chronic pain: a case report. Can J Anaesth. 2014;61:826–31.
8. Cruciani RA, Knotkova H, editors. Handbook of methadone prescribing and buprenorphine therapy. New York: Springer; 2013.
9. Ingelheim B. Buprenorphine sublingual tablets prescribing information. Columbus: Roxane Laboratories; 2015.
10. McCormick Z, Chu S, Chang-Chien G, Joseph P. Acute pain control challenges with buprenorphine/naloxone therapy in a patient with compartment syndrome secondary to McArdle's disease: a case report and review. Pain Med. 2013;14:1187–91.
11. Suboxone.com [Internet]. Richmond, VA: Indivior Inc; 2015. Available from http://www.suboxone.com. Accessed 5 Oct 2015.
12. Substance abuse and mental health services administration [Internet]. Rockville, MD: SAMHSA. Available from http://www.samhsa.gov. Accessed 7 Oct 2015.
13. Huxtable CA, Roberts LJ, Somogyi AA, Macintyre PE. Acute pain management in opioid-tolerant patients: a growing challenge. Anaesth Intensive Care. 2011;39:804–23.
14. Childers JW, Arnold RM. Treatment of pain in patients taking buprenorphine for opioid addiction #221. J Palliat Med. 2012;15(5):613–4.
15. Kornfeld H, Manfredi L. Effectiveness of full agonist opioids in patients stabilized on buprenorphine undergoing major surgery: a case series. Am J Ther. 2010;17:523–8.
16. Jones HE, Johnson RE, Milio L. Post-cesarean pain management of patients maintained on methadone or buprenorphine. Am J Addict. 2006;15:258–9.
17. Harrington C, Zaydfudim V. Buprenorphine maintenance therapy hinders acute pain management in trauma. Am Surg. 2010;76:397–9.
18. Book SW, Myrick H, Malcolm R, Strain EC. Buprenorphine for postoperative pain following general surgery in a buprenorphine-maintained patient. Am J Psychiatry. 2007;164:979.
19. Alford DP, Compton P, Samet JH. Acute pain management for patients receiving maintenance methadone or buprenorphine therapy. Ann Intern Med. 2006;144:127–34.
20. Chern SYS, Isserman R, Chen L, Ashburn M, Liu R. Perioperative pain management for patients on chronic buprenorphine: a case report. J Anesth Clin Res. 2012;3:1–4.

Sensory and Motor Deficit with High Amplitude Stimulation in Spinal Cord Stimulators

50

Shaan Sudhakaran and Magdalena Anitescu

50.1 Case Description

A 66-year-old male with failed back surgery syndrome is evaluated for severe chronic back pain. The patient's medical history is consistent with an L4–L5 fusion for his spondylolisthesis 15 years ago that improved his symptoms at that time. Three years later, he sustained a work-related injury, which resulted in a T7 vertebral compression fracture. He underwent T6–T8 fusion with instrumentation, but he continued to have severe lumbar and thoracic pain. He was treated in several pain clinics and underwent multiple thoracic and lumbar epidural steroid injections without sustained relief.

His pain is reported as severe, 8/10 on a numerical rating scale. Back pain is accompanied by bilateral chronic radicular pain and constant paresthesia, exacerbated when he walks and sometimes associated with foot drop. He cannot walk more than two blocks because of pain and suffers from mechanical instability with one to two falls every few months. His medications include 1800 mg extended-release gabapentin nightly, baclofen 10 mg three times a day, oxycodone/acetaminophen 7.5 mg/325 mg every 6 h as needed, and meloxicam 7.5 mg twice a day. He denies any unintentional weight loss, fever, night sweats, or chills and does not have bowel or bladder symptoms.

Other medical history includes non-specific autoimmune disease, treated with chronic low dose prednisone by a rheumatologist. On review of systems, he admits to fatigue, myalgias, gait issues, weakness, and intermittent numbness.

S. Sudhakaran, M.D. • M. Anitescu, M.D., Ph.D. (✉)
Department of Anesthesia and Critical Care,
University of Chicago Medical Center,
5841 S. Maryland Ave., MC 4028, Chicago, IL, USA
e-mail: ssudhakaran@dacc.uchicago.edu;
MAnitescu@dacc.uchicago.edu

On physical examination, his strength is 5/5 throughout upper and lower extremities. His range of motion at the hip including flexion and extension is slightly limited. He has mild tenderness to palpation over the T6-T8 vertebral bodies and mild paravertebral muscle tenderness in this area.

Because the conservative medical regimen has failed, the patient is evaluated for placement of a spinal cord stimulator. After rigorous screening, the patient was deemed an ideal candidate. Oral opioid medication was discontinued 10 days before the placement of the spinal cord stimulator. Leads were placed at T8 and T10 for the stimulator trial. An inadvertent dural tear occurred during insertion, but there were no symptoms. Pain scores during the 1-week trial decreased to 2/10, and mobility and ambulation improved. A permanent stimulator system was placed 2 weeks after conclusion of the trial with leads positioned at T8–T10 (Fig. 50.1).

At the conclusion of placement, the patient's electrodes were programmed and the patient was educated on adjusting pulse width and amplitude. After the adjustment session, the patient increased the amplitude to higher values. He was unable to walk because of a wide, fixed, spastic gait with instability. Lying down did not improve the symptoms. A CT brain scan was ordered to rule out a cerebrovascular disorder. Amplitude setting was widely deviated from the initial PACU settings on interrogation (Fig. 50.2).

The amplitude was 7.5 mA (maximum 10.5), adjusted by the patient who did not sense the stimulation while prone. When the stimulator was turned off, sensation and motor control returned almost immediately. Physical examination demonstrated normal gait and no focal neurologic deficits. Thoracic radiography showed no migration of the leads (Fig. 50.1). After adjustment of the settings, the patient's symptoms improved dramatically and he was discharged home. His pain remained low 2–3/10 on a numeric rating scale.

M. Anitescu et al. (eds.), *Challenging Cases and Complication Management in Pain Medicine*,
https://doi.org/10.1007/978-3-319-60072-7_50

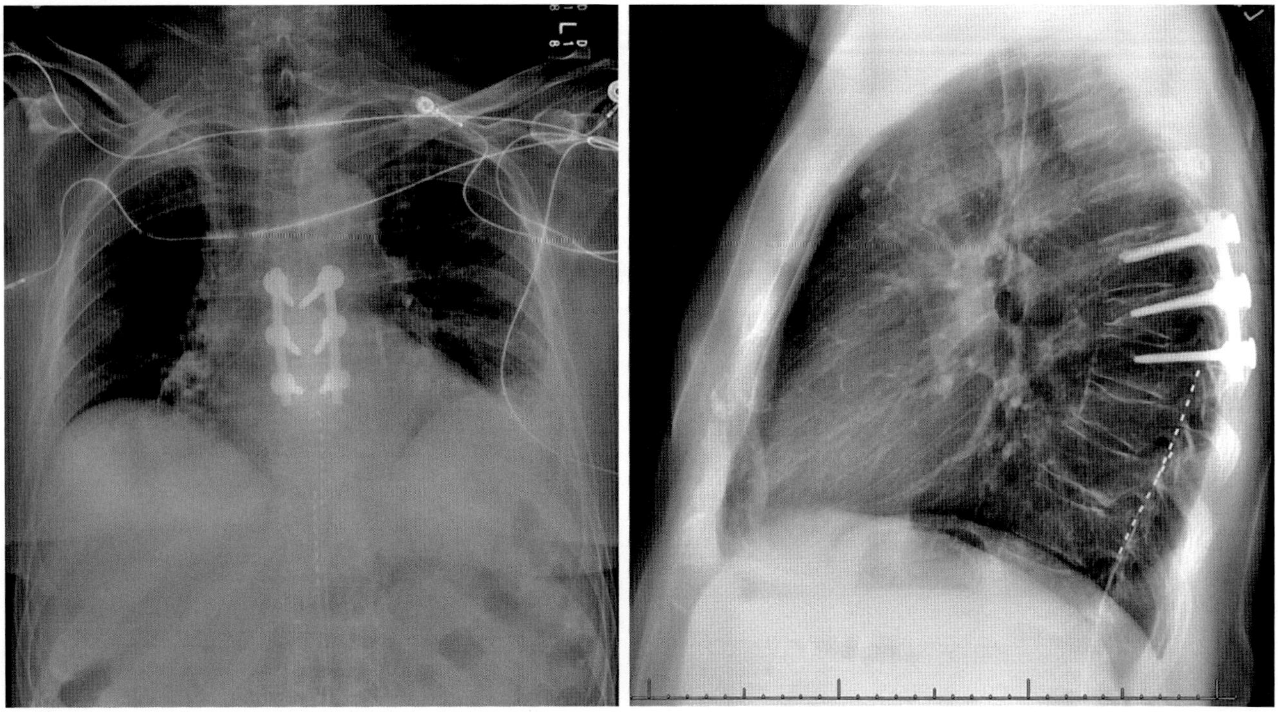

Fig. 50.1 (**a**, **b**) AP and lateral view chest X-ray: Termination of electrodes at T8 and T10 confirms the absence of obvious lead migration. Images from personal library

Group Report

Group A

(# Indicates Adaptivestim Enabled)

Rate range (Hz) :	2 - 35 -85
Cycling on/off (?/?)	off
SoftStart/stop (s)	4
TargetMyStim	off

A1 :

			Amp (v)	pw (μs)
|0	|8			
|1	|9			
|2	|10		-----	-----
|3	|11	Upper	10.5	450
|4-	|12			
|5+	|13	Programmed	2.6	450
|6+	|14			
|7-	|15	Lower	0.0	450
		Resolution	0.05	na

Fig. 50.2 Print out from the implanted stimulator with the set programmed amplitude of 2.6 V that the patient increased during the event to 7.5 V. As seen the adaptive stim has not been yet activated for this patient. This created the need for increase of the amplitude with the side effects described in the text when position was changed from sitting to standing. Symptoms resolved with resetting of the system to lower amplitudes and activation of the position change device. Image from personal library

50.2 Case Discussion

Spinal cord stimulators were first used to treat pain in 1967. The gate theory mechanism of pain hypothesized that the substantia gelatinosa in the dorsal horn of the spinal cord modulates transmission of sensory stimuli. Large fibers inhibit and small fibers activate the gate [1]. At first, neuromodulator devices were placed directly on the dorsal column to stimulate large fibers to inhibit pain transmission. As technology advanced over the next few decades, devices became smaller, safer and more efficacious.

Indications for spinal cord stimulation therapy are failed back surgery syndrome, complex regional pain syndrome, peripheral neuropathy, ischemic limb pain, phantom limb pain, and chronic angina pectoris. Before placement, patients undergo rigorous screening criteria including a minimal response to conservative therapy for at least 6 months and a psychiatric evaluation to exclude somatoform disorders. Prescription or illicit drugs must be discontinued. Finally, there must be no secondary gain or litigation involved with the case.

The larger needle (14G) used to reach the epidural space in SCS tends to increase the risk of unintended intravascular cannulation or damage of vascular structures in the epidural space. Patients older than 65 years who take antiplatelet or anticoagulant medications are at highest risk for spinal hematoma. Symptoms include sharp, transient back and leg pain that can lead to flaccid paralysis. Symptoms tend to develop over hours after implantation, which is consistent with this patient's presentation.

Epidural abscess is another complication of stimulator placement. In such cases, symptoms of fever, malaise, and back pain develop 1–3 days after placement. Flaccid (early) or spastic (late) paralysis can be experienced, depending on the effect on the spinal cord. Strict aseptic surgical techniques may limit this complication. Imaging studies help to clarify the diagnosis. Our patient did not experience these complications.

About one of three spinal cord stimulator insertions will produce a complication [2]. Surgical revision is required for 23% of patients. The most common reasons are lead migration, lead connection failure, and lead breakage [3]. Lead migration occurs within the first few days after implantation and more often with percutaneous leads than with surgically placed paddle leads. The most common reasons for stimulator removal are infection, equipment malfunction, and unsatisfactory pain relief. Infection was found in 4.6%, and it may be deep or superficial. True hardware malfunction was found in 10% of implantations. Malfunctions can be discovered in the pulse generator, leads, or wires. In the event of a dural puncture on electrode placement, the lead malfunctions temporarily, and the patient may experience a post-dural puncture headache [4]. Patients most likely to respond to stimulators have allodynia [5]. After a 1-week trial that decreases pain by 50%, a permanent system is implanted.

The amplitude of a stimulus is the magnitude of the current or voltage that is delivered at the electrode. It is measured in milliamps or volts. In our patient, the Medtronic spinal cord stimulator was designed to vary the amplitude by varying the voltage of the system. The range of value spanned from 2.5 to 10.5 V. Another modifiable variable is pulse width, which is the duration of the stimulus (in microseconds). Decreasing pulse width is thought to increase the gap in activation thresholds between large and small nerve fibers. Stimulation of dorsal cord fibers generates paresthesias of many dermatomes caudal to the level of the stimulating cathode. There is poor correlation between cathode placement and desired location of paresthesias attributed to variations in cord geometry and dorsal volume of cerebrospinal fluid.

In the period immediately following placement, the patient generally titrates amplitude above the perception threshold and below the discomfort threshold. As amplitude increases, paresthesia intensity increases along with coverage expansion. The discomfort threshold is the level at which the amplitude results in pain, loss of sensation, or motor stimulation. This level is usually ~1.5 times the paresthesia perception threshold [6]. There is significant variation with stimulation amplitude and patient positioning. The spinal cord is free to move within the fluid dural sac and varies with gravity. The distance between the electrodes and spinal cord decreases when the patient is supine and increases when prone. Although an adaptive system that senses patient position exists, this feature is not usually turned on immediately in the postoperative period. Prior to insertion, the patient has an in-depth discussion with the physician regarding the complexity of the variables that go into maintaining analgesia with a spinal cord stimulator. The presence of a system that senses the position of the spine in rapport to the stimulating leads is essential in ensuring optimal pain treatment in the patients with these implantable devices; however, in many situations, this system is not activated immediately postoperatively, allowing tissue healing and limiting erroneous programming in the presence of immediate postoperative changes (presence of residual tissues and blood in the epidural space); this feature is usually turned on at the 1-week postoperative visit; generally, patients adapt to using the complex systems very easily; however, limited understanding of the complex processes involved in the settings of the electronic device can predispose patients to side effects and complications as it was in this case; therefore a better and detailed discussions need to take place at multiple visits in order to ease the patients and their families in a proper understanding and utilization of this device.

Conclusion

Spinal cord stimulator systems provide excellent results in a variety of intractable pain syndromes. While many implantable systems exists, the physicians should choose a device that would be the best fit for the patient and her/his condition. Detailed discussions with the patient regarding modifying parameters before and immediately after the implantation will ensure best outcome in the immediate and distant postoperative period. This case delineates a complication less described in clinical practice, primarily related to the parameters that patients are able to adjust. As seen in our case description, this adverse event can easily mimic more severe complications such as stroke and epidural hematoma alerting physician to promptly intervene; we hope that by being aware of this possible complications, physicians will include it in their evaluations, to hopefully reduce unnecessary diagnostic testing. However, physicians should keep in mind more grave complications that can occur with the spinal cord stimulator system implantation and treat those instances with increase care.

Key Points

- A high amplitude setting on a spinal cord stimulator can result in a sensory and motor deficit, but the deficit is not permanent.

- Amplitude must be adjusted on spinal cord stimulators relative as the distance from spinal cord to electrode changes.
- The discomfort threshold is usually 1.5 times the amplitude of the perception threshold.

References

1. Moayedi M, Davis KD. Theories of pain: from specificity to gate control. J Neurophysiol. 2013;109:5–12.
2. Turner JA, Loeser JD, Deyo RA, Sanders SB. Spinal cord stimulation for patients with failed back surgery syndrome or complex regional pain syndrome: a systematic review of effectiveness and complications. Pain. 2004;108(1–2):137–47.
3. Jeon YH. Spinal cord stimulation in pain management: a review. Korean J Pain. 2012;25(3):143–50.
4. Eldrige JS, Weingarten TN, Rho RH. Management of cerebral spinal fluid leak complicating spinal cord stimulator implantation. Pain Pract. 2006;6:285–8.
5. Kunnumpurath S, Srinivasagopalan R, Vadivelu N. Spinal cord stimulation: principles of past, present and future practice: a review. J Clin Monit Comput. 2009;23:333–9.
6. Molnar G, Panken C, Kelley K. Effects of spinal cord movement and position changes on neural activation patterns during spinal cord stimulation (abstract). San Antonio, TX: American Academy of Pain Medicine; 2010.

Anterior Epidural Space Lead Placement

51

Maunuk V. Rana and Simon Willis

51.1 Case Description

A 62-year-old male diagnosed with failed back surgery syndrome (FBSS) with major complaints of refractory diffuse lower back pain and bilateral lower extremity radicular pain underwent a permanent spinal cord stimulator implantation after having pain relief of greater than 75% on trial stimulation. The eight-contact leads were implanted using a dual lead percutaneous approach with cylindrical type lead tips placed parallel to one another at the T8 vertebral level of the posterior epidural space with verification under fluoroscopic guidance. The leads were placed no greater than 2 mm off the physiologic midline and anchored to the supraspinous fascia using interrupted 2.0 nonabsorbable suture with silicon anchors. Additionally, tension in the leads was minimized with strain relief loops for each lead in the midline incision as well as at the site of the implantable pulse generator (IPG). The IPG was placed in the right flank at the posterior superior gluteal region with lead wires tunneled to the pocket. Intra- and postoperative testing revealed and confirmed 100% paresthesia coverage of the areas of pain. The patient noted good, consistent relief during the first week after completion of the procedure.

Around the 11th postoperative day, the patient began experiencing a gradual return of right lower extremity pain in the same distribution prior to implantation with a disappearance of paresthesias down the same leg, as well as a new sensation of involuntary right-sided abdominal muscle contractions with rib pain noted along the left rib in the T8 dermatomal distribution during stimulation. Upon return to the clinic he denied any fever, night sweats, weight loss, malaise, weakness, loss of bowel or bladder control, nor worsening of presurgical pain. Vital signs taken in the office were within normal limits except for a mildly elevated blood pressure at 150/90. Physical examination demonstrated clean closure margins of the surgical site with sutures intact and a wound without any erythema, warmth, or drainage. There were no signs of swelling or fluctuance on palpation over incisions. There were no alterations in motor strength and reflex testing compared to pretrial and permanent SCS implantation exams. Muscle twitching of his abdomen was visible, worse at the upper right abdominal area during stimulation cycles. The appearance of clean, non-erythematous, non-dehiscing surgical sites as well as the lack of fever, other constitutional symptoms, and tenderness to palpation made clinical infection lower on the list of differentials. This included epidural abscess, IPG or connector tract infections, and superficial wound infection. No palpable fluctuance or swelling at or near the surgical incisions also pointed away from a diagnosis of epidural abscess or epidural hematoma.

Changes in coverage patterns of stimulation, abnormal muscle contractions, and new onset of pain along the distribution of the lower thoracic ribs pointed to a diagnosis involving dysfunction of the leads and connector system or malfunctioning of the implanted instrumentation. Possible etiologies in a differential regarding the leads and connector system included lead migration, lead malfunction, and wire kinks, breaks, or detachment. Possible differentials involving the instrumentation included issues with battery quality, including battery life and charging capacity, as well as malfunctioning of the overall SCS system. In the office the neurostimulator battery was interrogated revealing no discrepancy in overall battery quality. Stimulator parameters

M.V. Rana, M.D. (✉)
Associate Professor, Department of Anesthesiology and Critical Care, The University of Chicago Medical Center, Burr Ridge, Chicago, IL 60527, USA
e-mail: mrana@dacc.uchicago.edu

S. Willis, M.D.
Department of Physical Medicine and Rehabilitation, Medstar Georgetown University Hospital/National Rehabilitation Hospital, 3800 Reservoir Rd NW, Washington, DC 20007, USA
e-mail: smwillis703@gmail.com

M. Anitescu et al. (eds.), *Challenging Cases and Complication Management in Pain Medicine*,
https://doi.org/10.1007/978-3-319-60072-7_51

including pulse width, amplitude, rate, and electrode selection were tried at different values and variations in the hopes of recapturing paresthesia coverage; however, upon alterations the patient noted a wider stimulation area around his lower thorax along with increasing intensity of pain, development of a buzzing sensation along his ribs, as well as worsening force of his muscle contractions. As symptoms worsened with changes in parameters in conjunction with the presence of muscle contractions, lead migration was felt to be causing his altered presentation, and the patient was sent for anteroposterior (AP) and lateral plain film radiographs to assess lead position.

Radiographs demonstrated a left lead at the T8 vertebral level in proper location in the posterior epidural space without noticeable kinks, bends, or breakages in the lead wires. On further review of the image, the right lead had appeared to have migrated laterally and anteriorly at the T8 level, ending with the lead tip settled into the anterior epidural space. The patient underwent a revision surgery a few days later, this time applying a "midline anchoring" technique involving the use of the plica mediana dorsalis instead of the conventional anchoring technique [1]. Intraoperative testing revealed paresthesia coverage bilaterally, masking the lower back and radicular pain, and he was seen 2 weeks postoperatively without any noted complications. He reported continued coverage at various other follow-up appointments and denied any further changes in stimulation pattern.

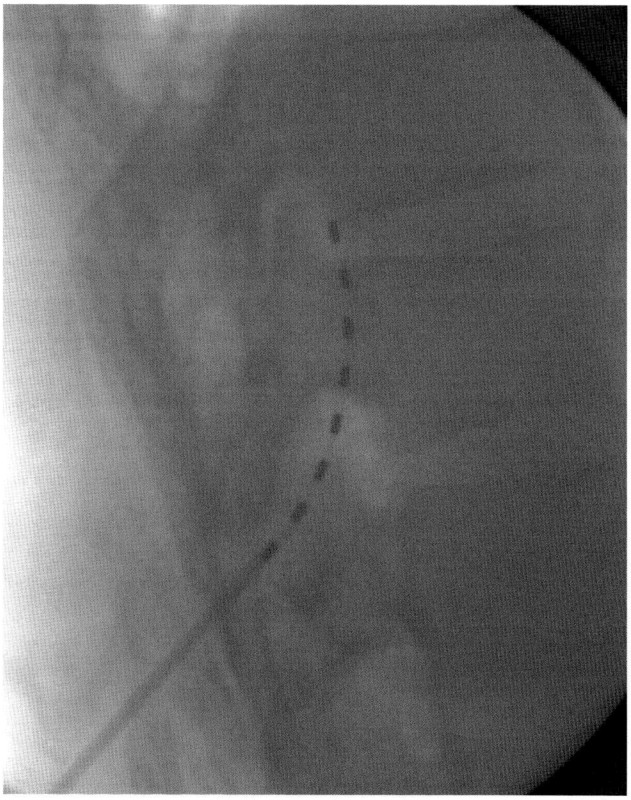

Fig. 51.1 Lateral view during placement of a stimulating lead showing anterior epidural space trajectory; the lead was withdrawn and repositioned in the posterior epidural space. During testing, patient experienced testicular paresthesia and abdominal wall discomfort with stimulation around T10, prompting quick repositioning and retesting. Image from personal library

51.2 Case Discussion

51.2.1 Background

Since the introduction of implanted electrode-induced electrical stimulation in 1967 by Dr. Norman Shealy and colleagues [2] for uncontrolled, chronic pain, SCS have been used to treat a variety of pain states with increasing success. Currently SCS is approved for treatment of complex regional pain syndrome (CRPS); failed back surgery syndrome; postherpetic neuralgia, peripheral vascular disease; visceral pain in the chest, abdomen, and pelvis; and peripheral neuropathy [3]. Traditional spinal cord stimulation, otherwise known as dorsal column stimulation, uses continuous pulsed electrical energy that is delivered to the spinal cord to inhibit or alter the interpretation of pain stimuli [4]. It utilizes two types of leads placed in the posterior epidural space: cylindrical which is placed using a percutaneous approach and paddle which historically has required implantation via laminotomy (Figs. 51.1 and 51.2).

In 2011 a surgical paddle-type lead was developed that could also be placed percutaneously [5]. Although the exact mechanisms are unknown, it is hypothesized that stimulation applied to the dorsal horn affects local neurophysiologic properties at the level of the neurotransmitters, promoting suppression of neuronal hyperexcitability, modification of sympathetic tone, as well as an inhibition of

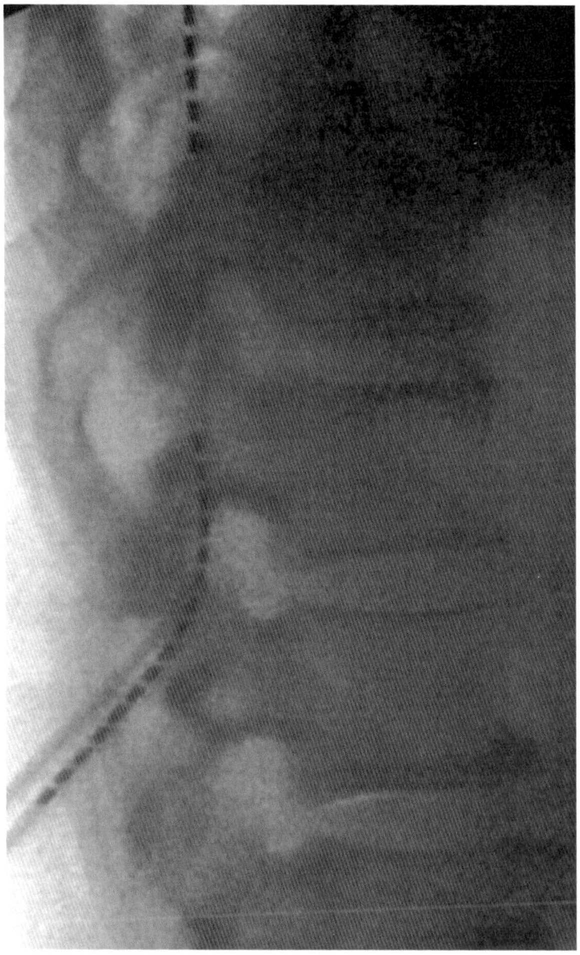

Fig. 51.2 Lateral view of a stimulating lead placement. This different system in the same patient shows posterior epidural space trajectory. Patient reports substituting pain with paresthesia of his lower back pain and bilateral legs. Image from personal library

orthodromic transmission of stimuli via an antidromic response [6–8].

51.2.2 Epidemiology and Etiology

Advancements in Neuromodulation have led to more efficient stimulation with safer trial and permanent implant techniques. Despite these enhancements, SCS is not without complications. Although uncommon, complications from spinal cord stimulators are secondary to technical limitations, biological circumstances, or, rarely, a combination of the two [9]. According to a literature review performed in 2004 [9], 27% of complications resulting from SCS implantation in 3679 patients over a 20-year period were of technical malfunction, 87% of which correlated to issues with leads. The most common complication observed postoperatively after stimulator implantation was lead migration with a rate of between 11 and 13.2% [9].

Lead movement is most commonly secondary to issues with anchoring techniques that have failed to maintain the posterior epidural lead location. Migration generally occurs in two patterns: vertical translation or horizontal shifts. For it to occur, both directional and tactile forces placed on the electrode must exceed the strength of the anchoring force. Many factors contribute to the anchoring forces placed on the leads including suture strength, technique, and placement. Other factors that play an integral part in the occurrence of lead migration involve the type of tissue used during the anchoring process, the angle and trajectory of the leads into the epidural space, areas of mobility in which the leads traverse, and the chosen area of placement of the hardware that comprises the remainder of the stimulator [10]. Historically, lead migration was more common with the percutaneous approach versus the laminectomy technique for SCS implantation, as well as a higher incidence when the battery is placed in the abdominal area versus placement in the gluteal region. Kumar and colleagues [10], however, concluded in a study that the more proximally the implanted pulse generator (IPG) is placed to the actual site of insertion of the lead wires, the lower the risk of lead migration. This observation likely reflects the increase in stress placed on the lead wires between the site of anchor and the IPG when these components are separated by a greater distance. This separation increases more during extension and flexion of the spine. Furthermore, in 2006, Rosenow and colleagues [11] found that lead migration rates in a cohort of 289 patients were actually higher in those that had undergone a surgical laminotomy for SCS implantation. Migration rates are also noted to be higher in cervical leads, occurring nearly twice as often as leads placed in the lower thoracic region, reflecting the variability in mobility of differing segments of the spine [10].

51.2.3 Anatomy

The dorsal column fibers of the spinal cord are organized in a lamellated fashion with a caudal to rostral pattern of sensation correlating with medial to lateral structures of the dorsal column [11]. The goal location for lead placement is in the posterior epidural space for direct stimulation to the dorsal column of the spinal cord or the dorsal nerve roots, without stimulation to the anterior motor horns. Stimulation directed at this section of the spinal cord aims to produce purely sensory changes, in the form of paresthesias, and thereby avoids any motor abnormalities. When appropriate placement is achieved, paresthesias produced should cover a pattern both ipsilaterally and caudally to the level of the lead. Muscle contractions, warm sensations, burning, or abnormal paresthesias after SCS placement likely indicates that stimulation is being applied external to the dorsal columns. Depending on the abnormalities observed as well as an in-depth understanding of spinal cord anatomy, the location of aberrant stimulation can be localized, allowing for a faster time between diagnosis of malfunction and corrective measures.

When lead migration or aberrant procedural placement occurs, the various spinal tracts can be activated during stimulation depending on spatial occupancy within the epidural space and proximity to traversing tracts. In the instance of corticospinal tract stimulation, patients present with complaints of muscle contractions, typically seen with lower frequencies than 60–90 Hz, both ipsilaterally and caudally to the level at which the stimulation is applied. Similarly, ventral stimulation of the spinal cord, including the ventral roots, would provoke muscle contractions ipsilateral and at the level of stimulation. If leads were to overlay autonomic pathways, patients could experience warmth and burning ipsilaterally and caudally to level of stimulation. Energy applied to the dorsal root fibers, seen more laterally in the spinal canal, would produce ipsilateral paresthesias; however, differing from dorsal column stimulation in that root activation is seen at lower stimulation potency. In the rare instance that the spinothalamic tracts were to be activated via lead position, warmth, pain, and burning would be observed in a contralateral and caudal fashion from the level of stimulation [11].

51.2.4 Technical Considerations and Prevention

Both trial and permanent percutaneous placement involve the introduction of the SCS leads, via fluoroscopic guidance, into the epidural space using a standard epidural needle or curved epidural needle. The leads are directed into the posterior or dorsal paramedian epidural space with skin point entry usually two levels below the midline epidural entrance. They are then threaded to a designated anatomic location, generally involving the region of the low thoracic cord, ranging between the T8 and T10 segments, for lower back and radicular leg pain. For patients who experience upper extremity symptoms, including cervicalgia, cervical leads can be placed between C2 and C7 depending on the predominant area of pain. When the desired level is reached in the permanent implant, an incision is made at the needle site, cutting down to the supraspinous fascia. Other surgeons will make a single midline incision initially, dissecting to the supraspinous process, placing the epidural needle into this accessed area. Regardless of the technique chosen, leads are then anchored as close as possible to the fascia entry site using nonabsorbable sutures, ideally with the tip of the anchor penetrating into the fascia.

Newer surgical techniques and technologies have allowed for decreased rates of lead migration due to technological advancements. A few measures used to prevent lead movement include the implementation of a 30° angle for needle entry, placement of the epidural needle at a minimum of two vertebral bodies distal to the target, using the spinal ligaments, most commonly the supraspinous fascia, as the point of anchor, and placing a strain relief loop at the site of lead entry to the ligament as well as at the generator site [13] have led to improved results. Mironer and colleagues [1] found that "midline anchoring" techniques utilizing the plica mediana dorsalis as the anchor point resulted in a decrease in lead migration from 23 to 6% after trial insertion and from 24 to 7% after implantation versus the standard technique. Since the advent and usage of multipolar and multichannel electrode systems, a significant decline in incidence of migration has been noted over more than a decade. Kumar et al. noted a 5% decline in the incidence of surgical revision in a 10-year case series, siting the variability of coverage that multichannel electrodes offered compared to monopolar systems as well as increased success of recapture with multichannel systems [9]. North et al. reported that in cases using simple bipolar leads, surgical revision rates were as high as 23%, while only 16% of those utilizing multichannel programmable devices required revision [14]. Furthermore, placing two separate leads increases success of recapture in instances of migration by expanding the number of viable electrodes as well as stimulation coverage area.

In recent years, new anchoring devices have been created in the hopes of replacing suturing methods for lead stabilization. The devices have been touted as both increasing anchoring forces as well as decreasing procedural times compared to standard methods of fixation [15]. One commercialized anchor produced by Boston Scientific Corporation (Valencia, CA, USA) reported a holding force of 2.9 times greater than that of their conventional silicone suture sleeve in cadaveric testing. Furthermore, they reported a decreased procedure time by an average of 34% [16]. A study performed by Bowman et al. found that these novel semi-automated devices provided more secure fixation of SCS leads when compared to standard suturing techniques in excised caprine spine [17]. However, before these devices can be adopted into standard of practice, further studies are required to assess their benefit in human subjects.

51.2.5 Diagnostic Measures

When assessing a patient with abnormal paresthesia coverage, changes in stimulation patterns, return of painful impulses, or abnormal muscle activity, it is imperative to first start with an assessment of the hardware and the SCS settings. An in-office evaluation can be performed to assess the functionality of the battery including if it has been properly charged as well as assessing battery quality, particularly the ability to carry a charge. Furthermore, the various settings of the SCS should be assessed to evaluate for optimal pain relief therapy including frequency or rate, pulse width, amplitude, and electrode selection. If the hardware is found to be within normal parameters and functioning at expected capacity, changes to SCS programming parameters should be attempted at different settings in the hopes of recapturing paresthesia coverage of the intended anatomy. Pulse width, measured in microseconds (μs), represents the duration of a stimulation pulse. Pulse width is generally set between 100 and 400 μs, and any alteration would, respectively, alter the patient's span of paresthesia coverage. Amplitude, measured in volts (V) or milliamperes (mA), represents the stimulation intensity or strength and is often regarded as the most important programmable parameter. Frequency, measured in Hertz (Hz), represents the cycles of pulses per second. Traditional SCS utilizes a frequency typically between 20 and 120 Hz, with lower rates producing a thumping sensation and higher rates producing a buzzing sensation [18]. In 2015 the FDA approved a newer high-frequency SCS which utilizes a frequency of 10,000 Hz. A study conducted in 2015 by Kapural et al., held a head-to-head comparison of the high-frequency SCS therapy versus the traditional SCS, demonstrating non-inferiority and superiority of the high-frequency stimulator [19]. The trial resulted in an 84.5 and 83.1% response rate for back pain and leg pain, respectively, in the high-frequency group compared to 43.8 and 55.5% in the traditional cohort. Electrode selection allows for various arrangements of lead contact, otherwise known as "current steering," which allows for enhanced ability to cover most areas of pain as well as expanded programming capabilities [20].

In the setting in which recapture is unable to be achieved, the next step involves radiographic imaging to assess lead placement. Live fluoroscopic imaging can be utilized if a C-arm is readily available for practitioners who have in-office fluoroscopy capabilities; otherwise, patients should be sent for plain films to include an AP and lateral X-ray of the thoracic or cervical spine, depending on the original target area of epidural placement. The radiographs are used to evaluate for any possible lead migration, kinking or breakage of the wires, or any other abnormalities that could be altering stimulation patterns. If a collection of fluid is suspected, such as an epidural hematoma or abscess, despite physical appearance and presentation, a CT scan can be used to better define fluid borders and volume. Otherwise CT and MRI offer little utility in the setting of lead migration as leads can be visualized on plain films, saving patients the added exposure to radiation.

51.2.6 Treatment

Currently corrective methods for lead migration involve attempting SCS reprogramming of system parameters for recapture, with surgical revision reserved in the instance that appropriate recapture of paresthesia is unable to be achieved. However, Jeon et al. [21] trialed a newly developed technique of correction using a guide wire from the SCS implant kit to assist the migrated lead back to its intended location. The technique involves threading a bent guide wire into the epidural space under fluoroscopic guidance, using a 14-gauge Tuohy needle, until it comes in contact with the rouge lead. The wire and the lead are then advanced together until the lead has been readjusted back into position at the location of optimal coverage. May et al. reported surgical revision rates secondary to lead migration of 4.5% [22]. Meanwhile, Barolat and colleagues reported revision rates as high as 13.6% [20]. Kumar and associates reported that in their 160 patient, 10-year case series, 11.3% of lead systems required surgical revision. In 1998, Kemler and Furnee reported patient costs of 360 and 1530 euros for repositioning of a lead and replacing a lead, respectively [23]. Similarly, in 1993, Bell and associates reported patient costs of $2700 and $5450 for the same procedures [24].

Key Concepts

- Lead migration is the most common complications observed with spinal cord stimulators. It represents 11–13% of all complications seen and most commonly occurs in the vertical or lateral directions. Although very rare, extreme lateralization of leads can cause movement anteriorly into the anterior epidural space causing very distressing symptoms to the patient.
- Lead migration should be suspected in patients who experience changes in paresthesia patterns, decrease in pain coverage, muscle contractions, or a developing sense of warmth and burning.
- A thorough understanding of spinal cord anatomy can help in identifying stimulation patterns and potential sites of lead migration.

- Prompt diagnoses can be made utilizing either live fluoroscopy or with standard AP and lateral plain films.
- SCS parameters, including pulse width, rate or frequency, electrode selection, and amplitude can be adjusted in an attempt to recapture paresthesia coverage of the patient's pain distribution. New technology, including multichannel electrode systems have allowed for easier recapture and decreased morbidity related to lead migration.
- If attempts at recapture are unsuccessful, the ultimate corrective measure for lead migration is revision surgery. Newer surgical anchoring techniques have lowered the rate of migration without compromising efficacy and function of the stimulator.

References

1. Mironer YE, et al. A new technique of "midline anchoring" in spinal cord stimulation dramatically reduces lead migration. Neuromodulation. 2004;7(1):32–7.
2. Shealy S, Mortimer JT, Reswick JB. Electrical inhibition of pain by stimulation of the dorsal columns: preliminary clinical report. Anesth Analg. 1967;46:489–91.
3. Mekhail NA, Mathews M, Nageeb F, Guirguis M, Mekhail MN, Cheng J. Retrospective review of 707 cases of spinal cord stimulation: indications and complications. Pain Pract. 2011;11:148–53.
4. Kumar K, Nath R, Wyant GM. Treatment of chronic pain by epidural spinal cord stimulation: a 10-year experience. J Neurosurg. 1991;75(3):402–7.
5. Lanza GA, Grimaldi R, Greco S, Ghio S, Sarullo F, Zuin G, De Luca A, et al. Spinal cord stimulation for the treatment of refractory angina pectoris: a multicenter randomized single-blind study (the SCS-ITA trial). Pain. 2011;152(1):45–52.
6. Holsheimer J, Buitenweg JR. Review: bioelectrical mechanisms in spinal cord stimulation. Neuromodulation. 2015;18(3):161–70.
7. Oakley JC, Prager JP. Spinal cord stimulation: mechanisms of action. Spine. 2002;27(22):2574–83.
8. Marchand S. Spinal cord stimulation analgesia: substantiating the mechanisms for neuropathic pain treatment. Pain. 2015;156(3):364–5.
9. Cameron T. Safety and efficacy of spinal cord stimulation for the treatment of chronic pain: a 20-year literature review. J Neurosurg Spine. 2004;100(3):254–67.
10. Kumar K, Wilson JR, Taylor RS, Gupta S. Complications of spinal cord stimulation, suggestions to improve outcome, and financial impact. J Neurosurg Spine. 2006;5(3):191–203.
11. Rosenow JM, Stanton-Hicks M, Rezai AR, Henderson JM. Failure modes of spinal cord stimulation hardware. J Neurosurg Spine. 2006;5(3):183–90.
12. Levy RM. Anatomic considerations for spinal cord stimulation. Neuromodulation. 2014;17(S1):2–11.
13. Deer TR, Douglas Stewart C. Complications of spinal cord stimulation: identification, treatment, and prevention. Pain Med. 2008;9(S1):S93–101.
14. North RB, Calkins S-K, Campbell DS, Sieracki JM, Piantadosi S, Daly MJ, Dey PB, Barolat G. Automated, patient-interactive, spinal cord stimulator adjustment: a randomized controlled trial. Neurosurgery. 2003;52(3):572–80.
15. North RB, Recinos VR, Attenello FJ, Shipley J, Long DM. Prevention of percutaneous spinal cord stimulation electrode migration: a 15-year experience. Neuromodulation. 2014;17(7):670–7.
16. Chen R, Surekha H, Anne P, Syed ZA. Improved efficiency and holding force with a novel mechanical SCS anchor. Poster presented at: 6th annual meeting of the Canadian Neuromodulation Society, Jacksons Point, ON; 15–17 June 2012.
17. Bowman RG, Caraway D, Bentley I. Comparison of a novel fixation device with standard suturing methods for spinal cord stimulators. Neuromodulation. 2013;16(5):454–8.
18. Abejón D, Cameron T, Feler C, Pérez-Cajaraville J. Electric parameters optimization in spinal cord stimulation. Study in conventional nonrechargeable systems. Neuromodulation. 2010;13(4):281–7.
19. Kapural L, Yu C, Doust MW, Gliner BE, Vallejo R, Sitzman BT, Amirdelfan K, et al. Novel 10-kHz high-frequency therapy (HF10 therapy) is superior to traditional low-frequency spinal cord stimulation for the treatment of chronic back and leg pain: the SENZA-RCT randomized controlled trial. Anesthesiology. 2015;123(4):851–60.
20. Barolat G, Oakley JC, Law JD, North RB, Ketcik B, Sharan A. Epidural spinal cord stimulation with a multiple electrode paddle lead is effective in treating intractable low back pain. Neuromodulation. 2001;4(2).
21. Jeon SY, Ji JY, Yoo SH, Chon JY, Jung SH, Moon HS. Percutaneous adjustment method for transversely migrated spinal cord stimulation leads: a technical report. J Anesth. 2015;29(6):953–6.
22. May MS, Banks C, Thomson SJ. A retrospective, long-term, third-party follow-up of patients considered for spinal cord stimulation. Neuromodulation. 2002;5(3).
23. Kemler MA, Furnée CA. Economic evaluation of spinal cord stimulation for chronic reflex sympathetic dystrophy. Neurology. 2002;59(8):1203–9.
24. Bell GK, Kidd D, North RB. Cost-effectiveness analysis of spinal cord stimulation in treatment of failed back surgery syndrome. J Pain Symptom Manag. 1997;13(5):286–95.

Epidural Emphysema After Placement of a Thoracic Epidural Catheter

52

Pavan Rao and Dalia Elmofty

52.1 Case Description

A 44-year-old female with a history of stage IIB cervical carcinoma is scheduled to undergo an anterior pelvic exenteration with epidural anesthesia and catheter placement for postoperative pain management. A T10-T11 epidural catheter is placed with the loss of resistance to air technique. On postoperative day 1, the patient complains of neck pain while sitting up in bed or lying down. Abdominal and neck pain worsens over the course of the day and the epidural catheter migrates out of the epidural space. Patient controlled analgesia (PCA) with hydromorphone is initiated overnight and the following day the epidural catheter is replaced uneventfully at the T9-T10 interlaminar space again with the loss of resistance to air technique. By that evening, abdominal pain lessens but neck pain worsens. There is a concern that the patient's symptoms are caused by an inadvertent dural puncture resulting in a postdural puncture headache. She does not exhibit the typical symptoms of a postdural puncture headache, which resolve in the supine position. Intravenous hydration, Fioricet™, and caffeinated beverages are initiated but symptoms do not resolve. A cervical spine radiograph is ordered to rule out a pathological cause for the symptoms. The report reveals findings suggestive of gas density within the posterior soft tissues of the neck and the epidural space (Fig. 52.1). Further imaging with computed tomographic scan of the head and neck (Fig. 52.2) reveals cervical vertebral level 1 through cervical vertebral level 4 epidural air exiting into the right paraspinal and posterior subcutaneous area of the neck. A small focus of epidural air also is seen in the thoracic spine (Fig. 52.3). It becomes apparent that ours is a rare case of epidural emphysema. Air could have entered into the epidural space from the epidural Tuohy needle, the

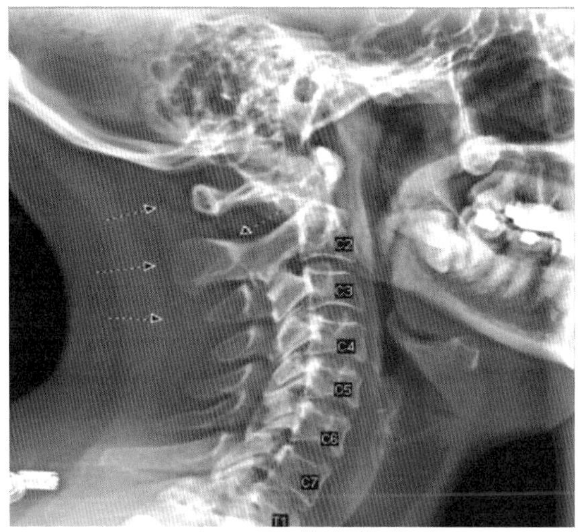

Fig. 52.1 Cervical spine x-ray with findings suggestive of gas density within the posterior soft tissues of the neck

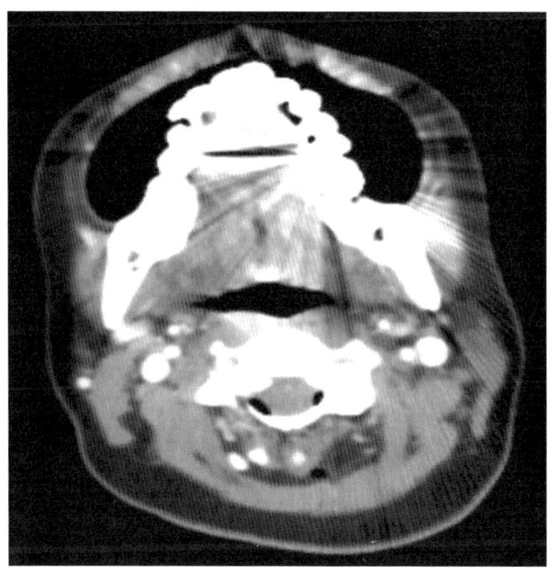

Fig. 52.2 Computed tomography scan with contrast of the head, neck, and soft tissue revealing cervical 1 through cervical 4 epidural air exiting into the right paraspinal and posterior subcutaneous tissue of the neck, tracking along fascial planes

P. Rao, M.D. • D. Elmofty, M.D. (✉)
Department of Anesthesia and Critical Care,
University of Chicago, 5841 S. Maryland Ave., M.C. 4028,
Chicago, IL 60637, USA
e-mail: DElmofty@dacc.uchicago.edu

M. Anitescu et al. (eds.), *Challenging Cases and Complication Management in Pain Medicine*,
https://doi.org/10.1007/978-3-319-60072-7_52

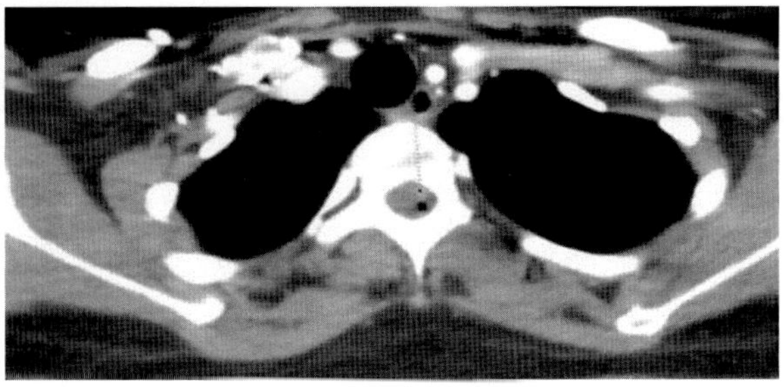

Fig. 52.3 Computed tomography scan with contrast of the thoracic spine revealing a small focus of epidural air is seen at thoracic 3 level

epidural catheter, or a gas-forming infection. The patient had no symptoms or signs of infection. The epidural tubing was inspected and no air was noted in the tubing. The epidural pump in-line air sensor and alarm have been activated to detect more than 2 mL of air in the tubing. From the computed tomography scan we estimate a total of 5–10 cm^3 of air noted in all compartments, with most of the air outside of the epidural space. This is likely from using the loss of resistance to air technique. Patient was administered continuous oxygen by face mask for 24 h; her neck pain decreased in intensity during this interval and completely resolved at discharge from the hospital time.

52.2 Case Discussion

Pneumorrhachis, also known as aerorachia, describes an uncommon phenomenon, the presence of gas in the spinal canal [1]. Pneumorrhachis is distinguished from pneumocephalus, the presence of intracranial gas [2]. Pneumorrhachis can be intradural or extradural. The extradural category also is known as epidural air, epidural pneumatosis, or epidural emphysema. Because of the lower resistance from loose connective tissue, as compared with the rich vascular network anteriorly, the epidural air usually collects in the posterior epidural space [3].

52.3 Etiology and Pathogenesis

Epidural emphysema has been described in association with the iatrogenic, traumatic, and nontraumatic clinical scenarios (Table 52.1) [3]. Iatrogenic causes of epidural emphysema are: (1) epidural anesthesia and using the widely applied loss of resistance to air technique, (2) inadvertent infusion of air through an epidural catheter, and (3) other surgical or diagnostic intervention invading the epidural space. Traumatic causes of epidural emphysema are penetrating spinal injury, skull fractures, or traumatic pneumothorax and pneumomediastinum. The air dissects through fascial planes into paraspinal connective tissue, along vascular and nerve root sheaths, and through the neural foramina into the epidural space [3]. The fascial plane in the mediastinum communicates with the fascial plane in the epidural space. Barotrauma increases pressure gradients and is the most common cause of clinically significant epidural emphysema [4]. Air can move through these tracts when a pressure gradient forms after high intrathoracic or intra-abdominal pressure is transduced to the epidural space. The air is then trapped when the skin and subcutaneous tissue act as a one-way valve. Nontraumatic epidural emphysema happens with epidural infections by a gas-forming organism or abscess formation, rupture of a vacuum disc, or spontaneous pneumothorax or pneumomediastinum. Degenerative discs may contain air. The presence of gas within an intervertebral disc is found in 2–3% of the population [5]. Herniation of the discs can lead to epidural emphysema. Similar to traumatic barotraumas, spontaneous pneumothorax and pneumomediastinum dissect air along fascial planes into neuroforamen to the epidural space.

Table 52.1 Causes of epidural emphysema

Iatrogenic: • Epidural anesthesia • Surgical and diagnostic interventions
Traumatic: 1. Penetrating spinal injury 2. Skull fracture 3. Traumatic pneumothorax or pneumomediastinum Air pathways • Conditions producing high intrathoracic pressure and barotrauma • Dissecting through paraspinal soft tissues through neural foramina in nerve root sheaths
Nontraumatic: • Infection by gas-producing organism • Vacuum disc phenomenon • Spontaneous pneumothorax or pneumomediastinum

52.4 Clinical Manifestations

Epidural emphysema, rarely symptomatic, can be associated with discomfort, pain, or neurological deficits. Symptoms arise when injected air acts as a space-occupying lesion to exert pressure on nervous structures to compress cord or nerve roots or increase intracranial pressure. Patients may complain of headache, nausea, and vomiting. More severe symptoms include vision and hearing changes, altered mental status, and seizures. Papilledema may be noted on physical examination. Cushing's triad may be seen with characteristic systolic hypertension and widened pulse pressure to increase cerebral perfusion pressure, reflex bradycardia, and irregular respiration caused by impaired brainstem function. In the most severe cases, patients may suffer from cord compression with neurologic deficits and symptoms of cauda equina syndrome such as loss of bowel or bladder function.

Patients undergoing epidural anesthesia who complain of a headache or neck pain afterwards are assumed to have a postdural puncture headache. According to the International Headache Society, a postdural puncture headache is a headache that worsens within 15 min after sitting or standing and improves within 15 min after lying down. It has at least one of the following characteristics: neck stiffness, tinnitus, hypacusia, photophobia, or nausea [6]. The headache must also start within 5 days of the dural puncture and usually resolves spontaneously within 1 week. A dural puncture leads to continued cerebrospinal fluid leak. The leak decreases intracranial pressure and leads to vascular expansion and downward traction on pain-sensitive intracranial structures such as veins, meninges, and the central nervous system. With epidural emphysema, symptoms are the result of intracranial hypertension. Interestingly, intracranial hypertension and hypotension have similar symptoms. Both lead to headache, nausea, vomiting, and vision and hearing changes. The vision changes, however, vary between intracranial hypertension and hypotension. With intracranial hypotension, patients with visual changes often have CN III, IV, or VI palsies. With intracranial hypertension, patients typically have a peripheral visual field deficit. When a patient with intracranial hypotension lies down, headaches improve. When a patient with intracranial hypertension lies down, headaches worsen. Patients with intracranial hypertension also may experience altered mental status, seizures, or Cushing's triad.

52.5 Diagnostic Methods

Often times, epidural emphysema is an incidental finding on radiographic imaging. Epidural emphysema may result in serious injuries or diseases, and the underlying etiology should be established. A plain radiograph is a simple, quick, and low-cost modality but not as useful in distinguishing the exact location, or the amount of gas. A computed tomography scan is a rapid and dependable diagnostic method to delineate the location and describe the size of the gas collection. It can also locate smaller pockets of gas. In some cases, however, it may be difficult to delineate intra- versus extradural gas. In these instances, magnetic resonance imaging may be more beneficial. If neurologic deficits are present, magnetic resonance imaging of the spinal cord, exiting nerves, and surrounding soft tissues will help identify areas of cord and nerve compression.

52.6 Prevention

Epidural emphysema after administration of epidural analgesia can be prevented by implementing precautionary measures. Instead of the loss of resistance to air technique, saline is used to locate the epidural space to eliminate small amounts of epidural air from accumulating. Small amounts of air rarely produce symptoms or require medical intervention. Epidural tubing is flushed to reduce the presence of air. Epidural pump in-line air sensors and alarms are activated to prevent administrating large amounts of air. All connections are secured and tightly fastened because a loose connection between the epidural and the drug infusion line may let in air distal to the in-line sensor.

52.7 Treatment

There are no established guidelines or standards of care for the treatment of epidural emphysema. Most cases of epidural emphysema are asymptomatic if gas entrapment is small. Mild symptoms such as nausea, vomiting, and headache may warrant conservative treatment such as a higher fractional inspired oxygen concentration to promote nitrogen washout and to decrease the size of the gas collection. With a nitrous oxide combination during general anesthesia, the volume of gas collections may increase. In cases with symptoms of increased intracranial hypertension, care should be taken to prevent increases in intracranial pressure. More severe symptoms may warrant 100% oxygen delivery in a hyperbaric chamber to increase the rate of gas absorption [7]. For patients with symptoms of cord compression, emergent surgical or epidural needle decompression is likely warranted. Monitoring may be determined on a case by case basis, with more frequent monitoring for cases with a neurologic deficit or delayed resolution of symptoms (Table 52.2).

Key Concepts

- Epidural emphysema is the presence of gas in the epidural space. Epidural emphysema is also known as epidural air or epidural pneumatosis.
- The causes of epidural emphysema are iatrogenic, traumatic, or nontraumatic.

Table 52.2 Extracranial epidural emphysema

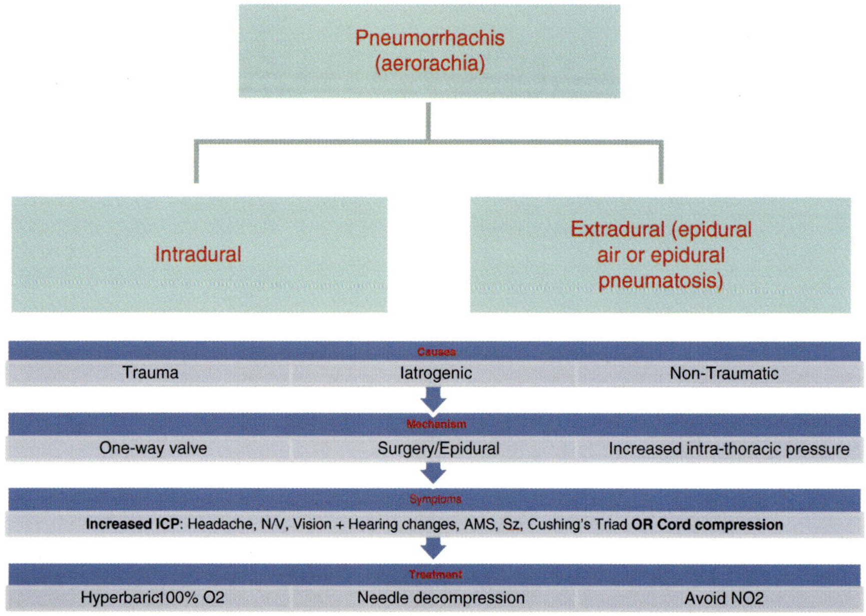

- Epidural emphysema is often asymptomatic; symptoms come from the mass effect of gas on the spinal canal.
- Epidural emphysema can be treated with observation, surveillance with imaging, supplemental oxygen, hyperbaric oxygen, or emergent needle or surgical decompression, depending on the severity of symptoms.
- Epidural emphysema and postdural puncture headache cause symptoms through intracranial hypertension and hypotension, respectively. Both these conditions have many symptoms in common.

References

1. Newbold R, Wiener M, Volger J. Traumatic pneumorrhachis. Am J Roentgenol. 1987;148:615–6.
2. Schirmer C, Heilman C. Pneumocephalus: case illustrations and review. Neurocrit Care. 2010;13:152–8.
3. Oertel M, Reinges M. Pathogenesis, diagnosis and management of pneumorrhachis. Eur Spine J. 2006;15(5):S636–43.
4. Cloran F, Bui-Mansfield LT. Extracranial epidural emphysema: pathway, aetiology, diagnosis and management. Br J Radiol. 2011;84(1002):570–5.
5. Ford LT, Gilula LA, Murphy WA, Gado M. Analysis of gas in vacuum lumbar disc. AJR Am J Roentgenol. 1977;128:1056–7.
6. International Headache Society. Post-dural (post-lumbar) puncture headache. IHS classification ICHD-II. 7.2.1. http://ihsclassification.org/en/02_classification/03_teil2/07.02.01_nonvascular.html. Accessed 1 Mar 2016.
7. Overdiek N, Grisales D, Gravenstein D. Subdural air collection: a likely source of radicular pain after lumbar epidural. J Clin Anesth. 2001;13:392–7.

Index

M. Anitescu et al. (eds.), *Challenging Cases and Complication Management in Pain Medicine*,
https://doi.org/10.1007/978-3-319-60072-7

D

E

T

Printed by Printforce, the Netherlands